W9-ANB-588

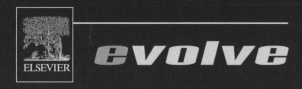

Leading and Managing in Nursing

THIRD EDITION

Patricia S. Yoder-Wise, RN, BC, EdD, CNAA, FAAN
Texas Tech University Health Sciences Center
Lubbock, Texas

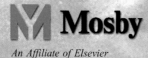

Mosby

An Affiliate of Elsevier

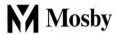

An Affiliate of Elsevier

11830 Westline Industrial Drive
St. Louis, Missouri 63146

Library of Congress Cataloging-in-Publication Data
Leading and managing in nursing / [edited by] Patricia S. Yoder-Wise—3rd ed.
      p. cm.
      Includes bibliographical references and index.
      ISBN-13: 978–0–323–01632–2   ISBN-10: 0–323–01632–4
      1. Nursing services—Administration. 2. Leadership. I. Wise, Pat. S. Yoder.
      RT89 .L43 2002
      362.1′73′068—dc21   2002033668

ISBN-13: 978–0–323–01632–2
ISBN-10: 0–323–01632–4

Acquisitions Editors: Tom Wilhelm/Susan Epstein
Developmental Editors: Eric Ham/Maria Broeker
Publishing Services Manager: John Rogers
Senior Project Manager: Beth Hayes
Design: Sheila Barrett/Graphic World Inc.
Design Coordinator: Kathi Gosche
Cover Art: Kathi Gosche

GW/QWV

Printed in China

Last digit is the print number: 9   8   7   6   5   4

Contributors

Michael R. Bleich, PhD, RN, CNAA
RWJ Executive Nurse Fellow
Associate Dean, Clinical and Community Affairs
Associate Professor, Nursing Administration
University of Kansas School of Nursing
Kansas City, Kansas
Executive Director and Chief Operating Officer
KU Health Partners, Inc.
Kansas City, Kansas
Chapter 1: Managing, Leading, and Following

Sharon A. Brigner, MS, RN
Senior Health Policy Analyst
National Committee to Preserve Social Security
    and Medicare
Washington, DC
*Chapter 27: Leading Through Professional
    Associations*

Carol Alvater Brooks, RN, DNSc, CNAA
Professor Emerita
Syracuse University
School of Nursing
Syracuse, New York
Chapter 6: Healthcare Organizations
*Chapter 9: Understanding and Designing
    Organizational Structures*

Brenda L. Cleary, RN, PhD, FAAN
Executive Director
North Carolina Center for Nursing
Raleigh, North Carolina
Chapter 14: Consumer Relationships

Christine R. Curran, PhD, RN, CNA
Assistant Professor
Director, Informatics Program
Director, Research Resources
School of Nursing
Columbia University
New York, New York
*Chapter 12: Managing Information
    and Technology: Caring and Communicating
    With Computers*

Karen Ann Dadich, RN, MN, CNS
Associate Professor
Texas Tech University Health Sciences Center
School of Nursing
Lubbock, Texas
Chapter 15: Care Delivery Strategies
*Chapter 26: Career Management: Putting Yourself
    in Charge*

Mary Ann T. Donohue, PhD, RN, APN
Administrative Director of Nursing for Psychiatric
    Services and Nursing Research
Hackensack University Medical Center
Hackensack, New Jersey
Psychotherapist, Private Practice
Ridgewood, New Jersey
Chapter 20: Conflict: The Cutting Edge of Change

Michael L. Evans, PhD, RN, CNAA, FACHE
Vice President for Learning and Chief Learning
    Officer
Texas Health Resources
Arlington, Texas
Chapter 2: Developing the Role of Leader

Jennifer Gray, RN, PhD
Assistant Professor
School of Nursing
The University of Texas at Arlington
Arlington, Texas
Chapter 23: Role Transition

Ginny Wacker Guido, JD, MSN, RN, FAAN
Associate Dean and Director, Graduate Studies
University of North Dakota
College of Nursing
Grand Forks, North Dakota
Chapter 4: Legal and Ethical Issues

Fran Hicks, RN, PhD, FAAN
Professor Emeritus
School of Nursing
University of Portland
Portland, Oregon
Chapter 10: Collective Action

Karen Kelly, EdD, RN, CNAA, BC
Associate Professor
School of Nursing
Southern Illinois University at Edwardsville
Edwardsville, Illinois
Chapter 25: Power, Politics, and Influence

Catherine M. Kirk, RN, BSN, MSN
Director
Acute Care Nursing Services
All Saints Healthcare System, Inc.
Racine, Wisconsin
Chapter 16: Staffing and Scheduling

Karren Kowalski, PhD, RN, FAAN
President
Kowalski and Associates, Consulting
Castle Rock, Colorado
Chapter 19: Building Teams Through Communication and Partnerships

Kristi D. Menix, RN, EdD, CNAA, BC
Education Consultant
Former Assistant Professor and CNE Nurse Planner
The University of Texas at Tyler
Tyler, Texas
Chapter 8: Leading Change

Dorothy A. Otto, RN, MSN, EdD
Associate Professor
The University of Texas Health Science Center-Houston
School of Nursing
Clinical Associate Professor
M.D. Anderson Cancer Center
Houston, Texas
Chapter 3: Developing the Role of Manager
Chapter 18: Cultural Diversity in Healthcare

Amy C. Pettigrew, BSN, MSN, DNS, RN
Associate Professor
University of Cincinnati College of Nursing
Cincinnati, Ohio
Chapter 24: Self-Management: Stress and Time

Cynthia Whittig Roach, RN, DSN
Associate Professor
Beth-El College of Nursing and Health Sciences of the University of Colorado at Colorado Springs
Colorado Springs, Colorado
Chapter 17: Selecting, Developing, and Evaluating Staff
Chapter 22: Managing Personal/Personnel Problems

Darlene Steven, RN, BScN, BA, MHSA, PhD
Professor, School of Nursing
Lakehead University
Thunder Bay, Ontario
Canada
Chapter 7: Strategic Planning, Goal Setting, and Marketing

Ana M. Valadez, RN, EdD, CNAA, FAAN
Associate Dean for the Undergraduate Program
Professor in the Roberts' Practiceship
School of Nursing
Texas Tech University Health Sciences Center
Lubbock, Texas
Chapter 3: Developing the Role of Manager
Chapter 18: Cultural Diversity in Healthcare

Darla J. Vale, DNSc, RN, CCRN
Chairperson and Associate Professor
Department of Nursing
College of Mount St. Joseph
Cincinnati, Ohio
Chapter 11: Managing Quality and Risk

Rose Aguilar Welch, RN, EdD
Associate Professor, Division of Nursing
California State University, Dominguez Hills
Carson, California
Chapter 5: Decision Making and Problem Solving

Deborah A. Wendt, RN, PhD
Associate Professor of Nursing
College of Mount St. Joseph
Cincinnati, Ohio
Chapter 11: Managing Quality and Risk

Donna Westmoreland, RN, BSN, MSN, PhD
Associate Professor
University of Nebraska Medical Center
Omaha, Nebraska
Chapter 13: Managing Costs and Budgets

K. Lynn Wieck, PhD, RN
Chief Executive Officer
Management Solutions for Healthcare
Katy, Texas
President
Texas Nurses Association
Austin, Texas
Chapter 2: Developing the Role of Leader

Patricia S. Yoder-Wise, RN, BC, EdD, CNAA, FAAN
Texas Tech University Health Sciences Center
Lubbock, Texas and Odessa, Texas
Chapter 21: Delegation: An Art of Professional Practice
Chapter 26: Career Management: Putting Yourself in Charge
Epilogue: Thriving in the Future

Photo Credits

Chapter 1 (opener), p. 1, courtesy *Chuck Dresner,* photographer
Chapter 3 (opener), p. 35, courtesy *Chuck Dresner,* photographer
Chapter 6 (opener), p. 91, (top) © *Patrick Watson,* photographer; (bottom), courtesy *Gretchen Halstead,* The Baptist Home. Rhinebeck, New York; (internal), p. 98, © *Patrick Watson,* photographer
Chapter 11 (opener), p. 173, courtesy *Chuck Dresner,* photographer
Chapter 12 (cover far left and opener), p. 191, courtesy *Corometrics Medical Systems,* Wallingford, Connecticut

Chapter 17 (opener), p. 293, courtesy *Chuck Dresner,* photographer
Chapter 19 (opener), p. 323, © *Linda Bartlett,* 1994.
Chapter 20 (opener), p. 349, courtesy *Chuck Dresner,* photographer
Chapter 23 (opener), p. 399, courtesy *Chuck Dresner,* photographer
Chapter 24 (opener), p. 413, courtesy *Chuck Dresner,* photographer

Acknowledgments

We are indebted to our reviewers, whose insightful comments and suggestions were invaluable in helping revise this book. The end result of their efforts, as in any peer-review process, is a stronger presentation. We are deeply grateful to the following people for their assistance:

Martha Baker, PhD, RN, CS, CCRN
Associate Professor
Missouri Southern State College
Joplin, Missouri

Martha Butler, PhD, RN
Nursing Program Director
Southwestern College
Winfield, Kansas

Gayle K. Campbell, BSN, RN
Health Science Coordinator
Georgian College, Midland Campus
Midland, Ontario
Canada

Mary L. Fisher, PhD, RN, CNAA
Associate Professor
Indiana University
Indianapolis, Indiana

Sandra L. Greeno, MSN, BSN, ADN, RN
Instructor
School of Nursing
University of Central Florida
Orlando, Florida

Glenda C. Johnson, RN, BSN, MSA
Nurse Educator
Louise Obici School of Professional Nursing
Suffolk, Virginia

Mary Jo Mattocks, RN, BSN, PhD
Assistant Professor
Montana State University Northern, Great Falls
  Campus
Great Falls, Montana

Claudia Louth Mitchell, RN, BSN, MSN
Professor of Nursing
Santa Barbara City College
Santa Barbara, California

Mary Moberly, RN
Staff Development Coordinator
Columbine Care Center West
Fort Collins, Colorado

Desma R. Reno, MSN, RN, CS, GCNS
Assistant Professor in Nursing
Outreach Coordinator, RN-BSN Program
Southeast Missouri State University
Cape Girardeau, Missouri

Kimberly Tucker, RN, BSN, CCRN
Director
Center for Advanced Medicine
Barnes-Jewish Hospital
St. Louis, Missouri

Marianne Walston, RN, MSN
Nursing Instructor
Louise Obici School of Nursing
Suffolk, Virginia

Melinda Warfield, MSM, BSN, RN, CAN, BC
Assistant Director of Nursing and Staff
  Development Coordinator
The Laurels of Kent
Lowell, Michigan

Special Acknowledgments

Many people helped make this book a reality. All of the contributing authors to this book worked within very tight time frames to accomplish their work. To them I extend my deepest appreciation for being responsive, making the necessary revisions, and sounding eager to hear from me whenever I emailed them. AOL, Federal Express, fax, and Kinko's remain household words!

Special thanks go to our new editors, Susan Epstein and Tom Wilhelm; to our developmental editors, Maria Broeker and Eric Ham, for answering questions, providing the "latest" version of whatever we were talking about, and doing all sorts of tasks that kept us on track; to those who exceeded our wildest expectations of involvement (you know who you are); and to Robert Thomas Wise, my husband and best friend, for being such a great sounding board and consistent supporter.

One final note: No learner can remain stagnant. The context in which nurses manage and lead is constantly changing, sometimes for the better, sometimes for the worse. The key to success is to keep learning, keep caring, and maintain our passion for nursing. That, if nothing else, must be instilled in our leaders of tomorrow. Lead on . . . ¡Adelanté!

Patricia S. Yoder-Wise
RN, BC, EdD, CNAA, FAAN
Texas Tech University Health Sciences Center
Lubbock, Texas

This book is dedicated to the
families and friends who supported all of us who created it,
to the faculty who use it to develop nursing's new leaders and managers,
and to the learners who have the vision and insight to
grasp today's reality and mold it into the
future of dynamic nursing leadership.

Lead on . . . ¡Adelanté!

Preface to the Instructor

Leading and managing are two essential expectations of all professional nurses, and they are more important than ever in today's rapidly changing healthcare system. To lead and manage successfully, nurses must possess not only knowledge and skills but also a caring and compassionate attitude. After all, leading and managing are about people.

Volumes of information on leadership and management principles can be found in nursing, healthcare administration, business, and forecasting literature. The numerous journals in each of these fields offer research and opinion articles focused on improving leaders' and managers' abilities. The first and second editions of this text demonstrated that learners, faculty, and registered nurses in practice found that a text that synthesized applicable knowledge and related it to contemporary practice was useful. Unlike clinical nursing textbooks, which offer exercises and assignments designed to provide opportunities for learners to apply theory to practice, nursing leadership and management textbooks traditionally have offered limited opportunities of this kind. We changed that tradition in 1995 by incorporating application exercises within the text and a skills workbook section for learners. Today, we are changing that tradition yet again by linking this text to a website where case studies can exemplify a chapter's point and provide even more recent references.

This book results from our continued strong belief in the need for a text that focuses on the nursing leadership and management issues of today and tomorrow in a distinctive way. We continue to find that we were not alone in this belief. Before the first edition, Mosby, primarily through the efforts of Darlene Como, solicited faculty members' and administrators' ideas to determine what they thought professional nurses most needed to know about leading and managing and what

kind of text would best help them obtain the necessary knowledge and skills. Their comprehensive list of suggestions remains relevant in this edition. This edition incorporated many reviewers from both service and education to be sure that the text conveys important and timely information to users as they focus on the critical roles of leading, following, and managing.

CONCEPT AND PRACTICE COMBINED

Innovative in both content and presentation, *Leading and Managing in Nursing* merges theory, research, and practical application in key leadership and management areas. Our overriding concern remains in this edition to create a text that, while well grounded in theory and concept, presents the content in a way that is real. Wherever possible, we have used real-world examples from the continuum of today's healthcare settings to illustrate the concepts. Because each chapter contributor has focused on synthesizing the assigned content, you will find no lengthy quotations in these chapters. Instead, we have made every effort to make the content as engaging, inviting, and interesting as possible. Reflecting our view of the real world of nursing leadership and management today, the following themes pervade the text:

- The focus of healthcare is shifting from the hospital to the community.
- Healthcare consumers and the healthcare workforce are becoming increasingly culturally diverse.
- Today, virtually every professional nurse leads and manages regardless of title or position.
- Consumer relationships play a central role in the delivery of nursing and healthcare.

- Communication, collaboration, team building, and other interpersonal skills form the foundation of effective nursing leadership and management.
- Change continues at a rapid pace in healthcare and society in general.

DIVERSITY OF PERSPECTIVES

The contributors have been recruited from diverse settings, roles, and geographic areas, enabling them to offer a broad perspective on the critical elements of nursing leadership and management roles. To help bridge the gap often found between nursing education and nursing practice, some contributors were recruited from academia; others, from practice settings. This blend not only contributes to the richness of this text but also conveys a sense of oneness in nursing. The historical "gap" between education and service must become a sense of a continuum and not a chasm.

AUDIENCE

This book is designed for undergraduate learners in nursing leadership and management courses, including those in BSN-completion courses. In addition, we know there are nurses in practice who had not anticipated formal leadership and management roles in their careers. The design of this text allows those persons to capitalize on their own real-life experiences as a way to develop greater understanding about leading and managing and the important role of following. Because today's learners tend to be more visually oriented than past learners, we have incorporated illustrations, boxes, and a functional full-color design to stimulate their interest and maximize their learning. In addition, numerous examples and "The Challenge" in each chapter remain to provide relevance to the real world of nursing.

ORGANIZATION

We have organized this text around issues that are key to the success of professional nurses in today's constantly changing healthcare environment.

First, it is important to understand the concepts of leading and managing and how the theories and foci differ from each other. For example, headship (holding a formal position or title) does not always

mean that person is demonstrating leadership. Next, nurses should understand key concepts as they relate to leading and managing. You will find key organizational information that ranges from a basic understanding about the kinds of organizations delivering care to the changing demands for quality, technology, and cost-effectiveness. Consumer relationships lead into considerations of how to deliver care and relationships with staff. Cultural diversity, again, does not focus so much on understanding diversities of patients (appropriate for clinical textbooks) as it does on understanding and valuing diversities in employees (critical to leading and managing). The text then transitions from the critical elements of teams and how they interact to accomplish work to the individual expectations and influences we must have throughout our careers.

The Epilogue conveys three key points: (1) We will all be required to exhibit leadership; (2) we must continue to develop ourselves professionally, or we will be irrelevant; and (3) we must focus on the future and what can influence nursing and how we transition ourselves and our profession.

Because repetition plays a crucial role in how well learners learn and retain new content, some topics appear in more than one chapter and in more than one section. We have also made an effort to express a variety of different views on some topics, as is true in the real world of nursing.

DESIGN

A functional full-color design continues to distinguish this text. As described in later sections, the design is used to emphasize and identify the text's many teaching/learning strategies, which are featured to enhance learning. Full-color photographs provide visual reinforcement of concepts, such as body language and the changes occurring in contemporary healthcare settings, while adding visual interest. Figures elucidate and graphically depict concepts and activities described in the text.

TEACHING/LEARNING STRATEGIES

The numerous teaching/learning strategies featured in this text are designed both to stimulate learners' interest and to provide constant reinforcement throughout the learning process. In addition, the visually appealing, full-color design itself serves a learning purpose. Color is used consistently throughout the text to help the reader identify the various chapter elements described in the following sections.

 ## CHAPTER OPENER ELEMENTS

- The introductory paragraph briefly describes the purpose and scope of the chapter.
- Objectives articulate the chapter's learning goals at the application level or higher.
- Questions to Consider stimulate learners to think about their personal viewpoint or experience with the topics and issues discussed in the chapter.
- The Challenge presents a contemporary nurse's real-world concern related to the chapter's focus.

ELEMENTS WITHIN THE CHAPTERS

Glossary Terms appear in bold type in each chapter. They are also listed in the "Terms to Know" at the end of the chapter. Definitions appear in the Glossary at the end of the text.

Exercises stimulate learners to think critically about how to apply chapter content to the workplace and other real-world situations. They provide experiential reinforcement of key leading and managing skills. Exercises are highlighted with a colored vertical rule and are numbered sequentially within each chapter to facilitate using them as assignments or activities.

Research and Literature Perspectives illustrate the relevance and applicability of current scholarship to practice. Perspectives always appear in boxes with an "open book" logo.

Theory Boxes provide a brief description of relevant theory and key concepts.

Numbered boxes contain lists, tools such as forms and work sheets, and other information relevant to chapter content that learners will find useful and interesting.

 ## END OF CHAPTER ELEMENTS

The Solution provides an effective method to handle the real-life situations set forth in The Challenge.

Chapter Checklists summarize key concepts from the chapter in both paragraph and itemized list form.

Tips offer practical guidelines for learners to follow before applying the information presented in each chapter.

Terms to Know are included as additional study/review aids.

References and Suggested Readings provide the learner with a list of key sources for further reading on topics found in the chapter.

 ## OTHER TEACHING/ LEARNING STRATEGIES

End-of-Text Glossary contains a comprehensive list of definitions of all boldfaced terms used in the chapters.

 ## ONLINE INSTRUCTOR LEARNING RESOURCES

Together with the text *Leading and Managing in Nursing,* the Evolve website contains online Instructor Learning Resources. With an image collection and test bank, this online resource offers practical teaching suggestions and strategies for presenting material in the text, making the most effective use of the workbook section in conjunction with the text, and testing. The Instructor's Learning Resources include a chapter-by-chapter test bank containing more than 250 multiple-choice questions, with answer keys at the end of each set of chapter questions. Also, more than 40 images of key illustrations from the text and other materials that instructors will find useful to present in the classroom are included.

Learner's Guide

As a professional nurse in today's changing health-care system, you will need strong leadership and management skills more than ever, regardless of your specific role. You will also need to be an independent, dependable follower. The third edition of *Leading and Managing in Nursing* not only provides the conceptual knowledge you will need but also offers practical strategies to help you hone the various skills so vital to your success as a leader and manager.

Because repetition is a key strategy in learning and retaining new information, you will find many topics discussed in more than one chapter. In addition, as in the real world of nursing, you will often find several different views expressed on a single topic. This repetition reinforces ideas and illustrates how one concept has multiple applications. Rather than referring you to another portion of the text, the key information is provided within the specific chapter.

To help you make the most of your learning experience, try the following strategy. Read the opening paragraph (on the title page of each chapter). This preview should create a context for your reading. The objectives suggest what your accomplishments should be by the time you conclude the chapter. Questions to consider form a way for you to think about your own relevant abilities and experiences. The Challenge allows you to "hear" a real-life situation and always poses the question, "What do you think you would do if you were this nurse?" (The Solution, at the end of the chapter, examines what one individual did in this situation and again asks you to think about how that fits for you and why.) The Introduction and subsequent content, like any text, provide critical information. For some learners,

it is useful to skim those headings and the box content to gain an overall sense of the concepts inherent in the chapter. For others, reading and reflecting from the beginning of the chapter to the end might be useful. The material in boxes (boxes, tables, Research and Literature Perspectives, and Theory boxes) is designed to augment understanding of the content in the text narrative. The checklist highlights the key points the chapter presented, and tips illustrate ways to apply the content just studied. After you complete each chapter, stop and think about what the chapter conveyed. What does it mean for you as a leader, follower, and manager? How do the chapter's content and your interaction with it relate to the other chapters you have already completed? How might you briefly synthesize the content for a nonnurse friend? Reading the chapter, restating its key points in your own words, and completing the text exercises and workbook activities will go far to help you make the content truly your own.

We think you will find leading and managing to be an exciting, challenging field of study, and we have made every attempt to reflect that belief in the design and approach of this edition.

LEARNING AIDS

The third edition of *Leading and Managing in Nursing* continues to incorporate important tools to help you learn about leading and managing and apply your new knowledge to the real world. The next few pages graphically point out how to use these study aids to your best advantage.

The vivid full-color chapter opener **photographs** and other photographs throughout the text help convey each chapter's key message while providing a glimpse into the real world of leading and managing in nursing.

The **introductory paragraph** tells you what you can expect to find in the chapter. To help set the stage for your study of the chapter, read it first and then summarize in your own words what you expect to gain from the chapter.

The list of **Objectives** helps you focus on the key information you should be able to apply after having studied the chapter.

The **Questions to Consider** challenge you to think critically about issues in the chapter. You might want to write down your answers both before and after reading the chapter, and then compare them.

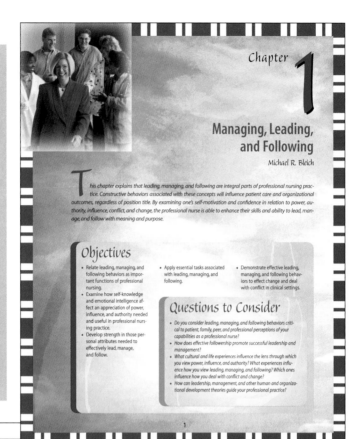

Chapter 1

Managing, Leading, and Following

Michael R. Bleich

This chapter explains that leading, managing, and following are integral parts of professional nursing practice. Constructive behaviors associated with these concepts will influence patient care and organizational outcomes, regardless of position title. By examining one's self-motivation and confidence in relation to power, authority, influence, conflict, and change, the professional nurse is able to enhance their skills and ability to lead, manage, and follow with meaning and purpose.

Objectives

- Relate leading, managing, and following behaviors as important functions of professional nursing.
- Examine how self-knowledge and emotional intelligence affect an appreciation of power, influence, and authority needed in professional nursing practice.
- Develop strength in those personal attributes needed to effectively lead, manage, and follow.
- Apply essential tasks associated with leading, managing, and following.
- Demonstrate effective leading, managing, and following behaviors to effect change and deal with conflict in clinical settings.

Questions to Consider

- Do you consider leading, managing, and following behaviors critical to patient, family, peer, and professional perceptions of your capabilities as a professional nurse?
- How does effective followership promote successful leadership and management?
- What cultural and life experiences influence the lens through which you view power, influence, and authority? What experiences influence how you view leading, managing, and following? Which ones influence how you deal with conflict and change?
- How can leadership, management, and other human and organizational development theories guide your professional practice?

The Challenge

From Rebecca M. Vaughn, RN, MSN
The University of Kansas School of Nursing, Kansas City, Kansas

As a former charge nurse for a 20-bed intensive care unit, it was my responsibility to manage the nursing staff and ensure the delivery of effective clinical and emotional care for patients and their families. I felt confident about my clinical competency, the positive rapport I held with the nursing staff, and the way systems were structured on our unit (i.e., documentation, patient/family education, medication administration, and RN/MD communications). Typically, the staffing ratio for this setting was 1:2 and the average daily census was 17.

One morning in early December, a 64-year-old male patient experienced a cardiac arrest and became unconscious during a dialysis treatment. Unit staffing and skill level were appropriate, and systems were functional for this "Code Blue" situation.

Several minutes into the process, a prominent member of the hospital administrative staff entered the room and proclaimed that this patient was a hospital "VIP" and that each employee should "focus their actions and attentions accordingly." Four well-trained RNs and one cardiology fellow looked to me for a response.

What do you think you would do if you were this nurse?

 INTRODUCTION

Too often, nurses new to the profession believe that their knowledge, skills, and abilities in performing clinical procedures are what make them appear professional to those receiving care, to their peers, or to the public. They may believe that leading and managing are left to those who hold management positions or that being a follower means blindly adhering to the directions of others. What many nurses fail to realize is that their professional nursing image and success are equally dependent on effective leading, managing, and following behaviors. These behaviors are the first lens through which patients, families, subordinates, and other professionals view them and gain confidence in their abilities. Effective leading, managing, and following behaviors are essential to functioning optimally in clinical settings today. Furthermore, nurses must be able to shift effortlessly among these roles within moments when necessary.

Many organizations face the challenge of making the best use of scarce nursing resources. They expect professional nurses to hone their leading, managing, and following behaviors to avert medical errors, achieve patient satisfaction, and promote positive patient outcomes. In addition, they expect professional nurses to contain unnecessary costs at the bedside or when overseeing care, contributing to quality improvement and other organizational activities, or interacting with other healthcare team members.

In this chapter and in Chapters 2 and 3, various perspectives of the concepts of leading (leadership), managing (management), and following (followership) are presented. There is overlap between and among these concepts, meaning that a nurse must lead, manage, and follow concurrently! The distinctiveness of each concept is highlighted for ease of understanding the differences.

Leadership refers to the use of personal traits and personal power to constructively and ethically influence patients, families, and others toward an end point vision or goal. Exact or predictable steps to achieve the goal are not known, must be decided along the way, or require adaptation from what is known. The nurse leader builds and develops relationships so that those being led are empowered to accomplish clinical or organizational goals. Effective leaders communicate a sense of direction, use principles to guide the process, and possess an air of self-assuredness that, in turn, evokes a sense of security in those associated with the task at hand and encourages reasonable risk taking. Leadership does not involve coercion or manipulation of others; the leader makes known to followers the goal or target being tackled. In coercive or manipulative relationships, this information is withheld from followers. Think of leadership in terms of delving into uncharted territory, dealing with and composing strategies as you go to handle details that could not be predicted in advance, while inspiring others to get the job done!

Management is a set of behaviors and activities that provides structure and direction in conducting

In **The Challenge**, practicing nurse leaders/managers offer their real-world views of a concern related to the chapter. Has a nurse you know had similar or dissimilar challenges?

Most chapters contain at least one **Research** or **Literature Perspective** box that you can identify by the "open book" logo. These boxes summarize articles of interest and point out their relevance and applicability to practice. Check the journal that the article came from to find a list of indexing terms to help you locate additional and even more recent articles on the same topic.

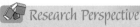 Research Perspective

Bowles, K. (2000). The relationship between critical-thinking skills and the clinical-judgment skills of baccalaureate nursing students. *Journal of Nursing Education, 39*(8), 373.

Although terms such as *critical thinking, problem solving, decision making, creativity,* and *clinical judgment* have been used interchangeably, the relationship among the concepts is unclear and studies have failed to demonstrate a consistent relationship among them.

Kathleen Bowles (2000) endeavored to answer the question: What is the relationship of critical thinking to the clinical judgment abilities of baccalaureate nursing students at the completion of the program? The sample for her study consisted of a convenience sample of nursing students from two baccalaureate programs in public universities in Northern California. The prelicensure students were in the last semester of the nursing program. Demographic data collected included age, cumulative grade point average (GPA), and total years in college. Instruments used to measure critical thinking and clinical judgment were the California Critical Thinking Skills Test (CCTST), form A, and the Clinical Decision Making in Nursing Scale (CDMNS). The CCTST was developed based on the definition of critical thinking adopted by the American Philosophical Association. Bowles used Tanner's definition of clinical judgment, which states clinical judgment includes decisions regard-

ing patient observations and data and resultant actions based upon analysis of them.

The sample consisted of 68 senior nursing students. Their ages ranged from 22 to 50 years, GPA ranged from 2.8 to 4.0, and number of years in college ranged from 4 to 12 years. Scores on the CCTST ranged from 8 to 27 (maximum possible is 34), with a mean score of 18.2 (standard deviation of 4.2). There was a low correlation but statistically significant relationship between the CCTST and CDMNS ($r = .21$, $p < .05$). There was no significant relationship between clinical judgment based on age, GPA, or number of years in college. However, a statistically significant relationship was noted between critical thinking skills and GPA ($r = .55$, $p = .00$).

IMPLICATIONS FOR PRACTICE

The nonrandom sampling and sample size limit the study. Nevertheless, the author concluded that the study findings support previous research that demonstrates a relationship between clinical judgment and critical thinking. Clearly, future research is needed to determine the relationship between these skills, as well as the best ways to measure and strengthen them.

menting the option, and evaluating the result. Box 5-1 contains a form that can be used to complete these steps.

A poor-quality decision is likely if the objectives are not clearly identified or if they are inconsistent with the values of the individual or organization. Lewis Carroll illustrates the essential step of defining the goal, purpose, or objectives in the following excerpt from *Alice's Adventures in Wonderland.*

One day Alice came to a fork in the road and saw a Cheshire Cat in a tree. "Which road do I take?" she asked. His response was a question: "Where do you want to go?" "I don't know," Alice answered. "Then," said the cat, "it doesn't matter."

Decision Models

The decision model that a nurse uses depends on the circumstances. Is the situation routine and predictable or complex and uncertain? Is the goal of the decision to make a decision conservatively that is just "good enough" (satisficing) or one that is optimal? Examples of decision models or theories are presented in the Theory box.

The following scenario illustrates decision theories. Staff nurses on a medical-surgical unit have complained that excessive time is spent documenting on numerous flowcharts and forms, often charting the same information in several places. Their frustration over charting is exacerbated by the inaccessibility of the medical records on the unit. A **satisficing decision** might involve the expedient option of

---

Theory Box

THEORIES FOR PLANNED CHANGE

KEY CONTRIBUTORS	KEY IDEA	APPLICATION TO PRACTICE
Six Phases of Planned Change Havelock (1973) is credited with this planned change model.	Change can be planned, implemented, and evaluated in six sequential stages. The model is advocated for the development of effective change agents and use as a rational problem-solving process. The six stages* are as follows: 1. Building a relationship 2. Diagnosing the problem 3. Acquiring relevant resources 4. Choosing the solution 5. Gaining acceptance 6. Stabilizing the innovation and generating self-renewal	Useful for low-level, low-complexity change.
Seven Phases of Planned Change Lippitt, Watson, and Westley (1958) are credited with this planned change model.	Change can be planned, implemented, and evaluated in seven sequential phases. Ongoing sensitivity to forces in the change process is essential. The seven phases† are as follows: 1. The client system becomes aware of the need for change. 2. The relationship is developed between the client system and change agent. 3. The change problem is defined. 4. The change goals are set and options for achievement are explored. 5. The plan for change is implemented. 6. The change is accepted and stabilized. 7. The change entities redefine their relationships.	Useful for low-level, low-complexity change.
Innovation-Decision Process Rogers (1995) is credited with formulating this process.	Change for an individual occurs over five phases when choosing to accept or reject an innovation/idea. Decisions to not accept the new idea may occur at any of the five stages. The change agent can promote acceptance by providing information about benefits and disadvantages and encouragement. The five stages‡ are as follows: 1. Knowledge 2. Persuasion 3. Decision 4. Implementation 5. Confirmation	Useful for individual change.

*Modified from Havelock, R. G. (1973). *The change agent's guide to innovation in education.* Englewood Cliffs, NJ: Educational Technology Publications.
†Modified from Lippitt, R., Watson, J., & Westley, B. (1958). *The dynamics of planned change.* New York: Harcourt Brace.
‡Modified from Rogers, E. M. (1995). *Diffusion of innovations* (4th ed.). New York: The Free Press.

Most chapters contain a **Theory Box** to highlight and summarize pertinent theoretical concepts.

Every chapter contains numbered **Exercises** that challenge you to think critically about concepts in the text and apply them to real-life situations.

Key Terms appear in boldface type throughout the chapter. (A list of all "Terms to Know" used in the chapter appears at the end of the chapter, and the Glossary at the end of the text contains a list of their definitions.)

The **boxes** in every chapter highlight key information such as lists and contain forms, worksheets, and self-assessments to help reinforce chapter content.

---

26   Leading and Managing in Nursing

knowledgeable, motivating, and competent and has a positive attitude and good people skills (Wieck, Prydun, & Walsh, in press). Bradford and Raines (1992) state, "The effective leader and motivator of the twentysomethings is a coach, mentor and guide who gets to know workers individually" (p. 124).

Successfully leading the emerging workforce means the leader must shape a vision and win the twenty-somethings to it. The vision must be one that excites them because fun and balance are an important part of their lives. A vision that is powerful enough can transform what would otherwise be routine drudgery into collectively focused energy, even sacrifice (Bennis, 1999).

The successful leader must mobilize the followers to act. The required actions must provide value to the followers (e.g., learning a new skill or attaining certification or recognition). The younger generations are happy to follow as long as they can retain the balance in their lives, have information about and input into the decisions that affect them, and see some benefit in the activity. Exemplary leadership is impossible unless the leader has a creative alliance with the followers (Bennis, 1999). It is the leader's challenge to provide this type of environment where younger-generation followers want to follow.

The Entrenched Workforce: The 1946 to 1965 Generation

Baby Boomers, born after World War II, see work life very differently compared with the emerging workforce. Boomer workers are much more likely to believe in the power of collective action, based on their successes with social movements in their formative years in the 1960s. They tend to mistrust authority and are very comfortable with the process of getting to a goal. They find the journey of getting to the goal almost as important as reaching the goal. They are tolerant of, even dependent on, meetings and ongoing discussions that the younger generation finds tedious and wasteful.

The preferred leader of the **entrenched workforce** shares some of the characteristics of the younger generation's leader, such as being motivational, honest, approachable, competent, and knowledgeable. However, Baby Boomers also expect their leader to be professional, be supportive, and have high integrity, a concept not even mentioned by the younger generation (Wieck, Prydun, & Walsh, in press).

Challenges for the entrenched workforce are sharing leadership with the younger generation, em-

powering them to lead in their own model rather than trying to make them into second-generation Baby Boomers, and retaining the younger leaders in leadership ranks. Many younger employees are opting out of traditional work roles to become entrepreneurs. They take their leadership potential with them where there are few older role models for them to follow. A risk for aging Boomers is that the best and the brightest potential leaders will lose interest in leading and will opt for personal satisfaction and wealth accumulation rather than leadership and service roles.

The challenges of generational acceptance is one of many facing twenty-first century leaders. Attention to the needs of both the leader and the follower will create an environment where everyone thrives.

Exercise 2-4
List the names of the people with whom you work most frequently. Determine to which workforce (emerging or entrenched) each belongs. Describe known benefits of the workplace that support each generation's view. (One list may be longer than the other.) What elements of benefits are present in the personnel policies and workplace practices that benefit each? What elements are absent?

SURVIVING AND THRIVING AS A LEADER

The key to leadership is to believe in the vision and to enjoy the journey. The leader has a responsibility to self and followers to stay healthy and enthusiastic for the mission of the group. Surviving and thriving as a leader is based on the rules in Box 2-2.

The Leader Must Maintain Balance

Time management is essential for an effective leader. Many new leaders, in their zeal to be accessible to their constituents, lose control of their

BOX 2-2

The Five Rules of Leaders

1. Maintain balance.
2. Generate self-motivation.
3. Build self-confidence.
4. Listen to constituents.
5. Maintain a positive attitude.

Chapter 3   **Developing the Role of Man**

Table 3-3   THE MANAGER'S COROLLARY TO THE COURAGE OF FOLLOWERS

Dimension of the Relationship (Follower)	Manager
Courage to assume responsibility	Demonstrates trust in individual autonomy
Courage to serve	Advocates for service role
Courage to challenge	Poses dilemmas to encourage behavior
Courage to participate in transformation	Designs opportunities to develop transformation abilities
Courage to leave by separating from a leader or group	Risks separation

Modified from Chaleff, L. (1995). *The courageous follower: Standing up to and for our leaders.* San Francisco: Berrett-Koehler.

agers of the twenty-first century. Valadez and Sportsman (1999) address the use of quantum theory when managing the environment. They offer three guiding principles to manage the healthcare environment: (1) The world is unpredictable; (2) the world is not independent of the observer; and (3) relationships among things are what counts, not the things themselves. The authors identify a critical role component for health professionals today, that is, manipulation of factors that may impair workers' ability to accomplish a goal.

Porter-O'Grady (1999) writes of quantum leadership having five expectations of the nurse manager. (1) Do not predict the future, for none of us can know it with certainty. Predicting the future can have negative consequences on the consumer as well as staff. (2) Learn to read the direction of change. The manager who closely monitors current trends and correlates them can forecast an accurate picture and offer some direction to the change. (3) Constant translation of meaning of information is necessary. Staff have access to numerous sources of information, and this can lead to sensory overload. It is the manager's responsibility to give staff positive reinforcement for their data-gathering efforts while at the same time assisting them to effectively narrow their data-retrieval efforts. (4) Assist staff members to learn self-management. Two key elements necessary for staff to function effectively in the new healthcare environment include being independent in their role functions and being interdependent in their relationships within the team. The manager's challenge is to instill independent traits in the staff and remove the long-standing idea that a manager's role is as a sage advisor who assumes a parent role. (5) Technological proficiency is not an option but an expectation. The staff's interdependent role necessitates a technologically proficient staff who can communicate with the team through wire and wireless modes, facsimiles, and new links. The manager's role includes holding staff accountable for the technological communication and providing them with the necessary skills to be proficient in technology.

To be successful in day-to-day operations, a manager must be concerned with relationships. Chaleff (1995) developed a model of followership to reorient individuals. "Courageous followership is built on the platform of courageous relationship. The courage to be right, the courage to be wrong, the courage to be different from each other. Each of us sees the world through our own eyes and experiences" (p. 4). Chaleff describes five dimensions of the relationship: the courage to assume responsibility, the courage to serve, the courage to challenge, the courage to participate in transformation, and the courage to leave by separating from a leader or group. Table 3-3 poses the possible corollary role of the manager for supporting this courage development in **followers**.

CONSUMER OF RESEARCH

The nurse manager's role calls for a twofold responsibility: that of being a participant in research and that of being an interpreter of research. Nursing literature, especially in nursing administration journals, reflects that nurse managers are contributing to research either by doing unit research or contributing to large-scale agency research projects. Likewise, the nurse manager also interprets published research findings that have implications for the staff or the patients and makes every effort

The **tables** that appear throughout the text provide convenient capsules of information for your reference.

The numerous full-color **illustrations** visually reinforce key concepts.

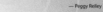

Figure 7-1   Key steps in strategic planning.

- Appraisal of the major opportunities and threats in the environment
- Identification and evaluation of the various strategies available to the organization to meet these opportunities and threats
- Selection of the best option that balances the organization's potential with the challenges of changing conditions, taking into account the values of its management and its social responsibilities
- Preparation of the strategy
- Implementation and evaluation of the strategy

Reasons for Planning

To survive the ongoing change and restructuring of the healthcare system, thoughtful and deliberate planning becomes a necessity. This process leads to success in the achievement of goals and objectives, gives meaning to work life, and provides direction for operational activities of the organization.

Furthermore, planning may result in efficient and effective use of resources and may assist in the formulation of visionary activities and the future direction of the agency. There are numerous reasons why nursing administrators should plan in a systematic manner: Knowledge regarding philosophy, goals, and external and internal operations of the organization are necessary; an understanding of the planning process is essential; and time must be divided on day-to-day operations rather than on short- and long-range plans.

Phases of the Strategic Planning Process

The strategic planning process is proactive, vision-directed, action-oriented, creative, innovative, and oriented toward change. "Healthcare providers increasingly are relying on strategic planning to guide the allocation of capital and other resources. Strategic planning helps identify and prioritize op-

---

The Solution

In any redesign effort, involving the staff is critical. I began by meeting with the staff and telling them why I wanted to begin a redesign process and what I hoped to accomplish from such efforts. I then set up redesign teams that have a great deal of staff involvement.

Involving the staff is critical for several reasons. First, the individuals who are actually taking care of patients most of the time think of the most creative solutions for redesign. Second, staff are more likely to embrace redesign activities if they feel that they have been actively involved in the process. Finally, staff can often anticipate issues or problems with these efforts and help develop solutions before the implementation of redesign.

If I worked in a unionized environment, my approach would not differ, except I would meet with the union representatives before initiating the redesign efforts. Again, I would explain what I hoped to accomplish through these efforts, answer any questions or concerns, and ask for their support of the project.

— Peggy Reiley

Would this be a suitable approach for you? Why?

CHAPTER CHECKLIST

Collectively, nurses possess the knowledge, skills, abilities, and numbers to influence decisions. Collective action may take many forms. Geographic and organizational contexts influence the formal and informal structures in which nurses participate. An organization's structure establishes the parameters for participation in decision making. Managers establish the context for participation. The decision to organize for the purpose of collective bargaining represents an important decision for nurses and for the organization in which they practice. A level of tension exists when an external group becomes a part of an organization's decision-making processes. External groups may enter as a new management consultant, as a part of a merger, as a new owner, or as a union representing registered nurses. The acceptance and appreciation of the external group are influenced by understanding the rationale for the group's entry and by the respect between the constituencies.

- The purposes of collective participation by nurses are to do the following:
  - Promote the practice of professional nursing
  - Establish and maintain standards of care
  - Allocate resources effectively and efficiently
  - Create satisfaction and support in the practice environment (Minarik & Catramabone, 1993)

- Increased autonomy and diversification decrease the following:
  - Fear of ridicule
  - Fear of punishment
  - Fear of loss of job
  - Fear of favors
- Governance strategies dictate levels of participation. The level of participation in decision making influences job satisfaction.
- Shared governance is characterized by partnerships, equity, accountability, and ownership.
- The framework for advocacy includes mutuality, facilitation, protection, and coordination. The manifestations of advocacy are as follows:
  - Ensuring relevant information
  - Enabling the selection of information
  - Disclosing a personal view
  - Providing support for making and implementing decisions
  - Helping determine personal values
- The goal of workplace advocacy is to equip nurses to practice in a rapidly changing environment.
- Collective bargaining is an effective mechanism used by nurses to obtain the right to participate in decisions regarding their practice.
- Represented nurses must be proven wrong or in error. Unrepresented nurses bear the burden of proving themselves to be correct.

Continued

Each chapter ends with these features:

The Solution provides an effective method to handle the situations presented in The Challenge.

The **Chapter Checklist** provides a quick summary of key points in the chapter. To help you keep in mind the broad themes of the chapter, read it immediately *before* you start reading the chapter.

The **Tips** offer guidelines to follow for each chapter before applying the information presented in the chapter.

The **Terms to Know** in every chapter include all the key terms used in that chapter. You might find it helpful to review this list before reading the chapter and to look up in the Glossary any definitions that are unfamiliar.

CHAPTER CHECKLIST—CONT'D

- Federal and state governments have enacted a number of employment laws that nurses must understand and follow when dealing with managerial issues. These include the following:
  - Equal Pay Act of 1963
  - Civil Rights Act
  - Age Discrimination Act of 1967
  - Americans with Disabilities Act of 1990
  - Affirmative Action
  - Equal Employment Opportunity Laws
  - Occupational Safety and Health Act
  - Employment-at-Will and Wrongful Discharge
  - Family and Medical Leave Act of 1993
  - Collective Bargaining
- Ethical theories and principles relate to moral actions and value systems and apply both to patient situations and to management situations.
  - Ethical theories justify existing moral principles and are considered universally applicable.
  - Ethical theories include the following:
    - Deontology
    - Teleology (utilitarianism)
    - Principlism
  - Ethical principles exert direct control over professional nursing practice and encompass basic premises from which rules are developed.
  - Ethical principles include the following:
    - Autonomy
    - Beneficence
    - Nonmaleficence
    - Veracity
    - Justice
    - Paternalism
    - Fidelity
    - Respect for others
  - The MORAL model is an easy acronym to remember in ethical decision making.
  - Ethics committees aid in assisting nurses to implement solutions in everyday clinical practice.

TIPS ON LEGAL AND ETHICAL ISSUES

- Before applying the information presented in the chapter, the following five tips are offered:
  - Read the state nurse practice act carefully to fully comprehend the allowable scope of practice within the given state.

- Consult with risk management, the institutional attorney, or the legal department for a fuller understanding of how federal employment laws pertain to the individual nurse manager.
- Cultivate a group of professional consultants, either within the institution or outside the institution, who can assist with legal-ethical questions. Professional consultants may have great insight into issues as they arise and can assist in preventing problems in the future.
- Discover who serves on the institutional ethics committee and develop friendships with selected members. Attend the meetings to see how ethical issues are addressed in the institution. Become an active part of the ethical rounds if they exist in the institution.
- Think before you act. Remember it is always easier to hesitate, even briefly, so that the better approach can be implemented than to try to retract or amend something already done or already verbalized.

TERMS TO KNOW

apparent agency	law
autonomy	liability
beneficence	liable
collective bargaining	malpractice
common law	MORAL model
confidentiality	negligence
corporate liability	nonmaleficence
deontological theories	nurse practice act
emancipated minors	paternalism
ergonomics	personal liability
ethics	principlism
ethics committees	privacy
expert witnesses	respect for others
failure to warn	respondeat superior
fidelity	standard of care
foreseeability	statute
indemnification	teleological theories
independent contractors	values
informed consent	veracity
justice	vicarious liability
labor unions	

Glossary

Absenteeism The rate at which an individual misses work on an unplanned basis. (Ch. 20)
Acceptance The second phase of the change process when change is willingly used.
Accommodation An unassertive, cooperative approach to conflict in which the individual neglects personal needs, goals, and concerns in favor of satisfying those of others. (Ch. 19)
Accountability The expectation of explaining actions and results. (Ch. 18)
Acknowledgment Recognition that an employee is valued and respected for what he or she has to offer to the work place, team, or group; acknowledgment may be verbal or written, public or private. (Ch. 17)
Absenteeism The rate at which an individual misses work on an unplanned basis. (Ch. 20)
Acceptance The second phase of the change process when change is willingly used.
Accommodation An unassertive, cooperative approach to conflict in which the individual neglects personal needs, goals, and concerns in favor of satisfying those of others. (Ch. 19)
Accountability The expectation of explaining actions and results. (Ch. 18)
Acknowledgment Recognition that an employee is valued and respected for what he or she has to offer to the work place, team, or group; acknowledgment may be verbal or written, public or private. (Ch. 17)
Absenteeism The rate at which an individual misses work on an unplanned basis. (Ch. 20)
Acceptance The second phase of the change process when change is willingly used.
Accommodation An unassertive, cooperative approach to conflict in which the individual neglects personal needs, goals, and concerns in favor of satisfying those of others. (Ch. 19)
Accountability The expectation of explaining actions and results. (Ch. 18)
Acknowledgment Recognition that an employee is valued and respected for what he or she has to offer to the work place, team, or group; acknowledgment may be verbal or written, public or private. (Ch. 17)
Absenteeism The rate at which an individual misses work on an unplanned basis. (Ch. 20)
Acceptance The second phase of the change process when change is willingly used.
Accommodation An unassertive, cooperative approach to conflict in which the individual neglects personal needs, goals, and concerns in favor of satisfying those of others. (Ch. 19)

Accountability The expectation of explaining actions and results. (Ch. 18)
Acknowledgment Recognition that an employee is valued and respected for what he or she has to offer to the work place, team, or group; acknowledgment may be verbal or written, public or private. (Ch. 17)
Absenteeism The rate at which an individual misses work on an unplanned basis. (Ch. 20)
Acceptance The second phase of the change process when change is willingly used.
Accommodation An unassertive, cooperative approach to conflict in which the individual neglects personal needs, goals, and concerns in favor of satisfying those of others. (Ch. 19)
Accountability The expectation of explaining actions and results. (Ch. 18)
Acknowledgment Recognition that an employee is valued and respected for what he or she has to offer to the work place, team, or group; acknowledgment may be verbal or written, public or private. (Ch. 17)
Absenteeism The rate at which an individual misses work on an unplanned basis. (Ch. 20)
Acceptance The second phase of the change process when change is willingly used.
Accommodation An unassertive, cooperative approach to conflict in which the individual neglects personal needs, goals, and concerns in favor of satisfying those of others. (Ch. 19)
Accountability The expectation of explaining actions and results. (Ch. 18)
Acknowledgment Recognition that an employee is valued and respected for what he or she has to offer to the work place, team, or group; acknowledgment may be verbal or written, public or private. (Ch. 17)

15

The **Glossary** at the end of the text lists alphabetically all the boldfaced terms from the chapters.

The **Workbook Section** is a built-in, perforated tool to help you self-assess and evaluate your learning and understanding of the content in the text.

CHAPTER **1** WORKBOOK

Managing, Leading, and Following

INTRODUCTION

Effective managers focus efficiently on objectives, tasks, procedures, and policies. Recently, however, the emphasis has been on leaders who provide vision, inspiration, and empowerment. Exactly what do these terms mean? Who should lead, manage, or follow, and when? The activities in this section are designed to help you recognize the differences between leading, managing, and following and to recognize how and why these behaviors are essential for organizations to move forward.

ACTIVITY 1-1

1. What words come to mind when you think of the word *leader*?

2. What words come to mind when you think of the word *follower*?

3. Analyze the differences between the two lists. Do you think of leaders in different ways than you think of followers?

4. Recall pairs of leaders-followers from politics, science, education, the media, or personal experience. As you recall these pairs of individuals, what made one the "leader" and the other the "follower"? How did the leader contribute to the follower's success? How did the follower contribute to the leader's success? Were there times when the leader functioned more as the follower? Were there times when the follower functioned more as the leader? What does this analysis tell you about the nature of leader-follower relationships?

Contents

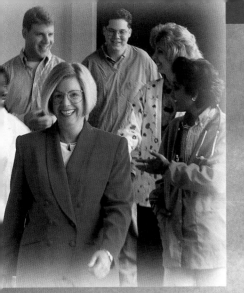

Managing, Leading, and Following

Michael R. Bleich

*T*his chapter explains that leading, managing, and following are integral parts of professional nursing practice. Constructive behaviors associated with these concepts will influence patient care and organizational outcomes, regardless of position title. By examining one's self-motivation and confidence in relation to power, authority, influence, conflict, and change, the professional nurse is able to enhance their skills and ability to lead, manage, and follow with meaning and purpose.

Objectives

- Relate leading, managing, and following behaviors as important functions of professional nursing.
- Examine how self-knowledge and emotional intelligence affect an appreciation of power, influence, and authority needed and useful in professional nursing practice.
- Develop strength in those personal attributes needed to effectively lead, manage, and follow.

- Apply essential tasks associated with leading, managing, and following.

- Demonstrate effective leading, managing, and following behaviors to effect change and deal with conflict in clinical settings.

Questions to Consider

- *Do you consider leading, managing, and following behaviors critical to patient, family, peer, and professional perceptions of your capabilities as a professional nurse?*
- *How does effective followership promote successful leadership and management?*
- *What cultural and life experiences influence the lens through which you view power, influence, and authority? What experiences influence how you view leading, managing, and following? Which ones influence how you deal with conflict and change?*
- *How can leadership, management, and other human and organizational development theories guide your professional practice?*

The Challenge

From Rebecca M. Vaughn, RN, MSN
The University of Kansas School of Nursing, Kansas City, Kansas

As a former charge nurse for a 20-bed intensive care unit, it was my responsibility to manage the nursing staff and ensure the delivery of effective clinical and emotional care for patients and their families. I felt confident about my clinical competency, the positive rapport I held with the nursing staff, and the way systems were structured on our unit (i.e., documentation, patient/family education, medication administration, and RN/MD communications). Typically, the staffing ratio for this setting was 1:2 and the average daily census was 17.

One morning in early December, a 64-year-old male patient experienced a cardiac arrest and became unconscious during a dialysis treatment. Unit staffing and skill level were appropriate, and systems were functional for this "Code Blue" situation.

Several minutes into the process, a prominent member of the hospital administrative staff entered the room and proclaimed that this patient was a hospital "VIP" and that each employee should "focus their actions and attentions accordingly." Four well-trained RNs and one cardiology fellow looked to me for a response.

 What do you think you would do if you were this nurse?

INTRODUCTION

Too often, nurses new to the profession believe that their knowledge, skills, and abilities in performing clinical procedures are what make them appear professional to those receiving care, to their peers, or to the public. They may believe that leading and managing are left to those who hold management positions or that being a follower means blindly adhering to the directions of others. What many nurses fail to realize is that their professional nursing image and success are equally dependent on effective leading, managing, and following behaviors. These behaviors are the first lens through which patients, families, subordinates, and other professionals view them and gain confidence in their abilities. Effective leading, managing, and following behaviors are essential to functioning optimally in clinical settings today. Furthermore, nurses must be able to shift effortlessly among these roles within moments when necessary.

Many organizations face the challenge of making the best use of scarce nursing resources. They expect professional nurses to hone their leading, managing, and following behaviors to avert medical errors, achieve patient satisfaction, and promote positive patient outcomes. In addition, they expect professional nurses to contain unnecessary costs at the bedside or when overseeing care, contributing to quality improvement and other organizational activities, or interacting with other healthcare team members.

In this chapter and in Chapters 2 and 3, various perspectives of the concepts of leading (leadership), managing (management), and following (followership) are presented. There is overlap between and among these concepts, meaning that a nurse must lead, manage, and follow concurrently! The distinctiveness of each concept is highlighted for ease of understanding the differences.

Leadership refers to the use of personal traits and personal power to constructively and ethically influence patients, families, and others toward an end point vision or goal. Exact or predictable steps to achieve the goal are not known, must be decided along the way, or require adaptation from what is known. The nurse leader builds and develops relationships so that those being led are empowered to accomplish clinical or organizational goals. Effective leaders communicate a sense of direction, use principles to guide the process, and possess an air of self-assuredness that, in turn, evokes a sense of security in those associated with the task at hand and encourages reasonable risk taking. Leadership does not involve coercion or manipulation of others; the leader makes known to followers the goal or target being tackled. In coercive or manipulative relationships, this information is withheld from followers. Think of leadership in terms of delving into uncharted territory, dealing with and composing strategies as you go to handle details that could not be predicted in advance, while inspiring others to get the job done!

Management is a set of behaviors and activities that provides structure and direction in conducting patient care and organizational functions where the norms and outcomes to be achieved are known and where a desired sequence to accomplish these outcomes is prescribed, either in writing or through historical practices embedded in the organization's culture. Management tasks are afforded to any staff member who bears responsibility for the work of others or who has the responsibility to ensure that an organizational process is carried out. *Management* can also refer to engaging individual skills and abilities to organize self-directed actions to accomplish goals within a predetermined time frame (as in completing all essential patient care activities for an assignment of patients by the end of a shift). In this chapter the term *management* does *not* usually refer to the top positions of authority (such as a Nursing Director or Patient Care Executive). Think of management as using power constructively as a professional to expediently guide the accomplishment of a task known to be necessary for clinical and organizational success (such as in assignment making or coordinating discharge planning with other disciplines). In management, a best way or a set of norms is introduced, made known to others, and used to accomplish goals.

Followership refers to the behaviors demonstrated by individuals with whom the leader or manager interacts. Followership is the healthy, assertive use of personal behaviors that contributes to patient, family, and healthcare team achievement. Followers move toward clinical and organizational outcomes while practicing *acquiescence* in certain tasks, such as direction setting, politicking, pacesetting, or planning, to the individuals leading or managing the team. Followership is *not* a passive process, but rather a set of behaviors that demonstrates collaboration, influence, and action *with* the leader.

When taken together, the behaviors that reflect leading, managing, and following are complementary to each other. By virtue of being professional nurses, all nurses will be in leading, managing, and

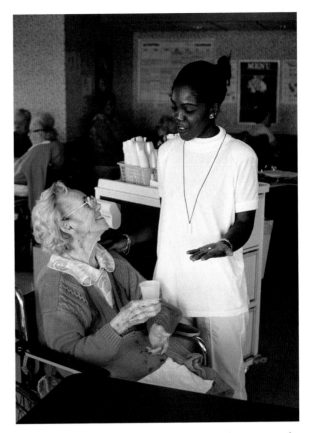

Many nurse leaders are motivated by a strong desire to care for those who cannot care for themselves.

following situations. Some positions, such as being a charge nurse or nurse manager, are formal positions requiring more leading and managing behaviors to establish organizational goals and objectives, oversee human resources, provide staff with performance feedback, facilitate change, and manage conflict to meet patient care and organizational requirements.

PERSONAL ATTRIBUTES NEEDED TO LEAD, MANAGE, AND FOLLOW

Leading, managing, and following require a different skill set from those associated with the technical aspects of nursing. Goleman (1995) and others refer to **emotional intelligence,** that is, possessing social skills, interpersonal competence, psychological maturity, and emotional awareness such that these skills then "help people harmonize" and become "increasingly valued in the workplace" (p. 160).

■ *Exercise 1–1*

Using the definitions of leadership, management, and followership, imagine that you are faced with a critically ill patient whose family members are spread throughout the country. Some family members are holding vigil at the bedside, while others are calling the patient care unit incessantly. You recognize the family's care and concern, yet you want to move out of a reactive stance to a practice position. How would you solve this problem as a leader? a manager? a follower? Which role are you most comfortable in? least comfortable? Which role leads to the best outcome for all parties?

Nurses have countless interactions within the course of a workday. Each of these interactions benefits from leading, managing, or following abilities within the five domains that comprise an emotionally intelligent practitioner:

- Having self-awareness (the ability to step outside and see oneself in the context of what is happening while recognizing and owning feelings associated with an event)
- Managing emotions (naming, claiming, and taming feelings such as fear, anxiety, anger, and sadness and taking appropriate actions to progress through feelings in a healthy manner; avoiding passive-aggressive and victim responses)
- Motivating oneself (focusing on a goal, often with delayed gratification, such that emotional self-control is achieved and impulses are stifled)
- Being empathetic (valuing differences in perspective and showing sensitivity to the experiences of others in a way that demonstrates ability to reveal another's perspective on a situation)
- Handling relationships (exhibiting social appropriateness and using social skills to help others manage emotions)

The emotionally intelligent nurse has credibility because of patient, family, and organizational awareness, collaborative capacity, insight into others, and commitment to self-growth. When coupled with performing clinical tasks and critical thinking, the nurse demonstrates expanded capabilities. The synergy associated with credibility and capability fuse to become markers of professional nursing. Without self-reflective skills, growth in emotional intelligence when leading, managing, or following is stymied, work becomes routinized, and the nurse often experiences a lack of synchrony with others. Box 1-1 reflects a composite of leadership and management attributes that build credibility and capability.

Exercise 1–2

Referring back to Exercise 1-1, how would a nurse with highly developed emotional intelligence lead, manage, or follow in reference to problem solving? Emotional intelligence is developed through insight into one's self, positive "self-talk," journal recording, and other methods that promote awareness of situations, biases, and the like. Develop a personal recipe for enhancing your own emotional intelligence.

THEORY DEVELOPMENT IN LEADING, MANAGING, AND FOLLOWING

Theories are useful because they generate direction and allow outcomes to be predicted. Although leadership, management, and followership theories are still evolving and have not reached a stage where, "if 'A' circumstance is present and 'B' intervention is applied, then 'C' outcome is guaranteed," useful theory has been developed that guides structures, methods, and variables used to drive successful outcomes. Unfortunately, theories that address human behavior in the context of organizational settings are complicated and limited in their absolute predictive power.

The development of leadership, motivation, and management theory rapidly evolved at the beginning of the twentieth century when industries flourished to achieve mass production. As large numbers of people migrated from rural communities to work together in these contained environments in urban settings, the factors that ensured successful production were examined. Theory development began with an examination of the influence of *charismatic leaders* on the workforce, followed by *motivational factors* that supported

---

BOX 1-1

Attributes of Leaders and Managers

Uses focused energy and stamina to accomplish a vision

Uses critical-thinking skills in decision making

Trusts personal intuition, then backs up intuition with facts

Accepts responsibility willingly and follows up on the consequences of actions taken

Identifies the needs of others

Deals with people skillfully: coaches, communicates, counsels

Demonstrates ease in standard/boundary setting

Examines multiple options to accomplish the objective at hand flexibly

Is trustworthy; handles information from various sources with respect for the source

Motivates others assertively toward the objective at hand

Demonstrates competence or is capable of rapid learning in the arena where change is desired

worker job satisfaction and, later, the *environmental determinants* that contributed to or deterred from achieving quotas.

Leadership theory emerged as a body of knowledge attempting to explain the traits and behaviors of leaders perceived to successfully influence situations, people, and events toward organizational goal attainment. Leadership theory has developed through the fields of sociology and psychology. The initial goal of leadership theory was to predict the qualities of leaders that would successfully influence others in meeting organizational outcomes (Research Perspective).

Because leadership is an interactive process, several motivational theories are closely tied to leadership theory. The motivational theories explain how individuals derive and sustain behaviors to accomplish a goal or how leaders and environmental factors influence how workers maintain production. Motivational theories have been developed primarily by the field of psychology.

Management theory constitutes the body of knowledge that describes how managers conduct activities to keep the organization operating effectively. Management theory describes myriad topics such as how work is organized, planning accomplished, change managed, and production quotas determined. Because of the diverse nature of activities that contribute to management theory development, representatives from a broad range

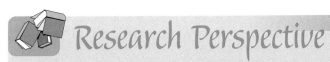

Research Perspective

Genrich, S. J., Banks, J. C., Bufton, K., Savage, M. E., & Owens, M. U. (2001). Group involvement in decision-making: A pilot study. *The Journal of Continuing Education in Nursing, 32*(1), 20-26.

Shared governance is a viable organizational design that has as a central tenet: nurses as active participants in decision making. Manthey and Miller (1994) suggest that professionals are given authority based on the complexity of decision making at four different levels: Level I, at which staff gather data only and pass the information along to other decision makers; Level II, at which staff collect data and offer recommendations to other decision makers; Level III, at which staff participate with managers in decision making; and Level IV, at which staff make independent decisions. Shared governance places decision making at Level IV, giving staff "power, authority, accountability, and final decision-making capacity" (Porter-O'Grady & Finnigan, 1984, p. 84).

Nurse researchers from the Baylor University School of Nursing linked shared governance with the Vroom-Yetton-Jago Leadership Theory. A convenience sample of 27 healthcare leaders was assembled to determine whether attending a 90-minute class on the use of the model would enhance group decision making, a process that is critical in the use of shared governance. Before and after attending the educational course titled "Group Involvement in Decision Making," participants were asked to read three case studies and identify the leadership style they would use in each scenario. The theory supports high-level decision making and addresses the obstacles and challenges associated with problem solving and leadership style from the perspectives of individual and group decision makers.

The results of the study suggest that high-level group decision making is achieved in healthcare organizations when staff are adequately prepared and developed in the areas of decision making, problem solving, and leadership.

IMPLICATIONS FOR PRACTICE

In today's healthcare environment, all members of the healthcare team are included in decision making to optimize efficiency and effectiveness. Opportunities for nurses to participate in high-level organizational decision making are increasing. Although nurses are skilled in making decisions unilaterally, they are even more productive with additional background and training related to group decision-making skills. Nurse leaders who are implementing shared governance models should not presume that development of staff is not an important part of the implementation strategy.

Theory Box

LEADERSHIP THEORIES

THEORY/CONTRIBUTOR	KEY IDEA	APPLICATION TO PRACTICE
Trait Theories Trait theories were first studied from 1900 to 1950. These theories are sometimes referred to as the *Great Man theory,* from Aristotle's philosophy extolling the virtue of being "born" with leadership traits. Stogdill (1948) is usually credited as the pioneer in this school of thought.	Leaders have a certain set of physical and emotional characteristics that are crucial for inspiring others toward a common goal. Some theorists believe that traits are innate and cannot be learned; others believe that leadership traits can be developed in each individual.	Self-awareness of traits is useful in self-development (e.g., developing assertiveness) and in seeking employment that matches traits (drive, motivation, integrity, confidence, cognitive ability, and task knowledge).
Style Theories Sometimes referred to as *group and exchange theories of leadership,* style theories were derived in the mid-1950s because of the limitations of trait theory. The key contributors to this renowned research were Shartle (1956), Stogdill (1963), and Likert (1961).	Style theories focus on what leaders do in relational and contextual terms. The achievement of satisfactory performance measures requires supervisors to pursue effective relationships with their subordinates, while comprehending the factors in the work environment that influence outcomes.	To understand "style," it is useful to obtain feedback from followers, superiors, and peers, such as through the Managerial Grid Instrument developed by Blake and Mouton (1985). Employee-centered leaders tend to be the leaders most able to achieve effective work environments and productivity.
Situational-Contingency Theories The situational-contingency theorists emerged in the 1960s and early to mid-1970s. These theorists believed that leadership effectiveness depends on the relationship among (1) the leader's task at hand, (2) his or her interpersonal skills, and (3) the favorableness of the work situation. Examples of theory development with this expanded perspective include Fiedler's (1967) Contingency Model, the Vroom-Yetton (1973) Normative Decision-Making Model, and House-Mitchell's (1974) Path-Goal theory.	Three factors are critical: (1) the degree of trust and respect between leaders and followers, (2) the task structure denoting the clarity of goals and the complexity of problems faced, and (3) the position power in terms of where the leader was able to reward followers and exert influence. Consequently, leaders were viewed as able to adapt their style according to the presenting situation. The Vroom-Yetton model was a problem-solving approach to leadership. Path-Goal theory recognized two contingent variables: (1) the personal characteristics of followers and (2) environmental demands. On the basis of these factors, the leader sets forth clear expectations, eliminates obstacles to goal achievements, motivates and rewards staff, and increases opportunities for follower satisfaction based on effective job performance.	The most important implications for leaders is that these theories consider the challenge of a situation and encourage an adaptive leadership style to complement the issue being faced. In other words, nurses must assess each situation and determine appropriate action based on the people involved.

Theory Box

LEADERSHIP THEORIES—cont'd

THEORY/CONTRIBUTOR	KEY IDEA	APPLICATION TO PRACTICE
Transformational Theories Transformational theories arose late in the last millennium when globalization and other factors caused organizations to fundamentally reestablish themselves. Many of these attempts were failures, but great attention was given to those leaders who effectively transformed structures, human resources, and profitability balanced with quality. Bass (1990), Bennis and Nanus (1985), and Tichy and Devanna (1986) are commonly associated with the study of transformational theory.	*Transformational leadership* refers to a process whereby the leader attends to the needs and motives of followers so that the interaction raises each to high levels of motivation and morality. The leader is a role model who inspires followers through displayed optimism, provides intellectual stimulation, and encourages follower creativity.	Transformed organizations are responsive to customer needs, are morally and ethically intact, promote employee development, and encourage self-management. Nurse leaders with transformational characteristics experiment with systems redesign, empower staff, create enthusiasm for practice, and promote scholarship of practice at the bedside.

Theory Box

MOTIVATIONAL THEORIES

THEORY/CONTRIBUTOR	KEY IDEA	APPLICATION TO PRACTICE
Hierarchy of Needs Maslow is credited with developing a theory of motivation, first published in 1943.	People are motivated by a hierarchy of human needs, beginning with physiological needs, then progressing to safety, social, esteem, and self-actualizing needs. In this theory, when the need for food, water, air, and other life-sustaining elements is met, the human spirit reaches out to achieve affiliation with others, which promotes the development of self-esteem, competence, achievement, and creativity. Lower-level needs will always drive behavior before higher-level needs will be addressed.	When this theory is applied to staff, leaders must be aware that the need for safety and security will override the opportunity to be creative and inventive, such as in promoting job change.
Two-Factor Theory Herzberg (1991) is credited with developing a two-factor theory of motivation, first published in 1968.	Hygiene factors, such as working conditions, salary, status, and security, motivate workers by meeting safety and security needs and avoiding job dissatisfaction. Motivator factors, such as achievement, recognition, and the satisfaction of the work itself, promote job enrichment by creating job satisfaction.	Organizations need both hygiene and motivator factors to recruit and retain staff. Hygiene factors do not create job satisfaction; they simply must be in place for work to get accomplished. If not, these factors will only serve to dissatisfy staff. Transformational leaders use motivator factors liberally to inspire work performance.

Continued

Theory Box

MOTIVATIONAL THEORIES—cont'd

THEORY/CONTRIBUTOR	KEY IDEA	APPLICATION TO PRACTICE
Expectancy Theory Vroom (1964) is credited with developing the expectancy theory of motivation.	Felt needs of individuals cause their behavior. In the work setting, this motivated behavior is increased if a person perceives a positive relationship between effort and performance. Motivated behavior is further increased if there is a positive relationship between good performance and outcomes or rewards, particularly when these are valued.	Expectancy is the perceived probability of satisfying a particular need based on past experience. Therefore nurses in leadership roles need to provide specific feedback about positive performance.
OB Modification Luthans (1973) is credited with establishing the foundation for Organizational Behavior Modification (OB Mod), based on Skinner's work on operant conditioning.	OB Mod is an operant approach to organizational behavior. OB Mod Performance Analysis follows a three-step ABC Model: A, antecedent analysis of clear expectations and baseline data collection; B, behavioral analysis and determination; and C, consequence analysis, including reinforcement strategies.	The leader uses positive reinforcement to motivate followers to repeat constructive behaviors in the workplace. Negative events that demotivate staff are negatively reinforced, so the staff is motivated to avoid certain situations that cause discomfort. Extinction is the purposeful nonreinforcement (ignoring) of negative behaviors. Punishment is used sparingly because the results are unpredictable in supporting the desired behavioral outcome.

of disciplines, including managers, psychologists, sociologists, and anthropologists, have contributed to its development.

Leadership, motivational, and management theories overlap, although they are presented as distinctive. Each area of theory development continues to evolve, incorporating new knowledge about organizational culture, structure, and function; motivation, development, and learning; conflict management; team functioning; change management; and other contemporary factors, such as globalization, diversity, generational differences, and gender equity.

The theory boxes in this chapter are organized to provide an orientation to the major schools of leadership and motivational theory development and to introduce those concepts that are applicable in healthcare settings. Management theories such as change theory are woven throughout this text.

What should be evident from the theories presented is that the pattern of leadership, management, and motivational research has been one of discarding, extending, and introducing and reintroducing ideas as the limitations or values of existing ideas materialized. Progression of different research orientations has guided the development of theory, yet no single theory fully addresses the totality of leading, managing, and following.

TASKS OF LEADING, MANAGING, AND FOLLOWING

When one is dealing with theory and concepts, it is sometimes easy for developing professionals to lose sight of the tangible behaviors that are needed to put these ideas into practice. Gardner (1990) recognized this when he set out to describe tasks of

Literature Perspective

Hanna, L. A. (1999). Lead the way. *Nursing Management, 30*(11), 37-39.

Effective leaders show objectivity, creativity, and knowledge. They develop personal leadership styles from existing models and personal experiences, and they use their strength to motivate staff, accomplish organizational goals, and develop future leaders.

Motivation comes from within the individual, rather than from his or her supervisors. Good motivators focus on employee desires, rather than on their fears. An individual's basic motivator is the desire to work, and that motivation is fed by expectations for financial rewards (e.g., salary, benefits, bonuses) and nonfinancial rewards (e.g., appreciation, recognition, autonomy, advancement, supplies).

Leaders can estimate employee motivation by observing personnel and their interactions in the institution. By achieving balance and identifying possible sources of interference, leaders gain insight into employees' attitudes toward their work, fellow workers, position status, and employers. Combining these observations with employee reactions to work hours, earnings, and institutional policies enables the leader to analyze motivation.

Employee behavior analysis elicits two types of evidence: (1) labor turnover, productivity, promptness, malingering, loitering, and absenteeism; and (2) employees' actions and reactions. Leaders must be alert to employees who exhibit an overall lack of interest, excessive absenteeism and patterns of unexcused time off, a lack of skills and understanding in the enforcement of rules, and intentional restriction of productivity.

IMPLICATIONS FOR PRACTICE

Today's leaders move with healthcare trends, developing tools to handle the motivational needs of staff. Strong leaders nurture the relationship between employees and organizations and promote satisfaction and teamwork. Their working knowledge of the environmental factors that influence staff behavior and individual development can help improve the workplace and boost motivation. To strengthen motivation, leaders must identify and eliminate negative responses such as lack of recognition, poor communication, inability to accept upper management, frustration from other departments, and working with inexperienced staff.

leadership in his book *On Leadership* (Box 1-2). The notion of describing tangible behaviors aligned with leading, managing, and following is introduced so that it is possible to distinguish between the tasks and the definitions of leadership, management, and followership presented earlier in the chapter.

Gardner's Tasks of Leadership

Envisioning Goals

Leading requires envisioning goals, not in isolation but in partnership with those being led. In the case of patient care, leading is required to help patients envision their life when a specific disease trajectory is unknown. It might be aimed at helping a patient envision walking again, participating in family events, or changing a lifestyle pattern. In the case of leading peers (not dissimilar to working with patients and family members), leader

competence, trustworthiness, self-assuredness, decision-making ability, and prioritization skills are needed to envision crafting solutions to problems. Imagine leading a change to an electronic medical record from a traditional paper record: The leader would need the aforementioned abilities to convince and persuade staff that this change is necessary and to proceed with setting direction. Envisioning goals is contingent upon trusting relationships, shared information, and agreement on mutual expectations.

Establishing **vision** is an important leadership concept. "Visioning" requires the leader to assess the current reality, determine and specify a desired end-point state, and then strategize to reduce the tension between the two states in a positive manner. If done well, the nurse and the patient or the nurse within an organization experience creative tension. *Creative tension* is positive tension that moves the

BOX 1-2

Gardner's Tasks of Leadership

1. Envisioning goals
2. Affirming values
3. Motivating
4. Managing
   - Planning and setting priorities
   - Organizing and institution building
   - Keeping the system functioning
   - Setting agendas and making decisions
   - Exercising political judgment
5. Achieving workable unity
6. Developing trust
7. Explaining
8. Serving as symbol
9. Representing the group
10. Renewing

From Gardner, J. W. (1990). *On leadership.* New York: Free Press.

patient toward the desired goal. For instance, if the nurse fails to engage the patient or fails to recognize the root cause of a clinical problem, then emotional tension (distress) results. *Emotional tension* drains the energy of those experiencing the change. Therefore exceptional visioning skills are an important function of leading. Visioning gives direction to accelerate change.

Affirming Values

Values are the inner forces that give purpose, direction, and precedence to life priorities. An organization, through its members, has composite values that are expressed through its mission and philosophy. Leaders have values that influence decision making and priority setting. People (either patients or peers being influenced by the leader) also have values that undergird their goals and are manifested through behavior. Values are a deep-seated, persuasive force driving how we choose to act and respond to others.

The word *value* conjures up an image of something that has worth; our values reflect through our actions those things of worth to us. A leader always seizes the opportunity to clarify and acknowledge the values that underlie the need to solve problems or create something new. This is because values are powerful forces that promote acceptance of change and drive achievement toward a goal.

Motivating

When we let our values drive our actions, values become a source of motivation. **Motivation** is tapping into what we value, personally and professionally, and reinforcing these factors to achieve growth and movement toward our vision. Motivators are the reinforcers that keep positive actions alive. They tap the inner drive, the reaction to feedback, and fuel the fires that generate our desire to engage in change. Theories of motivation identify and describe the forces that motivate people. Examples of motivation theory are presented in the motivational theory box.

Managing

The ability to manage is an important subset of leading, especially when the leader holds a position of influence in an organization (e.g., a nurse manager). It has been said that some individuals in management positions are effective managers, but that does not guarantee that they are effective leaders. Likewise, a charismatic leader may not necessarily be a good manager. Ideally, those charged with managing are also good leaders and good followers, for there are few organizational positions that require one set of behaviors over the other. Good leaders need management skills and abilities, and good managers need leading skills and abilities. The tasks of management are discussed later in this chapter.

Achieving Workable Unity

Another challenge of leading is to achieve workable unity between and among the parties being affected by change and to avoid, diminish, or resolve conflict so that the desired vision can be achieved (see Chapter 20). It is essential for leaders to acquire conflict-resolution skills. When a dispute occurs, whether because of conflicting values or interests, it is useful to follow a defined set of principles for conflict resolution. In their classic work, Ury, Brett, and Goldberg (1988) describe a highly effective approach for restoring unity and movement toward positive change, as shown in Box 1-3.

Developing Trust

A hallmark task of leadership is to behave in a way that is trustworthy. When leaders are clear with others about "where we are headed" and that the way to achieve high levels of performance is through building on strengths rather than entrapment of poor performance, followers develop trust in the leader. Inherent in this concept is the behavior of telling the truth. It is possible that a leader cannot

BOX 1-3

Principles of Conflict Resolution

1. Put the focus on interests:
   Examine the real issues of all parties.
   Be expedient in responding to the issues.
   Use negotiation procedures and processes such as ethics committees and other neutral sources.
2. Build in "loop-backs" to negotiation:
   If resolution fails, allow for a "cooling off" period before reconvening.
   Review the likely consequences of not proceeding with all parties so that they understand the full consequences of failure to resolve the issue.
3. Build in consultation *before* and feedback *after* the negotiations:
   Build consensus and use political skills to facilitate communication before confrontation, if anticipated, occurs.
   Work with staff or patients after the conflict to learn from the situation and to prevent a similar conflict in the future.
   Provide a forum for open discussion.
4. Provide the necessary motivation, skills, and resources:
   Make sure that the parties involved in conflict are motivated to use procedures and resources that have been developed; this requires ease of access and a nonthreatening mechanism.
   Ensure that those working in the dispute have skills in problem solving and dispute resolution.
   Provide the necessary resources to those involved to offer support, information, and other technical assistance.

Modified from Ury, W., Brett, J., & Goldberg, S. (1988). Getting disputes resolved: *Designing systems to cut the costs of conflict*. San Francisco: Jossey-Bass.

of the communication? Information that addresses the listener's self-interest must be presented.

3. Provide the opportunity for dialogue and feedback. Face-to-face communication is preferred because it affords immediate feedback to the leader and offers the opportunity to clarify information. Written feedback, especially email, is useful to reinforce key messages or to follow up on inquiries, but it is increasingly becoming a primary method of communication.
4. Know that it is possible to give too much information, which can temporarily paralyze the listener and divert energy away from key responsibilities.
5. Be willing to repeat information in many different ways, at different times. The more diverse the group being addressed, the more important it is to avoid complex terms, concepts, or ideas. Information should be kept simple. Remember, people hear a message when they are ready to hear it, not before.
6. Always explain *why* something is being asked or is changing. The values behind the communication should be reinforced.
7. Acknowledge loss and provide the opportunity for honest communication about what will be missed, especially if change is involved.
8. Be sensitive to nonverbal communication. It may be necessary in complex situations to have someone reinterpret key points and provide feedback about the clarity of the message after the meeting. Leaders must use every opportunity for explaining as a vehicle to fine-tune communication skills. (See Chapter 19 for more on communication.)

share all information, but it is unwise to misdirect others in their thinking and actions. Trustworthiness is apparent in actions and communications.

Explaining

Leading and managing require a willingness to communicate and explain—again and again. The art of communication requires the leader to do the following:

1. Know what information needs to be shared.
2. Know the parties who will receive the information. What will they "hear" in the process

Serving as Symbol

Every leader has the opportunity to be an ambassador for those they represent. Nurses may symbolically be present for patients and families, represent their department at an organizational event, or be involved in community public relation events. Serving as a symbol reflects unity and collective identity.

Representing the Group

More than being present symbolically, there are many opportunities for leaders to represent the group through active participation. Progressive organizations are creating more opportunities for employee participation, involvement, and innovation (such as those organizations that are vying for **Magnet Recognition**). Employees may be invited to participate on human resource committees, safety and security task forces, improvement committees, and other nursing department groups. Nurses are able to give their "voice" in each of these leadership opportunities. Decision making is often decentralized, and layers of management are compressed, giving each nurse more leadership accountability. In an environment of rapid change, the use of high-technology decision support, the skill set possessed by healthcare professionals, and the need for rapid organizational change have created many opportunities for collective problem solving. Leaders should treat these newfound opportunities with respect and honestly try to represent the group with openness and integrity. Ultimately, leaders must demonstrate an understanding of the organization's objectives and contribute to its mission and purpose.

Renewing

Leaders can generate energy within and among others. A true leader does not just expend the energy of the group or allow the group to lose its focus. In organizations and nursing practice, there is a constant need to find a balance between problem solving (energy expending) and vision setting (energy producing). When changes are made based on vision, they can be met with renewed spirit and purpose, if well led. Taking time in staff meetings to celebrate individual accomplishments or creating a "Hall of Honor" to post photos, letters, and other forms of positive feedback renews the spirit of workers.

Furthermore, leaders must take care of themselves—eat a balanced diet, get adequate sleep and exercise, and participate in other wellness-oriented activities—to maintain their perspective and the necessary energy level. Likewise, they must ensure that their constituents are given similar opportunities for renewal. Gardner (1990) states that, "The consideration leaders must never forget is that the key for renewal is the release of human energy and talent" (p. 136). This requires focused energy and personal well-being.

Gardner's leadership tasks are presented in Table 1-1 to provide a contrast between staff nurse leaders and leaders who hold formal middle-level and executive-level management positions. Note that each role represents the interests of the organization, even though the locus of attention is different.

Bleich's Tasks of Management

The ability to manage is very much aligned with how an organization structures its key systems and processes to deliver service. In the legendary *I Love Lucy* television series, the episode in which Lucy and Ethel work in a candy factory serves as a classic example of the role and energy that workers exude to achieve an acceptable work product. Recall the extraordinary effort of wrapping each piece of candy to specification as it passed by on a conveyor belt. The *process* was designed such that two workers stood side-by-side, each taking an alternating piece of candy and a wrapper, and wrapped the candy according to specifications. Simple and clear. Yet when worker productivity was challenged (poor directions, a nonsupportive supervisor, and limited worker training to the task at hand), the workers "gamed" the system to give the appearance of success! If you recall, the supervisor suggested that "one more mess up" would result in firing. The supervisor—who never truly observed, coached, or gave feedback to her workers—ends up declaring, "Speed it up!" and hilarity ensues as the rate of production approaches near-bedlam, thereby yielding even more errors.

This example highlights the roles of managing and following. Healthcare delivery is composed of processes of care far more complex than the candy factory example (observe a dietary tray line sometime, though!), and targeted behaviors are associated with each. A **process of care** specifies the desired sequence of steps that have been designed to achieve clinical standardization. Nurses are challenged to give medications, perform clinical procedures, administer blood, conduct patient education, and complete documentation of care, each an example of a process of care in the care delivery system. Effective managing depends on recognizing that these systems and processes exist, that efficiency and effectiveness is built in (or not built in) to these systems, and that there are prescribed roles for individual workers to comprehend. Data-driven outcome measurements are critical to good management. Likewise, honest feedback, coaching, and mentoring are also key elements. Rewards for individual and team effectiveness reinforce desired behaviors. Box 1-4 lists tasks of management essential to effective functioning.

Many healthcare settings have a dire need to reallocate managers' time so the patient care delivery system can be designed in more effective, efficient, patient-oriented, and staff-friendly ways. Workforce

Table 1-1 CONTRASTING LEADING/MANAGING BEHAVIORS OF NURSES IN CLINICAL, MANAGEMENT, AND EXECUTIVE POSITIONS

Gardner's Task	Behaviors		
	Clinical Position	**Management Position**	**Executive Position**
Envisioning goals	Visioning patient outcomes for single patients/families; assisting patients in formulating their vision of future well-being	Visioning patient outcomes for aggregates of patient populations and creating a vision of how systems support patient care objectives; assisting staff in formulating their vision of enhanced clinical and organizational performance	Visioning community health and organizational outcomes for aggregates of patient populations to which the organization can respond
Affirming values	Assisting the patient/family to sort out and articulate personal values in relation to health problems and the effect of these problems on lifestyle adjustments	Assisting the staff in interpreting organizational values and strengthening staff members' personal values to more closely align with those of the organization; interpreting values during organizational change	Assisting other organizational leaders in the expression of community and organizational values; interpreting values to the community and staff
Motivating	Relating to and inspiring patients/families to achieve their vision	Relating to and inspiring staff to achieve the mission of the organization and the vision associated with organizational enhancement	Relating to and inspiring management, staff, and community leaders to achieve desired levels of health and well-being and appropriate use of clinical services
Managing	Assisting the patient/family with planning, priority setting, and decision making; making sure that organizational systems work in the patient's behalf	Assisting the staff with planning, priority setting, and decision making; making sure that systems work to enhance the staff's ability to meet patient care needs and the objectives of the organization	Assisting other executives and corporate leaders with planning, priority setting, and decision making; ensuring that human and material resources are available to meet health needs
Achieving workable unity	Assisting patients/families to achieve optimal functioning to benefit the transition to enhanced health functions	Assisting staff to achieve optimal functioning to benefit transition to enhanced organizational functions	Assisting multidisciplinary leaders to achieve optimal functioning to benefit patient care delivery and collaborative care
Developing trust	Keeping promises to patients and families; being honest in role performance	Sharing organizational information openly; being honest in role performance	Representing nursing and executive views openly and honestly; being honest in role performance

Table 1-1 CONTRASTING LEADING/MANAGING BEHAVIORS OF NURSES IN CLINICAL, MANAGEMENT, AND EXECUTIVE POSITIONS—cont'd

Gardner's Task	Behaviors		
	Clinical Position	Management Position	Executive Position
Explaining	Teaching and interpreting information to promote patient/family functioning and well-being	Teaching and interpreting information to promote organizational functioning and enhanced services	Teaching and interpreting organizational and community-based health information to promote organizational functioning and service development
Serving as symbol	Representing the nursing profession and the values and beliefs of the organization to patients/families and other community groups	Representing the nursing unit service and the values and beliefs of the organization to staff, other departments, professional disciplines, and the community at large	Representing the values and beliefs of the organization and patient care services to internal and external constituents
Representing the group	Representing nursing and the unit in task forces, total quality initiatives, shared governance councils, and other groups	Representing nursing and the organization on assigned boards, councils, committees, and task forces, both internal and external to the organization	Representing the organization and patient care services on assigned boards, councils, committees, and task forces, both internal and external to the organization
Renewing	Providing self-care to enhance the ability to care for staff, patients, families, and the organization served	Providing self-care to enhance the ability to care for staff, patients, families, and the organization served	Providing self-care to enhance the ability to care for patients, families, staff, and the organization served

issues are commonly associated with the work environment. Leaders will help guide workplace transformation, but managers must sustain the spirit of clinical system functioning.

■ *Exercise 1–3*

Examine one structured process in the delivery of patient care from start to finish (e.g., food ordering, preparation, and delivery). Who is responsible for each step in the process? Who has the responsibility and authority for managing the process? What data are evident in the organization to measure how well the process is working?

Images associated with followers tend to conjure up associations with workers who are passive, uninspired, not intellectual, and waiting for direc-

tion. Nothing could be further from what is needed in healthcare workers today. The relationship between followers and leaders or managers is complicated. Burns (2000) states, "It would seem so simple at first glance—that leaders lead and followers follow. But we know it is much more complicated. When the leader dreams the dream or takes the initiative or issues the call, does the follower even hear the leader?" (p. 11). There are also times when the leader is the follower and vice versa.

On any given work shift there may be a charge nurse who holds a leading-managing role. During this shift this nurse assesses resources needed, sees the unit as a complete entity, notes where patients may be admitted or discharged, and delegates according to this "big picture" view. Throughout the

BOX 1-4

Bleich's Tasks of Management

1. Identifies systems and processes for which the manager has responsibility and accountability
2. Verifies minimum and optimum standards/specifications for staff to achieve
3. Validates the knowledge, skills, and abilities of available staff; capitalizes on strengths and strengthens areas in need of development
4. Devises and communicates a comprehensive "big picture" plan for the division of work, honoring the complexity and variety of assignments made at an individual level
5. Eliminates barriers/obstacles to work effectiveness
6. Measures the equity of workload and uses data to support judgments about efficiency and effectiveness
7. Offers rewards and recognition to individuals and teams
8. Recommends ways to improve systems and processes
9. Involves others in decision making when appropriate or relevant

BOX 1-5

Bleich's Tasks of Followership

1. Is individually accountable while working within the context of organizational systems and processes; does not change the way work is done for personal gain or short cuts
2. Honors the standards and specifications required to deliver acceptable care/service
3. Offers knowledge, skills, and abilities to accomplish the task at hand
4. Collaborates willingly with leaders and managers; avoids passive-aggressive or nonassertive responses to work assignment
5. Includes data collection as part of daily work activities as a self-guide to efficiency and effectiveness and to contribute to outcome measurement
6. Demonstrates accountability for individual actions within the team effort
7. Takes reasonable risks as an antidote for fearing change or unknown circumstances
8. Gives feedback on the efficiency and effectiveness of systems and processes that affect outcomes of care/service; values well-designed work
9. Gives and receives feedback to other team members, leaders, and managers to enhance a culture of nurturance and support

shift, critical clinical events arise that are better led by one of the senior staff nurses. Seamlessly, the charge nurse and senior staff nurse begin to shift their relationship so that the functioning of the unit is balanced. Assignments are temporarily adjusted, and talents and skills of individual nurses are deployed to patients and families in need, all with little or no fanfare. Yet examine the complexity, respect, and team achievement factors at play.

To be an effective follower requires effort to willingly and earnestly be led, to share time and talents, and to synergistically create and innovate solutions to problems or to take direction from the manager as needed while asserting oneself in the tasks that need accomplishment and to honor and respect the need for structured work activities that, despite their structured nature, are not devoid of critical-thinking decision making (Box 1-5).

Followers complement leaders and managers with their skills. Followers and leaders fill in the gaps that exist to build on each other's cognitive, technical, physical, and emotional strengths. Followers, through their attitude, offer respite in times of stress and minimize catastrophic situations. A follower responds to feedback, and the data provide a compass used to measure achievement and improve working conditions. As mentioned earlier, the follower acquiesces to the skills and abilities of the leader or manager to promote teamwork. This does not mean that the follower does not have the skills and abilities of the leader or manager; the follower may be thrust into one of those roles when circumstances demand. Box 1-5 lists the tasks of followership.

LEADING, MANAGING, AND FOLLOWING IN A DIVERSE ORGANIZATION

The healthcare industry is spiraling through unparalleled change, often away from the traditional industrial models that have reigned throughout the twentieth century. The culture in most healthcare organizations today is more ethnically diverse; has an expansive educational chasm from non–high school graduates to doctoral-prepared clinicians; has multiple generations of workers with varying values and expectations of the workplace; involves the increased use of technology to support all aspects of service functioning; and challenges workers, patients, families, and communities environmentally with medical waste, antibiotic-resistant strains of microorganisms, and other risks.

These and other variables make leading, managing, and following increasingly challenging. Occasionally, a leader must address the needs of a diverse community of those seeking care. Language and cultural barriers create the opportunity for misunderstanding. Those who manage the systems and processes of care may find a temporary workforce, individuals who are unfamiliar with organizational standards of care and practice,

as their primary resource. Followers may have leaders of other generations with values different from their own, so the opportunity for conflict is omnipresent.

Developing the leading, managing, and following skills and abilities noted throughout this chapter will sustain professional nurses to adapt to and accept differences as a positive rather than a negative force in daily work life. Building on gender strengths; generational values, gifts, and talents; cultural diversity; varying educational and experiential perspectives; and a mobile and flexible workforce is rewarding. It is also rewarding to be led in different ways, to experience the strength of a good manager, and to achieve positive outcomes as a follower knowing that the team approach generated a successful work experience.

The Solution

This situation required me to move into a *leadership* mode. As a team, we were *managing* the situation with expertise, skill, and determination. Upon entering the room, I *followed* the lead of the patient's primary nurse and I used my critical-thinking skills to complement the actions and behaviors of the rest of the team.

When we were informed of our patient's "VIP" status, I continued to work collaboratively with my staff to revive and stabilize our patient's heart. Serving as a *leader* and symbol of continuity of care, I redirected the team's energy by verbally confirming my confidence in their abilities.

After this situation, I met with the nursing staff to debrief and discuss the events encompassing the patient's

cardiac arrest. This transfer of information enabled me to clarify perceptions, to determine opportunities to improve or enhance the methods for delivering patient care, and to ascertain a method for the skillful communication of perceptions of the ICU nursing staff to the head nurse and other members of the hospital administrative staff.

— Rebecca M. Vaughn

 Would this approach be suitable for you? Why?

CHAPTER CHECKLIST

This chapter addresses the attributes and tasks of leading, managing, and following and presents the case that professional nurses require the knowledge, skill, and ability to move in and out of these roles with ease, whether in clinical or management positions. Emotional intelligence is defined in terms of self-understanding, and the argument is made that emotional intelligence is as critical to professional practice as are cognitive and

technical skills. Healthcare organizations are experiencing major change and are increasingly diverse in those being served and those serving; diversity presents new challenges and opportunities for leaders, managers, and followers.

- The personal attributes needed for effective leading and managing include the following:
  - Focused energy and stamina to accomplish the vision

- Ability to make decisions in an intelligent manner
- Willingness to use intuition, backed up with facts
- Willingness to accept responsibility and to follow up
- Sincerity in identifying the needs of others
- Skill in dealing with people, for example, through coaching, communicating, or counseling
- Comfortable standard and boundary setting
- Flexibility in examining multiple options to accomplish the objective at hand
- Trustworthiness and a good "steward of information"
- Assertiveness in motivating others toward the objective at hand
- Demonstrable competence and quick learning in the arena where change is desired

- The tasks of leading and managing include the following:
  - Envisioning goals
  - Affirming values
  - Motivating
  - Managing
    - Planning and priority setting
    - Organizing and institution building
    - Keeping the system functioning
    - Setting agendas and making decisions
    - Exercising political judgment
  - Achieving workable unity
  - Developing trust
  - Explaining
  - Serving as symbol
  - Representing the group
  - Renewing
- The tasks for managing include the following:
  - Identifies systems and processes

- Verifies minimum and optimum standards/specifications
- Validates the knowledge, skills, and abilities of available staff
- Devises and communicates a comprehensive "big picture" plan
- Eliminates barriers/obstacles to work effectiveness
- Measures the equity of workload
- Offers rewards and recognition to individuals and teams
- Recommends ways to improve systems and processes
- Involves others in decision making

- The tasks for following include the following:
  - Recognizes how individual responsibilities fit into organizational systems
  - Honors the standards and specifications
  - Offers knowledge, skills, and abilities
  - Collaborates willingly with leaders and managers
  - Includes data collection as part of daily work activities
  - Demonstrates accountability for individual actions
  - Takes reasonable risks
  - Gives feedback on the efficiency and effectiveness of systems
  - Gives and receives feedback to other team members, leaders, and managers

TERMS TO KNOW

emotional intelligence	followership
leadership	Magnet Recognition
management	management theory
motivation	process of care
values	vision

REFERENCES

Bass, B. M. (1990). From transactional to transformational leadership: Learning to share the vision. *Organizational Dynamics, 18*, 19-31.

Bennis, W. G., & Nanus, B. (1985). *Leaders: The strategies for taking charge.* New York: Harper & Row.

Blake, R. R., & Mouton, J. S. (1985). *The managerial grid III.* Houston: Gulf Publishing.

Burns, J. M. (2000). Leadership and followership: Complicated relationships. In B. Kellerman & L. R. Matusak (Eds.), *Cutting edge leadership 2000.* College Park: The James Academy of Leadership.

Fiedler, F. A. (1967). *A theory of leadership effectiveness.* New York: McGraw-Hill.

Gardner, J. W. (1990). *On leadership.* New York: Free Press.

Genrich, S. J., Banks, J. C, Bufton, K., Savage, M. E., & Owens, M. U. (2001). Group involvement in decision making: A pilot study. *The Journal of Continuing Education in Nursing, 32*(1), 20-26.

Goleman, D. P. (1995). *Working with emotional intelligence.* New York: Bantam Books.

Hanna, L. A. (1999). Lead the way. *Nursing Management, 30*(11), 37-39.

Herzberg, F. (1991). One more time: How do you motivate employees? In M. J. Ward & S. A. Price (Eds.), *Issues in nursing administration: Selected readings*. St. Louis: Mosby.

House, R. J., & Mitchell, T. R. (1974, Autumn). Path-goal theory of leadership. *Journal of Contemporary Business, 3*, 81-97.

Likert, R. (1961). *New patterns of management.* New York: McGraw-Hill.

Luthans, F. (1973). *Organizational behavior.* New York: McGraw-Hill.

Manthey, M., & Miller, D. (1994). Empowerment through levels of authority. *Journal of Nursing Administration, 24*(7/8), 23.

Maslow, A. (1943). A theory of human motivation. *Psychological Review, 50*, 370-396.

Porter-O'Grady, T., & Finnigan, S. (1984). *Shared governance for nursing*. Rockville, MD: Aspen.

Shartle, C. L. (1956). *Executive performance and leadership.* Englewood Cliffs, NJ: Prentice Hall.

Stogdill, R. M. (1948). Personal factors associated with leadership: A survey of the literature. *Journal of Psychology, 25*, 35-71.

Stogdill, R. M. (1963). *Manual for the leader behavior description questionnaire, form XII.* Columbus: The Ohio State University, Bureau of Business Research.

Tichy, N. M., & Devanna, M. A. (1986). *The transformational leader.* New York: John Wiley & Sons.

Ury, W., Brett, J., & Goldberg, S. (1988). *Getting disputes resolved: Designing systems to cut the costs of conflict.* San Francisco: Jossey-Bass.

Vroom, V. H. (1964). *Work and motivation.* New York: John Wiley & Sons.

Vroom, V. H., & Yetton, P. (1973). *Leadership and decision-making.* Pittsburgh: University of Pittsburgh Press.

SUGGESTED READINGS

Bass, B. M., & Avolio, B. J. (1994). *Improving organizational effectiveness through transformational leadership.* Thousand Oaks, CA: Sage Publications.

Bolman, L. G., & Deal, T. E. (1995). *Leading with soul.* San Francisco: Jossey-Bass.

Boston, C., & Forman, H. (1994). A time to listen: Staff and manager views on education, practice, and management. *Journal of Nursing Administration, 24*, 16-18.

Boyle, D. K., Bott, M. J., Hansen, H. E., Woods, C. Q., & Taunton, R. L. (1999). Managers' leadership and critical care nurses' intent to stay. *American Journal of Critical Care, 8*, 361-371.

Bridges, W. (1991). *Managing transitions: Making the most of change.* Reading, MA: Addison-Welsey.

Clegg, A. (2000). Leadership: Improving the quality of patient care. *Nursing Standard, 14*, 43-45.

Cohen, A. R., & Bradford, D. L. (1989). *Influence without authority.* New York: John Wiley & Sons.

Covey, S. (1991). *Principle-centered leadership.* New York: Summit.

Dixon, D. L. (1999). Achieving results through transformational leadership. *Journal of Nursing Administration, 29*, 17-21.

Gladwell, M. (2000). *The tipping point.* Boston: Little, Brown.

Grossman, R. J. (2000). Emotions at work: Health care organizations are just beginning to recognize the importance of developing a manager's emotional quotient, or interpersonal skills. *Health Forum Journal, 43*, 18-22.

Hesselbein, F., Goldsmith, M., & Beckhard, R. (1996). *The leader of the future.* San Francisco: Jossey-Bass.

Kellerman, B. (1999). *Reinventing leadership: Making the connection between politics and business.* New York: State University of New York Press.

Lentz, S. (1999). The well-rounded leader: Knowing when to use consensus and when to make a decision is crucial in today's competitive health care market. *Health Forum Journal, 42*, 38-40.

McDaniel, R. R. (1997). Strategic leadership: A view from quantum and chaos theories. *Health Care Management Review, 22*, 21-37.

McNeese-Smith, D. (1996). Increasing employee productivity, job satisfaction, and organizational commitment. *Hospital and Health Services Administration, 41*, 160-175.

McNichol, E. (2000). How to be a model leader. *Nursing Standard, 14*, 24.

Northouse, P. G. (2001). *Leadership theory and practice* (2nd ed.). Thousand Oaks, CA: Sage Publications.

Perra, B. M. (2000). Leadership: The key to quality outcomes. *Nursing Administration Quarterly, 24*, 56-61.

Pugh, D. S., & Hickson, D. J. (1997). *Writers on organizations* (5th ed.). Thousand Oaks, CA: Sage Publications.

Rainey, H. G., & Watson, S. A. (1996). Transformational leadership and middle management: Towards a role for mere mortals. *International Journal of Public Administration, 19*, 764-800.

Trott, M. C., & Windsor, K. (1999). Leadership effectiveness: How do you measure up? *Nursing Economics, 17*, 127-130.

Useem, M. (1998). *The leadership moment.* Times Business: Random House.

Van Wynen, E. A. (1997). Information processing styles: One size doesn't fit all. *Nurse Educator, 22*, 44-50.

Weeks, D. (1994). *The eight essential steps to conflict resolution.* New York: G. Putney Sons.

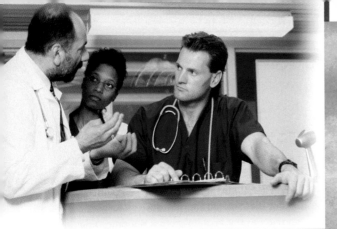

Chapter 2

Developing the Role of Leader

K. Lynn Wieck

Michael L. Evans

*T*his chapter focuses on leadership and its value in advancing the profession of nursing. Leadership development is explained with examples of how to survive and thrive in a leadership position. The differences between the emerging and entrenched workforce generations are explored, and desired leader characteristics for the emerging workforce are described. Leadership in a variety of situations, such as clinical settings, community venues, organizations, and political situations, are described. This chapter provides an introduction to the opportunities, challenges, and satisfaction of leadership.

Objectives

- Analyze the role of leadership in creating a satisfying working environment for nurses.
- Evaluate transactional and transformational leadership techniques for effectiveness and potential for positive outcomes.
- Explain the leadership challenges in dealing with generational differences.
- Compare and contrast leadership and management roles and responsibilities.
- Describe leadership development strategies and how they can promote leadership skills acquisition.

- Analyze leadership opportunities and responsibilities in a variety of venues.

- Explore strategies for making the leadership opportunity positive for both the leader and the followers.

Questions to Consider

- *Is there a difference between being a manager and being a leader?*
- *Is there one best way to lead?*
- *Are some people just born to be leaders, or can leadership be taught and learned?*
- *What are the special leadership challenges of the "twenty-something" generation?*
- *How can the leader keep from "burning out"?*
- *What kinds of opportunities are available for nurses to lead if they are not a member of the "management team"?*

The Challenge

Rosemary Luquire, PhD, RN, CNAA
Senior Vice President, Patient Care & Chief Quality Officer, St. Luke's Episcopal Health System, Houston, Texas

Houston, known as the Bayou City, is accustomed to frequent flooding. Located 60 miles from the Gulf of Mexico, tropical storms and hurricanes are not uncommon for the region. On Tuesday, June 5, 2001, Tropical Storm Allison moved across the city and dropped 2.5 inches of rain, causing some street flooding. St. Luke's Episcopal Hospital, a 948-bed tertiary hospital (26 stories high) in the Texas Medical Center, established an Emergency Command Center in accordance with its emergency preparedness plan. Tropical Storm Allison then moved northward, and the skies cleared. On Friday, June 8, the storm turned and moved back over Houston, creating massive flooding and loss of power throughout the Texas Medical Center. Between 5 PM on June 8 and 5 AM on June 9, 14 inches of rain fell; 36 inches of rain fell within 24 hours in northern Houston. The Bayou City was completely overwhelmed with this "500-year flood" as families fled to their rooftops to be saved by emergency personnel.

On the evening of Friday, June 8, St. Luke's had approximately 600 patients, 110 of whom were critically ill patients; many were on life support devices such as ventilators. I arrived at the hospital before flooding isolated the Texas Medical Center. I was the only senior executive on site. The evening staff was asked to stay and provide patient care as the storm precluded the arrival of any additional help. In the early morning hours, facilities notified me that the facility would lose all electrical power within an hour. Amid an environment of crisis, isolation, and uncertainty, critical decisions needed to be made quickly. Should patients be evacuated? Who should be evacuated while elevators were still functioning? How could the safety of patients and staff be ensured? When everything is a priority, how do you decide what is truly a priority?

 What do you think you would do if you were this nurse?

WHAT IS A LEADER?

A leader is an individual who works with others to develop a clear vision of the preferred future and to make that vision happen. Oakley and Krug (1994) call that type of **leadership** *enlightened leadership,* or the ability to elicit a vision from people and to inspire and empower those people to do what it takes to bring the vision into reality. Leaders bring out the best in people.

Leadership is a very important concept in life. Great leaders have been responsible for helping society move forward and for articulating and accomplishing one vision after another throughout time. Dr. Martin Luther King, Jr., called his vision a dream, and it was developed because of the input and lived experiences of countless others. Mother Teresa called her vision a calling, and it was developed because of the suffering of others. Steven Spielberg calls his vision a finished motion picture, and it is developed with the collaboration and inspiration of many other people. Florence Nightingale called her vision nursing, and it was developed because people were experiencing a void that was a barrier to their ability to regain or establish health.

The manager is concerned with doing things correctly in the present. The role of manager is very important in work organizations. Managers make sure that operations run smoothly and that well-developed formulas are applied to staffing situations, economic decisions, and other daily operations. The manager is not as concerned with developing creative solutions to problems as using prescriptive formulas to address today's expected and unexpected situations (Kerfoot, 1998). Covey (1992) believes that a well-managed entity may be proceeding correctly but, without leadership, may be proceeding in the wrong direction.

The roles of manager and leader are often considered interchangeable, but they are actually quite different. The manager may also be a leader, but the manager is not required to have leadership skills within the context of moving a group of people toward a vision. Other terms are used in place of *manager* and *leader,* such as *maintenance leader* and *innovation leader* (Trice & Beyer, 1992).

Management can be taught and learned using traditional teaching techniques. Leadership, on the other hand, is learned over time through experience in life situations (Kerfoot, 1998). According to Koestenbaum (1991), leadership is relevant for everyone, but in practice, only a few understand it and even fewer choose it.

Management and leadership are both important in the healthcare environment. The problem facing healthcare organizations is that they are overmanaged and underled (Atchison, 1990). Because we can teach new managers but our leaders are developed over time and through experience, it is important that we value, support, and provide our leaders with the one thing vital for good leadership—good followership. According to Trice and Beyer (1992), leadership requires more than leaders; it is a social process involving leaders and followers interacting in certain situations. Followers need three qualities from their leaders: direction, trust, and hope (Bennis, 1989). The trust is reciprocal. Leaders who trust their followers are, in turn, trusted by them.

Covey (1992) identifies eight characteristics of effective leaders. Effective leaders are continually engaging themselves in lifelong learning. They are service-oriented and concerned with the common good. They radiate positive energy. For people to be inspired and motivated, they must have a positive leader. Effective leaders believe in other people. They lead balanced lives and see life as an adventure. Effective leaders are synergistic; that is, they see things as greater than the sum of the parts. Finally, effective leaders engage themselves in self-renewal.

Exercise 2–1

List Covey's eight characteristics of effective leaders on the left side of a piece of paper. Next to each word list any examples of your activities or attributes that reflect the characteristic. Some areas may be blank; others will be full. Think about what this means for you personally.

Healthcare organizations are complex. In fact, healthcare is complex. Continual learning is essential to stay abreast of new knowledge, to keep the organization moving forward, and to continue delivering the best possible care. There is an emphasis on organizations becoming learning organizations, providing opportunities and incentives for individuals and groups of individuals to learn continuously over time. A learning organization is one that is continually expanding its capacity to create its future (Senge, 1994). Leaders are responsible for building organizations in which people continually expand their ability to understand complexity and to clarify and to improve a shared vision of the future—"that is, they are responsible for learning" (p. 340).

Leadership as an Important Concept for Nurses

Nurses must have leadership to move forward in harmony with changes in society and in healthcare. Within work organizations, certain nurses are designated as managers. These individuals are important to ensuring that care is delivered in a safe, efficient manner. Nurse leaders are also vital in the workplace to elicit input from others and to formulate a vision for the preferred future.

Moreover, leadership is key for nursing as a profession. The public depends on nurses to advocate for the public's needs and interests. Nurses must step forward into leadership roles in their workplace, in their professional associations, and in legislative and policy-making arenas.

Nurse leadership is vital. Nurses depend on their leaders to set goals for the future and the pace for achieving them. The public depends on nurse leaders to move the consumer advocacy agenda forward.

Leadership as a Primary Determinant of Workplace Satisfaction

Nurse satisfaction within the workplace is an important construct in nursing administration and healthcare administration. If nurses are not satisfied with the working environment, they are less likely to work at their highest level and are more likely to leave the organization and go elsewhere (Stamps, 1997). Turnover is extremely costly to any work organization in terms of money, expertise, and knowledge, as well as care quality.

The leader, not the manager, inspires others to work at their highest level. The presence of strong leadership sets the tone for achievement in the work environment. Because effective leadership is the basis for an effective workplace, attention must be paid to nurturing and supporting leaders in healthcare organizations and developing leaders for the future (Kerfoot, 1998).

■ *Exercise 2–2*

Follower behavior nurtures and supports—or deteriorates—leader behavior. Identify the behavior you exhibited during your most recent clinical experience. What was supportive? What did not support the leader?

THE PRACTICE OF LEADERSHIP

Leadership Approaches

How one approaches leadership depends on experience and expectations. Many leadership styles have been described. Two of the most popular approaches are transactional leadership and transformational leadership.

Transactional Leadership

A transactional leader is the traditional "boss" image. In a **transactional leadership** environment, employees understand that there is a superior who makes the decisions with little or no input from subordinates. Transactional leadership relies on three methods to move followers: (1) offering rewards to staff or followers for desired work, (2) monitoring work performance and correcting followers when a problem is noted, and (3) waiting until a problem occurs and then dealing with the issue retrospectively (Dunham-Taylor, 2000). Transactional leadership relies on the power of organizational position and formal authority to reward and punish performance. Followers are fairly secure about what will happen next and how to "play the game" to get where they want to be. A transactional leader uses a *quid pro quo* style to accomplish work (e.g., I'll do *x* in exchange for your doing *y*). The transactional leader is more likely to opt for status quo and is usually found in stable environments.

Transformational Leadership

A transformational leader is one who seeks and welcomes input from followers as goals are formulated and decisions are made. The **transformational leadership** style is described by Markham (1998) as collaborative, consultative, and consensus seeking and as ascribing power to interpersonal skills and personal contact. Covey (1992) states, "The goal of transformational leadership is to transform people and organizations in a literal sense, to change them in mind and heart; enlarge vision, insight and understanding; clarify purposes; make behavior congruent with beliefs, principles, or values; and bring about changes that are permanent, self perpetuating, and momentum-building" (p. 287).

Kouzes and Posner (1997) identify five key practices in transformational leadership: (1) challenging the process, which involves questioning the way things have been done in the past and thinking creatively about new solutions to old problems; (2) inspiring shared vision or bringing everyone together to move toward a goal that all accept as desirable and achievable; (3) enabling others to act, which includes empowering people to believe that their extra effort will have rewards and will make a difference; (4) modeling the way, meaning that the leader must take an active role in the work of change; and (5) encouraging the heart by giving attention to those personal things that are important to people, such as saying "thank you" for a job well done and offering praise after a long day. This type of leader seems particularly suited to the nursing environment. The Research Perspective box suggests that this type of leader increases nurse satisfaction. Transformational leaders have been found to be "more effective and satisfying" than transactional leaders (Bass, 1998). However, transformational leadership is hard work. It takes investment of time and energy to bring out the best in people.

Leadership is the ability to influence people to work to meet certain goals. Marriner-Tomey (1993) points out that leaders need to be hardy. Hardiness is a personality trait that can enable and empower a leader to withstand and adapt to change and stress. She defines hardy leaders as those who are in control, committed to leadership, and able to view change as a challenge. In the chaos of healthcare, nurse leaders face constant change and many challenges.

Barriers to Leadership

Leadership demands a commitment of effort and time. Many barriers exist to both leading and following. Good leadership and good followership go hand in hand, and both make the mission or the organization stronger. However, there are barriers to leadership.

False Assumptions

Some people have false assumptions about leaders and leadership. For example, some believe that position and title are equivalent to leadership. Having the title of Chief Executive Officer or Chief Nursing Officer does not guarantee that a person will be a good leader. Inspired and forward-moving organizations often select these executives specifically because of their ability to forge a vision and lead others toward it. However, a good executive is not

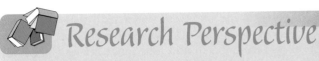

Research Perspective

Dunham-Taylor, J. (2000). Nurse executive transformational leadership found in participative organizations. *Journal of Nursing Administration, 30*(5), 241-250.

Transformational leaders have been found to increase nurse satisfaction in healthcare settings. Transformational leaders empower the workgroup to achieve a vision, whereas the transactional leader monitors work performance and corrects it as needed. In this study, nurse executives ($n = 396$) were asked to describe leadership characteristics, personal power level, and hospital organizational climate. At the same time, three of their staff members ($n = 1115$) were asked to describe their perceptions of the nurse executives' leadership style. Nurse executives who rated themselves as transformational leaders found this claim substantiated by their staff, although the nurse executives tended to rate themselves higher than their staff members. Staff who rated their executive as more of a transformational leader also reported more satisfaction, more effectiveness,

and more extra effort put forth in their job. Staff satisfaction decreased as the executive was rated as transactional. Higher transformational scores were seen as the nurse executive possessed higher educational degrees. Furthermore, the larger hospitals tended to be more participative and to attract the transformational nurse executive.

IMPLICATIONS FOR PRACTICE

Nurse executives who function in a transformational leadership style tend to have more satisfied employees. The existing cadre of transformational leaders need to serve as mentors and role models to other nurse executives, as well as for young nurses, so that the next generation of nurse executives will assume a transformational leadership style. An empowering, receptive environment is essential to the recruitment and retention of young nurses.

---

necessarily a good leader. Furthermore, assuming a management or administrative role does not automatically confer the title of leader on an individual. Leadership is an earned honor and an action-oriented responsibility.

Others believe that workers who do not hold official management positions cannot be leaders. Some nursing units are managed by the head nurse but led by the ward secretary or unit clerk. Leaders are those who do the best job of sharing their vision of where the followers want to be and how to get there. Many new nurse managers make the mistake of assuming that along with their new job comes the mantle of leadership. Leadership is an earned right and privilege.

Time Constraints

Leadership requires a time commitment; it does not just happen. The leader must fully comprehend the situation at hand, investigate and research options, assume the responsibility to communicate the vision to others, and continually reevaluate the organization or the team to ensure that the vision remains relevant and attainable. All of these activities take time. The twenty-first cen-

tury has been described as the period of doing more with less. Everyone is busy. Finding time to lead is therefore a barrier for many who have inspirational ideas but lack time to develop the skills needed to lead effectively.

Exercise 2–3

Define a clinical or management issue that sparks your passion. Assume you have 6 weeks to make a difference. Create a plan identifying your leadership tasks, the support required from others, and the time frame to move the issue toward resolution. Think about what your message is and how and when you will deliver it. Think about what you would do if no one was responsive to your issue. Think about why the issue may be important for you but not for others.

LEADERSHIP DEVELOPMENT

Leadership effectiveness depends on mastering the art of persuasion and communication. Success depends on persuading followers to accept a vision by using convincing communication techniques and making it possible for the followers to achieve the shared goals. There are several important leader-

Leadership Development Tasks

1. Select a mentor.
2. Lead by example.
3. Accept responsibility.
4. Share the rewards.
5. Have a clear vision.
6. Be willing to grow.

ship tasks that, when used effectively, will help ensure success (Box 2-1).

Select a Mentor

A **mentor** is someone who models behavior, offers advice and criticism, and coaches the novice to develop a personal leadership style. A mentor should have the qualities of a teacher, resource person, encourager, and provider of experience in day-to-day care practice (Earnshaw, 1995). Where do you find a mentor? Usually, a mentor is someone who has experience and some success in the leadership realm of interest, such as in a clinical setting or in an organization. A respected faculty member, a nurse manager or director, an organizational officer, or an active member may be a mentor. Mentorship is a two-way street. The mentor must agree to work with the novice leader and must have some interest in the novice's future development. A mentor must be close enough geographically to allow both observation and practice of leadership behaviors, as well as timely feedback. A mentor should provide advice, feedback, and role modeling. In addition, the mentor has a right to expect assistance with projects, respect, loyalty, and confidentiality. In a mentoring relationship, aspiring leaders soak up knowledge and experience and should expect to return it by serving as a mentor to a young aspiring leader in the future.

Lead by Example

An effective leader knows the most effective and visible way to influence people is to lead by example. Desired behavior can be modeled. For example, if an organization has a vision of becoming a political player in the state or community, the leader should be seen engaging in political activities. If the goal is to have improved relationships between followers, the leader must exhibit respect and patience with followers. Great leaders create civilized work environments (Kerfoot, 1999). A key skill to de-

velop is the ability to understand that the leader serves the followers. The effective leader does not send members to do a job, but rather leads them toward a mutual goal as a team.

Accept Responsibility

Even when the outcome is below expectations, the leader is ultimately responsible for the organization or activity. Leaders sometimes react in strange ways when negative outcomes occur. Sometimes the leader seeks to blame others or make excuses for undesirable or unintended outcomes. Some refuse to accept any responsibility at all. In accepting responsibility, the leader needs to know that there is reward in victory and growth in failure. No one plans to fail, but an effective leader sees failures as opportunities to learn and grow so that previous failures are never repeated. This is called *experience*. People who cannot accept any personal responsibility and become demoralized by their perfectionist attitude toward life when failure occurs will not progress as leaders (Kerfoot, 1998).

Share the Rewards

An effective leader is as eager to share the glory as to receive it. The more respect and trust are shared with others, the more they are returned to the leader. Followers who believe their major task is to make the leader look good will soon tire of the task. Empowerment, or giving power to others, has been found to result in more power gained (Fullam et al., 1998). Followers who think the leader is working to make them look good will follow eagerly. Followers form a network and a support base for the leader.

Have a Clear Vision

Leaders see beyond where they are and see where they are going. Strong leaders are proactive and futuristic. The effective leader knows why the journey is necessary and takes the time and energy to inspire others to go along. Failing to have a vision is a slow trip to irrelevance (Wieck, 2000). The ability to communicate and promote the vision is a vital part of achieving it. Effective leaders share their vision and empower followers to come along to achieve it. They also share their leadership skills and successes toward achievement of a goal.

Be Willing to Grow

It is a misconception to think that growth for the person or the organization is automatic. Complacency leads to stagnation. Leaders must continually read

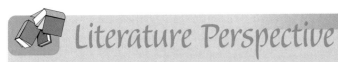

Literature Perspective

Drucker, P. F. (1999). *Management challenges for the 21st century*. New York: HarperBusiness.

Peter F. Drucker has written about leadership and management for more than a half a century. In his recent book about the twenty-first century, Drucker focuses on the priorities of new millennium workers. Tomorrow's workers will be knowledge workers who require a different kind of leadership style. They expect to be treated as associates rather than as subordinates. After their initial orientation period, the knowledge worker expects to know more about the job than the supervisor. The challenges and issues of leading tomorrow's workforce are already in the arena of ideas; those corporations and leaders who face these challenges today will dominate tomorrow. Those who do not will fall behind and may not survive. Using a team approach will continue to be an effective way to get the work of organizations done, but the new paradigm will be flexibility and change. There is no longer one right way to do things, nor is there one right organization. A primary challenge will be using the best of all leadership and management practices to create an environment that will attract and retain tomorrow's knowledge worker.

IMPLICATIONS FOR PRACTICE

Healthcare has been slower to respond to the changing needs and expectations of the new worker. Dominated by an aging leadership cohort, healthcare will have to refocus on challenging and appreciating the knowledge worker while creating an environment that allows the knowledge worker to be more marketable and more self-directed. The new workforce wants to be led instead of managed; Drucker's concepts for a new workplace will allow that to happen.

---

about new ideas and approaches, experiment with new concepts, and capitalize on a changing world. Continued education contributes to self-confidence by contributing to skills and knowledge needed for success (Allen, 1998). Growth takes risk, planning, investment, and work. Setting goals that complement the vision will help the aspiring leader know where to invest time and energy to grow into the desired role.

Leadership development is a lifetime endeavor. Effective leaders are constantly striving to improve their leadership skills. The good news is that leadership skills can be learned and improved. A commitment to improvement strengthens the leader's ability to lead effectively and elevates the bar for followers to achieve. The best leaders bring out the best in their followers, as seen in the Literature Perspective.

DEVELOPING LEADERS IN THE EMERGING WORKFORCE

Generational differences have always created challenges in the workplace. At the dawn of the twenty-first century, the workplace found an **emerging workforce** with vastly different goals, priorities, and work preferences than their Baby Boomer parents. Helping each generation understand and tolerate others is often a delicate orchestration of needs and wants, incentives and motives. Transgenerational leadership must focus on building an understanding and acceptance of each other.

The Emerging Workforce: The 1965 to 1985 Generation

Bradford and Raines (1992) said that the twenty-something generation "wants to be led, not managed." This cohort, born between 1965 and 1976, represents the smallest workforce entry pool since 1930, with just 44 million, compared with the 77 million Baby Boomers preceding them and the 70 million Generation Ys following them. They have a mindset and work ethic that Baby Boomers do not understand. Their younger siblings, the Generation Ys, who were born between 1977 and 1985, share many of the same approaches to work but bring their own challenges with no brand loyalty and a blatant disregard for status symbols.

In looking at what these emerging workforce members want in their leaders, a recent study of a national sample of student nurses indicates they want a leader who is receptive to people, a team player, honest, a good communicator, approachable, knowledgeable, motivating, and competent and has a positive attitude and good people skills (Wieck, Prydun, & Walsh, in press). Bradford and Raines (1992) state, "The effective leader and motivator of the twentysomethings is a coach, mentor and guide who gets to know workers individually" (p. 124).

Successfully leading the emerging workforce means the leader must shape a vision and win the twenty-somethings to it. The vision must be one that excites them because fun and balance are an important part of their lives. A vision that is powerful enough can transform what would otherwise be routine drudgery into collectively focused energy, even sacrifice (Bennis, 1999).

The successful leader must mobilize the followers to act. The required actions must provide value to the followers (e.g., learning a new skill or attaining certification or recognition). The younger generations are happy to follow as long as they can retain the balance in their lives, have information about and input into the decisions that affect them, and see some benefit in the activity. Exemplary leadership is impossible unless the leader has a creative alliance with the followers (Bennis, 1999). It is the leader's challenge to provide this type of environment where younger-generation followers want to follow.

The Entrenched Workforce: The 1946 to 1965 Generation

Baby Boomers, born after World War II, see work life very differently compared with the emerging workforce. Boomer workers are much more likely to believe in the power of collective action, based on their successes with social movements in their formative years in the 1960s. They tend to mistrust authority and are very comfortable with the process of getting to a goal. They find the journey of getting to the goal almost as important as reaching the goal. They are tolerant of, even dependent on, meetings and ongoing discussions that the younger generation finds tedious and wasteful.

The preferred leader of the **entrenched workforce** shares some of the characteristics of the younger generation's leader, such as being motivational, honest, approachable, competent, and knowledgeable. However, Baby Boomers also expect their leader to be professional, be supportive, and have high integrity, a concept not even mentioned by the younger generation (Wieck, Prydun, & Walsh, in press).

Challenges for the entrenched workforce are sharing leadership with the younger generation, empowering them to lead in their own model rather than trying to make them into second-generation Baby Boomers, and retaining the younger leaders in leadership ranks. Many younger employees are opting out of traditional work roles to become entrepreneurs. They take their leadership potential with them where there are few older role models for them to follow. A risk for aging Boomers is that the best and the brightest potential leaders will lose interest in leading and will opt for personal satisfaction and wealth accumulation rather than leadership and service roles.

The challenges of generational acceptance is one of many facing twenty-first century leaders. Attention to the needs of both the leader and the follower will create an environment where everyone thrives.

Exercise 2-4

List the names of the people with whom you work most frequently. Determine to which workforce (emerging or entrenched) each belongs. Describe known benefits of the workplace that support each generation's view. (One list may be longer than the other.) What elements of benefits are present in the personnel policies and workplace practices that benefit each? What elements are absent?

SURVIVING AND THRIVING AS A LEADER

The key to leadership is to believe in the vision and to enjoy the journey. The leader has a responsibility to self and followers to stay healthy and enthusiastic for the mission of the group. Surviving and thriving as a leader is based on the rules in Box 2-2.

The Leader Must Maintain Balance

Time management is essential for an effective leader. Many new leaders, in their zeal to be accessible to their constituents, lose control of their

BOX 2-2

The Five Rules of Leaders

1. Maintain balance.
2. Generate self-motivation.
3. Build self-confidence.
4. Listen to constituents.
5. Maintain a positive attitude.

lives. A good strategy for retaining or regaining control is to get control of communication. Good leaders use the simplest and fastest method of communication that makes them accessible but does not tie them down. The keys to success are setting priorities and keeping in control. Planned telephone time or email are excellent ways to keep control of time. Attending to matters as they come up, handling each question or piece of mail only one at a time, and focusing on the task at hand without distractions are just some of the time management strategies used by effective managers. Saving time, like wasting time, is a learned habit and can therefore be unlearned.

The Leader Must Generate Self-Motivation

Leaders who expect their followers to provide them with motivation, to be grateful for the time spent on followers' needs, and to offer frequent and lavish praise are in for a painful awakening. Followers in organizations, work situations, and elected constituencies feel they have earned the right to criticize the leader by being followers. Followers will have an opinion about everything. Sometimes the comments are favorable, and sometimes they are unfavorable. The reason that self-motivation is so essential is because the leader can expect very little external motivation. Most leaders are risk-takers and self-starters who are enthused by and believe in the vision they have created. Enthusiasm leads to an energized base that is a hallmark of a vibrant healthy organization.

The Leader Must Work at Building Self-Confidence

An effective leader must have self-confidence. This confidence comes from an acceptance of self despite imperfections. Self-confidence is a self-perpetuating virtue. Effective leaders perform an honest self-appraisal on a regular basis and work to feel good about the job they are doing. A leader who is surrounded by people who enhance the leader's own characteristics makes a formidable leadership team and strengthens self-confidence in the ability to lead.

The more confident a leader feels, the more likely it is success will follow. Success builds self-confidence. Two important factors are related to developing self-confidence. One is avoiding the tendency to become arrogant. The other is maintaining self-confidence despite setbacks.

The Leader Must Listen to the Constituents

Followers always have something to say. Leaders must listen to their constituents and determine whether action is indicated. Active listening, looking the person in the eye, and offering questioning probes are all ways to show an interest in what a person is saying. However, listening does not obligate the leader to any course of action. Clear boundaries must be communicated. A smart leader listens to all sides and makes decisions based on the vision and direction that is best for the group.

The Leader Must Have a Positive Attitude

Attitude is vital to leadership success. No one wants to follow a pessimist anywhere. People expect the leader to have the answers, to know where the organization is going, and to take the initiative to get the group to their goal. A positive attitude can be a great ally in sharing and maintaining the vision. Attitude is a choice, not a foregone conclusion. The effective leader uses positive thinking and positive messages to create an environment in which followers believe in the organization, the leader, and themselves. The problems and challenges in healthcare demand that nurses seek and fill leadership positions in a positive and future-oriented manner.

Exercise 2-5

Using the five rules for leaders, create a personal description of how you maintain balance, generate self-motivation, build self-confidence, listen to constituents, and maintain a positive attitude.

THE NURSE AS LEADER

Leadership Within the Workplace

The Staff Nurse as Leader

A common misconception is that leaders within the workplace are the managers. Leaders within the workplace are not necessarily those who are entrusted with the role and title of manager. The workplace manager is one who is a maintenance thinker. The goal of a maintenance thinker is to ensure that day-to-day operations run efficiently (Kerfoot, 1998). The manager is concerned about budgets, financial performance, staffing, employee evaluations, and employee education and training. All of these important activities are paramount concerns of the manager of an operational unit in healthcare. In contrast, the workplace leader is one who has the ability to envision a preferred future for the quality of the working environment. Nurse satisfaction is a construct that is measured and taken seriously by enlightened employers (Evans, 1999). A valued leader in the nursing workplace is a nurse who has ideas for increasing the level of workplace satisfaction for nurses on the work team. Leaders are those who creatively pose solutions to problems and capitalize on opportunities in the workplace. Leaders help create the future (Kerfoot, 1998). Nurses who believe that they have good ideas for future improvements should volunteer for opportunities to lead. Examples of these opportunities are negotiating committees in those environments with collective bargaining (Foley, 1999) and in professional practice councils in those environments with shared governance structures in place (Porter-O'Grady, 1999). If the hospital or other workplace has no formalized mechanism for nurse input into organizational decision making, staff nurses who are leaders should clarify their vision and work to make it happen.

Developing leadership skills for staff nurses can happen in several ways. Besides volunteering for leadership roles within the workplace, professional involvement with organizations outside of the workplace can help in the development of leadership skills (Kerfoot, 1999). In addition, establishing a mentoring relationship with a trusted leader in the workplace can be beneficial (Vance, 1999). It is important to remember that leadership can be developed and that staff nurse leaders can help establish workplaces that are satisfying and rewarding.

The Nurse Manager as Leader

Management and leadership, although different constructs, can be a strong combination for success. The nurse in the role of manager ensures that the day-to-day elements of the workplace are done correctly. Just as the effective manager pays attention to employee selection, hiring, orientation, continuing employee development, and financial accountability, in the role of leader, the manager raises the level of expectations and helps employees reach their highest level of potential excellence. A primary role of the leader is to inspire (Atchison, 1990).

Developing with staff nurses a shared vision of the preferred future is a goal of the nurse manager in the role of leader. Staff members tend to resist change that is thrust upon them. When they have a role in setting an agenda for change, they are far more likely to be invested in the eventual success of the workplace change (Oakley & Krug, 1994).

An essential element of success for the nurse manager as a leader is the inclusion of staff nurses in decision making. Including staff nurses in the process of formulating a vision for the preferred workplace of the future is a satisfier (Stamps, 1997). The nurse manager inspires staff by involving them in changing the workplace to make it more satisfying. In so doing, the nurse manager also develops personal leadership skills.

The Nurse Executive as Leader

A primary goal of the nurse executive is leadership within the workplace. The nurse executive has an outstanding opportunity to shape the future of professional practice within a working environment by creating opportunities for staff nurses and managers to have optimal input into organizational decision making relating to the future. The nurse executive thus helps create a shared vision of the preferred future.

The concept of empowerment is important to the role of leadership for the nurse executive in a work organization. Empowerment theory suggests that the role of leader rather than the role of manager motivates people to greatest efficiency and effectiveness (Stamps, 1997). To empower people, power must be given away or shared with others in the organization. Staff nurses may be encouraged to have input into decisions or may be given additional information about how decisions are made. The ability to make changes in the organization is a powerful tool. Nurses must believe that their input and ideas are considered when change occurs. Having input in decisions, having some control over the environment, and receiving feedback about actions taken or not taken all contribute to a feeling of being empowered to have control over one's practice and one's life.

The importance of managers and executives being leaders rather than managers is a recurring theme in more recent nursing management books (Tappen, 2000). The fact is both management and leadership skills in the nurse executive are essential. The ability to balance the day-to-day operating knowledge with the ability to lead a nursing service organization into the future is a winning combination.

The Nursing Student as Leader

Students have many opportunities to learn and practice leadership skills. The goals for leadership at the student level should be kept within a realistic framework. Allowing the student to practice novice leadership skills within the security of an educa-

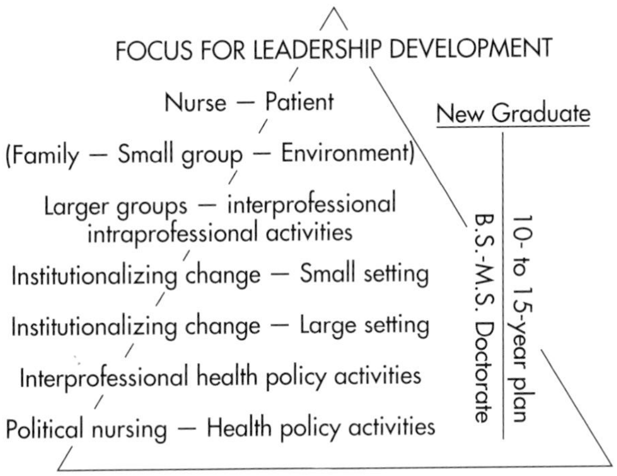

FOCUS FOR LEADERSHIP DEVELOPMENT

Nurse — Patient   New Graduate

(Family — Small group — Environment)

Larger groups — interprofessional intraprofessional activities

Institutionalizing change — Small setting

Institutionalizing change — Large setting

Interprofessional health policy activities

Political nursing — Health policy activities

B.S.-M.S. Doctorate

10- to 15-year plan

Figure 2-1 A leadership trajectory. (From Fagin, C. [2000]. *Essays on nursing leadership.* New York: Springer.)

tional program is a reasonable expectation. Novice leadership skills that contribute to future leadership success involve learning how to work in groups, deal with difficult people, resolve conflict, reach consensus on an action, and evaluate actions and outcomes objectively (Figure 2-1).

Fagin (2000) describes a 10- to 15-year leadership development plan for neophyte nurses that builds on their leadership skills from their beginning nurse-patient experiences. The reality of student development toward true leadership expertise takes place over a long period and should not be expected during the first year or two of nursing school or nursing practice. Nevertheless, every leader started somewhere. Movement toward an increasingly complex leadership experience allows for the new nurse to move from leading and planning with an individual to working with groups, such as families or communities. Further leadership development occurs during interactions with larger groups, instituting changes through research and application of new techniques, and moving toward health policy and political activities. With increasing educational achievement and career experience comes increasing complexity of leadership capabilities.

Most countries have some type of national student nurses' association, as well as regional, state, and school-based associations. These types of organizations offer an opportunity for student nurses to become involved in service to their future profession. Programs of study in schools of nursing are appropriately heavy on nursing theory and clinical

practice. Through involvement in the student association, the nursing student is able to understand the bigger picture of nursing as a profession.

The best way to begin involvement is to become active in the local chapter of the student association. If the student is interested in student association activities, there are opportunities to serve on committees or in elected positions on the board of directors at local, regional, state, and national levels. Examples of leadership development at the national level include serving on liaison committees with nurse leaders; attending leadership development educational programs; attending and leading events at local, state, and national meetings and conventions; and interacting with the leaders of complementary professional nursing organizations.

Organizational Leadership in Organizations

The American Nurses Association and State Affiliates

In the United States the best and most important step to take in becoming a leader within the nursing profession is to join a professional organization. Many nurses today take part in several organizations. However, membership in the American Nurses Association (ANA) and the state constituent member associations is essential for career growth and mobility, as well as demonstration of the commitment for professional nurses to deliver safe and competent care (Skaggs & deVries, 1998).

The best place to begin developing leadership skills in the professional association is to be involved in the local district level of the state association (Skaggs & deVries, 1998). Volunteering for committee memberships is a valued and useful way to learn and to grow within the association.

After becoming established and known in the local association, running for elected office in the local district association is the way many leaders within professional associations start their leadership careers. It is not unusual to be unsuccessful in the first attempt at running for an elective office in the professional association, but persistence can do two things: It can help with name recognition, and it can let members know that you are serious about being an association leader.

Many of the leaders within the ANA, after having begun their association leadership in the district association, later held office in the state constituent member associations. Volunteering for committee assignments and running for elected office in the state association establish leadership interest within the professional association. Leadership efforts at the national association level are usually more successful after establishing a record of successful leadership in the state constituent member association.

This pathway of professional involvement and leadership, from the student association to the district association to the state association and to the national association, may seem like a linear progression to more global opportunities for leadership in the profession. However, many very successful nursing leaders conceptualize the progression as circular rather than linear. Many well-known leaders who have held high office in the ANA do not then retire from professional involvement, but rather take their experience and expertise to return to offices and committee appointments at the district level and at the state levels.

Professional Specialty Organizations

Professional nursing specialty organizations play an important role in disseminating information to members in such areas as clinical practice (e.g., Oncology Nursing Society), role area (e.g., American Organization of Nurse Executives), and interest groups (e.g., Southern Nursing Research Society). Many of the professional specialty organizations maintain a national or regional presence rather than having state or local chapters. Some of them do have local chapters (e.g., Association of Operating Room Nurses), especially in the larger, more populated areas across the country. The major impact of the professional specialty organization is information sharing and dissemination, discussion of mutual clinical or role concerns, and education regarding the latest technical innovations in the field. Leadership opportunities are available to present posters or papers at local, regional, or national conferences, as well as to serve on committees and boards.

Leadership in the Community

Nurses as Community Opinion Leaders

Nurses are valued and respected members of their communities. As trusted professionals, nurses have an opportunity to serve as catalysts in leadership opportunities in the community. In partnership with others in the community, nurses can help build a more just, more peaceful, and more healthful society. Nurses are actualizing these possibilities in communities everywhere (Gottschalk & Baker, 1998).

Many avenues are available for nurses to serve as community opinion leaders. Attendance at civic gatherings, such as city commission and school board meetings, is an excellent way to be aware of what is happening and to offer input from a nursing perspective. For instance, when the school board begins deliberating whether the budget will accommodate a registered nurse for every school or whether to replace them with a trained clerk who can record vaccinations, a nursing voice in the audience could clarify the importance of school nurses to a school population. Writing letters to the editor of a newspaper and participating in public forums give the nurse an avenue to share expertise and mold community opinion.

Nurses as Community Volunteers

Many opportunities exist for volunteer participation in the community. Nurses bring a unique leadership skill set to community activities. The ability to understand complex systems and the understanding of interpersonal dynamics and communication techniques constitute knowledge that is valuable in community volunteer opportunities.

Leadership in mobilizing volunteers for health fairs, screening activities, and educational events is a community need that nurses can and do fill. Such activities promote health and advance the health of the community in important ways. Nurses can also lead efforts to engage others in the community in volunteer activities. In addition, nurses can organize individuals in the community to help develop a vision for the future of the community's health, healthcare opportunities, and healthcare delivery.

From the perspective of the nurse as a community leader, there is a unique opportunity to work with schools, city or county governments, and other community entities to formulate a vision for improving the health of the community through disease prevention and health promotion. The nurse can be a catalyst for a community to recognize present problems and to develop a plan to reach a preferred future.

Leadership Through Appointed and Elected Office

Nurses are valuable leaders in elected and appointed offices at the local, state, and national levels. Because of the trustworthiness of nurses in general, nurses should be able to mobilize resources to raise monies, develop support, and get elected to offices. The numbers of nurses in offices at all three levels of government are continually growing. The ANA Political Action Committee (PAC) and the state constituent member association PACs provide assistance to nurses who want to run for office. Nurses who are elected members of governmental bodies are able to exert their leadership to shape the vision of the government to help meet the needs of the citizens.

Local Offices

Leadership opportunities in elected or appointed positions in the local government include school boards, city councils, and community boards dealing with various community initiatives. At the local level, nurses who serve on elected or appointed boards and councils bring a unique perspective even when the major focus of the entity appears to be totally unrelated to healthcare. Leadership in this case is casting a vision of a healthy thriving community.

State Offices

Leadership opportunities at the state level in elected or appointed positions include being elected to state legislatures or appointment to state boards, such as the state board of nursing or the state board of health. The state constituent member association of the ANA often has a role in recommending names

of qualified members to be considered for appointment to various boards and committees in the state. Nurses who are members have the highest likelihood of being supported or recommended by the state association or national association.

National Offices

A few nurses have been successful in getting elected to the U.S. Congress as representatives. No nurse has yet been elected U.S. Senator, but many opportunities exist for nurses to be appointed to federal boards and commissions. The ANA and the state constituent member associations often play a role in putting forth nominations of members for appointment to such bodies.

The Leadership Challenge

The nurse is in a trusted role as nurturer and provider of care to the most vulnerable in our society. Nurses who choose leadership roles have many of the needed talents to serve their followers and their profession. Visionary and responsible leadership is vital to the future success of nursing as an art and a science. Professional nursing has been blessed with excellent leaders in the past and will continue to be led by the visionary nurse leaders of tomorrow.

The Solution

The following priorities were set:
- Patient safety
- Occupant safety
- Return to normal function as quickly as possible

Unit nursing staff were instructed to review their emergency preparedness manuals the evening of June 8 and ensure that they had flashlights and water. They were instructed to divide into teams and watch each other's patients, allowing some of the staff to rest. It was clear that the staff needed to pace themselves because it would be hours before additional personnel would arrive. Staff were reassured by frequent rounds made by the supervisors and calls to the units from the Command Center.

As water rushed into the basement of the facility, the departments of pharmacy and radiology moved their supplies higher and dry cereal, breads, and milk were obtained from the cafeteria to sustain patients over the coming hours. The

Network Services Department (hospital telephone and page operators) was relocated to higher ground. At 3 AM, as a power shortage became imminent, the decision to triage stable patients who were on life support devices was made. These patients were located on four different floors and were evacuated, starting at the highest floor and working down before elevators lost power. Patients were transferred to an adjacent medical tower building that had an outpatient ambulatory surgery center linked to the hospital via a skybridge. Anesthesiologists, residents, respiratory therapists, and nurses worked collaboratively to triage patients. Some critical care patients were evacuated down stairwells as elevators failed. All critically ill patients who were too unstable to evacuate were placed on ventilators with battery backup. It became apparent that power was needed quickly to maintain ventilator support because batteries would be drained. As soon as roads were passable, ex-

Continued

The Solution—cont'd

ternal diesel generators were obtained and connected to provide power to ventilators, which then created the need to test for carbon dioxide levels. A human chain was created to deliver medical supplies, water, food, and lights to staff.

Staff were educated to deliver IVs without pumps and take blood pressures the old fashioned way, with a manometer and a flashlight. Food was provided to patients and staff from volunteer agencies such as the Salvation Army. Patient and staff comfort was difficult to maintain in an un–air-conditioned, 26-story tower in the summertime. Patients were triaged for discharge; all admissions were carefully screened by a medical director and nurses because the City of Houston was short 3000

hospital beds for an extended period. Nine days after the flood, all beds and essential services were functioning and the hospital was open for all admissions.

Nurses often have not learned the necessary skills for triage and disaster response. An understanding of emergency plans and quick critical thinking skills are imperative to surviving a natural disaster.

— Rosemary Luquire

Would this be a suitable approach for you? Why?

CHAPTER CHECKLIST

The role of the nurse leader is to share a vision and provide the means for followers to reach it. When the group succeeds, the leader succeeds. Members of different generations have different expectations and different needs from those of a leader. Various leadership opportunities are available; it is up to the nurse to take advantage and contribute to the progress of the nursing profession.

- Excellent leadership in any working environment can improve recruitment and retention efforts and result in satisfied employees.
- Two leadership approaches contrast the leader role:
  - Transactional leaders rely on the power of the organizational position to reward or punish performance in order to control employees.
  - Transformational leaders ascribe power to interpersonal skills and personal contact in transforming people to make them want to progress.
- Key elements to becoming an effective leader can be learned and practiced:
  - Select an effective and willing mentor.
  - Lead by example through role modeling.
  - Share the rewards with followers.
  - Have a clear vision that followers can support.
  - Be willing to grow and change to meet current needs.

- The emerging workforce (born 1965 to 1976) want a leader who has good people skills and a nurturing attitude. The entrenched workforce (born 1946 to 1965) wants a leader who is tolerant of the process of change and who exhibits high integrity and professionalism.
- There are many opportunities to lead in nursing. To thrive in a leadership position, the nurse must do the following:
  - Maintain balance.
  - Generate self-motivation.
  - Build self-confidence.
  - Listen to constituents.
  - Have a positive attitude.

TIPS FOR BECOMING A LEADER

If you want to become an effective leader, here are some tips.

- Take advantage of leadership opportunities and practice your leadership skills.
- Expect to stumble occasionally, but learn from your mistakes and continue. Every leader has made mistakes. The truly inspired leaders have learned from them and moved forward.
- Get some help—a caring mentor is the best way to develop leadership ability. The mentor can give you

the benefit of experience and will serve as a resource to get feedback on actions and to explore options.

- Take risks. A person does not become a leader by maintaining the status quo. Leaders forge a vision and bring followers forward. However, change involves risks. Don't be fool-hardy, but don't be complacent either.

TERMS TO KNOW

emerging workforce
entrenched workforce
mentor
transactional leadership
transformational leadership

REFERENCES

Allen, D. (1998). How nurses become leaders: Perceptions and beliefs about leadership development. *Journal of Nursing Administration, 28*(9), 15-20.

Atchison, T. A. (1990). *Turning health care leadership around.* San Francisco: Jossey-Bass.

Bass, B. (1998). *Transformational leadership: Industry, military, and educational impact.* Mahwah, NJ: Lawrence Erlbaum Associates.

Bennis, W. (1989). *On becoming a leader.* Reading, MA: Addison-Wesley.

Bennis, W. (1999). The end of leadership: Exemplary leadership is impossible without full inclusion, initiatives, and cooperation of followers. *Organizational Dynamics, 28*(1), 71-80.

Bradford, L. J., & Raines, C. (1992). *Twenty-something: Managing and motivating today's new work force.* Denver: Merrill-Alexander Publishing.

Covey, S. R. (1992). *Principle-centered leadership.* New York: Simon & Schuster.

Dunham-Taylor, J. (2000). Nurse executive transformational leadership found in participative organizations. *Journal of Nursing Administration, 30*(5), 241-250.

Earnshaw G. J. (1995). Mentorship: The students' view. *Nurse Education Today, 15*(4), 274-279.

Evans, M. L. (1999). Nursing's role and outcomes in practice and advanced practice. In C. A. Anderson (Ed.), *Nursing student to nursing leader: The critical path to leadership development.* Albany, NY: Delmar.

Fagin, C. (2000). *Essays on nursing leadership.* New York: Springer Publishing.

Foley, M. (1999). Developing leadership as a staff nurse. In C. A. Anderson (Ed.), *Nursing student to nursing leader: The critical path to leadership development.* Albany, NY: Delmar.

Fulham, C., Lando, A., Johansen, M., Reyes, A., & Szaloczy, D. (1998). The triad of empowerment: Leadership, environment, and professional traits. *Nursing Economics, 16*(5), 254-257.

Gottschalk, J., & Baker, S. S. (1998). Contemporary issues in the community. In D. Mason and J. K. Leavitt (Eds.), *Policy and politics in nursing and health care* (3rd ed.). Philadelphia: WB Saunders.

Kerfoot, K. (1998). Management is taught, leadership is learned. *Dermatology Nursing, 10*(3), 226-227.

Kerfoot, K. (1999). The art of leading with grace. *Dermatology Nursing, 11*(3), 222-223.

Koestenbaum, P. (1991). *Leadership: The inner side of greatness.* San Francisco: Jossey-Bass.

Kouzes, J., & Posner, B. (1997). *The leadership challenge.* San Francisco: Jossey Bass.

Markham, G. (1998). Gender in leadership. *Nursing Management, 3*(1), 18-19.

Marriner-Tomey, A. (1993). *Transformational leadership in nursing.* St. Louis: Mosby.

Oakley, E., & Krug, D. (1994). *Enlightened leadership.* New York: Simon & Schuster.

Porter-O'Grady, T. (1999). Workplace advocacy, shared governance, and collective bargaining: Rights and opportunity. In C. A. Anderson (Ed.), *Nursing student to nursing leader: The critical path to leadership development.* Albany, NY: Delmar.

Senge, P. M. (1994). *The fifth discipline: The art and practice of the learning organization.* New York: Doubleday.

Skaggs, B. J., & deVries, C. M. (1998). You and your professional organization. In D. J. Mason & J. K. Leavitt (Eds.), *Policy and politics in nursing and health care* (3rd ed.). Philadelphia: WB Saunders.

Stamps, P. L. (1997). *Nurses and work satisfaction: An index for measurement.* Chicago: Health Administration Press.

Tappen, R. M. (2000). *Nursing leadership and management: Concepts and practice* (4th ed.). Philadelphia: FA Davis.

Trice, H. M., & Beyer, J. M. (1992). *The cultures of work organizations.* Englewood Cliffs, NJ: Prentice Hall.

Vance, C. (1999). Mentoring: The nursing leader and mentor's perspective. In C. A. Anderson (Ed.), *Nursing student to nursing leader: The critical path to leadership development.* Albany, NY: Delmar.

Wieck, K. L. (2000). A vision of nursing: The future revisited. *Nursing Outlook, 48*(1), 7-8.

Wieck, K. L., Prydun, M., & Walsh, T. (in press). What Emerging Workforce nurses want in their leaders. *Journal of Nursing Scholarship.*

SUGGESTED READINGS

Barger, S. E. (2000). Professional practice: The practice of leadership. *Journal of Professional Nursing, 16*(2), 72.

Bower, F. L. (2000). *Nurses taking the lead: Personal qualities of effective leadership*. St. Louis: Mosby.

Labarre, P. (2000, March). Do you have the will to lead? *FastCompany*, 222-230.

Northouse, P. G. (2001). *Leadership: Theory and practice* (2nd ed.). Thousand Oaks, CA: Sage Publishers.

Shtogren, J. A. (Ed.). (1999). *Skyhooks for leadership*. New York: American Management Association.

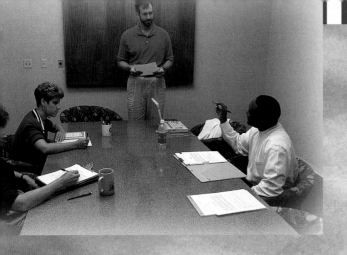

3

Developing the Role of Manager

Ana M. Valadez
Dorothy A. Otto

T his chapter identifies key concepts related to the roles of nurse manager. It describes basic manager functions, illustrates management principles that are inherent in the role of professional practice, and identifies descriptive competencies for the nurse manager. Role development is crucial to forming the right questions to ask in a management or clinical situation that will help the practitioner identify problems and anticipate needs. This chapter provides an overview for the further development of practical skills.

Objectives

- Analyze roles and functions of a nurse manager.
- Analyze the relationship of the nurse manager with others.
- Analyze management of health-care settings.
- Evaluate management resource allocation/distribution.
- Evaluate behaviors of professionalism of the nurse manager.

Questions to Consider

- Why do you want to be a nurse manager?
- In what type of practice setting would you like to be a nurse manager?
- How do you manage current resources?
- Do you yearn for having increased involvement in key decisions, changing systems, working with people, or improving patient care?
- How will your clinical expertise be used in the setting?

The Challenge

Joyce Burdett, RN, BSN
Nurse Manager, Covenant Health System, Lubbock, Texas

In this day and time, I have several challenges. The nursing shortage, although critical in itself, also creates other sideline challenges, one of them being staff and patient education. I have lost my clinical specialist for the unit. Now there is no one who is specifically responsible for inpatient staff and patient education. We do give our new employees material specific to oncology, and we do provide a chemo certification class every few months. The nurses try hard to provide the patients with the education they need, but all of the unit education is very much a hit-and-miss situation. Before the critical nurse shortage, I actually used to have two people responsible for the unit's educational needs. The assistant nurse manager did the staff education, and the clinical specialist did the patient teaching. So we are actually short two unit positions that were specifically designated to do the unit teaching. The unit has been without educational support for about 3 months.

 What do you think you would do if you were this nurse?

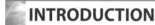 **INTRODUCTION**

Chapter 1 provided a general overview of leading and managing. This chapter looks at management from different perspectives. The underpinnings of role theory began with management theory, a science that has undergone numerous changes in the last 10 decades. In the early 1990s the theory of scientific management was embraced, a theory based on the idea that there is one best way to accomplish a task. Practice in the 1930s through the 1970s was dominated by participative, humanistic leadership theories. Although changes in healthcare delivery no doubt are affecting the roles of nurse managers, the relevance of role theory remains a constant. Conway's (1978) definition, "**role theory** represents a collection of concepts and a variety of hypothetical formulations that predict how actors will perform in a given role, or under what circumstances certain types of behaviors can be expected" (p. 17), is still appropriate today.

The evolutionary process of management theories has affected how managers address workers' concerns and needs. The beginning management theories discounted concern for workers' psychological needs and focused on productivity and efficiency. When theories relating to human relations came about, workers' needs and motivations became focal points for the nurse manager. Conversely, situational theories, such as Path-Goal the-ory, focused on the environment, clarifying the relationship between the pathway employees take and the outcome or goal they wish to obtain.

What is involved in management? Styles (1982) says that significant self-examination should be a requisite for one who desires to become a nurse **manager** through the process of career development. In self-appraisal, the potential nurse manager might ask: Do I have career goals that include gaining experience and education to become a nurse manager? What specific knowledge, skills, and personal qualities do I need to develop to be most effective in practice? What support systems have I established? If changes need to be made, they must be matched with changes in healthcare agencies and within the larger social system. A nurse manager must recognize the need for growth within, which then translates into improvement of one's practice. A prerequisite for self-actualization is a bond between the nurse and the community, for a nurse manager's patients and staff make up the community. Consider also, what is the **role** of the nurse manager? Practicing nurse managers illustrate role perceptions. Some nurse managers would cite decision making and problem solving as major roles, for which maintaining objectivity is sometimes a special challenge. Others would identify collaboration, especially with other departments, to enhance quality patient outcomes. Truly effective care is the result of efforts by the total healthcare team.

Table 3-1 BASIC MANAGER FUNCTIONS AND NURSE MANAGER FUNCTIONS

Basic Manager Functions	Nurse Manager Functions
Establishes and communicates goals and objectives	Delineates objectives and goals for assigned area Communicates objectives and goals effectively to staff members who will help attain goals
Organizes, analyzes, and divides work into tasks	Assesses and evaluates activities on assigned area Makes sound decisions about dividing up daily work activities for staff
Motivates and communicates	Stresses the importance of being a good team player Provides positive reinforcement
Analyzes, appraises, and interprets performance and measurements	Completes performance appraisals of individual staff members Communicates results to staff and management
Develops people, including self	Addresses staff development continuously through mentoring and preceptorships Furthers self-development by attending educational programs and seeking specialty certification credentialing

From Drucker, P. F. (1974). *Management tasks, responsibilities and practices.* New York: Harper & Row.

Effective collaboration includes honesty, directness, and listening to others' points of view. However, management is more complex than this.

THE MANAGEMENT ROLE

Management is a generic function that includes similar basic tasks in every discipline and in every society. However, before the nurse manager can be effective, he or she must be well grounded in nursing practice. Drucker (1974) identifies five basic functions of a manager:

- Establishes objectives and goals for each area and communicates them to the persons who are responsible for attaining them
- Organizes and analyzes the activities, decisions, and relations needed and divides them into manageable tasks
- Motivates and communicates with the people responsible for various jobs through teamwork
- Analyzes, appraises, and interprets performance and communicates the meaning of measurement tools and their results to staff and superiors
- Develops people, including self

Table 3-1 shows how these basic management functions apply to the nurse manager.

Managers develop efforts that focus on the individual. Their aim is to enable the person to develop his or her abilities and strengths to the fullest and to achieve excellence. According to Hershey and Blanchard (1977), "People differ not only in their ability to do, but also in their will to do or their motivation. . . . Commitment to a goal increases when people are involved in their own goal setting" (pp. 16, 25). Thus a manager has a role in helping people develop goals that are realistic. Goals should be set high enough, yet be attainable. Active participation, encouragement, and guidance from the manager and from the organization are needed for the individual's developmental efforts to be fully productive. Nurse managers who are successful in motivating staff are often providing an environment that facilitates accomplishment of goals resulting in personal satisfactions.

The nurse manager must possess qualities similar to those of a good leader: knowledge, integrity, ambition, judgment, courage, stamina, enthusiasm, communication skills, planning skills, and administrative abilities. The arena of management versus leadership has been addressed by numerous authors, and although there are differences in points of view, there are some similarities between managers and leaders.

Managers address complex issues by planning, budgeting, and setting target goals. They meet their goals by organizing, staffing, controlling, and solv-

Table 3-2 LEADER, MANAGER, AND FOLLOWER TRAITS

Leader Traits	Manager Traits	Follower Traits
Values commitments, relationships with others, and esprit de corps in the organization	Emphasizes organizing, coordinating, and controlling resources (e.g., space, supplies, equipment, people)	Perceives the needs of both the leader and other staff
Provides a vision that can be communicated and has a long-term effect on the organization that moves it in new directions	Attends to short-term objectives/goals	Demonstrates cooperative and collaborative behaviors
Communicates the rationale for changing paths; charts new paths that lead to progress	Maximizes results from existing resources	Exerts the power to communicate through various channels
Endorses and thrives on taking risks that bring about change	Interprets established policy, procedures, and mandates	Remains fully accountable for actions while relinquishing some autonomy and conceding certain authority to the leader
Demonstrates a positive feeling in the workplace and relates the importance of workers	Moves cautiously; dislikes uncertainty	Exhibits willingness to both lead and follow peers, as the situation warrants, allowing for competency-based leadership
	Enforces policy mandates, contracts, etc. (acts as a gatekeeper)	Assumes responsibility to understand what risks are acceptable for the organization and what risks are unacceptable

ing problems. By contrast, **leaders** set a direction, develop a vision, and communicate the new direction to the staff. Managers address complexity, whereas leaders address change. Another way of looking at management in contrast to leadership and followership is to look at the common traits of each. Table 3-2 compares the characteristics of a leader with those of a manager and a follower.

▪ *Exercise 3-1*

In a small group, discuss how patients pay for services of hospitals, clinics, hospices, or private provider offices. Hypothesize about what portion of those costs represents nursing care. How does a manager contribute to cost-effectiveness?

According to Gladwell (2001), little events can have a major effect. The role of nurse managers is to define those events and use them to "tip" the unit or group to a new level of performance. The key is for the manager to build a team of individuals so that new connections are formed. The nurse manager is also the environmentalist of the unit. In other words, the manager is always assessing the context in which people practice to determine how changes there can affect people's performance. No changes occur within an organization that are not visible in the larger societal context. Thus we see violence in the workplace today, just as we see it in society as a whole. The nurse manager can define that "what happens out there" could, and likely will, happen within an organization's confines. Clearly, one of the roles a manager must fulfill is translating what is happening in a societal sense into the possibilities of the organization. This requires that the nurse manager be involved in strategic planning that can translate to all with whom the manager works.

Quantum theory elucidates the complexity and unpredictability of events. Because nurse managers will continue to practice in an unstable, rapidly changing healthcare environment, quantum theory may be the most significant theory for nurse man-

Table 3-3 THE MANAGER'S COROLLARY TO THE COURAGE OF FOLLOWERS	
Dimension of the Relationship (Follower)	**Manager**
Courage to assume responsibility	Demonstrates trust in individual autonomy
Courage to serve	Advocates for service role
Courage to challenge	Poses dilemmas to encourage behavior
Courage to participate in transformation	Designs opportunities to develop transformation abilities
Courage to leave by separating from a leader or group	Risks separation

Modified from Chaleff, I. (1995). *The courageous follower: Standing up to and for our leaders.* San Francisco: Berrett-Koehler.

agers of the twenty-first century. Valadez and Sportsman (1999) address the use of quantum theory when managing the environment. They offer three guiding principles to manage the healthcare environment: (1) The world is unpredictable; (2) the world is not independent of the observer; and (3) relationships among things are what counts, not the things themselves. The authors identify a critical role component for health professionals today, that is, manipulation of factors that may impair workers' ability to accomplish a goal.

Porter-O'Grady (1999) writes of quantum leadership having five expectations of the nurse manager. (1) Do not predict the future, for none of us can know it with certainty. Predicting the future can have negative consequences on the consumer as well as staff. (2) Learn to read the direction of change. The manager who closely monitors current trends and correlates them can forecast an accurate picture and offer some direction to the change. (3) Constant translation of meaning of information is necessary. Staff have access to numerous sources of information, and this can lead to sensory overload. It is the manager's responsibility to give staff positive reinforcement for their data-gathering efforts while at the same time assisting them to effectively narrow their data-retrieval efforts. (4) Assist staff members to learn self-management. Two key elements necessary for staff to function effectively in the new healthcare environment include being independent in their role functions and being interdependent in their relationships within the team. The manager's challenge is to instill independent traits in the staff and remove the long-standing idea that a manager's role is as a sage advisor who assumes a parent role. (5) Technological proficiency is not an option but an expectation. The staff's interdependent role necessitates a technologically proficient staff who can communicate with the team through wire and wireless modes, facsimiles, and new links. The manager's role includes holding staff accountable for the technological communication and providing them with the necessary skills to be proficient in technology.

To be successful in day-to-day operations, a manager must be concerned with relationships. Chaleff (1995) developed a model of followership to reorient individuals. "Courageous followership is built on the platform of courageous relationship. The courage to be right, the courage to be wrong, the courage to be different from each other. Each of us sees the world through our own eyes and experiences" (p. 4). Chaleff describes five dimensions of the relationship: the courage to assume responsibility, the courage to serve, the courage to challenge, the courage to participate in transformation, and the courage to leave by separating from a leader or group. Table 3-3 poses the possible corollary role of the manager for supporting this courage development in **followers.**

CONSUMER OF RESEARCH

The nurse manager's role calls for a twofold responsibility: that of being a participant in research and that of being an interpreter of research. Nursing literature, especially in nursing administration journals, reflects that nurse managers are contributing to research either by doing unit research or contributing to large-scale agency research projects. Likewise, the nurse manager also interprets published research findings that have implications for the staff or the patients and makes every effort to incorporate the findings into unit activities so that both staff and patients can benefit. Nurse managers, as first-line managers, are also in the position of identifying best nursing practices that can be researched through collaborative efforts of service and educational institutions.

MENTORING

A manager also should be concerned about preparing successors. Although mentoring individuals for the purpose of attaining greater heights in career development is not a new concept, the use of mentors for women was not addressed until the late 1970s. Vance and Olson (1998) refer to a mentor as one who is a wise advocate prepared to offer another person guidance, encouragement, and sage advice over an extended period. A model of mentoring for nurse manager positions is one way of ensuring continuity and stability not only for the unit workplace but also (and more important) for the patient as the consumer of healthcare. Nurse managers who are mentoring others for a management position should encourage nurses not only to seek new experiences but also to document in their portfolio experiences that will give a potential employer a word portrait of their management skills (Bell, 2001). Salient portfolio components for an aspiring nurse manager might include (1) employee activities that added value to the employee's present position, such as leading a task force addressing quality improvement; (2) personal development, such as attending workshops on workplace violence; (3) budgetary experiences, such as budget developing for staff development activities; (4) verbal and written communication skills, such as giving presentations to the local PTA on safety responsibilities of parents and holding offices, such as secretary to a nursing organization; and (5) recognition or commendation awards, such as being named employee of the month for a cost-saving idea that proved invaluable to the unit.

ORGANIZATIONAL CULTURE

In the ever-changing environment of healthcare, nurse managers need to know the **organizational culture** of their hospitals and how it supports their unit's mission and goals. Jones and Redman (2000) reported on the organizational culture of three hos-

pitals undergoing work redesign. The authors used the Competing Values Framework (Cameron & Quinn, 1994) questionnaire for measuring organizational culture. Their results showed that one hospital underwent extensive organizational reengineering, including architectural changes. Yet that hospital did better than the other two hospitals. Nurse and patient satisfaction remained stable. The hospital's balanced cultural orientation before changes were implemented helped greatly in adapting to outside environmental changes. By contrast, the two hospitals that did not engage in extensive reengineering projects did not fare well. Nurse dissatisfaction prevailed and one of the hospitals also experienced patient dissatisfaction. Other findings revealed that organizations with unbalanced cultures are unable to adapt to organizational changes. The Competing Values Framework incorporates specific strategies for promoting desired cultural values and decreasing the undesirable ones. Although not all managers will have the experience of leading a total organizational redesign, it is likely that they will have experiences on a more limited scale.

DAY-TO-DAY MANAGEMENT CHALLENGES

The nurse manager who meets the day-to-day management challenges must be able to achieve an acrobatic balance of three sources of demand: upper management requests, consumer demands, and staff needs. The manager has to ensure that the staff have opportunities for providing upper management with input regarding changes that affect them and also has to make unit and staff needs known to upper management. The consumers of health services today are much better educated and accustomed to providing input into decisions that affect them. The nurse manager needs to respect their requests, yet maintain care in the broad context of safety and efficiency. The staff need recognition and independence when carrying out their roles and responsibilities. The nurse manager needs to have a sense of when to relinquish control, thus allowing decision making at the point of service.

The Research Perspective box describes interviews with a midlevel nurse manager following a patient-focused redesign.

As Covey (1989) writes: "Our character, basically, is a composite of our habits. . . . Because they

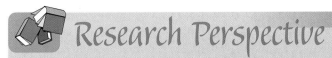

Research Perspective

Ingersoll, G. L., Cook, J., Fagel, S., Applegate, M., & Frank, B. (1999, May). The effect of patient-focused redesign on midlevel nurse managers' role responsibilities and work environment. *Journal of Nursing Administration, 29*(5), 21-27.

This descriptive study was conducted in two tertiary care hospitals in the Midwest. Nine midlevel nurse managers were interviewed 9 to 12 months after the agencies had implemented a patient focus redesign. The midlevel managers who were interviewed were responsible for several patient care units and answered directly to senior nurse executives. The study findings revealed several emerging themes: expanded role responsibilities, decreased self-esteem, environmental uncertainty, and concerns about the delivery of care.

IMPLICATIONS FOR PRACTICE

Midlevel manager roles are expanding, especially as senior nursing executives take on the responsibility of corporate- or system-level activities. Often, midlevel managers have assumed their position because of their effectiveness as first-line managers. Their new position as midlevel manager requires considerable role expansion and demonstrates a critical need of further development. Such development should include concepts related to advanced leadership and skills in planning and financial management.

are consistent, often unconscious patterns, they constantly, daily, express our character and produce our effectiveness . . . or ineffectiveness" (p. 46). Nurse managers also must be credible clinicians in the areas they manage. A critical factor in being an excellent nurse manager is understanding how to ensure optimal patient outcomes, involve families or significant others in the plan of care, and allocate resources and technology in a fair and ethical manner. The nurse manager-clinician is confronted with complex and ambiguous patient care situations. Sometimes decisions are made to meet one important patient care need at the expense of another. That is an important message to convey to staff.

Exercise 3–2

Select a nurse manager and a staff nurse follower in one of your clinical facilities. Observe them over a certain time (e.g., 4 to 8 hours). Compare and contrast the styles they exhibit. Is power shared or centralized? Are interactions positive or negative? What is the nature of their conversations? How does your summation of this observation relate to managerial, leadership, and followership characteristics?

Workplace Violence

Nurse managers continue to be responsible for ensuring the safety of their staff and patients. Workers

in high-risk areas such as the emergency room require special attention. For the nurse manager, "special attention" translates to his or her staff receiving adequate on-the-job training. Such training may include effective techniques relating to crisis intervention and the handling of highly agitated people who may be armed. Violence at home can also affect a worker's outlook and productivity. Nurse managers may have to address this problem if it exists on their unit. Because the nurse manager's workforce may include a majority of women, information that addresses violence against women should be readily available. The Position Statement on Violence Against Women, revised and adopted by the American Nurses Association (ANA) Board of Directors (2000), is a good source for the nurse manager to refer to when addressing domestic violence that may affect his or her staff.

MANAGING HEALTHCARE SETTINGS

Wilson and Porter-O'Grady (1999) speak of a world undergoing a major social transformation. It is difficult to comprehend the implications of such rapid change. For nurse managers, some of these changes, such as technology, quantum theory, and fiscal constraints that require downsizing of staff while maintaining quality, are but a few of the challenges they face. Bennis (2000) equates managing people to herding cats, which of course is impossible to do. However, using other techniques such as persuasion and gently leading often yields effective management results. Why is it so hard to manage people? According to Bennis, the people being led have options, educational knowledge, and a vast menu of technological resources. In essence, people are informed and have access to information previously accessible only to managers.

Healthcare settings are changing rapidly. They are an exciting, "full of opportunity" experience, yet there is flux in relation to where and how nurses will practice. Nurse managers may be redefining their role as case managers. The paradigm of patient care is shifting from in-hospital settings to patient-directed outpatient and community settings and from acute care disease treatment models to health promotion/disease prevention models. Regardless of how managers' roles are transforming, the manager's job is to link all of the resources together to be sure the work and goals are achieved.

The Pew Health Professions Commission, in its report *Reforming Health Care Workforce Regulation* (1995b), addressed transformations in our healthcare systems that will affect the nurse manager's role and self-accountability. Managed care in a cost-conscious environment places greater quality care demands on all healthcare providers. In addition, the Pew Health Commission report *Critical Challenges: Revitalizing the Health Professions for the Twenty-first Century* (1995a) envisioned a healthcare system for the end of the century that has notable changes. Prevailing trends that encompass the new healthcare system delineate a more inclusive definition of health, diversified healthcare systems, a commitment toward improving health for entire populations, and a shift of focus from disease and treatment to prevention, education, and management of care. The professional nurse who manages care in this healthcare era will have to bring a new cadre of skills into a dynamic, rapidly changing managerial role.

High technology will continue to modify nurse managers' roles. For example, because of the ability to perform more complex surgery through surgicenters, nurse managers will find themselves practicing with short-term or ambulatory care admissions. A key to successful management is interdependence. Covey (1989) makes a salient point when he addresses interdependence as a necessity to achieve life goals, whether familial or organizational. A critical

component of interdependence is collaboration, which uses the different strengths of each person. Collaboration requires one to be flexible and broadminded and to have a strong self-concept. Sullivan and Decker (2001) addressed the concept of collaboration from the perspective of conflict management. When collaboration is used to solve a conflict, the energies of all parties are focused on solving the problem versus defeating the opposing party.

The staff often look to the nurse manager to lead them in addressing workplace issues with higher levels of administration. To do this, the nurse manager must possess two sets of skills: (1) the ability to address power sources in one's work environment and define power-based strategies, such as in organizing a following of other nurse managers with similar concerns, and (2) the ability to effectively place pressure on the power holders so that needed changes can occur. Employees' "buy in" to a change sometimes needs to be thought out carefully. A study by Ingersoll, Kirsch, Merk, and Lightfoot (2000) explored the relationship of organizational culture and readiness for change. The authors examined the three components of the social system of an organization: commitment, readiness, and culture. Data were collected by surveying employees in two hospitals that were directly affected by a work redesign. More than 2000 surveys were distributed; 684 returned surveys were usable. Of the three constructs studied, readiness to change was the strongest predictor of commitment to the organization. This finding has significant meaning for the nurse manager because employee "disconnect" is likely to occur if workers feel the resources are lacking to do their job well. Consequently, workers may experience withdrawal from and lack of commitment to the organization. Nurse managers face the challenge of keeping employees connected.

Blanchard's and O'Connor's book *Managing by Values* (1997) provides a framework for stability, continuity, and growth in today's business world that is characterized by increasing change. Accordingly, the "managing by values" (MBV) process involves three phases: (1) clarification of mission/purpose and values, (2) communication of the mission and values, and (3) alignment of daily practices with the mission and values. Blanchard and O'Connor identify three core values as acts of life: achieving, connecting, and integrating. Achieving is a natural behavior for nurses, who are able to set goals beyond day-to-day survival. In connecting, nurses establish relationships with their patients, staff, or other healthcare professionals. The process of integrating brings achieving and connecting together to form purposes and values and to put them into daily nursing practice. When was the last time you defined or redefined your purpose in your personal and professional life? "Being values-aligned does not occur without changes in our daily habits, practices, and attitudes. When aligned around shared values and united in a common purpose, ordinary people accomplish extraordinary results and give their organization a competitive edge" (p. 144).

A way of demonstrating that employees are valued is by recognizing staff through various means. Employees who have gone beyond the scope of their job to meet the needs of the patient, department, or institution deserve recognition. An award may reflect the institution's philosophy, beliefs, and mission, as exemplified in one institution's "Quality Credo"—communication, competent performance, personal leadership, respect, and teamwork.

▪ Exercise 3-3

The Vice-President for Patient Care Services for the local health department has just undergone a tremendous challenge because of a natural disaster of flooding in their vicinity. Many of the staff, despite their own family needs, assisted flood victims with their needs, which ranged from crisis care to adequate follow-up of chronic disorders. The Vice-President for Patient Services wants to establish a recognition program for the staff who gave endless hours to their community. How would you approach establishing this recognition program? What resources would you need, and where would you go to seek the needed resources?

MANAGING RESOURCES

Each of these concepts is addressed in depth elsewhere in this book, but the key point is that the manager must manage each and integrate each with the others. The practice settings of tomorrow will no doubt continue to include in-hospital care; however, numerous innovative practice models operating from a community-based framework also may be found. Predictors of effective outcomes to ensure quality patient care include rationed and multi-tiered distribution of healthcare services, such as health maintenance organizations (HMOs), preferred provider organizations (PPOs), or independent private payment plans; very precise outcome-oriented quality assurance measures, such as critical pathways; and concerted efforts to control spiraling

health costs by increasing productivity and efficiency of healthcare providers. Other practice models, differentiated practice, shared governance, and restructured work environments make use of all levels of healthcare personnel.

The manager is responsible for managing all resources designated to the unit of care. This includes all personnel, professional and nonprofessional, under the manager's span of control. The wise manager quickly determines that a unit must function economically and, in so doing, realizes that there are many opportunities to reshape how nursing is delivered. Budget and personnel have always been considered critical resources. However, as technology improves, informatics must be integrated with budget and personnel as a critical resource element. Basing practice on research findings, networking through the Internet with other nurse managers, sharing concerns and difficulties, and being willing to step outside of tradition can assist future managers in decisions about resource utilization.

MANAGED CARE

Managed care, a healthcare delivery option introduced in the 1980s, has clearly affected the role and responsibilities of all nurses (Sportsman & Valadez 2001). This is especially true of nurses working in managerial positions. The goal of managed care is to provide services needed by patients efficiently and at an appropriate cost. In essence, this goal requires nurse managers to know and incorporate business principles into patient care practices. Nurse managers who know business principles become one of the conduits for ensuring safe, effective, affordable care.

CASE MANAGEMENT

Case management, a method used to provide care for many years in outpatient service areas, is now, because of managed care, an option of care in acute care settings (Sullivan & Decker, 2001). The key to effective case management is coordination of care, with identified time frames for accomplishing appropriate care outcomes. The nurse manager is often the overseer of the case managers, and in some settings, the nurse manager is the immediate supervisor of the case managers. Case management involves components of case selection, multidisciplinary assessment, collective planning, coordination of events, negotiation, and evaluation and documentation of the outcomes of patient status in measures of cost and quality. Case managers are employed in acute care settings, rehabilitation facilities, subacute facilities, community-based programs, home care, and insurance companies. These managers must possess a broad range of personal, interpersonal, and management skills.

 ## INFORMATICS

Informatics is in a stage of constant change, and it highlights for nurse managers two roles that have prevailed: educator and research translator. Both of these roles have become easier to accomplish because informatics has given quick and ready access to current and retrospective clinical patient data. The accessibility and use of the Internet facilitates the education of staff, patients, and their families. Nurse managers have taken advantage of informatics to gain quick access to patient classification systems that denote acuity of care and access to personnel hours that relate directly to patient acuity. A manager must ensure that the staff's data input is

accurate and must also demonstrate leadership in synthesizing how the data are used to deliver care. In addition, managers must be early adapters of the technology to demonstrate its value in performance.

BUDGETS

Budgetary allocations, whether they are related to the number of dollars available to manage a unit or in full-time equivalent employee formulas, may be the direct responsibility of nurse managers. For highly centralized organizations, only the administrative group at the executive level decides on the budgetary allocations. As healthcare organizations adopt "flat" organizational structures and decentralize responsibilities to the patient care areas, nurse managers allocate fiscal resources for their designated unit. In the decentralized organizational model, nurse managers must have the business and financial skills to be able to prepare and justify a detailed budget that reflects the short- and long-term needs of the unit.

Perhaps the most important aspect of a budget is the provision for a mechanism that allows some self-control, such as decision making at the point of service (POS), which does not require prior hi-

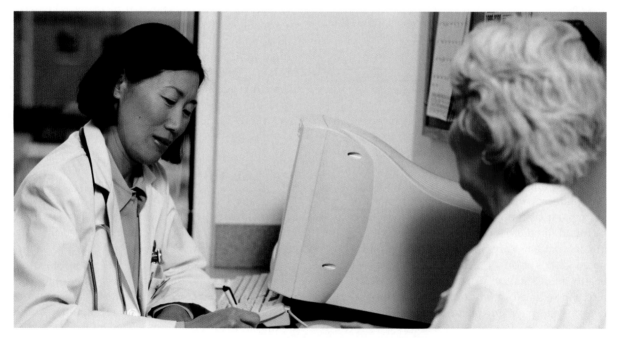

Patient care is shifting from in-hospital settings to outpatient and community settings.

erarchical approval and a rationale for budgetary spending.

■ Exercise 3-4

Visit a city health department or an adult day-care facility. What type of information system is used? Are both paper (hard copy) and computer sources used? What can you assume about the budget based on the physical appearance of the setting? Does any equipment appear dated? How do the employees (and perhaps volunteers) function? Do they seem motivated? Ask two or three to tell you, in a sentence or two, the purpose (vision or mission) of the organization. Can you readily identify the nurse manager? What does the manager do to manage the three critical resources of personnel, finances, and technological access?

QUALITY INDICATORS

The nurse manager is consistently concerned with the quality of care that is being delivered on his or her unit. The **quality indicators** developed by the ANA, such as the National Database of Nursing Quality Indicators (NDNQI) (http://nursingworld. org/readroom/fssafe99.htm), are good resources for the nurse manager. The NDNQI are specifically concerned with patient safety and aspects of quality of care that may be affected by changes in the delivery of care. The 10 quality indicators address staff mix and nursing hours for acute care setting as well as other care components. The NDNQI project is designed to assist healthcare organizations in identifying links between nursing care and patient outcomes.

PROFESSIONALISM

Nurse managers must set examples of professionalism, which include academic preparation, roles and function, and increasing autonomy. The ANA's classic "Nursing's Social Policy Statement" (1995) provides significant ideals for all nurses, specifically autonomy, self-regulation, and accountability. Nurses are guided by a humanistic philosophy that includes the highest regard for self-determination, independence, and choice in decision making, whether for staff or for patients. The policy statement can be used by the nurse manager as a framework for a broader understanding of nursing's connection with society and nursing's accountability to those who

receive nursing care that facilitates "health and healing" in a caring relationship. For example, a nurse manager's professional philosophy should include the patient's rights. These rights have traditionally identified such basic elements as human dignity, integrity, honesty, confidentiality, privacy, and informed consent. Additional basic rights now include self-determination through advance directives (living wills, directives to physicians and family or surrogates, medical power of attorney) and the right to healthcare accessibility.

■ Exercise 3-5

Donna D., a young nurse on a surgical orthopedic unit, has been asked several times during her 12-hour day shift for some medication for pain by one of her patients, Mr. Jones, who had foot surgery 3 days ago. Donna D.'s assessment of Mr. Jones leads her to believe that he is not having that much pain. Although the patient does have an oral medication order for pain, Donna D. independently decides to administer a placebo by subcutaneous injection and documents her medication intervention. Mr. Jones does not receive any relief from this subcutaneous medication. When Donna D. is relieved by the 12-hour night nurse, she gives the nurse a report of her intervention concerning Mr. Jones' pain. The following morning, the night nurse reports Donna D.'s medication intervention to you, the nurse manager. You will have to address Donna's behavior. What will you do? What resources will you use to handle Donna D.'s behavior? How will you demonstrate professionalism?

Professionalism is all-encompassing; the way a manager interacts with personnel, other disciplines, patients, and families reflects a professional philosophy. Professional nurses are ethically and legally accountable for the standards of practice and nursing actions delegated to others. Conveying high standards, holding others accountable, and shaping the future of nursing for a group of healthcare providers are inherent behaviors in the role of a manager.

The **Nursing Licensure Compact** is another aspect of professionalism that is being legislated by an increasing number of states. This legislation allows a nurse to have a single licensure that is recognized by the "compact" states, thus facilitating mobility across states. Although the compact promotes better compliance with rules and regulatory processes of boards of nursing, nurse managers will probably assume additional responsibility to ensure that a nurse practicing in a "compact" state maintains a home state license in only one state at a time and that the nurse meets the requirement for licensure in the designated home state (*RN Update*, October 1999).

The nurse manager is the closest link to the direct care staff. That individual sets the tone, creates the environment, and manages within the context while providing professional role modeling to develop future managers and leaders.

The Solution

Of course, the ideal solution is to hire someone for each position, but I do not see that happening in the near future. We are trying to tap into the Joe Arrington Cancer Treatment and Research Center. The Center has a very large education department, and we are looking into whether we can use them not only for staff education, which they are doing already with the chemotherapy classes, but also for patient teaching. Although the Center works primarily with outpatients, it is also involved in inpatient care. The unit often admits patients who are on research protocols prescribed by the Arrington Center.

The nurses from the Center do get involved with these patients' care and teaching. I think this cooperative educational venture has a lot of possibilities, and it will happen, but it will take some time to determine a realistic plan. We already have addressed this alternative plan in a couple of committees.

— Joyce Burdett

 Would this be a suitable approach for you? Why?

CHAPTER CHECKLIST

The role of the nurse manager is multifaceted and complex. Integrating clinical concerns with management functions, synthesizing leadership abilities with management requirements, and addressing human concerns while maintaining efficiency are the challenges facing a manager. Thus the nurse manager's role is to ensure effective operation of a defined unit of service and to contribute to the overall mission of the organization and quality of care by working through others.

- There are five basic functions of a manager:
  - Establishing and communicating goals and objectives
  - Organizing and analyzing activities and decisions and dividing them into tasks
  - Motivating and communicating with others
  - Analyzing, appraising, and interpreting performance
  - Developing people
- A nurse manger is responsible for the following:
  - Relationships with those above themselves, peers, and staff for whom they are accountable
  - Professionalism
  - Management of resources

TIPS FOR IMPLEMENTING THE ROLE OF NURSE MANAGER

Aspects of the role of the nurse manager include being a leader as well as a follower. To implement the role, the nurse manager must profess to the following:

- Management philosophy that values people
- Commitment to patient-focused quality care outcomes that address customer satisfaction
- Desire to learn healthcare changes and their effect on his or her role and functions

TERMS TO KNOW

case management	organizational culture
followers	quality indicators
leaders	quantum theory
managed care	role
manager	role theory
Nursing Licensure Compact	

REFERENCES

American Nurses Association. (1995). *Nursing's social policy statement* (NP-107).Washington, DC: American Nurses Publishing.

American Nurses Association Board of Directors. (2000, March). *Position statement: Violence against women.* Washington, DC: American Nurses Association.

An open letter to all RNs with a Texas license. (1999, October). *RN Update: A Quarterly Publication of the Board of Nurse Examiners for the State of Texas, 30*(4), 1-3.

Bell, S. K. (2001, Winter). Professional nurse's portfolio. *Nursing Administration Quarterly, 25*(2), 69-73.

Bennis, W. (2000). *Managing people is like herding cats.* Provo, UT: Executive Excellence Publishing.

Blanchard, K., & O'Connor, M. (1997). *Managing by values.* San Francisco: Berrett-Koehler.

Cameron, K. S., & Quinn, R. E. (1994). *PRISM5: Changing organizational culture: A competing values workbook.* Ann Arbor, MI: University of Michigan. Cited in Jones, K. R., & Redman, R. W. (2000, December). Organizational culture and work redesign: Experiences in three organizations. *Journal of Nursing Administration, 30*(12), 604-610.

Chaleff, I. (1995). *The courageous follower: Standing up to and for our leaders.* San Francisco: Berrett-Koehler.

Conway, M. E. (1978). Theoretical approaches to the study of roles. Cited in Hardy, M. E. & Conway, M. E. (1978). *Role theory: Perspectives for health professionals.* New York: Appleton-Century-Crofts.

Covey, S. R. (1989). *The 7 habits of highly effective people.* New York: Simon & Schuster.

Drucker, P. F. (1974). *Management tasks, responsibilities and practices.* New York: Harper & Row.

Gladwell, M. (2001). *The tipping point: How little things can make a big difference.* Boston: Little, Brown.

Hershey, P., & Blanchard, K. H. (1977). *Management of organizational behavior* (3rd ed.). Englewood Cliffs, NJ: Prentice Hall.

Ingersoll, G. L., Cook, J., Fagel, S., Applegate, M., & Frank, B. (1999, May). The effect of patient-focused redesign on midlevel nurse managers' role responsibilities and work environment. *Journal of Nursing Administration, 29*(5), 21-27.

Ingersoll, G. L., Kirsch, J. C., Merk, S. E., & Lightfoot, J. (2000, January). Relationship of organizational culture and readiness for change to employee commitment to the organization. *Journal of Nursing Administration, 30*(1), 11-20.

Jones, K. R., & Redman, R. W. (2000, December). Organizational culture and work design: Experiences in three organizations. *Journal of Nursing Administration, 30*(120), 604-610.

Pew Health Professions Commission. (1995a). *Critical challenges: Revitalizing the health professions for the twenty-first century.* San Francisco: The Commission.

Pew Health Professions Commission. (1995b). *Reforming health care workforce regulation: Policy considerations for the 21st century.* San Francisco: The Commission.

Porter-O'Grady, T. (1999, October). Quantum leadership: New roles for a new age. *Journal of Nursing Administration, 29*(10), 37-42.

Sportsman, S., & Valadez, A. M. (2001). Managed care and the law. Chapter 14. Cited in O'Keefe, M. E. *Nursing practice and the law: Avoiding malpractice and other legal risks.* Philadelphia: F.A. Davis.

Styles, M. M. (1982). *On nursing toward a new endowment.* St. Louis: Mosby.

Sullivan, E. J., & Decker, P. J. (2001). *Effective leadership and management in nursing* (5th ed.). Upper Saddle River, NJ: Prentice Hall.

The National Database of Nursing Quality Indicators (NDNQI) http://nursingworld.org/readroom/fssafe99.htm.

Valadez, A. M., & Sportsman, S. (1999, July/August). Environmental management: Principles from quantum theory. *Journal of Professional Nursing, 15*(4), 209-213.

Vance, C., & Olson, R. K. (1998). *The mentor connection in nursing.* New York: Springer.

Wilson, C. K., & Porter-O'Grady, T. (1999). *Leading the revolution in health care, advancing systems, igniting performance* (2nd ed.). Gaithersburg, MD: Aspen Publishers.

SUGGESTED READINGS

Aiken, L. H., & Patrician, P. A. (2000, May/June). Measuring organizational traits of hospitals: The revised nursing work index. *Nursing Research, 49*(3), 146-153.

Blank, R., & Slipp, S. (1994). *Voices of diversity: Real people talk about problems and solutions in a workplace where everyone is not alike.* New York: AMACON (American Management Association).

Canadian Nurses Association. (1997, March). *Code of ethics for registered nurses.* Ottawa, Ontario K2P 1E2: The Association.

Dunhan-Taylor, J. (2000, May). Nurse executive transformational leadership found in participative organizations. *Journal of Nursing Administration, 30*(5), 241-250.

Greenberg, J., & Baron, R. A. (2000). *Behavior in organizations* (7th ed.). Upper Saddle River, NJ: Prentice Hall.

Hardy, M. E., & Conway, M. E. (1988). *Role theory: Perspectives for health professionals* (2nd ed.). Norwalk, CT: Appleton & Lange.

Krejci, J. W. (1999, March). Changing roles in nursing. *Journal of Nursing Administration, 29*(3), 21-29.

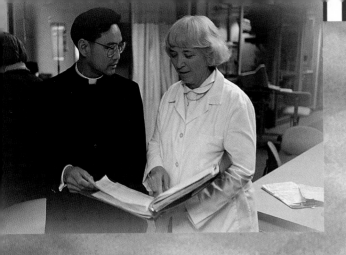

4

Legal and Ethical Issues

Ginny Wacker Guido

This chapter highlights and explains key legal and ethical issues as they pertain to managing and leading. Malpractice, informed consent, types of liability, selected federal and state employment laws, ethical theories, and ethical principles are discussed. This chapter provides specific guidelines for avoiding legal liability and guides the reader in applying ethical decision-making models in everyday clinical practice settings.

Objectives

- Examine nurse practice acts, including the legal difference between licensed registered nurses and licensed practical (vocational) nurses.
- Apply various legal principles, including malpractice, privacy, confidentiality, reporting statutes, and doctrines that minimize one's liability, to leading and managing roles in professional nursing.
- Analyze ethical theories, including deontology, teleology (utilitarianism), and principlism.
- Analyze ethical principles, including autonomy, beneficence, nonmaleficence, veracity, justice, paternalism, fidelity, and respect for others.
- Apply an ethical decision-making model to an ethical dilemma.

- Apply managers' rights and responsibilities from a legal and an ethical perspective to selected examples.
- Examine legal implications of resource availability versus service demand from a manager's perspective.

- Analyze key aspects of employment law and give examples of how these laws benefit professional nursing practice.
- Apply five guidelines that a nurse manager or leader can implement to encourage a professional, satisfying work setting.

Questions to Consider

- *What are the most common potential legal liabilities for nurse managers? How can they be avoided or minimized?*
- *What is the role of the nurse manager in incorporating ethical principles into ongoing relationships with employees?*
- *What federal employment laws affect nurse managers' work settings?*
- *What is the role of the nurse manager in determining which course of action to implement when a legal or ethical dilemma arises?*

The Challenge

Nancy Joyner BA, BSN, RN, CHPH
Case Manager, Altru Home Services Hospice, Grand Forks, North Dakota

One of the most important tenants of the philosophy of hospice is to neither prolong life nor hasten death. An issue that hospice nurses often confront concerns nutritional and hydration support for patients in the terminal stages of their illnesses. Questions that arise include whether the patient should have artificial hydration or nutrition to provide comfort in light of the fact that such additional hydration may cause more distress and an exacerbation of the primary disease state. For example, giving intravenous fluids may cause congestive heart failure or pulmonary edema to develop, thus hastening death.

A recent case example illustrates this concern. An elderly patient had deteriorated to the extent that she was able to use only mouth swabs soaked in water for her primary hydration. Family members were concerned that she was not eating and was not able to swallow fluids; thus the patient was not able to receive the hydration that she needed to sustain life. They equated this lack of hydration with the belief that the patient was starving to

death. Family members approached the hospice nurse to begin intravenous fluids. The hospice nurse spent some time with the family, explaining that the additional fluids would cause congestive heart failure to develop, ultimately hastening death. The congestive heart failure would also add to the patient's discomfort and restlessness. The family members rejected this concept and insisted that the physician be contacted for an order to begin intravenous fluids. The physician supported the family, stating that hospice needs to "treat the family and not the patient," and he ordered a bolus of intravenous fluids. The patient died shortly afterward, leaving the family members relieved that they had done something to assist the patient and the hospice nurse knowing that the primary tenant of hospice had been violated.

 What do you think you would do if you were this nurse?

INTRODUCTION

The role of professional nursing has expanded rapidly within the past few years to include increased expertise, specialization, autonomy, and accountability from both legal and ethical perspectives. This expansion has forced new concerns among nurse managers and leaders and a heightened awareness of the interaction of legal and ethical principles. Areas of concern include professional nursing practice, legal issues, ethical principles, labor-management interactions, and employment. Each of these areas is individually addressed in this chapter.

PROFESSIONAL NURSING PRACTICE

Nurse Practice Acts

The scope of nursing practice, those actions and duties that are allowable by a profession, is defined and guided individually by each state in the nurse practice act and by **common law.** Common law is

"derived from principles rather than rules and regulations and consists of broad and comprehensive principles based on justice, reason, and common sense" (*Bishop v. United States*, 1971, p. 418). Common law principles govern most interactions affecting nursing; they are based on a traditional justice perspective rather than a caring relationship. The state **nurse practice act** is the single most important piece of legislation for nursing because it affects all facets of nursing practice. Furthermore, the act is the law within the state, and state boards of nursing cannot grant exceptions, waive the act's provisions, or expand practice outside the act's specific provisions.

Nurse practice acts and common law define three categories of nurses: licensed practical or vocational nurses (LPNs and LVNs, respectively), licensed registered nurses (RNs), and advanced practice nurses. The acts, along with common law, set educational and examination requirements, provide for licensing by individuals who have met these requirements, and define the functions of each category of nurse, both in general and in specific terminology. The nurse practice act must be read to ascertain what actions are allowable for the three categories of nurses. Some states have separate acts for licensed RNs and LPNs/LVNs. If two acts exist, they must be reviewed at the same time to ensure that all allowable actions are included in one of the two acts and that there is no overlap between the acts. State acts are not consistent in defining or delineating advanced nursing roles.

Each practice act also establishes a state board of nursing. The main purposes of state boards of nursing are twofold. One purpose is to ensure enforcement of the act, serving to regulate those who come under its provisions and prevent those not addressed within the act from practicing nursing. The second purpose is to protect the public, ensuring that those who present themselves as nurses are licensed to practice within the state. The National Council of State Boards of Nursing (NCSBN) serves as a central clearinghouse, further ensuring that individual state actions against a nurse's license are recorded and enforced in all states in which the individual nurse holds licensure.

Because each state has its own nurse practice act and state courts hold jurisdiction on the common law of the state, all nurses are well advised to know and understand the provisions of the state's nurse practice act. This is especially true in the areas of diagnosis and treatment; states vary greatly on whether nurses can diagnose and treat or merely assess and evaluate. An acceptable action in one state may be the practice of medicine in a bordering state.

Thus nurses must know applicable state **law** and use the nurse practice act for guidance and appropriate action. Nurse managers have this same basic responsibility to apply legal principles in their practice. They are also responsible for monitoring the practice of employees under their supervision and for ensuring that personnel maintain current and valid licensure.

Exercise 4–1

Read your state's nurse practice act, which includes rules and regulations that the state board of nursing has promulgated for the profession. You may need to read two acts if RNs and LPNs/LVNs come under different licensing boards. Does your state address advanced practice? How do the definitions of nursing vary for RNs, LPNs/LVNs, and advanced practice nurses? Using these definitions, formulate three lists showing which tasks or assignments you would delegate to each category of nurses, referencing the nurse practice act as needed.

Negligence and Malpractice

Negligence denotes conduct that is lacking in care and typically concerns nonprofessionals. Many experts equate negligence with carelessness, a deviation from the **standard of care** that a reasonable person would deliver. **Malpractice,** sometimes referred to as *professional negligence,* concerns professional actions and is the failure of a person with professional education and skills to act in a reasonable and prudent manner. Issues of malpractice have become increasingly important to the nurse as the authority, accountability, and autonomy of nurses have increased. Usually, six elements must be presented in a successful malpractice suit. All of these factors must be proven before the court will find **liability** against the nurse or institution. Table 4-1 outlines these elements. To understand how the law applies each element of malpractice to specific court cases, the following scenario is offered.

A nurse, employed by a state medical center, has been assigned to care for Mrs. J., a patient admitted for a right hip replacement. Mrs. J. is 69 years old, in relatively good health, and mentally competent. She is scheduled to have surgery tomorrow and requires assistance in ambulating to and from the bathroom. While caring for Mrs. J., a nurse fails to obtain the assistance of a second person when walking Mrs. J. to the bathroom and the patient falls. Mrs. J. sustains a broken left hip and a mild concussion. She will be hospitalized for several additional days because she must undergo bilateral hip replacement and physical therapy. In addition, she will spend 2 days in the neurological step-down unit because of the concussion.

Elements of Malpractice

Duty Owed the Patient

The first element is duty owed the patient, which involves both the existence of the duty and the nature of the duty. That a nurse owes a duty of care to a patient is usually not hard to establish. Often, this is established merely by showing the valid employment of the nurse within the institution. The more difficult part is the nature of the duty, which involves standards of care that represent the minimum requirements for acceptable practice. In the preceding scenario, the applicable standard of care is taken from the institution policy and procedure manual and concerns the standard of care owed a patient regarding safety. Standards of care are established by reviewing the institution's policy and procedure manual, the individual's job description, and the practitioner's education and skills, as well as pertinent standards es-

Table 4-1 ELEMENTS OF MALPRACTICE

Elements	Examples
Duty owed the patient	Failure to monitor a patient's response to treatment
Nature of the duty	Existence of the duty
Breach of the duty owed	Failure to communicate change in patient status to the primary healthcare provider
Foreseeability	Failure to ensure minimum standards are met
Causation	Failure to provide adequate patient education
Injury	Fractured hip and head concussion after a patient fall
Damages	Additional hospitalization time; future medical and nursing care needs and costs

tablished by professional organizations, journal articles, and standing orders and protocols. Several sources may be used to determine the applicable standard of care. The American Nurses Association (ANA), as well as a cadre of specialty organizations, publishes standards for nursing practice.

The overall framework of these standards is the nursing process. In 1988 the ANA first published Standards for Nurse Administrators, a series of nine standards incorporating responsibilities of nurse administrators across all practice settings. Accreditation standards, especially those published yearly by the Joint Commission on Accreditation of Healthcare Organizations (JCAHO), also assist in establishing the acceptable standard of care for healthcare facilities. In addition, many states have healthcare standards that affect individual institutions and their employees.

Breach of the Duty of Care Owed the Patient

The second element required in a malpractice case is proven breach of the duty of care owed the patient. Once the standard of care is established, the breach or falling below the standard of care is easy to show. However, the standard of care may differ depending on whether the injured party is trying to establish the standard of care or whether the hospital's attorney is establishing an acceptable standard of care for the given circumstances. The injured party will attempt to show that the acceptable standard of care is a much higher standard of care than that shown by the defendant hospital and staff. **Expert witnesses** give testimony in court to determine the applicable and acceptable standard of care on a case-by-case basis and to assist the judge and jury in understanding nursing standards of care. In

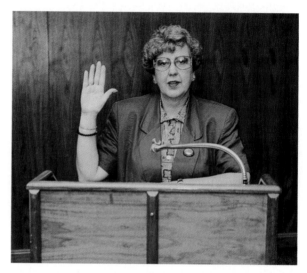

Nurses sometimes serve as expert witnesses whose testimony helps the judge and jury understand the applicable standards of nursing care.

the scenario involving Mrs. J., the injured party's expert witness would quote the institution policy manual, and the nurse's expert witness would note any viable exceptions to the stated policy.

A case example, *Sabol v. Richmond Heights General Hospital* (1996), shows this distinction. A patient was admitted to a general acute care hospital for treatment after attempting to commit suicide by drug overdose. While in the acute care facility, the patient became increasingly paranoid and delusional. A nurse sat with the patient and tried to calm him. Restraints were not applied because the staff feared this would compound the situation by raising his level of paranoia and agitation. The patient got out of bed, knocked down the nurse who was in his room, fought his way past two nurses in the hallway, ran off the unit, and jumped from a third-story window, fracturing his arm and sustaining other relatively minor injuries.

Expert witnesses for the patient introduced standards of care pertinent to psychiatric patients, specifically those hospitalized in psychiatric facilities or in acute care hospitals with separate psychiatric units. The court ruled that the nurses in this general acute care situation were not professionally negligent in this patient's care. The court stated that the nurses' actions were consistent with basic professional standards of practice for medical-surgical nurses in an acute care hospital. They did not have, nor were they expected to have, specialized psychiatric nursing training and would not be judged as if they did.

Foreseeability

The third element needed for a successful malpractice case, **foreseeability,** involves the concept that certain events may reasonably be expected to cause specific results. The nurse must have prior knowledge or information that failure to meet a standard of care may result in harm. The challenge is to show what was foreseeable given the facts of the case at the time of the occurrence, not when the case finally comes to court. In the scenario regarding Mrs. J., it was foreseeable that the patient could fall and harm herself if fewer than two people attempted to assist with ambulation.

Causation

The fourth element of a malpractice suit is causation, which means that the nurse's actions or lack of actions directly caused the patient's harm; the patient did not merely experience some type of harm. There must be a direct relationship between the failure to meet the standard of care and the patient's injury.

Injury

The resultant injury, the fifth malpractice element, must be physical, not merely psychological or transient. In other words, there must be some physical harm incurred by the patient before malpractice will be found against the healthcare provider. In the given scenario, Mrs. J. came to harm as a direct result of ambulating to the bathroom, and she incurred both a broken hip and a concussion.

Damages

Finally, the injured party must be able to prove damages, the sixth element of malpractice. Damages are

vital because malpractice is nonintentional. Thus the patient must show financial harm before the courts will allow a finding of liability against the defendant nurse or hospital. Mrs. J., in the given scenario, would be able to show additional hospital costs related to the second hip replacement surgery, physical therapy needs, and admission to the step-down unit.

A nurse manager must know the applicable standards of care and ensure that all employees of the institution meet or exceed them. The standards must be reviewed periodically to ensure that the staff members remain current and attuned to advances in technology and newer ways of performing tasks. If standards of care appear outdated or absent, the appropriate committee within the institution is notified so that timely revisions can be made. Finally, the nurse manager must ensure that all employees meet the standards of care. This may be done by (1) performing or reviewing all performance evaluations for evidence that standards of care are met, (2) randomly reviewing patient charts for standards of care documentation, and (3) inquiring of employees what constitutes standards of care and appropriate references for standards of care within the institution.

Exercise 4-2

Read a policy and procedure manual at a community nursing service with which you are familiar. Are any policies outdated? Find out who is in charge of revising and writing policies and procedures for the agency. Take an outdated policy and revise it, or think of an issue that you determine should be included in the policy and procedure manual and write such a policy. Does your rewritten or new policy define standards of care? Where would you find criteria for ensuring that your policy and procedures fit a national standard?

LIABILITY: PERSONAL, VICARIOUS, AND CORPORATE

Personal liability defines each person's responsibility and accountability for individual actions or omissions. Even if others can be shown to be **liable** for a patient injury, each individual retains personal accountability for his or her actions. The law sometimes allows other parties to be liable for certain causes of negligence. Known as **vicarious,** or substituted, **liability,** the doctrine of **respondeat superior** (let the master answer) makes employers accountable for the negligence of their employees. The rationale underlying the doctrine is that the employee would not have been in a position to have caused the wrongdoing unless hired by the employer and that the injured party will be allowed to suffer a double wrong merely because most employees are unable to pay damages for their wrongdoings. Nurse managers can best avoid these issues by ensuring that the staff they supervise know and follow hospital policy and procedure and deliver competent nursing care.

Nurses often believe that the doctrine of vicarious liability shields them from personal liability; the institution may be sued, but not the individual nurse or nurses. However, patients injured because of substandard care have the right to sue both the institution and the nurse. In addition, the institution has the right under **indemnification** to sue the nurse for damages paid an injured patient. The principle of indemnification is applicable when the employer is held liable based solely on the actions of the staff member's negligence and the employer pays monetary damages because of the employee's negligent actions.

Corporate liability is a newer trend in the law and essentially holds that the institution has the responsibility and accountability for maintaining an environment that ensures quality healthcare delivery for consumers. Corporate liability issues include negligent hiring and firing issues, failure to maintain safety in the physical environment, and lack of a qualified, competent, and adequate staff. Nurse managers play a key role in assisting the institution to avoid corporate liability. For example, the nurse manager is normally delegated the duty to ensure that staff members remain competent and qualified, that personnel within their supervision have current licensure, and that incompetent, illegal, or unethical practices are reported to the proper persons or agencies.

CAUSES OF MALPRACTICE FOR NURSE MANAGERS

Nurse managers are charged with maintaining a standard of competent nursing care within the institution. Several potential sources of liability for malpractice among nurse managers may be identified; guidelines to prevent or avoid these pitfalls should be developed.

Delegation and Supervision

The field of nursing management involves supervision of various personnel who directly provide nursing care to patients. The nurse manager retains personal liability for the reasonable exercise of delegation and supervision activities. The failure to delegate and supervise within acceptable standards of professional nursing practice may constitute malpractice. In addition, in a newer trend in the law, failure to delegate and supervise within acceptable standards may extend to direct corporate liability for the institution.

However, nurse managers are not liable merely because they have a supervisory function. The degree of knowledge concerning the skills and competencies of those one supervises is of paramount importance. The doctrine of "knew or should have known" is a legal standard in delegating tasks to the individuals one supervises. If it can be shown that the nurse manager delegated tasks appropriately and had no reason to believe that the assigned nurse was not competent to perform the task, then the nurse manager has no personal liability. The converse is also true; if it can be shown that the nurse manager was aware of incompetence in a given employee or that the assigned task was outside the employee's capabilities, the nurse manager does become potentially liable for the subsequent injury to a patient.

Nurse managers have a duty to ensure that the staff members under their supervision are practicing in a competent manner. The nurse manager must be aware of the staff's knowledge, skills, and competencies and should know whether they are maintaining their competencies. Knowingly allowing a staff member to function below the acceptable standard of care subjects both the nurse manager and the institution to potential liability. In *Sparks Regional Medical Center v. Smith* (1998), the Arkansas Court of Appeals upheld an $80,000 civil judgment against a hospital in favor of a female patient who was sexually assaulted by a male nurse. Before the incident in question, the court noted that this nurse had been counseled for sexually explicit conversations with female patients. The nurse was verbally warned but was not restricted from contact with vulnerable patients, nor was any attempt made to monitor his activities more closely. This, said the court, was negligence in supervising an employee.

Some nurse practice acts also legislate fines and discipline for the nurse manager who assigns tasks or patient care loads that make a nursing assignment unsafe. Means of ensuring continuing competency are expected and may include continuing education programs and assignment of a staff member to work with a second staff member to improve technical skills.

Duty to Orient, Educate, and Evaluate

Most healthcare institutions have continuing education departments to orient nurses new to the institution and to supply inservice education addressing new equipment, procedures, and interventions to existing employees. Nurse managers also have a duty to orient, educate, and evaluate. Nurse managers and their representatives are responsible for the daily evaluation of whether nurses are performing competent care. The key to meeting this requirement is reasonableness. Nurse managers should ensure that they promptly respond to all allegations, whether by patients or staff, of incompetent or questionable nursing care. Nurse managers should thoroughly investigate allegations, recommend options for correcting the situation, and follow up on recommended options and suggestions.

In *Bunn-Penn v. Southern Regional Medical Corporation* (1997), a male emergency center technician was accused of sexually assaulting a female patient. Before this incident, nurses had complained to the nurse manager that the male technician seemed too eager to assist female patients and that he stayed too long with female patients while they were undressing. The nurse manager spoke to the technician about these concerns. The nurse manager gave him detailed instructions regarding how he was to conduct himself in the future. She then monitored his activities carefully and noted no further evidence of inappropriate behavior. In finding that there was no liability on the part of the hospital, the court was positive in its praise of the nurse manager, noting that she had fulfilled her duty by counseling and monitoring the employee and in acting promptly when the issues were first presented to her. The court also noted that the nurse manager had monitored this employee for an 18-month period and had filed in his personnel folder favorable periodic reviews.

Failure to Warn

A newer area of potential liability for nurse managers is **failure to warn** potential employers of staff incompetencies or impairment. Information about suspected addictions, violent behavior, and incompetency is of vital importance to subsequent employers. If the institution has sufficient information and suspicion to warrant the discharge of an employee or force a resignation, subsequent employers should be advised of those issues.

One means of supplying this information is through the use of *qualified privilege* to certain communications. In general, qualified privilege concerns communications made in good faith between persons or entities with a need to know. Most states now recognize this privilege and allow previous employers to give factual, objective information to subsequent employers.

Staffing Issues

Three different issues arise under the general term *staffing*. These include maintaining adequate numbers of staff members in a time of advancing patient acuity and limited resources, floating staff from one unit to another, and using temporary or "agency" staff to augment hospital staffing. Each area is addressed separately.

Accreditation standards, specifically those of JCAHO and the Community Health Accreditation Program (CHAP), as well as other state and federal standards, mandate that healthcare institutions provide adequate staffing with qualified personnel. This applies not only to the number of staff but also to the legal status of the staff. For instance, some areas of an institution, such as critical care areas, postanesthesia care areas, and emergency centers, must have greater percentages of RNs than LPNs/LVNs. Other areas, such as the general nursing areas and some long-term-care areas, may have equal or lower percentages of RNs to LPNs/LVNs or nursing assistants. Whether understaffing exists in a given situation depends on the number of patients, care acuity scores, and number and classification of staff. Courts determine whether understaffing existed on an individual case basis.

A leading case concerning understaffing is *Harrell v. Louis Smith Memorial Hospital* (1990). This case concerned the ability of an emergency center staff to adequately diagnose and intervene appropriately with a patient who had experienced a myocardial infarction. The court concluded that the hospital was required to provide staff competent to exercise a reasonable degree of care and skill when delivering healthcare to patients.

California was the first state to adopt legislation that mandates fixed nurse-to-patient ratios (California staffing bill, 1999). Previously, California regulations required set ratios only for critical care units and neonatal intensive care units. The intent was to expand ratios to all areas of acute care organizations.

Although the institution is ultimately accountable for staffing issues, nurse managers may also incur some potential liability because they directly oversee the number of personnel assigned to a unit on a given shift. For nurse manager liability to occur, it must be shown that the resultant injury to a patient was a direct result of the short staffing and not the result of inappropriate or incompetent actions of individual staff members. To prevent nurse manager liability, he or she must show that sufficient numbers of competent staff were available to meet nursing needs.

Exercise 4-3

Judy Jones, RN, has worked in the emergency center for several years. She is currently advanced cardiac life support (ACLS) certified, as are the other emergency care nurses. The hospital policy requires ACLS certification for employment in critical care areas. A new hospital policy expressly forbids the intubation of patients by nurses; only physicians may intubate patients. A crisis occurred in the emergency center one evening and Judy Jones intubated (successfully) a patient in full cardiac arrest. What would you do about this issue?

Guidelines for nurse managers in short-staffing issues include alerting hospital administrators and upper-level managers of concerns. First, however, the nurse manager must do whatever is under his or her control to alleviate the circumstances, such as approving overtime for adequate coverage, reassigning personnel among those areas he or she supervises, and restricting new admissions to the area. Second, nurse managers have a legal duty to notify the chief operating officer, either directly or indirectly, when understaffing endangers patient welfare. One way of notifying the chief operating officer is through formal nursing channels, for example, by notifying the nurse manager's direct supervisor. Upper management must then decide how to alleviate the short staffing, either on a short-term or on a long-term basis. Appropriate measures could be closing a unit or units, restricting elective surgeries, or hiring new staff members. Once the

nurse manager can show that he or she acted appropriately, used sound judgment given the circumstances, and alerted his or her supervisors of the serious nature of the situation, the institution becomes potentially liable for staffing issues.

Floating staff from unit to unit is the second issue that concerns overall staffing. Institutions have a duty to ensure that all areas of the institution are staffed adequately. Thus units temporarily overstaffed because of low patient census or a lower patient acuity ratio usually float staff to units less well staffed. Although floating nurses to areas with which they have less familiarity and expertise can increase potential liability for the nurse manager, leaving another area understaffed can also increase potential liability.

Before floating staff from one area to another, the nurse manager should consider staff expertise, patient care delivery systems, and patient care requirements. Nurses should be floated to units as comparable to their own unit as possible. This requires the nurse manager to match the nurse's home unit and float unit as much as is possible or to consider negotiating with another nurse manager to cross-float a nurse. For example, a manager might float a critical care nurse to an intermediate care unit and float an intermediate care unit nurse to a general unit. Or the manager might consider floating the general unit nurse to the postpartum unit and floating a postpartum nurse to labor and delivery. Open communications regarding staff limitations and concerns, as well as creative solutions for staffing, can alleviate some of the potential liability involved and create better morale among the floating nurses. A positive option is to cross-train nurses within the institution so that nurses are familiar with two or three areas and can competently float to areas in which they have been cross-trained.

One legal case shows that employees also have some responsibility in the area of cross-training. In *David W. Francis v. Memorial General Hospital* (1986), an intensive care nurse refused to float to an orthopedic unit because he felt that he was unqualified to act as a charge nurse on that unit. The hospital offered to orient him, but he declined and was subsequently terminated. The court sided with the employer, noting that the employee's unwillingness to be oriented or to even try working with hospital administration undermined his case.

The use of temporary or "agency" personnel has created increased liability concerns among nurse managers. Until recently, most jurisdictions held that such personnel were considered **independent contractors** and thus the institution was not liable for their actions, although their primary employment agency did retain potential liability. Today, courts have begun to hold the institution liable under the principle of **apparent agency.** *Apparent authority* or *apparent agency* refers to the doctrine whereby a principal becomes accountable for the actions of his or her agent. Apparent agency is created when a person (agent) holds himself or herself out as acting in behalf of the principal; in the instance of the agency nurse, the patient is unable to ascertain whether the nurse works directly for the hospital (has a valid employment contract) or is working for a different employer. At law, lack of actual authority is no defense. This principle applies when it can be shown that a reasonable patient believed that the healthcare worker was an employee of the institution. If it appears to the reasonable patient that this worker is an employee of the institution, the law will consider the worker an employee for the purposes of corporate and vicarious liability.

One case, however, seems to uphold the idea that temporary nurses are independent contractors in cases of liability. In *Hansen v. Caring Professionals, Inc.* (1997), the Appellate Court in Illinois held that a temporary nurse was an independent contractor and not an employee of the temporary nursing agency. The court cited the nurse's filing of a Form 1099 (rather than a W-2 form), the payment of her own employment taxes, and the payment of her own workers' compensation coverage as proof of her independent employment status. However, the hospital did have potential liability because it controlled which patients would be assigned to the agency nurse and directly supervised the agency nurse's clinical performance. Classification may be unimportant; what is important is that the hospital, and thus the nurse manager, may be sued for incompetent care when an agency nurse gives less than competent nursing care.

These trends in the law make it imperative that the nurse manager consider the temporary worker's skills, competencies, and knowledge when delegating tasks and supervising the worker's actions. If there is reason to suspect that the temporary worker is incompetent, the nurse manager must convey this fact to the agency. The nurse manager must also either send the temporary worker home or reassign the worker to other duties and areas. The same screening procedures should be performed with temporary workers as are used with new institution employees.

Additional areas that nurse managers should stress when using agency or temporary personnel include ensuring that the temporary staff member is given a brief but thorough orientation to institution policies and procedures, is made aware of resource materials within the institution, and is made aware of documentation procedures. It is also advisable for nurse managers to assign a resource person to the temporary staff member. This resource person serves in the role of mentor for the agency nurse and serves to prevent potential problems that could arise merely because the agency staff member does not know the institution routine or is unaware of where to turn for assistance. This resource person also serves as a mentor for critical decision making for the agency nurse.

PROTECTIVE AND REPORTING LAWS

Protective and reporting laws ensure the safety or rights of specific classes of individuals. Most states have reporting laws for suspected child and older adult abuse and laws for reporting certain categories of diseases and injuries. Examples of reporting laws include reporting cases of sexually transmitted diseases, abuse of residents in nursing and convalescent homes, and suspected child abuse. Nurse managers are often the individuals who are responsible for ensuring that the correct information is reported to the correct agencies, thus avoiding potential liability against the institution.

Many states now also have mandatory reporting of incompetent practice, especially through nurse practice acts, medical practice acts, and the National Practitioner Data Bank. In addition, the National Council of State Boards of Nursing has developed an Electronic License Verification System (ELVIS) that monitors nurses' licensure status in all states and U.S. territories for discipline issues, competency ratings, and renewals. Reporting of incompetent practice often is restricted to issues of chemical abuse, and special provisions prevail if the affected nurse voluntarily undergoes drug diversion or chemical dependency rehabilitation. Mandatory reporting of incompetent practitioners is a complex process, involving both legal and ethical concerns. Nurse managers must know what the law requires, when reporting is mandated, to whom the report must be sent, and what the individual institution expects of its nurse managers. When in doubt, the nurse manager should seek clarification from the state board of nursing and hospital administration.

INFORMED CONSENT

Informed consent is the authorization by the patient or the patient's legal representative to do something to the patient; it is based on legal capacity, voluntary action, and comprehension. Legal capacity is usually the first requirement and is determined by age and competency. All states have a legal age for adult status defined by **statute.** Competency involves the ability to understand the consequences of actions or the ability to handle personal affairs. State statutes mandate who can serve as the representative for a minor or incompetent adult. The following types of minors may be able to give valid informed consent: **emancipated minors,** minors seeking treatment for substance abuse or communicable diseases, and pregnant minors. Voluntary action, the second requirement, means that the patient was not coerced by fraud, duress, or deceit into allowing the procedure or treatment.

Comprehension is the third requirement and the most difficult to ascertain. The law states that the patient must be given sufficient information, in terms he or she can reasonably be expected to comprehend, to make an informed choice. Information that must be included appears in Box 4-1.

Inherent in the doctrine of informed consent is the right of the patient to informed refusal. Patients must clearly understand the possible consequences of their refusal. In recent years, most states have enacted statutes to ensure that the competent adult has the right to refuse care and that the healthcare provider is protected should the adult validly refuse care.

Issues of informed consent among nurses often concern the actual signing of the informed consent document, not the teaching and information that make up informed consent. Many nurses serve as witnesses to the signing of the informed consent document and are attesting only to the voluntary nature of the patient's signature. There is no duty on the part of the nurse to insist that the patient repeat what has been said or what he or she remembers. Should the patient ask questions that alert the nurse to the inadequacy of true comprehension on the patient's part or express uncertainty while signing the document, the nurse has an obligation to inform the primary healthcare provider and appropriate persons that informed consent has not been obtained.

Exercise 4–4

A patient is admitted to your surgical center for minor surgery: a breast biopsy under local anesthesia. The surgeon has previously informed the patient of the surgery risks, options, desired outcomes, and possible complications. You give the surgery permit form to the patient for her signature. She readily states that she knows about the surgery and has no additional questions. She signs the form with no hesitation. Her husband, who is visiting with her, states he is worried because she will be awake during the procedure and he is afraid that something may be said to alarm her. What do you do at this point? Do you alert the surgeon that informed consent has not been obtained? Do you request that the surgeon revisit the patient and reinstruct her about the surgery? Or do you not need to do anything more once the patient has signed the form?

BOX 4-1

Information Required for Informed Consent

- An explanation of the treatment/procedure to be performed and the expected results of the treatment/procedure
- Description of the risks involved
- Benefits that are likely to result because of the treatment/procedure
- Options to this course of action, including absence of treatment
- Name of the person(s) performing the treatment/procedure
- Statement that the patient may withdraw his/her consent at any time

PRIVACY AND CONFIDENTIALITY

Privacy is the patient's right to protection against unreasonable and unwarranted interference with the patient's solitude. This right extends to protection of personality as well as protection of one's right to be left alone. Within a medical context, the law recognizes the patient's right to protection against (1) appropriation of the patient's name or picture for the institution's sole advantage, (2) intrusion by the institution on the patient's seclusion or affairs, (3) publication of facts that place the patient in a false light, and (4) public disclosure of private facts about the patient by the hospital or staff. **Confidentiality** is the right to privacy of the medical record.

Institutions can reduce potential liability in this area by allowing access to patient data, either written or oral, only to those with a "need to know." Persons with a need to know include physicians and nurses caring for the patient, technicians, unit clerks, therapists, social service workers, and patient advocates. Usually, this need to know extends to the house staff and consultants. Others wishing to access patient data must first ask the patient for permission to review a record. Administration of the institution can access the patient record for statistical analysis, staffing, and quality-of-care review.

The nurse manager is cautioned to ensure that staff members both understand and abide by rules regarding patient privacy and confidentiality. "Interesting" patients should not be discussed with others, and all information concerning patients should be given only in private and secluded areas. All nurses may need to review the current means of giving reports to oncoming shifts and policies about telephone information. Many institutions have now added to the nursing care plan a place to list persons to whom the patient has allowed information to be given. If the caller identifies himself or herself as one of those listed persons, the nurse can give patient information without violating the patient's privacy rights. Patients are becoming more knowledgeable about their rights in these areas, and some have been willing to take offending staff members to court over such issues.

The patient's right of access to his or her medical record is another confidentiality issue. Although the patient has a right of access, individual states mandate when this right applies. Most states give the right of access only after the medical record is completed; thus the patient has the right to review the record after discharge. Some states do give the right of access while the patient is hospitalized, so individual state law governs individual nurses' actions. When supervising a patient's review of his or her record, the nurse manager or representative should explain only the entries that the patient questions or about which the patient requests further clarification. The nurse makes a note in the record after the session indicating that the patient has viewed the record and what questions were answered.

Patients also have a right to copies of the record, at their expense. The medical record belongs to the institution as a business record, and patients never have the right to retain the original record. This is also true in instances in which a subpoena is obtained to secure an individual's medical record for court purposes. A hospital representative will verify that the copy is a "true and valid" copy of the original record.

An issue that is closely related to the medical record is that of incident reports or unusual occurrence reports. These reports are mandated by JCAHO and serve to alert the institution to risk management and quality assurance issues within the setting. As such, incident reports are considered internal documents and thus not discoverable (open for review) by the injured party or attorneys representing the injured party. In most jurisdictions where this question has arisen, however, the courts have held that the incident report was discoverable and thus open to review by both sides of the suit.

It is therefore prudent for nurse managers to complete and to have staff members complete incident reports as though they will be open records. It is advisable to omit any language of guilt, such as, "The patient would not have fallen if Jane Jones, RN, had ensured the side rails were in their up and locked position." This document should contain only pertinent observations and all care given the patient, such as x-ray films that were obtained for a potential broken bone, medication that was given, and consultants who were called to examine the patient. It is also advisable not to note the occurrence of the incident report in the official record because that incorporates the incident report "by reference," and there is no way to keep the report from being seen by the injured party or attorneys for the injured party.

POLICIES AND PROCEDURES

Risk management is a process that identifies, analyzes, and treats potential hazards within a given setting. The object of risk management is to identify potential hazards and eliminate them before anyone is harmed or disabled. Risk management activities include writing policies and procedures. Written policies and procedures are a requirement of JCAHO. These documents set standards of care for the institution and direct practice. They must be clearly stated, well delineated, and based on current practice. Nurse managers should review the policies and procedures frequently for compliance and timeliness. If policies are absent or outdated, the nurse manager must request the appropriate person or committee to either initiate or update the policy.

■ *Exercise 4-5*

You are assigned some risk management activities in the nursing facility where you work. In investigating incident reports that were filed by your staff, you discover that this is the third patient this week who has fallen while attempting to get out of bed and sit in a chair. How would you handle this issue? Decide how you would start a more complete investigation of this issue. For example, is it a facilitywide issue or one that is confined to one unit? Does it affect all shifts or only one? What safety issues are you going to discuss with your staff, and how are you going to discuss these issues? Do these falls involve the same staff member? Design a unit inservice class for the staff concerning incident reports and patient safety.

EMPLOYMENT LAWS

The federal and individual state governments have enacted laws regulating employment. To be effective and legally correct, nurse managers must be familiar with these laws and how individual laws af-

fect the institution and labor relations. Many nurse managers have come to fear the legal system because of personal experience or the experiences of colleagues, but much of this concern may be directly attributable to uncertainty with the law or partial knowledge of the law. By understanding and correctly following federal employment laws, nurse managers may actually decrease their potential liability by complying with both federal and state laws. Table 4-2 gives an overview of key federal employment laws.

Equal Employment Opportunity Laws

Several federal laws have been enacted to expand equal employment opportunities by prohibiting discrimination based on gender, age, race, religion, handicap, pregnancy, and national origin. These laws are enforced by the Equal Employment Opportunity Commission (EEOC). All states have also enacted statutes that address employment opportunities, and the nurse manager should consider both when hiring and assigning nursing employees.

The most significant legislation affecting equal employment opportunities today is the amended 1964 Civil Rights Act (1978). Section 703 (a) of Title VII makes it illegal for an employer "to refuse

Table 4-2 SELECTED FEDERAL LABOR LEGISLATION

Year	Legislation	Primary Purpose of the Legislation
1935	Wagner Act; National Labor Act	Unions, National Labor Relations Board established
1947	Taft-Hartley Act	Equal balance of power between unions and management
1948	1962 Executive Order 10988	Public employees could join unions
1963	Equal Pay Act	Became illegal to pay lower wages based on gender
1964	Civil Rights Act	Protected against discrimination based on race, color, creed, national origin, etc.
1967	Age Discrimination	Act Protected against discrimination based on age
1970	Occupational Safety and Health Act	Ensured healthy and safe working conditions
1974	Wagner Amendments	Allowed nonprofit organizations to unionize
1990	Americans with Disabilities Act	Barred discrimination against workers with disabilities
1991	Civil Rights Act	Addressed sexual harassment in the workplace
1993	Family and Medical Leave Act	Allowed work leaves based on family and medical needs
1999	Ergonomics Program Standard	Addressed the issue of work-related musculoskeletal Disorders
2000	Ergonomics Program Standard Repealed	

Modified from Marquis, B. S., & Huston, C. J. (2000). *Leadership roles and management functions in nursing* (3rd ed.). Philadelphia: Lippincott.

to hire, discharge an individual, or otherwise to discriminate against an individual, with respect to his compensation, terms, conditions, or privileges of employment because of the individual's race, color, religion, sex, or national origin." Title VII was also amended by the Equal Opportunities Act of 1972, so it applies to private institutions with 15 or more employees, state and local governments, **labor unions,** and employment agencies.

The Civil Rights Act was signed into law in 1991. This act further broadened the issue of sexual harassment in the workplace and supersedes many of the sections of Title VII. Sections of the new legislation define sexual harassment, its elements, and the employer's responsibilities regarding harassment in the workplace, especially prevention and corrective action. The Civil Rights Act is enforced by the EEOC created in the 1964 act; its powers were broadened in the 1972 Equal Employment Opportunity Act. The primary activity of the EEOC is processing complaints of employment discrimination. There are three phases: investigation, conciliation, and litigation. Investigation focuses on determining whether provisions of Title VII have been violated by the employer. If the EEOC finds "probable cause," an attempt is made to reach an agreement or conciliation between the EEOC, the complainant, and the employer. If conciliation fails, the EEOC may file suit against the employer in federal court or issue to the complainant the right to sue for discrimination under its auspices, including those relating to staffing practices and sexual harassment in the workplace. The EEOC defines sexual harassment broadly, and this has generally been upheld in the courts. Nurse managers must realize that it is the duty of employers (management) to prevent employees from sexually harassing other employees. The EEOC issues policies and practices for employers to implement both to sensitize employees to this problem and to prevent its occurrence; nurse managers should be aware of these policies and practices and seek guidance in implementing them if sexual harassment occurs in their units.

Employers may seek exceptions to Title VII on a number of premises. For example, employment decisions made on the basis of national origin, religion, and gender (never race or color) are lawful if such decisions are necessary for the normal operation of the business, although the courts have viewed this exception very narrowly. Promotions and layoffs based on bona fide seniority or merit systems are permissible (*Herrero v. St. Louis*

University Hospital, 1997), as are exceptions based on business necessity.

Age Discrimination in Employment Act of 1967

The Age Discrimination in Employment Act of 1967 made discrimination against older men and women by employers, unions, and employment agencies illegal. A 1986 amendment to the law prohibits discrimination against persons older than 40 years. The practical outcome of this act has been that mandatory retirement is no longer allowed in the American workplace.

As with Title VII, there are some exceptions to this act. Reasonable factors other than age may be used when terminations become necessary; such reasonable factors may include a performance evaluation system or certain limited occupational qualifications, for example, the tedious physical demands of a specific job.

Americans With Disabilities Act of 1990

The Americans with Disabilities Act (ADA) of 1990 provides protection to persons with disabilities and is the most significant civil rights legislation since the Civil Rights Act of 1964. The purpose of the ADA is to provide a clear and comprehensive national mandate for the elimination of discrimination against individuals with disabilities and to provide clear, strong, consistent, enforceable standards addressing discrimination in the workplace. The ADA is closely related to the Civil Rights Act and incorporates the antidiscrimination principles established in Section 504 of the Rehabilitation Act of 1973.

The act has five titles; Table 4-3 shows the pertinent issues of each title. The ADA has jurisdiction over employers, private and public; employment agencies; labor organizations; and joint labor-management committees. It defines disability broadly. With respect to an individual, a disability is (1) a physical or mental impairment that substantially limits one or more of the major life activities of such individual, (2) a record of such impairment, or (3) being regarded as having such an impairment (Americans with Disabilities Act, 1990). The overall effect of the legislation is that persons with disabilities will not be excluded from job opportunities or adversely affected in any aspect of employment unless they are not qualified or are otherwise unable to perform the job. The ADA thus protects qualified individuals with disabilities in regard to job application proce-

Table 4-3	AMERICANS WITH DISABILITIES ACT OF 1990
Title	**Provisions**
I	Employment: defines the purpose of the act and who is qualified under the act as having a disability
II	Public services: concerns services, programs, and activities of public entities as well as public transportation
III	Public accommodations and services operated by private entities: prohibits discrimination against persons with disabilities in areas of public accommodations, commercial facilities, and public transportation services
IV	Telecommunications: intended to make telephone services accessible to individuals with hearing or speech impairments
V	Miscellaneous provisions: certain insurance matters; incorporation of this act with other federal and state laws

From Americans with Disabilities Act (1990).

dures, hiring, compensation, advancement, and all other employment matters.

The number of lawsuits filed under the ADA since its enactment has been extensive. Recent cases have assisted in defining disability eligibility. The following findings have been decided in court regarding disabilities: (1) A nurse with a lifting disability is not qualified for protection under the ADA (*Thompson v. Holy Family Hospital*, 1997), (2) erratic behavior does not give notice to the employer that the individual has a mental impairment (*Webb v. Mercy Hospital*, 1996), (3) depression and anxiety are not disabling conditions (*Cody v. Cigna Healthcare of St. Louis, Inc.*, 1998), (4) a nurse taking medications for depression is not disabled (*Wilking v. County of Ramsey*, 1997), (5) migraine headaches and latex allergies are not disabilities (*Howard v. North Mississippi Medical Center*, 1996), and (6) pregnancy is not a disability (*Jessie v. Carter Health Care Center, Inc.*, 1996).

The ADA requires an employer or potential employer to make reasonable accommodations to employ persons with a disability. The law does not mandate that individuals with disabilities be hired before fully qualified persons who do not have a disability; it does mandate that those with disabilities not be disqualified merely because of an easily accommodated disability.

This last point was well illustrated by the court in *Zamudio v. Patia* (1997). The court stated that the employer would be required to inform Ms. Zamudio when a position became available for which the rea-

sonable accommodation she required could be met. She would be allowed to apply, but "as a disabled employee seeking reasonable accommodation she did not have to be given preference over other employees without disabilities who might have better qualifications or more seniority" (p. 808).

Moreover, the court will not impose job restructuring on an employer if the person needing accommodation qualifies for other jobs not requiring such accommodation. In *Mauro v. Borgess Medical Center* (1995), the court refused to impose accommodation on the employer hospital merely because the affected employee desired to stay within a certain unit of the institution. In this case, an operating surgical technician who tested positive for human immunodeficiency virus (HIV) was offered an equivalent position by the hospital in an area where there would be no patient contact. He refused the transfer, desiring accommodation within the operating arena, and was denied such accommodation by the Michigan court.

The act also provides for essential job functions. These are defined by the ADA as those functions that the person must be able to perform to be qualified for employment positions. Courts have assisted in determining these essential job functions. For example, in *Jones v. Kerrville State Hospital* (1998), the court found that an essential job function for a psychiatric nurse is the ability to restrain patients. In *Laurin v. Providence Hospital and Massachusetts Nurses Association* (1998), the ability to work rotating shifts was held to be an essential job function.

The act also specifically excludes the following from the definition of *disability:* homosexuality and bisexuality, sexual behavioral disorders, gambling addiction, kleptomania, pyromania, and current use of illegal drugs (Americans with Disabilities Act, 1990). Moreover, employers may hold alcoholic persons to the same job qualifications and job performance standards as other employees, even if the unsatisfactory behavior or performance is related to the alcoholism (Americans with Disabilities Act, 1990). As with other federal employment laws, the nurse manager should have a thorough understanding of the law as it applies to the institution and his or her specific job description and should know whom to contact within the institution structure for clarification as needed.

Affirmative Action

The policy of affirmative action (AA) differs from the policy of equal employment opportunity (EEO). AA policy enhances employment opportunities of protected groups of people; EEO policy is concerned with implementing employment practices that do not discriminate against or impair the employment opportunities of protected groups. Thus AA can be seen in conjunction with several federal employment laws; for example, in conjunction with the Vietnam Era Veterans' Re-adjustment Act of 1974, AA requires that employers with government contracts take steps to enhance the employment opportunities of veterans with disabilities and other veterans of the Vietnam era.

Equal Pay Act of 1963

The Equal Pay Act makes it illegal to pay lower wages to employees of one gender when the jobs (1) require equal skill in experience, training, education, and ability; (2) require equal effort in mental or physical exertion; (3) are of equal responsibility and accountability; and (4) are performed under similar working conditions. Courts have held that unequal pay may be legal if it is based on seniority, merit, incentive systems, or a factor other than gender. The main cases filed under this law in the area of nursing have been by nonprofessionals.

Occupational Safety and Health Act

The Occupational Safety and Health Administration (OSHA) Act of 1970 was enacted to ensure that healthful and safe working conditions would exist in the workplace. Among other provisions, the law requires isolation procedures, placarding areas containing ionizing radiation, proper grounding of electrical equipment, protective storage of flammable and combustible liquids, and the gloving of all personnel when handling bodily fluids. The statute provides that if no federal standard has been established, state statutes prevail. Nurse managers should know the relevant OSHA laws for the institution and his or her specific area. Frequent review of new additions to the law must also be undertaken, especially in this era of acquired immunodeficiency syndrome (AIDS) and infectious diseases, and care must be taken to ensure that necessary gloves and equipment, as specified, are available on each unit.

A newer area in the OSHA standards, the Ergonomics Program Standard, was issued on November 14, 2000, and took effect on January 16, 2001. This standard was created to address the issue of work-related musculoskeletal disorders (MSDs) that result when there is a physical mismatch between the physical capacity of the worker and the physical demands of the workplace. Approximately 1.8 million workers in the United States report work-related MSDs, including carpal tunnel syndrome, tendinitis, and back injuries; 600,000 workers report loss of time from work for these work-related injuries (U.S. Department of Labor, 2001). **Ergonomics,** the science of fitting the job to the worker, is seen as one solution to this issue.

The standard requires that the employer provide the following basic information to all employees: (1) common MSDs and their signs and symptoms, (2) the importance of reporting MSDs as soon as possible, (3) how to report MSDs in the workplace, (4) risk factors and job and work activities associated with MSD hazards, and (5) a brief description of OSHA's ergonomics standard. The six elements of the complete ergonomics program include (1) management leadership and employee training, (2) hazard information and reporting, (3) job hazard analysis and control, (4) employee training, (5) MSD management, and (6) program evaluation. The first two elements are required for all jobs that carry a potential risk for MSDs, even if no MSD has been reported, and had to be fully implemented by October 14, 2001 (OSHA Regulations, 1999).

Projected to cost employers $4.5 billion annually, the standard was repealed by the U.S. Senate and House of Representatives on March 6 and 7,

2001. President George W. Bush signed the joint resolution of Congress on March 20, 2001, stating that "Joint Resolution 6 . . . repeals an unduly burdensome and over broad regulation dealing with ergonomics. . . . There needs to be a balance between and an understanding of the costs and benefits associated with Federal regulations. In this instance, though, in exchange for uncertain benefits, the ergonomics rule would have cost both large and small employers billions of dollars and presented employers with overwhelming compliance challenges." He further pledged to "pursue a comprehensive approach to ergonomics that addresses the concerns surrounding the ergonomics rule repealed today" (Bush, 2001, paragraphs 2 and 3).

Family and Medical Leave Act of 1993

The Family and Medical Leave Act of 1993 was passed because of the large numbers of single-parent and two-parent households in which the single parent or both parents are employed full-time, placing job security and parenting at odds. The law also supports the growing demands that aging parents are placing on their working children. The act attempts to balance the demands of the workplace with the demands of the family, allowing employed individuals to take leaves for medical reasons, including the birth or adoption of children and the care of a spouse, child, or parent who has serious health problems.

Essentially, the act provides job security for unpaid leave while the employee is caring for a new infant or other family healthcare needs. The act is gender-neutral and allows both men and women the same leave provisions.

To be eligible under the act, the employee must have worked for at least 12 months and worked at least 1250 hours during the preceding 12-month period. The employee may take up to 12 weeks of unpaid leave. The act allows the employer to require the employee to use all or part of any paid vacation, personal leave, or sick leave as part of the 12-week family leave. Employees must give the employer 30 days notice, or such notice as is practical in emergency cases, before using the medical leave.

Employment-at-Will and Wrongful Discharge

Historically, the employment relationship has been considered a "free will" relationship. Employees were free to take or not take a job at will, and employers were free to hire, retain, or discharge employees for any reason. Many laws, some federal but predominantly state, have been slowly eroding this at-will employment relationship. Evolving case law provides at least three exceptions to the broad doctrine of employment-at-will.

The first exception is a public policy exception. This exception involves cases in which an employee is discharged in direct conflict with established public policy (Pozgar, 1999). Some examples include discharging an employee for serving on a jury, reporting employers' illegal actions (better known as "whistleblowing"), and filing a workers' compensation claim.

Several recent court cases attest to the number of terminations in healthcare settings that serve as retaliation for the employer. More commonly known as "whistleblowing" cases, the healthcare provider in these cases is terminated for one of three distinct reasons: (1) speaking out against unsafe practices, (2) reporting violations of federal laws, or (3) filing lawsuits against employers. In *Roulston v. Tendercare (Michigan), Inc.* (2000), a social services director was dismissed after she confronted the director of nursing for what the social services director termed *patient abuse*. The social services director had reported instances of patient abuse to the state Department of Consumer and Industry Services and the Health Care Fraud Unit of the state attorney general's office. The nursing director first attempted to debate the definition of patient abuse, then told the social services director that she had better start thinking like everyone else who worked at the nursing home. The court was satisfied that the social services director's lawsuit against the nursing home for retaliation was appropriate.

In *Fleming v. Correctional Healthcare Solutions, Inc.* (2000), a nurse in a correctional facility was dismissed for reporting financial mismanagement. The nurse was terminated for insubordination, and she sued her former employer for retaliation under the New Jersey whistleblower act. The court upheld her right to sue for wrongful dismissal. Similarly, the court in *UTMB v. Hohman* (1999) allowed a nurse to bring suit for wrongful dismissal when she was discharged for reporting a physician's alleged abuses.

The court in *Taylor v. Memorial Health Systems, Inc.* (2000) enumerated the conditions that must be present to file a valid employer retaliation lawsuit. (1) The whistleblower must disclose or threaten to disclose an allegation in writing and under oath to the state department of professional regulation. (2) The allegation must have been about an activity, policy, or practice of the employer that is or was a violation of a state or federal law, rule, or regulation. (3) The employee must have given the employer written notification and reasonable time to correct the problem. (4) The employee must have suffered retaliation in the form of some actual harm (*Taylor v. Memorial Health Systems, Inc.*, 2000, p. 755). Although states may vary slightly on these elements, this court essentially outlines the elements to consider when contemplating a whistleblower lawsuit.

The second exception to wrongful discharge involves situations in which there is an implied contract. The courts have generally treated employee handbooks, company policies, and oral statements made at the time of employment as "framing the employment relationship" (*Watkins v. Unemployment Compensation Board of Review*, 1997). For example, in *Trombley v. Southwestern Vermont Medical Center* (1999), the court found that the employee handbook outlined the procedure for progressive discipline, mandating that such procedure be followed before a nurse could be terminated for incompetent nursing care.

The third exception to wrongful discharge is a "good faith and fair dealing" exception. The purpose of this exception is to prevent unfair or malicious terminations, and the exception is used sparingly by the courts. An older case illustrates its use. In *Fortune v. National Cash Register Company* (1977), an employee was discharged just before a final contract was signed between his employer and another company for which the employee would have received a large commission. The court held that he was discharged in bad faith, solely to prevent payment of his commission by National Cash Register.

Nurse managers are urged to know their respective state laws concerning this growing area of the law. Managers should review institution documents, especially employee handbooks and recruiting brochures, for unwanted statements implying job security or other unintentional promises. Managers are also cautioned not to say anything during the preemployment negotiations and interviews that might be construed as implying job security or other unintentional promises to the potential employee. To prevent successful suits for retaliation by whistleblowers, nurse managers should carefully monitor the treatment of an employee after a complaint is filed and ensure that performance evaluations are performed and placed in the appropriate files. The nurse manager should also take steps to correct the whistleblower's complaint or refer the complaint to upper management so that it can effectively be addressed.

Exercise 4-6

Mary Sanchez is the nurse manager for a busy home health-care agency. She overhears staff members discussing the quality of nursing care that they are forced to deliver to patients because of the number of patients served by the home healthcare agency and limited number of staff. The nurses are especially critical of the number of vacancies for RNs. She fears that the staff may file a formal complaint with the state. What should she do to prevent the filing of such a complaint? If a complaint is filed, what advice would you give Mary Sanchez?

Collective Bargaining

Collective bargaining, also called *labor relations*, is the joining together of employees for the purpose of increasing their ability to influence the employer and improve working conditions. Usually, the employer is referred to as management and the employees, even professionals, are labor. Those persons involved in the hiring, firing, scheduling, disciplining, or evaluating of employees are considered management and may not be included in a collective bargaining unit. Those in management could form their own group but are not protected under these laws. Nurse managers may or may not be part of management; if they have hiring and firing authority, they are part of management.

Collective bargaining is defined and protected by the National Labor Relations Act and its amendments; the National Labor Relations Board (NLRB) oversees the act and those who come under its auspices. The NLRB ensures that employees are able to choose freely whether they want to be represented by a particular bargaining unit, and it serves to prevent or remedy any violation of the labor laws. Chapter 10 provides a further analysis of this concept.

PROFESSIONAL NURSING PRACTICE: ETHICS

Ethics Theories

Ethics is a science relating to moral actions and one's value system. Many nurses envision ethics as dealing with principles of morality and thus what is right or wrong. A broader conceptual definition of ethics is that ethics is concerned with motives and attitudes and the relationship of these attitudes to the good of the individual. "Ethics has to do with actions we wish people would take, not actions they must take" (Hall, 1990, p. 37). Thus **values** are interwoven with ethics; values are personal beliefs about the truth and worth of thoughts, objects, and behavior.

Ethics may be distinguished from the law because ethics is internal to an individual, looks to the good of an individual rather than society as a whole, and concerns the "why" of one's actions. The law, comprising rules and regulations pertinent to society as a whole, is external to oneself and concerns one's actions and conduct. The difference is thus between what the person did or failed to do and why the person acted how he or she did. Ethics concerns the good of an individual within society, whereas law concerns society as a whole. Law can be enforced through the courts and statutes, whereas ethics are enforced via **ethics committees** and professional codes.

Today, ethics and legal issues often become entwined, and it is difficult to separate ethics from legal concerns. Legal principles and doctrines assist the nurse manager in decision making, and ethical theories and principles are often involved in those decisions. Thus the nurse manager must be cognizant of both areas in everyday management concerns.

Many different ethical theories have evolved to justify existing moral principles; these theories are considered normative because they are universally applicable theories of right and wrong. Most normative approaches to ethics fall under the three broad categories of deontological theories, teleological theories, and principlism.

Deontological (from the Greek *deon*, or "duty") **theories** derive norms and rules from the duties human beings owe to one another by virtue of commitments made and roles assumed. Generally, deontologists hold that a sense of duty consists of rational respect for the fulfilling of one's obligations to other human beings. The greatest strength of this theory is its emphasis on the dignity of human beings. Deontological theory looks not to the end or consequences of an action, but to the intention of the action. It is one's good intentions, the intentions to do a moral duty, that ultimately determine the praiseworthiness of the action. Deontological ethics have sometimes been subdivided into situation

ethics, wherein the decision making takes into account the unique characteristics of each individual, the caring relationship between the person and the caregiver, and the most humanistic course of action given the circumstances.

Teleological (from the Greek *telos*, for "end") **theories** derive norms or rules for conduct from the consequences of actions. "Right" consists of actions that have good consequences, and "wrong" consists of actions that have bad consequences. Teleologists disagree, however, about how to determine the goodness or badness of the consequences of actions. This theory is often referred to as *utilitarianism;* what makes an action right or wrong is its utility, and useful actions bring the greatest amount of good into existence. An alternative way of viewing this theory is that the usefulness of an action is determined by the amount of happiness it brings. Utilitarian ethics can then be subdivided into rule and act utilitarianism. Rule utilitarianism seeks the greatest happiness for all; it appeals to public agreement as a basis for objective judgment about the nature of happiness. Act utilitarianism tries to determine which course of action in a particular situation will bring about the greatest happiness or the least harm and suffering to a single person. As such, act utilitarianism makes happiness subjective (Guido, 2001).

A third ethical theory has slowly been evolving and, although not yet given the full status of a theory, it does assist nurses and healthcare providers struggling with difficult ethical issues. Called **principlism,** this emerging theory incorporates existing ethical principles and attempts to resolve conflicts by applying one or more ethical principles. Ethical principles actually control ethical decision making much more than ethical theories do because principles encompass the basic premises from which rules are developed. Principles are moral norms that nurses demand and strive to implement daily in clinical settings. Each of the principles can be used individually, although it is much more common to see two or more ethical principles used in concert.

Ethical theories are important because they form the essential base of knowledge from which to proceed, rather than giving easy, straightforward answers. Without ethical theories, decisions revolve on personal emotions and values. Because most nurses do not ascribe to either deontology or teleology exclusively, principlism is growing in popularity.

BOX 4-2

Ethical Principles

- Autonomy
- Beneficence
- Nonmaleficence
- Veracity
- Justice
- Paternalism
- Fidelity
- Respect for others

Ethical Principles

Ethical principles that the nurse manager should consider when making decisions include the eight items listed in Box 4-2. Each of these principles can be used alone, although it is much more common to see more than one ethical principle affecting a nurse's clinical practice. The principle of **autonomy** addresses personal freedom and the right to choose what will happen to one's own person. The legal doctrine of informed consent is a direct reflection of this principle. The principle underlies the concept of progressive discipline because the employee has the option to meet delineated expectations or take full accountability for his or her actions. This principle also underlies the professional nurse's clinical practice because autonomy is reflected in individual decision making about patient care issues and in group decision making about unit operations decisions.

The principle of **beneficence** states that the actions one takes should promote good. In caring for patients, *good* can be defined in many ways, including allowing a person to die without advanced life support. Good can also prompt the nurse to encourage the patient to undergo extensive, painful treatment procedures, especially if these procedures will increase both the quality and quantity of life. This principle is used when nurse managers accentuate the employee's positive attributes and qualities rather than focusing on the employee's failures and shortcomings. Nurse managers also use this principle when they encourage staff members to excel to their fullest potential.

The corollary of beneficence, the principle of **nonmaleficence,** states that one should do no harm. Many nurses find it difficult to follow this principle when performing treatments and procedures that bring discomfort and pain to patients. Thus the principle of beneficence may be chosen because even pain and suffering can bring about good for the patient. For a nurse manager following this principle, performance evaluation should emphasize the employee's good qualities and give positive direction for growth. Destroying the employee's self-esteem and self-worth would be considered doing harm under this principle.

Veracity concerns telling the truth and incorporates the concept that individuals should always tell the truth. The principle also compels that the truth be told completely. Nurse managers use this principle when they give all the facts of a situation truthfully and then assist employees to make decisions. For example, with low patient censuses, employees must be told all the options and then be allowed to make their own decisions about floating to other units, taking vacation time, or taking a day without pay if the institution has such a policy.

Justice is the principle of treating all persons equally and fairly. This principle usually arises in times of short supplies or when there is competition for resources or benefits. This principle is considered with holiday and vacation time and paid attendance at national or local conferences; overall performance should be considered, rather than who is next on the list to attend a conference or to be allowed time off.

The principle of **paternalism** allows one person to make decisions for another and often is seen as a negative or undesirable principle. Paternalism assists persons to make decisions when they do not have sufficient data or expertise. Staff members often use some degree of paternalism when they help patients and their family members decide whether surgical procedures should be undertaken or whether medical management is a better option. Paternalism becomes undesirable when the entire decision is taken from the patient or employee. Nurse managers use this principle in a positive manner by assisting employees in deciding major career moves and plans.

Fidelity means keeping one's promises or commitments. Staff members know not to make commitments that they may not be able to keep, such as assuring the patient that no code will be performed before consulting with the patient's physician for such an order. Nurse managers abide by this principle when they follow through on any promises they have previously made to employees, such as a promised leave, a certain shift to be worked, or a promotion to preceptor within the unit.

Theory Box

WATSON'S THEORY OF CARING

THEORY/CONTRIBUTOR	KEY IDEA	APPLICATION TO PRACTICE
Theory of Caring (Jean Watson)	Caring is a moral ideal rather than a task-oriented behavior, whose goal is the preservation of human dignity and humanity in the healthcare system. Caring transcends time and space and has spiritual dimensions. Nurses have the responsibility to facilitate clients' and peers' development.	This can be accomplished by teaching, providing situational support, and recognizing coping skills and adaptation to the environment.

From Watson, J. (1988). *Nursing: Human science and human care—A theory of nursing.* New York: National League for Nursing.

Many think the principle of **respect for others** is the highest principle and incorporates all other principles. Respect for others acknowledges the right of individuals to make decisions and to live by these decisions. Respect for others also transcends cultural differences, gender issues, and racial concerns. Nurse managers positively reinforce this principle daily in their actions with employees, patients, and peers because they serve as role models for staff members and others in the institution. Nurses also reinforce these principles when they incorporate Watson's Theory of Caring in their interactions with patients and peers (see the Theory box).

■ *Exercise 4-7*

The community has been suffering from a severe nursing shortage made worse by a particularly virulent flu that has affected many of the staff members. Upper management is aware of the severity of the shortage and has decreased bed census by 20%; only emergency surgery is being performed until the crisis abates. You are considering reassigning a portion of your critical care staff, including dialysis and emergency care nurses, to the general medical and surgical floors because the crisis is most severe on the general units. None of the staff has been cross-trained specifically to the general units. From an ethical standpoint, how would you begin to achieve this task? How would you select which nurses to reassign and which nurses to retain in the unit? Would you involve the nurses themselves in the decision-making process? Why or why not?

Ethical Decision-Making Framework

Ethical decision making involves reflection on the following: who should make the choice; possible options or courses of action; available options; consequences, both good and bad, of all possible options; rules, obligations, and values that should direct choices; and desired goals or outcomes. When making decisions, nurses need to combine all of these elements using an orderly, systematic, and objective method; ethical decision-making models assist in accomplishing this goal.

There are various models for ethical decision making. Perhaps the easiest model to remember and implement is the **MORAL model** (Box 4-3) developed by Thiroux in 1977 and further developed for nursing by Halloran in 1982. Many nurses prefer this method because the letters of the acronym remind the user of the steps of the process.

Ethical decision making is always a process. To facilitate this process, the nurse manager must use all available resources, including the institutional ethics committee, and communicate with and support all those involved in the process. Some decisions are easier to reach and support. It is important to allow sufficient time for the process so that a supportable option can be reached. The Research Perspective box shows how nurse administrators make ethical decisions in clinical situations.

BOX 4-3

MORAL Model for Ethical Decision Making

M   Massage the dilemma. Identify and define the issues in the dilemma. Consider the options of all the major players in the dilemma and their value systems. This includes patients, family members, nurses, physicians, clergy, and any other interdisciplinary healthcare members.

O   Outline the options. Examine all the options, including those that are less realistic and conflicting. This stage is designed only for considering options and not for making a final decision.

R   Resolve the dilemma. Review the issues and options, applying basic principles of ethics to each option. Decide the best option based on the views of all those concerned in the dilemma.

A   Act by applying the chosen option. This step is usually the most difficult because it requires actual implementation, whereas the previous steps allow only for dialogue and discussion.

L   Look back and evaluate the entire process, including the implementation. No process is complete without a thorough evaluation. Ensure that those involved are able to follow through on the final option. If not, a second decision may be required and the process must start again at the initial step.

Modified from Thiroux, J. (1977). *Ethics: Theory and practice.* Philadelphia: Macmillan; and Halloran, M. C. (1982). Rational ethical judgments utilizing a decision making tool. *Heart and Lung, 11,* 566-570.

Ethics Committees

With the increasing numbers of ethical dilemmas in patient situations and administrative decisions, healthcare providers are using hospital ethics committees for guidance. Such committees can provide both long-term and short-term assistance. Ethics committees can provide structure and guidelines for potential problems, serve as open forums for discussion, and function as true patient advocates by placing the patient at the core of the committee discussions.

To form such a committee, the involved individuals should begin as a bioethical study group so that ethical principles and theories can be explored

by all potential members. The composition of the committee should include nurses, physicians, clergy, clinical social workers, nutritional experts, pharmacists, administrative personnel, and legal experts. Once the committee has become active, individual patients or patients' families and additional representatives of members of the healthcare delivery team may be invited to committee deliberations.

Ethics committees traditionally follow one of three distinct structures, although some institutional committees blend the three structures. The autonomy model facilitates decision making for competent patients. The patient benefit model uses substituted judgment (what the patient would want for himself or herself if capable of making these issues known) and facilitates decision making for the incompetent patient. The social justice model considers broad social issues and is accountable to the overall institution.

In most settings the ethics committee already exists because there are complex issues dividing healthcare workers. In many centers, ethical rounds, conducted weekly or monthly, allow staff members who may later become involved in ethical decision making to begin reviewing all the issues and to become more comfortable with ethical issues and their resolution.

Future Ethical Concerns for Nurses

Issues of concern in the near future involve autonomy and independent practice among nurses, quality of care in home and community settings, and development of nurses as leaders in the healthcare delivery field. Issues that continue to permeate ethical concerns for nurses include the patient's refusal of healthcare, issues surrounding death and dying, nurses' ability to be patient advocates in today's healthcare structure, and the ability to perform competent, quality nursing care in a system that rewards only cost-saving measures and that employs increasingly fewer professional nurses. Nursing must begin to address potential issues in a timely manner, or the profession will be unable to address them when needed (Edwards & Roemer, 1996).

Nurses need to begin now to look at the issues, professional values, and expectations they face and decide the issues for which they will fight and those that are acceptable as they are. Once these issues are identified, strategies for promoting quality nursing care can be delineated.

Research Perspective

Smith, M. K., Janzen, S. K., Schaefer, S., & Hixon, A. K. (2001). Administrative support for addressing staff nurses' ethical concerns regarding staffing. *Journal of Nursing Administration, 31*(3), 103-104.

The need for this study arose when the executive of a large Department of Veterans Affairs hospital was made aware by the hospital ethics committee that staff nurses had linked ethical concerns to staffing issues. The ethics committee had conducted a survey to identify staff nurses' ethical concerns. With a 47% return rate, the most frequently occurring ethical concern was whether the distribution of nursing staff was adequate to meet patients' needs. The executive was committed to addressing this issue.

The research team decided to use a focus group approach because focus groups are a sound choice for gathering data when the study concerns complex behaviors and diversity of opinions. The project team, consisting of the nurse executive, two nurse practitioners who were members of the ethics committee, and the institution's quality improvement expert, conducted 60-minute focus meetings. Group size was limited to 10 participants, and participants represented medical-surgical, rehabilitation, nursing home, psychiatric, ambulatory care, operating room, and intensive care staff nurses.

Five themes emerged from the focus groups: (1) lack of control over fluctuation in daily workload, making it difficult to ensure adequate staffing when nurses were absent; (2) inability to effectively meet workload demands—if the appropriate staff mix was not available, nurses were forced to choose between completing routine care, such as daily baths, and providing patient education; (3) nurses setting priorities to meet workload demands found conflicting issues related to quality of care and meeting critical customer service needs—nurses reported that increased patient turnover interfered with timeliness of meeting patient needs, such as the delayed delivery of requested pain medications; (4) decreased team communication and interdisciplinary team effectiveness—the nurses identified a desire for greater family involvement in the treatment planning process; (5) nursing staff's emphasis on promoting quality patient care rather than complaining about heavy workload. Staff nurse participants valued extra time to provide emotional support to patients and families. The focus was not on having to work harder, but on the need to provide the best quality care to patient.

Using these five themes, the nurse executive developed an action plan to support staff in addressing their ethical concerns. Strategies included developing a core staffing plan with the ability to expand upward when workloads increased, enhancing effective communication through interdisciplinary team building, and recording positive nursing efforts in the electronic nursing bulletin.

IMPLICATIONS FOR PRACTICE

The use of focus groups successfully clarified ethical concerns identified by the staff nurses. The process allowed nurses to better define and understand perceptions and to communicate these perceptions to upper management. The involvement of the nurse executive in the process and development of an action plan to address issues demonstrated administration's commitment to resolving ethical concerns of staff members.

The Solution

Several members of the hospice staff met with the ethics committee. They had requested a meeting to assist them in deciding how to best assist patients and families before a second such incident occurred and also to resolve their own feelings about the situation. Following the meeting with the ethics committee, the hospice nurses worked with legal counsel and patient educators in developing guidelines for educating patients, family members, hospice staff, and physicians involved in hospice care. They also developed teaching brochures and pamphlets, written at a tenth grade level, using language patients and family members could easily understand, and these materials are now used to educate and support family members.

Since this incident, the hospice staff members have been much more proactive rather then reactive. Edu-

cational materials are discussed, questions are answered, and the family is informed that an ethics committee meeting may be convened if they desire such a meeting. Staff members continue to reassure family members that the primary concern is the comfort and welfare of the patient. Since this approach has been used, there have been no repeats of such instances. Rather, family members know that we are trying to do the very best for the patient and respecting the dying process by not prolonging life unnecessarily nor hastening death, but allowing each person to die with dignity.

— Nancy Joyner

 Would this be a suitable approach for you? Why?

CHAPTER CHECKLIST

This chapter addresses the issues of legal and ethical interactions with regard to nurse managers. Legislative and legal controls have been established to clarify the boundaries of professional practice and to protect consumers. Thus there are some definite answers and guidelines to assist practitioners from the legal and legislative areas. These controls are constantly evolving, and the nurse manager must continually be aware of these changes as they affect the scope of the practice. Ethics has no such answers. Nor are there rules and guidelines that cover all aspects of human life. Thus nurse managers must explore value systems and become expert in using ethical models, incorporating both ethical theories and principles. The use of a systematic, humanistic approach reduces bias, facilitates decision making, and allows the best working conditions possible from an ethical standpoint.

- Understanding and using legal and ethical principles are key strategies to be integrated into the role of an effective nurse manager.
- Nurse practice acts define the scope of acceptable practice for licensed registered nurses and licensed practical (vocational) nurses.

- Legal principles, if effectively integrated into all aspects of nursing management, minimize one's potential legal liability.
  - Malpractice is the failure of a person with professional education and skills to act in a reasonable and prudent manner.
  - Causes of malpractice for nurse managers include the following:
    - Issues of delegation and supervision
    - Duty to orient, educate, and evaluate
    - Failure to warn
    - Staffing issues
  - Liability may be classified as personal, vicarious, corporate, or strict product.
  - Protective and reporting laws ensure the safety or rights of specific groups of people.
  - Informed consent is the authorization by the patient or the patient's legal representative to do something to the patient.
  - Privacy and confidentiality rights protect the patient from unreasonable and unwanted interference and secure the privacy of the patient's medical record.

Continued

CHAPTER CHECKLIST—CONT'D

- Federal and state governments have enacted a number of employment laws that nurses must understand and follow when dealing with managerial issues. These include the following:
  - Equal Pay Act of 1963
  - Civil Rights Act
  - Age Discrimination Act of 1967
  - Americans with Disabilities Act of 1990
  - Affirmative Action
  - Equal Employment Opportunity Laws
  - Occupational Safety and Health Act
  - Employment-at-Will and Wrongful Discharge
  - Family and Medical Leave Act of 1993
  - Collective Bargaining
- Ethical theories and principles relate to moral actions and value systems and apply both to patient situations and to management situations.
  - Ethical theories justify existing moral principles and are considered universally applicable.
  - Ethical theories include the following:
    - Deontology
    - Teleology (utilitarianism)
    - Principlism
  - Ethical principles exert direct control over professional nursing practice and encompass basic premises from which rules are developed.
  - Ethical principles include the following:
    - Autonomy
    - Beneficence
    - Nonmaleficence
    - Veracity
    - Justice
    - Paternalism
    - Fidelity
    - Respect for others
  - The MORAL model is an easy acronym to remember in ethical decision making.
  - Ethics committees aid in assisting nurses to implement solutions in everyday clinical practice.

TIPS ON LEGAL AND ETHICAL ISSUES

- Before applying the information presented in the chapter, the following five tips are offered:
  - Read the state nurse practice act carefully to fully comprehend the allowable scope of practice within the given state.

- Consult with risk management, the institutional attorney, or the legal department for a fuller understanding of how federal employment laws pertain to the individual nurse manager.
- Cultivate a group of professional consultants, either within the institution or outside the institution, who can assist with legal-ethical questions. Professional consultants may have great insight into issues as they arise and can assist in preventing problems in the future.
- Discover who serves on the institutional ethics committee and develop friendships with selected members. Attend the meetings to see how ethical issues are addressed in the institution. Become an active part of the ethical rounds if they exist in the institution.
- Think before you act. Remember it is always easier to hesitate, even briefly, so that the better approach can be implemented than to try to retract or amend something already done or already verbalized.

TERMS TO KNOW

apparent agency	law
autonomy	liability
beneficence	liable
collective bargaining	malpractice
common law	MORAL model
confidentiality	negligence
corporate liability	nonmaleficence
deontological theories	nurse practice act
emancipated minors	paternalism
ergonomics	personal liability
ethics	principlism
ethics committees	privacy
expert witnesses	respect for others
failure to warn	respondeat superior
fidelity	standard of care
foreseeability	statute
indemnification	teleological theories
independent contractors	values
informed consent	veracity
justice	vicarious liability
labor unions	

REFERENCES

American Nurses' Association. (1988). *Standards for nurse administrators*. Kansas City, MO: Author.

Americans with Disabilities Act of 1990, 42 U.S.C. § 12101 *et seq.* (1990).

Bishop v. United States, 334 F. Supp. 415 (D.C. Tex. 1971).

Bunn-Penn v. Southern Regional Medical Corporation, 488 S.E. 2d. 747 (Ga. App. 1997).

Bush, G. W. (2001). *Ergonomics*. Retrieved March 27, 2001. http://osha-slc.gov/ergonomics-standard/.

California staffing bill signed into law: Nurses happy, hospitals disappointed. (1999). Legislative Network for Nurses, 16(21), 163.

Civil Rights Act of 1964, § 703 et seq. (1978).

Cody v. Cigna Healthcare of St. Louis, Inc., 139 F.3d 595 (8th Cir. 1998).

David W. Francis v. Memorial General Hospital, 726 P.2d 852 (New Mexico, 1986).

Edwards, P. A., & Roemer, L. (1996). Are nurse managers ready for the current challenges of health care? Journal of Nursing Administration, 26(9), 11-17.

Fleming v. Correctional Healthcare Solutions, Inc., 751 A.2d 1035 (N.J. 2000).

Fortune v. National Cash Register Company, 272 Mass. 96, 264 N.E.2d 1251 (1977).

Guido, G. W. (2001). Legal and ethical issues in nursing (3rd ed.). Upper Saddle River, NJ: Prentice Hall.

Hall, J. K. (1990). Understanding the fine line between law and ethics. *Nursing 90, 20*(10), 37.

Halloran, M. C. (1982). Rational ethical judgments utilizing a decision making tool. *Heart and Lung, 11*, 566-570.

Hansen v. Caring Professionals, Inc., 676 N.E.2d 1349 (Ill. App. 1997).

Harrell v. Louis Smith Memorial Hospital, 397 S.E. 2d 746 (Georgia, 1990).

Herrero v. St. Louis University Hospital, 109 F.3d 481 (8th Cir. 1997).

Howard v. North Mississippi Medical Center, 939 F. Supp. 505 (N.D. Miss. 1996).

Jessie v. Carter Health Care Center, Inc., 926 F. Supp. 613 (E.D. Ky 1996).

Jones v. Kerrville State Hospital, 142 Fed.3d 263 (5th Cir. 1998).

Laurin v. Providence Hospital and Massachusetts Nurses Association, 150 F.3d 52 (1st Cir 1998).

Marquis, B. S., & Huston, C. J. (2000). *Leadership roles and management functions in nursing* (3rd ed.). Philadelphia: Lippincott.

Mauro v. Borgess Medical Center, 4:94 CV 05 (Michigan 1995).

OSHA Regulations (1999). Standards. 29 CFR Standard 1910.900.

Pozgar, G. D. (1999). *Legal aspects of health care administration* (7th ed.). Gaithersburg, MD: Aspen Press.

Roulston v. Tendercare (Michigan), Inc., 608 N.W.2d 525 (Mich. App. 2000).

Sabol v. Richmond Heights General Hospital, 676 N. E.2d 958 (Ohio App. 1996).

Smith, M. K., Janzen, S. K., Schaefer, S., & Hixon, A. K. (2001). Administrative support for addressing staff nurses' ethical concerns regarding staffing. *Journal of Nursing Administration, 31*(3), 103-104.

Sparks Regional Medical Center v. Smith, 976 S.W.2d 396 (Ark. App. 1998).

Taylor v. Memorial Health Systems, Inc., 770 So.2d 752 (Fla. App. 2000).

Thiroux, J. (1977). *Ethics: Theory and practice*. Philadelphia: Macmillan.

Thompson v. Holy Family Hospital, 122 F.3d 537 (9th Cir. 1997).

Trombley v. Southwestern Vermont Medical Center, 738 A.2d 103 (Vt. 1999).

U.S. Department of Labor, Occupational Safety and Health Administration. (2001). *Ergonomics*. Retrieved March 27, 2001. http://www.inventoryops.com/ergonomics.htm.

UTMB v. Hohman, 6 S. W.3d 767 (Tex. App. 1999).

Watkins v. Unemployment Compensation Board of Review, 689 A.2d 1019 (Pa. Commonwealth 1997).

Watson, J. (1988). *Nursing: Human science and human care—A theory of nursing*. New York: National League for Nursing.

Webb v. Mercy Hospital, 102 F.3d 958 (8th Cir. 1996).

Wilking v. County of Ramsey, 983 F. Supp. 848 (D. Kan. 1997).

Zamudio v. Patia, 956 F. Supp. 803 (N.D. Ill. 1997).

SUGGESTED READINGS

Anthony, M. K., Standing, T., & Hertz, J. E. (2000). Factors influencing outcomes after delegation to unlicensed assistive personnel. *Journal of Nursing Administration, 30*(10), 474-481.

Crow, K., Matheson, L., & Steed, A. (2000). Informed consent and truth telling: Cultural directions for healthcare providers. *Journal of Nursing Administration, 30*(3), 148-152.

Curtin, L. (2001). The first 10 principles for the ethical administration of nursing services. *Nursing Administration Quarterly, 25*(1), 7-13.

Diers, D., Torre, C., Jr., Heard, D. M., Bozzo, J., & O'Brien, W. (2000). Bring decision support to nurse managers. *Computers in Nursing, 18*(3), 137-142.

Dingman, S. K., Williams, M., Warnick, M., & Fosbinder, D. (1999). Implementing a caring model to improve patient satisfaction. *Journal of Nursing Administration, 29*(12), 30-37.

Donnelly, P. L. (2000). Ethics and cross-cultural nursing. *Journal of Transcultural Nursing, 11*(2), 119-26.

Fiesta, J. (1999). Greater need for background checks. *Nursing Management, 30*(11), 26.

Krairiksh, M., & Anthony, M. K. (2001). Benefits and outcomes of staff nurses' participation in decision making. *Journal of Nursing Administration, 31*(1), 16-23.

LaDuke, S. (2000). Nurses' perceptions: Is your nurse uncomfortable or incompetent? *Journal of Nursing Administration, 30*(4), 163-165.

Spetz, J. (2001). What should we expect from California's minimum nurse staffing legislation? *Journal of Nursing Administration, 31*(3), 132-140.

Steckler, S. L. (2000). Nursing case law update. *Journal of Nursing Law, 7*(1), 55-64.

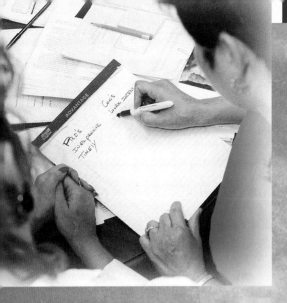

Decision Making and Problem Solving

Rose Aguilar Welch

This chapter describes the key concepts related to problem solving and decision making. The relationship between these essential skills and critical thinking is also explored. This chapter explains the primary steps of the problem-solving and decision-making processes and offers analytical tools that are helpful in planning and visualizing decision-making activities. It also presents strategies for individual or group problem solving and decision making. These strategies may be applied to both personal and professional situations.

Objectives

- Use a decision-making format to list options to solve a problem, identify the pros and cons of each option, rank the options, and select the best option.
- Evaluate the effect of faulty information gathering on a decision-making experience.
- Investigate the decision-making style of a nurse leader/manager.

- Design a flowchart for a personal or professional project.
- Increase skills in problem solving and decision making.

- Investigate resources on the Internet that focus on critical thinking, problem solving, and decision making.

Questions to Consider

- *Why are problem-solving and decision-making skills important for professional nursing practice?*
- *How can you enhance your skills in problem solving and decision making?*
- *What is the relationship between critical-thinking ability and skill in problem solving and decision making?*

The Challenge

Vickie Lemmon, RN, MSN
Public Health Nursing Supervisor, Ventura County Public Health, Ventura, California

Healthcare managers today are faced with numerous and complex issues that pertain to providing quality services for patients within a resource-scarce environment. Stress levels among staff can escalate when problems are not resolved, leading to a decrease in morale, productivity, and quality service. This was the situation I encountered recently when I became the Nurse Manager for the AIDS Center. Staff expressed frustration and dissatisfaction with staffing, workload, and team communications. This was evidenced by high staff turnover, customer complaints, and unmet deadlines for reports, data collection,

and documentation. I had not worked as a case manager in this program. It was hard for me to determine how to address the problems the staff presented to me. I wanted to be fair, yet felt that I did not have enough information to make changes immediately. I needed to find a way to resolve these problems, or I would soon be left without a program to serve the needs of the patients in my county.

 What do you think you would do if you were this nurse?

INTRODUCTION

Problem solving and **decision making** are vital abilities for nursing practice. Not only are these processes involved in managing and delivering care, but also they are essential for engaging in planned change. Myriad technological, social, political, and economic changes have had a dramatic effect on healthcare and nursing. Increased patient acuity, shorter hospital stays, increased technology, and the continuing shift from inpatient to ambulatory and home healthcare are some of the changes that require nurses to make rational and valid decisions that achieve results. Moreover, increased diversity in employment settings and types of healthcare providers demands efficient and effective decision making and problem solving. In addition to the focus on achieving people-oriented and cost-effective results, more emphasis is now placed on involving patients in decision making and problem solving and using multidisciplinary teams.

Professional nursing organizations have affirmed that competency in decision making and problem solving is essential to nursing practice. The reader can review select position and policy statements by referring to the Internet resources in Table 5-1 (or conduct a search using the organization's name or go to this text's website).

Nurses must possess the basic knowledge and skills required for effective problem solving and decision making. These competencies are especially

important for nurses with leadership and management responsibilities.

Problem solving and *decision making* are not synonymous terms. However, the processes for engaging in both behaviors are similar. Both skills require **critical thinking**, which is a higher cognitive process, and both can be improved with practice.

Decision making is a purposeful and goal-directed effort that uses a systematic process to choose among options. Not all decision making begins with a problem situation. Instead, the hallmark of decision making is the identification and selection of options or alternatives. For example, the nurse manager of a home healthcare agency is strategizing ways to empower the nursing staff. The options under consideration include allowing the staff to make out the schedule, perform self-evaluations, or have more input in the formulation of agency policy.

Problem solving, which includes a decision-making step, is focused on trying to solve an immediate problem, which can be viewed as a gap between "what is" and "what should be." In addition, there is the dissatisfaction that the problem creates for individuals/groups. For example, a nurse educator complains to a unit manager that the staff nurses rarely attend the inservice classes or continuing education programs that are offered. In attempting to address this issue, the parties gather and examine information in an effort to define the problem and identify possible solutions.

Table 5-1 PROFESSIONAL NURSING ORGANIZATIONS

Organization	URL
American Nurses Association	www.nursingworld.com Click on or search "Position Statements." Click on or search "Ethics and human rights." Click on or search "Nursing and the Patient Self Determination Act."
Australian Nursing Council, Inc.	www.anci.org.au Click on or search "Competency Standards."
Canadian Nurses Association	www.cna-nurses.ca Click on or search "Policy Statements." Click on or search "Evidence-based Decision Making and Nursing Practice."

As previously mentioned, effective problem solving and decision making are predicated on an individual's ability to think critically. Although critical thinking has been defined in numerous ways, the National Council for Excellence in Critical Thinking Instruction defines it as the "intellectually disciplined process of actively and skillfully conceptualizing, applying, analyzing, synthesizing, or evaluating information gathered from, or generated by, observation, experience, reflection, reasoning or communication, as a guide to belief and action" (Paul, 1995, p. 110). Critical thinking is not an isolated process. It is manifested whenever a nurse asks "why," "what," or "how." A nurse who questions why a patient is restless is thinking critically. Compare the analytical abilities between a nurse who assumes a patient is restless because of anxiety related to an upcoming procedure and a nurse who asks if there could be another explanation and proceeds to investigate possible causes.

It is important for managers to assess their staff members' ability to think critically and enhance their knowledge and skills through staff development programs, coaching, and role modeling. Establishing a positive and motivating work environment can enhance attitudes and the disposition to think critically.

Creativity is essential for the generation of options or solutions. Creative individuals are able to conceptualize new and innovative approaches to a problem or issue by being more flexible and independent in their thinking.

The model depicted in Figure 5-1 demonstrates the relationship among clinical judgment, decision making, problem solving, creativity, and critical thinking. Some researchers believe that critical

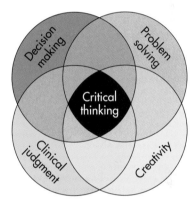

Figure 5-1 Problem-solving and decision-making model. (Modified from Sullivan, E. J., & Decker, P. J. [1992]. *Effective management in nursing.* Menlo Park, CA: Addison-Wesley.)

thinking is the concept that interweaves and links the others. An individual, through the application of critical-thinking skills, engages in problem solving and decision making in an environment that can promote or inhibit these skills. It is the manager's task to model these skills and promote them in others. The Research Perspective box summarizes a research study that explored the relationship between critical thinking and clinical judgment.

DECISION MAKING

The phases of the decision-making process include defining objectives, generating options, identifying advantages and disadvantages of each option, ranking the options, selecting the option most likely to achieve the predefined objectives, imple-

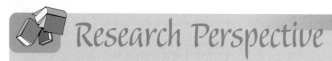

Research Perspective

Bowles, K. (2000). The relationship between critical-thinking skills and the clinical-judgment skills of baccalaureate nursing students. *Journal of Nursing Education, 39*(8), 373.

Although terms such as *critical thinking, problem solving, decision making, creativity,* and *clinical judgment* have been used interchangeably, the relationship among the concepts is unclear and studies have failed to demonstrate a consistent relationship among them.

Kathleen Bowles (2000) endeavored to answer the question: What is the relationship of critical thinking to the clinical judgment abilities of baccalaureate nursing students at the completion of the program? The sample for her study consisted of a convenience sample of nursing students from two baccalaureate programs in public universities in Northern California. The prelicensure students were in the last semester of the nursing program. Demographic data collected included age, cumulative grade point average (GPA), and total years in college. Instruments used to measure critical thinking and clinical judgment were the California Critical Thinking Skills Test (CCTST), form A, and the Clinical Decision Making in Nursing Scale (CDMNS). The CCTST was developed based on the definition of critical thinking adopted by the American Philosophical Association. Bowles used Tanner's definition of clinical judgment, which states clinical judgment includes decisions regarding patient observations and data and resultant actions based upon analysis of them.

The sample consisted of 68 senior nursing students. Their ages ranged from 22 to 50 years, GPA ranged from 2.8 to 4.0, and number of years in college ranged from 4 to 12 years. Scores on the CCTST ranged from 8 to 27 (maximum possible is 34), with a mean score of 18.2 (standard deviation of 4.2). There was a low correlation but statistically significant relationship between the CCTST and CDMNS ($r = .21$, $p < .05$). There was no significant relationship between clinical judgment based on age, GPA, or number of years in college. However, a statistically significant relationship was noted between critical thinking skills and GPA ($r = .55$, $p = .00$).

IMPLICATIONS FOR PRACTICE

The nonrandom sampling and sample size limit the study. Nevertheless, the author concluded that the study findings support previous research that demonstrates a relationship between clinical judgment and critical thinking. Clearly, future research is needed to determine the relationship between these skills, as well as the best ways to measure and strengthen them.

menting the option, and evaluating the result. Box 5-1 contains a form that can be used to complete these steps.

A poor-quality decision is likely if the objectives are not clearly identified or if they are inconsistent with the values of the individual or organization. Lewis Carroll illustrates the essential step of defining the goal, purpose, or objectives in the following excerpt from *Alice's Adventures in Wonderland*.

> One day Alice came to a fork in the road and saw a Cheshire Cat in a tree. "Which road do I take?" she asked. His response was a question: "Where do you want to go?" "I don't know," Alice answered. "Then," said the cat, "it doesn't matter."

Decision Models

The decision model that a nurse uses depends on the circumstances. Is the situation routine and predictable or complex and uncertain? Is the goal of the decision to make a decision conservatively that is just "good enough" (satisficing) or one that is optimal? Examples of decision models or theories are presented in the Theory box.

The following scenario illustrates decision theories. Staff nurses on a medical-surgical unit have complained that excessive time is spent documenting on numerous flowcharts and forms, often charting the same information in several places. Their frustration over charting is exacerbated by the inaccessibility of the medical records on the unit. A **satisficing decision** might involve the expedient option of

BOX 5-1

Decision-Making Format

Objective: _____

Desired outcome: _____

Options:

_____
_____
_____
_____

Analysis of options:

Option	Advantages	Disadvantages

Rank priority of options (1 being most preferred)

_____
_____

Select the best option (Implementation Plan)

_____
_____

Evaluation plan

_____
_____

Theory Box

DECISION MODEL THEORIES

THEORY/CONTRIBUTOR	KEY IDEA	APPLICATION TO PRACTICE
Normative or prescriptive	Used when information is objective, and routine decisions are involved or the problem is structured. Options are known and predictable	Situations that fall under this category can be handled using agency policy, standard procedures, or analytical tools.
Descriptive or behavioral	Used when information is subjective, non-routine, and unstructured. Uncertainty exists because options or outcomes are either unknown or unpredictable.	Situations that fall under this category are best handled by gathering more data, using past experience, using creative approaches, or following a group process.
Satisficing	Decision maker selects the solution that minimally meets the objective or standard for a decision. It is the more conservative method compared to an optimized approach.	This process is the most expedient and may be the most appropriate when time is an issue.
Optimizing	Decision maker selects the solution that maximally meets the objective or standard for a decision. Usually, this process involves accessing the pros and cons of each known option and listing benefits and costs associated with each option. The goal is to select the most ideal solution.	This process is more likely to result in a better decision, but it takes longer.

Based on Lancaster, J., & Lancaster, W. (1982). *Concepts for advanced nursing practice: The nurse as a change agent.* St. Louis: Mosby; and Sullivan, E. J., & Decker, P. J. (1992). *Effective management in nursing.* Menlo Park, CA: Addison-Wesley.

separating the nursing forms from the medical record and placing them on a clipboard for easy access. However, an **optimizing decision** might involve creating a multidisciplinary task force to investigate the feasibility of streamlining forms or instituting computerized documentation.

Decision-Making Styles

The decision-making style of a nurse manager is similar to the leadership style that the manager is likely to use. A manager who leans toward an autocratic style may choose to make decisions independent of the input or participation of others. This has been referred to as the "decide and announce" approach, an authoritative style. On the other hand, a manager who uses a democratic or participative approach to management involves the appropriate personnel in the decision-making process. Participative management has been shown to increase work performance and productivity, decrease employee turnover, and enhance employee satisfaction.

Any decision style can be used appropriately or inappropriately. Like the tenets of situational leadership theory, the situation and circumstances should dictate which decision making style is most appropriate.

In their classic book, *Leadership and Decision-Making*, Vroom and Yetton (1973) provide a useful model for defining the most appropriate leadership style based on the characteristics of the problem. Eight variables or "decision rules" assist the decision maker in selecting which of the five leadership styles is most appropriate:

1. The importance of the decision quality to institutional success
2. The degree to which the manager possesses the information and skills to make the decision
3. The degree to which the followers have the necessary information to generate a quality decision
4. The degree to which the problem is structured
5. The importance of follower commitment
6. The likelihood that an autocratic decision would be accepted
7. The strength of follower commitment to institutional goals
8. The likelihood of follower conflict over the final decision

The autocratic method results in more rapid decision making and is appropriate in crisis situations or when groups are likely to accept this type of decision style. However, followers are generally more supportive of consultive and group approaches. Although these approaches take more time, they are more appropriate when conflict is likely to occur, when the problem is unstructured, or when the manager does not have the knowledge or skills to solve the problem.

■ *Exercise 5–1*

Interview colleagues about their most preferred decision-making style. What barriers or obstacles to effective decision making have your colleagues encountered? What strategies are used to increase the effectiveness of the decisions made?

Factors Affecting Decision Making

Numerous factors affect individuals and groups in the decision-making process. The perception of the situation can be influenced by internal and external factors. Internal factors include variables such as the decision maker's physical and emotional state, personal philosophy, biases, values, interests, experience, knowledge, and attitudes. External factors include environmental conditions, time, and resources. Decision-making options are externally limited when time is short or when the environment is characterized by a "we've always done it this way" attitude.

Values affect all aspects of decision making, from the statement of the problem through the evaluation. Values are determined by one's cultural, social, and philosophical background. Values and beliefs provide the foundation for one's ethical stance. "An ethical foundation will encourage strong, ethical decision-making" (Peer & Rakich, 1999, p.7).

Dr. Michael McDonald, Director of the Centre for Applied Ethics at the University of British Columbia, provides a "Framework for Ethical Decision-Making" (http://www.ethics.ubc.ca/mcdonald/decisions.html). The steps for engaging in ethical decision making are similar to the steps described earlier; however, alternatives or options identified in the decision-making process are evaluated with the use of ethical resources. Resources that can facilitate ethical decision making include institutional policy; principles such as autonomy, nonmaleficence, beneficence, veracity, paternalism, respect, justice, and fidelity; personal judgment; trusted co-workers; institutional ethics committees; and legal precedent.

Certain personality factors, such as self-esteem and self-confidence, affect whether one is willing to take risks in solving problems or making decisions. Ask yourself, "Do I prefer to let others make the decisions? Am I more comfortable in the role of 'follower' than leader? If so, why?" Characteristics reported in the literature of an effective decision maker include courage, a willingness to take risks, self-awareness, energy, creativity, sensitivity, and flexibility.

Exercise 5-2

Identify a current or past situation that involved resource allocation, end-of-life issues, conflict among healthcare providers or patient/family/significant others, or other ethical dilemma. Describe how the internal and external factors previously described influenced the decision options, the option selected, and the outcome.

Group Decision Making

There are two primary criteria for effective decision making. First, the decision must be of a high quality; that is, it achieves the predefined goals, objectives, and outcomes. Second, those who are responsible for its implementation must accept the decision. Variables that influence the quality of decisions include the following:

- Was the information used factual, complete, and relevant to the situation?

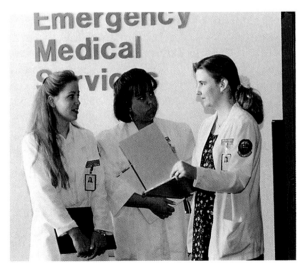

To be part of the solution, followers must be part of the problem-solving process.

- What were the behavioral characteristics of the decision makers?
- Were they able to process the data?
- Is the decision defensible in that the solution generated can be justified?
- Did the benefits of the decision outweigh the risks that were involved?
- How well did the decision solve the problem or meet the identified need/outcome?

Higher-quality decisions are more likely to result if groups are involved in the problem-solving and decision-making process. When individuals are allowed input into the process, they tend to function more productively and the quality of the decision is generally superior. Taking ownership of the process and outcome provides a smoother transition. Multidisciplinary teams should be used in the decision-making process, especially if the issue, options, or outcome involve other disciplines.

Research findings suggest that groups are more likely to be effective if members are actively involved, the group is cohesive, communication is encouraged, and members demonstrate some understanding of the group process. In deciding to use the group process for decision making, it is important to consider group size and composition. If the group is too small, there will be a limited number of options generated and fewer points of view expressed. Conversely, if the group is too large, it may lack structure and consensus becomes more difficult. Homogeneous groups may be more compatible; however, heterogeneous groups may be more successful in problem solving. Research has demonstrated that the most productive groups are those that are moderately cohesive.

For groups to be able to work effectively, the group facilitator or leader should carefully select members on the basis of their knowledge and skills in decision making and problem solving. Individuals who are aggressive, are authoritarian, or manifest self-oriented behaviors tend to decrease the effectiveness of groups.

Furthermore, the leader should provide a non-threatening and positive environment in which group members are encouraged to actively participate. Using tact and diplomacy, the facilitator can control aggressive individuals who tend to monopolize the discussion and can encourage more passive individuals to contribute by asking direct, open-ended questions. Providing positive feedback, such as "You raised a good point"; protecting members and their suggestions from attack; and keeping the group focused on the task are strategies that create an environment conducive to problem solving.

Gregory-Dawes (1999) challenges decision makers to actively solicit and encourage the free exchange of information from others. Moreover, she stresses the importance of going beyond the "because we've always done it that way" response, which can hinder creativity and uphold the status quo.

The advantages of group decision making are numerous. The adage "two heads are better than one" illustrates that when individuals with different knowledge, skills, and resources collaborate to solve a problem or make a decision, the likelihood of a quality outcome is increased. More ideas can be generated by groups than by individuals functioning alone. In addition, when followers are directly involved in this process, they are more apt to accept the decision because they have an increased sense of ownership or commitment to the decision. Implementing solutions becomes easier when individuals have been actively involved in the decision-making process. Involvement can be enhanced by making information readily available to the appropriate personnel, requesting input, establishing committees and task forces with broad representation, and using group decision-making techniques.

The group leader must establish with the participants what decision rule will be followed. Will the group strive to achieve consensus (100% agreement) or will the majority rule? In determining which decision rule to use, the group leader should consider the necessity for quality and acceptance of the decision. Achieving both a high-quality and an acceptable decision is possible, but it requires more involvement and approval from individuals affected by the decision.

Groups will be more committed to an idea if it is derived by consensus rather than as an outcome of individual decision making or majority rule. Consensus requires that all participants agree to go along with the solution. Although achieving consensus requires considerable time, it results in both high-quality and high-acceptance decisions and reduces the risk of sabotage.

Majority rule can be used to compromise when 100% agreement cannot be achieved. This method saves time, but the solution may only partially achieve the goals of quality and acceptance. In addition, majority rule carries certain risks. First, if the informal group leaders happen to fall in the minority opinion, they may not support the decision of the majority. Certain members may go so far as to build coalitions to gain support for their position and block the majority choice. After all, the majority may represent only 51% of the group. In addition, group members may support the position of the formal leader even though they do not agree with the decision because they fear reprisal or they wish to obtain the leader's approval. In general, as the importance of the decision increases, so does the percentage of group members required to approve it.

To secure the support of the group, the leader should maintain open communication with those affected by the decision and be honest about the advantages and disadvantages of the decision. The leader should also demonstrate how the advantages outweigh the disadvantages, suggest ways the unwanted outcomes can be minimized, and be available to assist when necessary.

Although group problem solving and decision making have distinct advantages, involving groups also carries certain disadvantages and may not be appropriate in all situations. As previously stated, group decision making requires more time. In some situations this may not be appropriate, especially in a crisis situation requiring prompt decisions.

Another disadvantage of group decision making relates to unequal power among group members. Dominant personality types may influence the more passive or powerless group members to conform to their points of view. Furthermore, individuals may expend considerable time and energy defending their positions, resulting in the primary objective of the group effort being lost.

Groups may be more concerned with maintaining group harmony than engaging in active discussion on the issue and generating creative ideas to address it. Group members who manifest a "group-think" mentality are so concerned with avoiding conflict and supporting their leader and other members that important issues or concerns are not raised. Failure to bring up options, explore conflict, or challenge the status quo results in ineffective group functioning and decision outcomes.

Strategies

Strategies exist to minimize the problems encountered with group problem solving and decision making. These strategies include brainstorming, nominal group techniques, focus groups, and the Delphi technique.

Brainstorming can be an effective method for generating a large volume of creative options. Often, the premature critiquing of ideas stifles creativity and idea generation. When members use inflammatory statements, euphemistically referred to as *killer phrases,* the usual response is for members to stop contributing. Killer phrases include statements such as "It will never work," "Administration won't go for it," "What a dumb idea," "It's not in the budget," "If it ain't broke, don't fix it," or "We tried that before."

The hallmark of brainstorming, a right-brain activity, is to list all ideas as stated without critique or discussion. The group leader or facilitator should encourage people to tag onto or spin off ideas from those already suggested. One idea may be piggybacked off others. Ideas should not be judged, nor should the relative merits or disadvantages of the ideas be discussed at this time. The goal is to generate ideas, no matter how seemingly unrealistic or absurd. It is important for the group leader or facilitator to cut off criticism and be alert for nonverbal behaviors signaling disapproval. Because the emphasis is on the volume of ideas generated, not necessarily the quality, solutions may be superficial and fail to solve the problem. Group brainstorming also takes longer, and the logistics of getting people together may pose a problem. If the facilitator allows the group to establish the rules for discussion, the aspects that stymie an open discussion often are eliminated by the group's "rules of engagement."

The nominal group technique, a method designed by Delbecq and Gustafson in the 1970s, allows group members the opportunity to provide input into the decision-making process. It also enhances group interaction and helps build consensus around issues (Moon, 1999). Although the group is physically present, participants are asked not to talk to each other as they write down their ideas to solve a predefined problem or issue. After a period of silent generation of ideas, generally no more than 10 minutes, each member is asked to share an idea, which is displayed on a chalkboard or flip chart. Comments and elaboration are not allowed during this phase. Each member takes a turn sharing an idea until all ideas are presented, after which discussion is allowed. Members may "pass" if they have exhausted their list of ideas. During the next step, ideas are clarified and the merits of each idea are discussed. In the third and final step, each member privately assigns a priority rank to each option. The solution chosen is the option that receives the highest ranking by the majority of participants. The advantage of this technique is that it allows

equal participation among members and minimizes the influence of dominant personalities. The disadvantages of this method are that it is time consuming and requires advance preparation. In addition, it requires that the group physically come together. Moon (1999) described using the nominal group technique in a physician's office to explore two questions: "What are five ways we could improve our current level of customer service?" and "What are five things we should be doing to make our practice stand out?" By using the nominal group technique, the group of 13 generated 47 ideas, which were rank-ordered to yield the top five for each question.

The purpose of focus groups is to explore issues and generate information. The groups meet face-to-face to engage in the discussion of issues and are facilitated by a group leader who serves as a moderator.

Another group decision making strategy is the Delphi technique. It involves systematically collecting and summarizing opinions and judgments from respondents, such as expert panels, on a particular issue through interviews, surveys, or questionnaires. Opinions of the respondents are repeatedly fed back to them with a request to provide more refined opinions and rationales on the issue or matter under consideration. Between rounds, the results are tabulated and analyzed so that the findings can be reported to the participants. This allows the participants to reconsider their responses. The goal is to achieve a consensus. An example of the Delphi technique appears in the Literature Perspective box. The hallmarks of the Delphi technique are the ability to ask open-ended questions, the allowance for anonymous feedback, and the ability to conduct qualitative and quantitative analysis (Bowles, N., 1999).

There are different variations on the Delphi technique. Nevertheless, the procedure generally calls for anonymous feedback, multiple rounds, and statistical analyses. One advantage of this technique is the ability to involve a large number of respondents because the participants do not need to assemble together. Indeed, participants may be located throughout the country or world. Also, the questionnaire or survey requires little time commitment on the part of the participant. This technique may actually save time because it eliminates the "off-the-subject" digressions typically encountered in committee meetings. In addition, the Delphi technique avoids the negative or unproductive verbal and nonverbal interactions that can occur when groups work together. Although the Delphi tech-

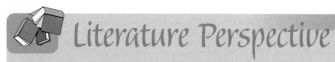

Literature Perspective

Sowell, R. L. (2000). Identifying HIV/AIDS research priorities for the next millennium: A Delphi Study with nurses in AIDS. *The Journal of the Association of Nurses in AIDS Care, 11*(3), 43-55.

Sowell (2000) described the use of the Delphi process to identify HIV/AIDS research priorities. A panel of experts, members of the Association of Nurses in AIDS Care (ANAC), participated in a three-round Delphi technique. The members were located throughout the United States, which made the Delphi process a feasible approach compared with face-to-face meetings. Participants identified and ranked research topics in HIV/AIDS in order of priority.

In Round One, 700 ANAC members were mailed a questionnaire, which consisted of two parts. The first part consisted of demographic questions, and the second part asked the respondents to identify research topics they considered important in the field of HIV/AIDS research. Of the members who received the questionnaire, 45% returned the survey ($n = 317$). Analysis of the data resulted in two lists of HIV/AIDS research topics. One list focused on general research, and the second focused on nursing research.

In Round Two, a second questionnaire was mailed to the individuals who returned the

Round One survey. The survey included the two lists of 12 research topics deemed as priorities, although they were listed randomly. Participants were asked to rank the items in order of importance, with 1 indicating most importance. Of the sample, 80% ($n = 252$) returned Round Two questionnaires.

In Round Three, researchers sought feedback from an additional panel of experts. Nurses attending the ANAC conference in San Diego, California, in fall 1999 were asked to rank order the five research topics and five nursing research topics produced from Round Two; 226 ANAC members in attendance at the conference participated (this number may have included individuals who participated in Round One or Two).

IMPLICATIONS FOR PRACTICE
The Delphi technique is a widely used and documented approach to group input. It is useful in reaching decisions requiring broad input.

---

nique has its advantages, using the Delphi technique may result in a lower sense of accomplishment and involvement because the participants are detached from the overall process and do not communicate with each other.

Decision-Making Tools
Several decision-making tools exist to aid a nurse manager in planning a decision-making process or selecting the best decision among the available options. The most common quantitative tools include decision grids and payoff tables. These tools are most appropriately used when information is available and options are known.

Decision grids facilitate the visualization of the options under consideration and allow comparison of options using common criteria. Criteria, which are determined by the decision makers, may include time required, ethical or legal considerations, equip-

ment needs, and cost (Figure 5-2). The relative advantages and disadvantages of the different options should be listed for each option.

Payoff tables require the manager to establish the cost-versus-benefit relationships and the probabilities of certain outcomes using current information and historical data. To illustrate, the manager of a hospital education department is evaluating whether it is better to retain the services of an outside consultant to coordinate an advanced cardiac life support course in the hospital or pay the per-person fees to send the staff elsewhere. The type of information this manager might compile includes a breakdown of the costs for both options, equipment needs, benefits of each option, the number of nurses needing the course, future training needs, and the feasibility of training hospital staff to conduct the course. Examples of these and other analytic tools can be reviewed at http://www.mindtools.com/pages2.html.

Options Under Consideration	Time	Cost	Legal/ethical Considerations	Equipment Needed

Figure 5-2   Decision grid.

Exercise 5–3

Design a decision grid for a current situation you are experiencing. Identify the components you need to explore in the decision-making process, such as cost, time, resources, advantages, and disadvantages, for the various options you are considering.

PROBLEM SOLVING

The steps for problem solving are similar to those for decision making; however, in this case the trigger for action is the existence of a "problem" or issue. Before attempting to solve a problem, a nurse must ask certain key questions:

1. Is it important?
2. Do I want to do something about it? (e.g., Do I "own" the problem?)
3. Am I qualified to handle it?
4. Do I have the authority to do anything?
5. Do I have the knowledge, interest, time, and resources to deal with it?
6. Can I delegate it to someone else?
7. What benefits will be derived from solving it?

If the answer to questions 1 through 5 is "no," why waste time, resources, and personal energy? At this juncture a conscious decision is made to ignore the problem, refer or delegate it to others, or consult or collaborate with others to solve it. On the other hand, if the answers are "yes," the nurse chooses to accept the problem and thus assume responsibility for it. Another way to look at whether to do something about a problem is to ask, Is the problem high volume? high cost? high risk? high interest? (Redick, 1999). Box 5-2 illustrates a model for approaching problem solving.

BOX 5-2

The FOCUS-PDCA Model

The FOCUS-PDCA model was developed by the Hospital Corporation of America. Redick (1999) described the application of the model to explore problems associated with inaccurate readings with the use of tympanic thermometers. Ramsey, Ormsby, and Marsh (2000) applied the model to reduce costs associated with cholecystectomy surgeries. The FOCUS-PDCA model is a performance improvement strategy and is an acronym for the following:

- **F**ind a process to improve.
- **O**rganize a team that knows the process.
- **C**larify current knowledge of the process.
- **U**nderstand causes of process variation.
- **S**elect the process to improve and start the "Plan-Do-Check-Act" phase.
- **P**lan the improvement.
- **D**o data collection, analysis, and improvement.
- **C**heck data for process improvement and customer outcome (e.g., results and lessons learned).
- **A**ct to hold, gain, and continue improvement (adopt, adjust, or abandon the change).

Methods of Problem Solving

The main principles for diagnosing a problem are know the facts, separate the facts from interpretation, be objective and descriptive, and determine the scope of the problem. Nurses also need to determine how to establish priorities for solving problems. For example, do you tend to work on problems that are encountered first, that appear to be the easiest, that take the shortest amount of time to solve, or that may have the greatest urgency?

Common methods for problem solving include trial and error, experimentation, and purposeful inaction ("do nothing") approaches. Often, inexperienced nurses use trial and error by trying one intervention after another until one method seems to address the problem. For example, patients' visitors have been complaining about the restrictive visiting hours in nursing units. Without an in-depth analysis of the problem, an inexperienced manager institutes different visiting policies until one seems to generate the least amount of complaints. Trial and error is the simplest technique, but it is often time consuming and may not be effective, especially if the problem is complex.

Scientific experimentation involves studying the situation under controlled conditions, often using trial periods or pilot projects. It is useful when additional information is needed to understand the problem further. Although the likelihood of achieving positive outcomes is greater, sufficient time is required for the experimental approach to be effective.

To use an experimentation approach in the preceding example, after gathering data on the specific nature of the visitors' complaints, the manager might institute one visiting policy in one unit and a different visiting policy in another unit. After a designated time, visitor satisfaction might be assessed through a survey, questionnaire, or interviews, and the results are then compared.

After identifying the problem, the decision maker must decide whether it is significant enough to require intervention and whether it is even within his or her control to do anything about it. Sometimes new managers believe they need to "solve" every problem brought to their attention. There are situations, such as some interpersonal conflicts, that are best resolved by the individuals who own the problem. Known as *purposeful inaction,* a "do nothing" approach might be indicated when other persons should resolve problems or if the problem is beyond the manager's control. Consider the following scenario:

> Mary complains to the nurse manager that Sam, a fellow nurse, was rude and abrupt with her during a hallway interchange. How should the nurse manager handle Mary's complaint? Should the manager discuss the problem with Sam? Should Mary be present during the discussion? What are the possible risks or benefits of such an approach? Alternatively, should the manager assist Mary in developing her communication skills so that Mary can solve the problem herself?

■ *Exercise 5-4*

Using the decision-making format presented in Box 5-1, list other options for this scenario and the advantages and disadvantages of each approach. Rank the options in order of most desirable to least desirable and select the best option. Determine how you would implement and evaluate the chosen option.

Some decisions are "givens" because they are based on firmly established criteria in the institution, which may be based on the traditions, values, doctrines, culture, or policy of the organization. Every manager has to live with mandates from persons higher in the organizational structure. Although managers may not have the authority to control certain situations, they may be able to influence the outcome. For example, because of losses in revenue, administration has decided to eliminate the clinical educator positions in a home health agency and place the responsibility for clinical education with the senior home health nurses. It is beyond the manager's control to reverse this decision. Nevertheless, the manager can explore the nurses' fear and concerns regarding this change and facilitate the transition by preparing them for the new role.

In these examples it is a misnomer to refer to the approach as *do nothing* because there is deliberate action on the part of the manager. This approach should not be confused with the laissez-faire (hands off) approach taken by a manager who chooses to do nothing when intervention is indicated.

Problem-Solving Process

Several models or approaches to problem solving exist. The traditional process for problem solving is illustrated in Figure 5-3. This figure gives the appearance of a sequential and linear process. However, like the nursing process, the problem-solving process is a dynamic one. These steps are described in more detail in the following section.

Define the Problem, Issue, or Situation

The most common cause for failure to resolve problems is the improper identification of the problem/issue; therefore problem recognition and identification are considered the most vital steps. The quality of the outcome depends on accurate identification of the problem. Problem identification is influenced by the information available; by the values, attitudes, and experiences of those involved; and by time. Sufficient time should be allowed for the col-

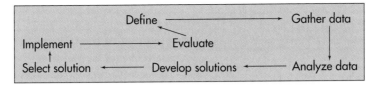

Figure 5-3   The problem-solving process.

lection and organization of data. All too often an inadequate amount of time is allocated for this essential step, resulting in unsatisfactory outcomes.

In work settings, problems often fall under certain categories that have been described as the four M's: manpower, methods, machines, and materials. A fishbone diagram, also known as a *cause-and-effect diagram,* is a useful model for categorizing the possible causes of a problem. The diagram graphically displays, in increasing detail, all of the possible causes related to a problem to try to discover its root causes. This tool encourages problem solvers to focus on the content of the problem and not be sidetracked by personal interests, issues, or agendas of team members. It also collects a snapshot of the collective knowledge of the team and helps build consensus around the problem. The "effect" is generally the problem statement, such as decreased morale, and is placed at the right end of the figure (the "head" of the fish). The major categories of causes are the main bones, and these are supported by smaller bones, which represent issues that contribute to the main causes (Figure 5-4).

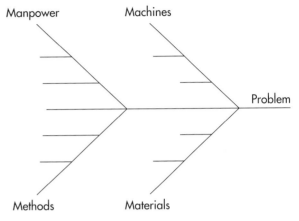

Figure 5-4   Fishbone diagram.

erly. Individuals charged with resolving this problem may discover that this is symptomatic of the underlying problem, perhaps inadequate staffing. Based on the proper identification of the problem in this scenario, a possible solution might be to assign the task of checking and stocking the emergency cart to the unlicensed personnel in the unit.

Gather Data

After the general nature of the problem is identified, individuals can focus on gathering and analyzing data to resolve the issue. Assessment, through the collection of data and information, is done continuously throughout this dynamic process. The data gathered consist of objective (facts) and subjective (feelings) information. Information gathered should be valid, accurate, relevant to the issue, and timely. Moreover, individuals involved in the process must have access to information and adequate resources to make cogent decisions. Generally, decisions based on "intuition" only should be avoided. Nursing lore places value on actions based on intangible and invisible "gut feeling" responses. However, in the era of evidence-based practice, reliance on intuition alone can cause problems. Research supports the use of systematic decision-making and problem-solving

> ### Exercise 5-5
>
> Given the following list of problems, identify which category they fall under (each problem may fit in more than one category): manpower, methods, machines, or materials.
> - Power struggles or "turf wars"
> - Poor communication
> - Legal or ethical issues
> - Work conditions (e.g., workload)
> - Unsatisfactory performance
> - Lack of training
> - Staff interactions and relationships
> - Lack of equipment
> - Inadequate staffing

It is important to differentiate between the actual problem and the symptoms of a problem. Consider the problem of an inadequately stocked emergency cart in which emergency medications are often missing and equipment fails to function prop-

approaches to promote effective patient outcomes (Lamond & Thompson, 2000). Decisions based on analytical approaches are more logical and defensible (Lauri et al., 2001).

Analyze Data

Data are analyzed to further refine the problem statement and identify possible solutions or options. It is important to differentiate a problem from the symptoms of a problem. For example, a nurse manager is dismayed by the latest continuous quality improvement (CQI) report indicating nurses are not documenting patient teaching. Is this evidence that patient teaching is not being done? Is lack of documentation the actual problem? Perhaps it is a symptom of the actual problem. On further analysis the manager may discover that the new computerized documentation system is not user-friendly. By distinguishing the problem from the symptoms of the problem, a more appropriate solution can be identified and implemented.

Develop Solutions

The goal of generating options is to identify as many choices as possible. Occasionally, the quality of outcomes is hampered by rigid "black and white" thinking. A nurse who is unhappy with his or her work situation and can think of only two options—stay or quit—is displaying this type of thinking.

Being flexible, open-minded, and creative is critical to being able to consider a range of possible options. Everyone has preconceived notions and ideas when confronted with certain situations. Putting these notions on hold and considering other ideas is beneficial, although it is difficult to do. However, asking questions such as the following can allow a person to consider other viewpoints:

- Am I jumping to conclusions?
- If I were [insert name of role model], how would I approach it?
- How are my beliefs and values affecting my decision?

Select a Solution

The decision maker should then objectively weigh each option according to its possible risks and consequences, as well as positive outcomes that may be derived. Criteria for evaluation might include variables such as cost, effectiveness, time, and legal or ethical considerations. The options should be ranked in the order in which they are likely to result in the desired goals or objectives. The solution selected should be the one that is most feasible and satisfactory and has the fewest undesirable consequences. Nurses must consider whether they are picking the solution because it is the best solution or because it is the most expedient. Being able to make cogent decisions based on thorough assessment of a situation is an important yardstick of a nurse's effectiveness.

Implement the Solution

The implementation phase should include a contingency plan to deal with negative consequences, should they arise. In essence, the decision maker should be prepared to institute "plan B" as necessary.

Evaluate the Result

Considerable time and energy are usually spent on identifying the problem or issue, generating possible solutions, selecting the best solution, and implementing the solution. However, not enough time is typically allocated for evaluation and follow-up. It is important to establish early in the process how evaluation and monitoring will take place, who will be responsible for it, when it will take place, and what the desired outcome is.

Take the previous example of the manager who instituted new visiting policies in response to visitor complaints. To ensure that this action was effective in solving the problem, an evaluation and monitoring plan should be developed in advance. In collaboration with the nursing staff, the manager would determine when follow-up surveys should be distributed; who will be responsible for their distribution, collection, and analysis; and how the findings will be communicated to appropriate personnel. Be prepared to make mistakes and take responsibility for them. The key is to learn from mistakes and use the experiences to help guide future actions.

Regardless of the model or approach taken, using a systematic approach helps one address issues in an organized and focused manner. All nurses, whether they are managers, leaders, or followers, need adequate problem-solving and decision-making skills to be effective in their roles. Additional strategies are listed at the end of the chapter for increasing problem-solving and decision-making effectiveness.

The Solution

In a previous job, I had used multidisciplinary process improvement teams (PITs), which consisted of key stakeholders, to initiate process improvement. I chose to give this concept a try in this setting. Our team consisted of the AIDS department staff, the infectious disease physician, the health officer, the public health clinic coordinator, and myself. I believed that a group approach to these problems would yield the most information and gain the greatest support for any changes that would be made. The team met weekly for an hour. We began by identifying our customers and key stakeholders and their expectations. This was extensive and took a few months to complete. Key stakeholders included the grantors of funds, as well as administration. The expectations were centered on data collection, reports, and documentation of services. Reviewing this helped the staff to understand why they were being asked to perform these functions. In addition, the team learned a great deal about each person's job expectations (there were a few surprises) and about the effect each person's job had on other people's ability to do their job. This was also enlightening.

Next the team brainstormed (divergent thinking) a list of issues. The numerous issues were then grouped according to similarity, and duplicates were eliminated. Multivoting was then used to determine the three highest-priority issues. Action plans were developed for the top three priorities and monitored weekly at the PIT meetings.

One year later I asked the team to list the problems they believed we had solved through our PIT's efforts. They listed (1) improved staffing, (2) increased staff morale and decreased turnover (all the positions were now filled), (3) better understanding of the job expectations and the rationale behind those expectations, and (4) improved teamwork. They have maintained enthusiastic support of the PIT and participation remains high. The team is still highly focused on problem solving. We have refocused our efforts on the patient services (primarily how to access funds to provide medical care to our patients) and streamlining documentation. These are formidable problems that will not be resolved quickly, but with the united efforts of the team, progress is being made. I have learned that when assuming leadership of a department in which one has no prior experience, a structured team approach to information gathering, assessment of data, identification of problems, and implementation of action plans can be highly effective in the resolution of priority problems.

— Vickie Lemmon

 Would this be a suitable approach for you? Why?

CHAPTER CHECKLIST

The ability to make good decisions and encourage effective decision making in others is a hallmark of nursing leadership and management. A nurse manager or leader is in a good position to facilitate effective decision making by individuals and groups. This requires good communication skills, conflict resolution and mediation skills, knowledge of the vagaries of group dynamics, and the ability to foster an environment conducive to effective problem solving, decision making, and creative thinking.

- ■ The main steps of the traditional problem-solving process are as follows:
  - Define the problem, issue, or situation.
  - Gather data.
  - Analyze data.
  - Develop solutions and options.
  - Select a solution with a desired outcome.
  - Implement the solution.
  - Evaluate the result.
- ■ A decision making format involves the following:
  - Listing options
  - Identifying the pros and cons of each option
  - Ranking the options in order of preference
  - Selecting the best option
- ■ If you want to make sound decisions or solve problems effectively, information gathered must be as follows:
  - Accurate
  - Relevant

Continued

CHAPTER CHECKLIST—cont'd

- Valid
- Timely
- The situation and circumstances should dictate the leadership style used by managers to solve problems and make decisions. Analytical tools that are helpful in planning and illustrating decision-making activities include the following:
  - Decision grids
  - Gap analysis exercises
  - Problem definition exercises
  - Fishbone analysis

TIPS FOR DECISION MAKING AND PROBLEM SOLVING

- Seek additional information from other sources, even if it does not support the preferred action.

- Learn how other people approach problem situations.
- Talk to colleagues and superiors who you believe are effective problem solvers and decision makers. Observe these positive role models in action.
- Research journal articles and relevant sections of textbooks to increase your knowledge base.
- Risk using new approaches to problem resolution through experimentation, and calculate the risk to self and others.

TERMS TO KNOW

creativity	optimizing decision
critical thinking	problem solving
decision making	satisficing decision

REFERENCES

Bowles, K. (2000). The relationship between critical thinking skills and the clinical judgement skills of baccalaureate nursing students. *Journal of Nursing Education, 39*(8), 373.

Bowles, N. (1999). The Delphi technique. *Nursing Standard, 13*(45), 32-36.

Gregory-Dawes, B. S. (1999). Why? Because we've always done it that way. *Association of Operating Room Nurses, 69*(2), 338-340.

Lamond, D., & Thompson, C. (2000). Intuition and analysis in decision making and choice. *Journal of Nursing Scholarship, 32*(4), 411-414.

Lancaster, J., & Lancaster, W. (1982). *Concepts for advanced nursing practice: The nurse as a change agent.* St. Louis: Mosby.

Lauri, S., Salantera, S., Chalmers, K., Ekman, S. L., Kim, H. S., Kappeli, S., & MacLeod, M. (2001). An exploratory study of clinical decision-making in five countries. *Journal of Nursing Scholarship, 33*(1), 83-90.

McDonald, M. (2001). A framework for ethical decision-making. Retrieved April 2, 2001, from http://www.ethics.ubc.ca/mcdonald/deicisions.html.

Moon, R. H. (1999). Finding diamonds in the trenches with the nominal group process. *Family Practice Management, 6*(5), 49.

Paul, R. W. (1995). *Critical thinking: How to prepare students for a rapidly changing world.* Santa Rose, CA: Foundations for Critical Thinking.

Peer, K. S., & Rakich, J. S. (1999). Ethical decision making in healthcare management. *Hospital Topics, 77*(4), 7-13.

Ramsey, C., Ormsby, S., & Marsh, T. (2000, December). Performance improvement strategies can reduce costs. *Healthcare Financial Management,* pp. 2-6.

Redick, E. L. (1999). Applying FOCUS-PDCA to solve clinical problems. *Dimensions of Critical Care Nursing, 18*(6), 30-34.

Sowell, R. L. (2000). Identifying HIV/AIDS research priorities for the next millennium: A Delphi study with nurses in AIDS care. *The Journal of the Association of Nurses in AIDS Care, 11*(3), 42-52.

Sullivan, E. J., & Decker, P. J. (1992). *Effective management in nursing.* Menlo Park, CA: Addison-Wesley.

Vroom, V. H., & Yetton, P. W. (1973). *Leadership and decision-making.* Pittsburgh: University of Pittsburgh Press.

SUGGESTED READINGS

Fralic, M. F., & Denby, C. B. (2000). Retooling the nurse executive for 21st century practice: Decision support systems. *Nursing Administration Quarterly, 24*(2), 19-28.

Gordon, J. M. (2000). Congruency in defining critical thinking by nurse educators and non-nurse scholars. *Journal of Nursing Education, 39*(8), 340-351.

INTERNET RESOURCES

California Academic Press: http://www.calpress.com

Center for Critical Thinking and Foundation for Critical Thinking at Sonoma State University: http://www.critical-thinking.org

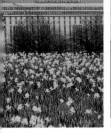
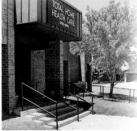
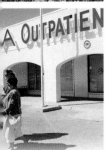
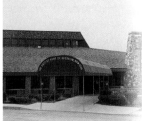

6

Healthcare Organizations

Carol Alvater Brooks

This chapter presents an overview of the healthcare organizations that exist or are emerging in a time of rapid change. Distinguishing characteristics of different types of organizations and issues that are altering these characteristics are presented. Economic, social, and demographic factors that are driving change are discussed. A major emphasis is placed on management and leadership responses that professional nurses must consider in planning the delivery of nursing care in the changing environment. Leaders, managers, followers, and professional nursing students engaged in active practice must be aware of the changing dynamics if they choose to anticipate new expectations or to be appropriately responsive.

Objectives

- Relate characteristics that are used to differentiate healthcare organizations.
- Classify healthcare organizations by major types.
- Analyze economic, social, and demographic forces that drive the development of healthcare organizations.
- Explain the implications of healthcare organizational evolution for nursing leadership and management roles.

Questions to Consider

- What are the changes that have taken place in healthcare organizations in your geographic region in the past 5 years?
- What changes have taken place in specific characteristics of ownership, service orientation, teaching status, and financing of healthcare organizations in your community?
- What economic, social, and demographic factors are forces driving the development of healthcare organizations in your community?
- What leadership and management functions are nurses performing in relationship to the evolution of healthcare organizations in your geographic region?

The Challenge

Beth A. Smith, RN, MSN, MBA
Director, Case Management, W.A. Foote Memorial Hospital, Jackson, Michigan

Our hospital system is faced with the challenge of caring for a large number of uninsured patients who do not receive basic healthcare. When they do seek healthcare, it is often because they have an advanced disease process that consequently requires high-cost treatment and support. One such patient was a 42-year-old uninsured, self-employed seasonal worker with no current income, assets, or support systems. He underwent a partial laryngectomy for his throat cancer. When he was ready to be discharged, he still required tube feedings, a tracheostomy with humidified air, IV antibiotics, and speech therapy. I needed to balance virtually nonexistent resources with great needs.

What do you think you would you do if you were this nurse?

INTRODUCTION

Healthcare organizations are a part of the healthcare system, which provides the totality of services offered by all of the health disciplines. Economic, social, and demographic factors affect the purpose and structuring of the system, which in turn affect the mission, philosophy, and structure of healthcare organizations.

In the past, healthcare organizations provided two general types of services: illness care (restorative) and wellness care (preventive). Illness care services help the sick and injured. Wellness care services promote better health and illness and accident prevention. Although most organizations (e.g., hospitals, clinics, public health departments, community-based organizations, physicians' offices) have provided both illness and wellness services, the focus has been on illness. Recent economic, social, and demographic changes have placed emphasis on the development of organizations that focus on the full spectrum of health, especially wellness and prevention, to meet consumers' needs in more cost-effective ways. Emphasis is being placed on the role of the nurse both as a designer of these restructured organizations and as a healthcare leader and manager within the organizations. For example, the way in which chronic illnesses and social illnesses are managed are dramatically different from a decade ago. Similarly, as population numbers increase and the demand for nurses exceeds the supply, we can anticipate more changes. In addition, benchmarking demands that any organization constantly consider its own practices and make appropriate changes, including those related to the organization's culture (Garry, 2000).

Nurses practice in many different types of healthcare organizations. Nursing roles develop in response to the same social, cultural, economic, legislative, and demographic factors that shape the organizations in which they work. As the largest group of healthcare professionals providing direct and indirect care services to consumers, nurses have an obligation to present a unified direction for the development of healthcare, social, and economic policies that shape healthcare organizations.

CHARACTERISTICS AND TYPES OF ORGANIZATIONS

The healthcare industry is made up of many types of organizations. The process of healthcare-system development is in a continual state of evolution. Questions, concerns, and decisions surround both the characteristics used to differentiate healthcare organizations and the types of organizations themselves.

Institutional Providers

Hospitals, long-term care facilities, and rehabilitation facilities have traditionally been classified as institutional providers. Major characteristics that differentiate institutional and other types of healthcare organizations are (1) services offered, (2) length of direct service provision, (3) ownership, (4) financial

Table 6-1 CONTINUUM OF HEALTHCARE ORGANIZATIONS

Type of Care	Purpose	Organization or Unit Providing Services
Primary	Entry into system Health maintenance Long-term care Chronic care Treatment of temporary nonincapacitating malfunction	Ambulatory care centers Physicians offices Preferred provider organizations Nursing centers Independent provider organizations Health maintenance organizations School health clinics
Secondary	Prevention of disease complications	Home healthcare Ambulatory care centers Nursing centers
Tertiary	Rehabilitation Long-term care	Home healthcare Long-term care facilities Rehabilitation centers Skilled nursing facilities Assisted living programs/retirement centers

provisions, (5) teaching status, (6) geographic location, and (7) accreditation and licensure status.

Services offered is a key characteristic used to differentiate institutional providers. Services range from those provided by specialty institutions limited to specific disease entities or population segments to institutions referred to as *general,* which provide a full range of services for all segments of the population. Examples of specialty hospitals are those limited to one type of patient population, such as psychiatric care, burn care, children's care, women's and infants' care, or oncology care. Another aspect of services is the duration of care. Some services are short term, such as those provided in acute care institutions where patients are discharged as soon as their conditions are stabilized. Others are long term, such as those provided by some geriatric organizations that provide care services from onset of impairments until death. Many institutions, however, are multiunit and have components of both short-term and long-term services. They may provide acute care, home care, hospice care, ambulatory clinic care, day surgery, and an increasing number of other services, such as day care for dependent children and adults or focused services, such as Meals-on-Wheels. *Healthcare networks* is a term used to refer to units connected with institutions that either are owned by the institutions or have cooperative agreements with the institutions to provide a full spectrum of wellness and illness services ranging from **primary care** (first-access care) to **secondary care** (disease-restorative care) through **tertiary care** (rehabilitative or long-term care). Table 6-1 describes the continuum of care and the units of healthcare organizations that provide services in the three phases of the continuum.

Ownership designated as either **private** or **public** is a second characteristic used to classify healthcare organizations. The Research Perspective suggests that knowing the ownership is important. Private institutions are those directed and supported by private citizens. Multihospital systems, which are defined as two or more institutional providers having common owners, represent a significant development that has taken place in the last two decades. Public institutions are government-owned organizations that provide health services to groups of people under the support and direction of the local, state, or federal government. Public institutions' services are often provided without cost to specially designated patients, such as veterans or prisoners. They may also be offered at a reduced rate to the medically indigent.

Exercise 6-1

Using the local telephone directory, determine the types and numbers of primary care, secondary care, and tertiary care services available. Table 6-2 is an example of a format for collecting data.

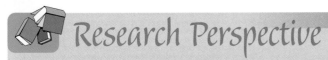

Research Perspective

Baker, C. M., Messmer, P. L., Gyurko, C. C., Domagala, S. E., Conly, F. M., Eads, T. S., Harshman, K. S., & Layne, M. K. (2000). Hospital ownership, performance, and outcomes: Assessing the state-of-the-science. *Journal of Nursing Administration, 30*(5), 227-240.

This study assessed the state-of-the-science surrounding hospital ownership, performance, and outcomes in acute care hospitals in the United States. As the size of the not-for-profit sector decreased and the size of the for-profit sector increased, hospital ownership warranted examination. A comprehensive, computerized search of the healthcare literature yielded 69 databased references published between 1995 and 1999. Hospital ownership affected hospital performance in relation to system operations, costs, price, and financial management practices and personnel issues. Organizational outcomes were similar among hospital ownership types in relation to increasing costs and overall mediocre efficiency. Organizational outcomes differed among hospital ownership types in relation to nursing staff mix and professional satisfaction. Hospital ownership status affected the type and magnitude of community benefits.

IMPLICATIONS FOR PRACTICE

Nurse researchers need to include hospital ownership as an important structural variable in their studies of hospital-based nursing. This study could form the basis for evaluating prospective employment situations to determine how similar a given hospital is in relation to those studied here.

These organizations must answer directly to the sponsoring government agency or boards and are indirectly responsible to elected officials and taxpayers who support them. Examples of these at the federal level are veterans, members of the military, Indian, and prisoner healthcare organizations. State-supported organizations may be health service teaching facilities, chronic care facilities, and prisoner facilities. Locally supported facilities include county- and city-supported facilities. Table 6-2 shows how several common healthcare organizations are classified.

Table 6-2 CHARACTERISTICS AND TYPES OF HEALTHCARE ORGANIZATIONS

Healthcare Organization	Characteristics					
	Type	Services	Own	Fin	Tchg	Multi
Veterans Administration	Instit	General	Fed	NP	Y	Y
Medical Center	Instit	General	State	NP	Y	Y
Community General	Instit	General	Private	NP	N	Y
Shriners Burn Hospitals	Instit	Specialty	Private	NP	N	N
Prepaid Health Plan	Ambu group HMO	General	Private	NP	N	N
Public Health Department	Commun	General	State	NP	N	N
Women's and Infants' Project	Commun	Specialty	State	NP	N	N
Geriatric Corporation	Instit	Long term	Private	NP	N	Y

Ambu, Ambulatory; *Commun,* community; *Fed,* federal; *Fin,* financing; *HMO,* health maintenance organization; *Instit,* institution; *Multi,* multiunit; *N,* no; *NP,* nonprofit; *Own,* ownership; *Tchg,* teaching status; *Y,* yes.

Financial provisions are classified by whether the institution operates on a for-profit or **not-for-profit** basis and are another characteristic that classifies organizations. Operating without profit means that funds are redirected into the organiza-

tion for maintenance and growth rather than as dividends to stockholders. These organizations are required to serve people regardless of their ability to pay. Not-for-profit organizations located in impoverished urban and rural areas are often economically disadvantaged by the amounts of uncompensated care that they provide. Some states, such as New York, have created charity pools to which all not-for-profit organizations in the state are required to contribute to offset financial problems of the disadvantaged institutions. Tax-exempt not-for-profit organizations that meet the health needs of the public may also be referred to as *voluntary agencies.* Historically, not-for-profit organizations have been tax exempt. The owners of such organizations include churches, communities, industries, and special interest groups such as labor unions. Ownership differs in various countries.

For-profit organizations are also referred to as *proprietary organizations.* These investor-owned hospitals serve only people who can pay for their services either directly or indirectly through organizations such as private or public insurers, known as **third-party payers.** Owners may be individuals, partnerships, corporations, or multisystems. Many for-profit organizations, like the not-for-profit ones, receive supplementary funds through private and public sources to provide special services and research. This funding allows them to provide financial assistance to patients who can afford ordinary care but are not in a position to finance catastrophic occurrences such as vital organ failure, birth of premature or sick infants, or transplant operations.

Investor-owned multihospital systems are becoming increasingly popular. Nursing homes, home care, psychiatric services, and health maintenance organizations (HMOs) are commonly units in such systems.

Teaching status is a fifth characteristic that is used to classify healthcare organizations. The term **teaching institution** is applied to academic health centers, those entities with a school of medicine, at least one other health profession school, and affiliated teaching hospitals that provide only the clinical portion of a health education institution's teaching program. Traditionally, these programs have received government reimbursement to cover the costs of the educational program that are not covered by typical fees for patient care. Costs include salaries of physicians who supervise students' care delivery and participate in educational programs such as teaching rounds and seminars. Currently, these expenses are reimbursed based on a formula that takes into consideration the cost of caring for the low-income and uninsured patients who populate academic teaching programs. Revisions in this reimbursement are occurring as states reduce subsidies for the education of physicians. Other countries, such as Canada, have experimented with primary healthcare reform.

Exercise 6-2

Return to the data you started in the first exercise and add financial and teaching status information.

Consolidated Systems

Healthcare organizations are being organized into **consolidated systems** both through the formation of for-profit or not-for-profit multihospital systems and through the development of **networks** of independently owned and operated healthcare organizations.

Consolidated systems tend to be organized along five levels. The first includes the large national hospital companies, most of which are investor owned. The second level involves large voluntary affiliated systems, which provide members with access to capital, political power, management expertise, joint venture opportunities, and links to health insurance services or, as in Canada, to a national healthcare coverage program. The third level involves regional hospital systems that cover a defined geographic area, such as an area of a state. The fourth level involves metropolitan-based systems. The fifth level is composed of the special interest groups that own and operate units organized along religious lines, teaching interests, or related special interests that drive their activities. This level often crosses over the regional, metropolitan, and national levels already described. Through the creation of multiunit systems, an organization has greater marketing, policy, and contracting potentials.

Accreditation is the final characteristic. Three private organizations play significant roles in both establishing standards and ensuring care delivery compliance with standards: the Joint Commission on Accreditation of Healthcare Organizations (JCAHO), The National Committee for Quality Assurance (NCQA), and the Community Health Assessment Program (CHAP) originally established by the National League for Nursing. Other countries have comparable organizations. All three organizations have met federal requirements for deemed status, which means that federal agencies will accept their inspection approvals as authorization for continuing payment of federal funds for services. Individual states, because of states rights provisions, make their own decisions regarding acceptance of the approval of these organizations. More information on these bodies can be obtained through their websites (http://jcaho.org, http://www.ncqa.org, and http://www. chapinc.org).

ACQUISITIONS AND MERGERS

The economic forces of capitated payments and **managed care** are causing healthcare organizations to reorganize, restructure, and reengineer to decrease waste and economic inefficiency. Many organizations are forming multiinstitutional alliances that integrate healthcare systems under a common organizational infrastructure. These alliances are accomplished through acquisitions or mergers. Acquisitions involve one organization directly buying another. Mergers involve combining two or more organizations and their assets to form a new entity. Mergers can also happen within organizations as departments or patient care units come together. People, structure, culture, and political issues or organizational change can be very traumatic and lead to dysfunctional outcomes if they are not managed. Barry-Walker (2000) found that the hours per patient day increased during and immediately after mergers of patient populations. Smart managers and administrators take such potentials into consideration when mergers are imminent. Diania et al. (1997) developed a model to facilitate the merger process based on transformation theory. Elements of structuring to meet the need generated by continuous restructuring are further discussed in Chapter 9. One of the complexities of mergers or buyouts is what to do with the monies set aside in the original organizational foundations. This issue becomes especially critical when there is a merger of a public institution with a for-profit one.

NETWORKS

Markets with 100,000 or more residents are generally served by one to three health networks. The networks usually follow one of three organizational models: public utilities, for-profit businesses, or loose alliances. Public utility models are organized and governed just like today's public utilities, for example, the county water department. Their aim is serving large regional populations. In most markets, two or three competing markets have emerged that require significant capital, causing many traditional not-for-profit providers to shift to for-profit status. Loose alliances take the shape of loosely connected "virtual" networks that emulate integrated health systems through contracts and linked computer systems.

AMBULATORY-BASED ORGANIZATION

Many health services are provided on an ambulatory basis. The organizational setting for much of this care has been the group practice or private physician's office. A growing form of group practice is prepaid group practice plans, referred to as managed care systems, which combine care delivery and financing and provide comprehensive services for a fixed prepaid fee. A goal of these services is to reduce the cost of expensive acute hospital care by focusing on out-of-hospital preventive care and illness follow-up care. Group practice plans take various forms. One form has a centralized administration that directs and pays salaries for physician practice (e.g., HMOs).

The HMO is a configuration of healthcare agencies that provide basic and supplemental health maintenance and treatment services to voluntary enrollees who prepay a fixed periodic fee without regard to the amount of services used. To be federally qualified, an HMO company must offer inpatient and outpatient services, treatment and referral for drug and alcohol problems, laboratory and radiological services, preventive dental services for children younger than 12 years, and preventive healthcare services in addition to physician services.

Independent practice associations (IPAs) (of professional associations [PAs]) are a form of group practice in which physicians in private offices are paid on a **fee-for-service** basis by a prepaid plan to deliver care to enrolled members. Preferred provider organizations (PPOs) operate similarly to IPAs; contracts are developed with private practice physicians, but fees are discounted from their usual and customary charges. In return, physicians are guaranteed prompt payment.

Nurse practitioners' leadership in managing patients in these group practices has contributed greatly to their success. Examples of this can be found by reviewing literature related to nurses' activities at Kaiser Permanente HMO and the Harvard Community Health Plan.

Numerous freestanding ambulatory centers are developing. These organizations include surgicenters, urgent care centers, primary care centers, and imaging centers.

■ *Exercise 6–3*
Again return to the data started in the first exercise and add information about the status of the multiunit systems that are in place.

Community Services

Community services, including public health departments, are focused on the treatment of the community rather than that of the individual. The historical focus of these organizations has been on control of infectious agents and provision of preventive services under the auspices of public health departments. Funds are allocated to local health departments by local, state, and federal governments for personal health services that include maternal and child care, care for communicable diseases such as acquired immunodeficiency syndrome (AIDS) and tuberculosis, services for children with birth defects, mental healthcare, and investigation of epidemiology and treatment of bioterrorism threats and attacks such as anthrax. Monies are also allocated for environmental services, such as ensuring that food services meet established standards, and for health resources, such as control of reproduction, promotion of safer sex, and breast cancer screening programs. Local health departments have been provided some autonomy in determining how to use funds that are not assigned to categorical programs.

School health programs whose funds are also allocated to them by local, state, and federal governments traditionally have been organized to control infectious disease outbreaks, to detect and refer problems that interfere with learning, to treat onsite injuries and illnesses, and to provide basic health education programs. Increasingly, schools are being seen as primary care sites for children.

Visiting nurse associations, which are voluntary organizations, have provided a large amount of the follow-up care for patients after hospitalization and for newborns and their mothers. Some are organized by cities, and others serve entire regions. Some operate for profit; others do not.

Other Services

Although hospitals, nursing homes, health departments, visiting nurse services, and private physicians' offices have made up the traditional primary service delivery organizations, it is important to recognize the increasing role being played by other organizations that may be freestanding or units of hospitals or other community organizations. These include subacute facilities and a proliferating number of home health agencies and hospices. This rapid growth was spurred by the implementation of the prospective payment system, which resulted in early discharge of many patients from acute care facilities. These patients require highly technical continuing nursing care to maintain a stable status. The focus of these organizations is on the care of individuals and their family and significant others, rather than a focus on the community as a whole. Many of these organizations are functioning as PPOs, and this is expected to be a continuing pattern in the future.

Nurse-Owned and Nurse-Organized Services

Nursing centers, which are nurse owned and operated and places where care is provided by nurses, are another form of community-based organization (Murphy, 1995). Many nursing centers are administered by schools of nursing and serve as a base for faculty practice and research and clinical experience for students. Others are owned and operated by groups of nurses. These centers have a variety of missions. Some focus on care for specific populations such as the homeless or on care for people with AIDS. Others have taken responsibility for university health services. Some have assumed responsibility for school health programs in the community, and others operate employee wellness programs, hospices, and home care services. Some are freestanding, and others are units of hospitals. Church-affiliated organizations, sometimes operating as parish or shul (a service of synagogues) nursing, are also examples of nurse-based organizations.

Self-Help Voluntary Organizations

Other organizations are the self-help/self-care organizations. These organizations also come in various forms. They are often composed of and directed by peers who are consumers of healthcare services. Their purpose is most often to enable patients to provide support to each other and raise community consciousness about the nature of a specific physical or emotional disease. AIDS support groups and Alcoholics Anonymous are two examples. Community geriatric organizations, frequently sponsored by healthcare organizations and offering multiple services for promoting wellness and rehabilitation, are increasing rapidly.

Home Health Organizations

Home health organizations have numerous configurations; they may be freestanding or owned by a hospital and may be for-profit or not-for-profit organizations. Professional nurses with expert skills in assessing patients' self-care competencies and in building structures to overcome patients' and families' social and emotional deficits in providing sick and palliative care are needed to meet home care needs. Home care agencies staffed appropriately with adequate numbers of professional nurses have the potential to keep elderly persons, those with disabilities, and persons with chronic illnesses comfortable and safe at home. An increasing number of restrictions on home care by managed care companies are threatening the adequate performance of this function.

Home care is the fastest growing segment in healthcare. The organizational design will likely change to the integration of a functional and divisional structure because the home health service industry is becoming more complex and changing rapidly. For example, reimbursement for home care is moving from a fee-for-service arrangement to contract pricing and capitation. The integration of clinical, financial, and human resources and patient outcome information are factors that will in-

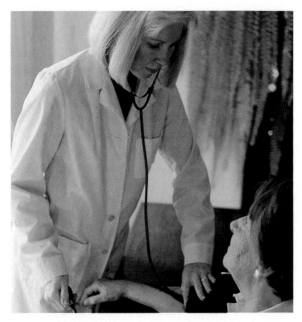

Visiting nurse associations provide follow-up care at home for many.

fluence the organizational design of the home care agency.

Subacute Facility

Because hospitals are discharging patients so quickly, a new kind of facility—the subacute facility—is emerging. Many of these new facilities are just old-style nursing homes refurbished with the high-tech equipment necessary to deal with patients who have just come out of surgery or who are still acutely ill and have complex medical needs. Others are newly built centers or new businesses that have taken over hospitals that were shut down in the merger mania of recent years.

Hospice

Hospices can be located on inpatient nursing units, such as the kind commonly found in Canada, the United Kingdom, and Australia, or in the home or residential centers in the community. The concept of hospice or palliative care was launched at St. Christopher Hospice in London. Hospices focus on confirming rather than denying the reality of death and thus provide care that ensures dignity and comfort.

Supportive and Ancillary Organizations

Organizations involved in the direct provision of healthcare are supported by a number of other organizations whose operations have a significant effect on provider organizations, as well as on the overall performance of the health system. These organizations include regulatory and planning organizations, third-party financing organizations, pharmaceutical and medical equipment supply corporations, and various educational and training organizations.

■ *Exercise 6–4*

Identify supportive and ancillary organizations operating in your community. Can you determine whether nurses are playing roles in those organizations and what functions are incorporated into existing nursing roles?

Regulatory and Planning Organizations

Regulatory and planning organizations set standards for the operation of healthcare organizations, ensure compliance with federal and state regulations developed by governmental administrative agencies, and investigate and make judgments regarding complaints brought by consumers of the services and the public. They are responsible for approving organizations for licensure. Compliance with established standards is necessary for authorization to receive Medicare and Medicaid funding from both state and federal governments. Public agencies sometimes approve private organizations as surveyors for compliance based on their ability to meet certain criteria. Nursing leaders have played active roles in establishing standards and ensuring that organizations comply with standards both in their roles as members of healthcare organizations providing direct and indirect services to patients and as members of, or advisors to, regulatory agencies.

In addition to roles of approving organizations to function as providers of care and to receive public funds for their services, regulatory and planning agencies influence decisions regarding capital construction, cost and charges for service, personnel standards, quality of services, and working conditions (among other things).

Peer-review organizations (PROs) are mandated by federal regulation to be organized in each state for the purpose of monitoring hospital service use and the quality of care received by Medicare patients. These organizations, like all others, are in a continuous state of evolutionary transformation brought about by the changing needs related to healthcare delivery. Nurses have played key roles in developing, implementing, and evaluating the review processes of these regulatory agencies.

Third-Party Financing Organizations

Organizations that provide for financing healthcare comprise another subset of supportive and ancillary organizations. The government, through the Centers for Medicare/Medicaid Services (CMS) (formerly the Health Care Financing Administration [HCFA]), finances a large portion of the population and represents the largest third-party organization involved in healthcare provision.

Private health insurance carriers, who account for most of the remaining financing, are composed of not-for-profit and for-profit components. Blue Cross and Blue Shield are examples of the not-for-profit components. The Blues have led the move of insurers from fee-for-service insurance to managed care. This has been both a cost-reduction mechanism and a marketing response to the managed care concept introduced by HMOs and the arrange-

ments discussed previously in relation to physician practice agreements. Commercial insurance companies represent the private sector.

Third-party financing organizations have major effects both on the actual delivery of healthcare and on shaping that delivery through political influence. Proposals of a single national payer system and of group insurance purchase by consumer-constituted health alliances are changes under consideration for these organizations. These proposals are generated by the constantly escalating percentage of the gross national product (GNP) that is devoted to healthcare costs and the increasing percentage of the population that is uninsured. Reconfiguration of the third-party payer system and its organizations will in turn bring about restructuring of healthcare organizations responsible for service delivery. An understanding of the interrelated changes in healthcare organizations can be gained by examining the results of the 1982 enactment by Congress of the Tax Equity and Fiscal Reimbursement Act (TEFRA), which introduced the prospective payment system for Medicare reimbursement. One of the results was the rapid development of home care organizations in response to the early discharges engendered by the system's financial incentives and the institution of financial penalties if patients had to be readmitted within certain time periods.

Pharmaceutical and Medical Equipment Supply Systems

About one tenth of all healthcare expenditures is allocated to drugs and medical equipment, and this is increasing. When other healthcare supply organizations, such as healthcare information system corporations, are considered, the estimated percentage may rapidly escalate toward the one-quarter mark. Nurses, as primary users of these products, play a significant role in healthcare organizations in setting standards for safe and efficient products that meet both consumers' and organizations' needs in a cost-effective manner. Supply organizations often seek nurses as customers and as participants in market surveys for the design of new products, services, and marketing techniques. Nurses are employed by these organizations as designers of new products, marketing representatives, and members of the sales and research staffs. Examples of the roles nurses play can be seen by studying organizations that employ nurses to design new products and market them through production and distribution of a newsletter and ongoing continuing-education presentations.

Professional Organizations

Professional organizations have the primary purposes to protect and enhance the interests of the service delivery organizations and their disciplines. These organizations, because of their tremendous influence on the healthcare delivery system, must be considered in any discussion of healthcare organizations. Professional organizations operate at the local, state, and national levels and perform a number of functions, including protection and support through political lobbying; education; and the development and maintenance of standards for caregivers, resources, environment, and care. Examples of these are the American Nurses Association, the American Medical Association, and the American Hospital Association. In addition to the professional organizations, labor organizations representing healthcare organization employees also play an increasing role in healthcare organization development.

FORCES THAT INFLUENCE HEALTHCARE ORGANIZATION DEVELOPMENT

The radical restructuring of the healthcare system that is required to reduce the continuing escalation of economic resources into the system and to make healthcare accessible to all citizens will necessitate ongoing changes in healthcare organizations. Healthcare organizations, functioning as corporate actors, are a major repository of power within the healthcare system. As previously discussed, healthcare expenditures represent a significant percentage of the GNP, and as federal and state governments continue to be major purchasers of care, the influence of healthcare corporate actors will increase. Healthcare expenditure is also a major portion of the budgets in countries with nationalized healthcare approaches. Demonstration of professional nursing organizations' ability to influence their environment has been shown by the many points from Nursing's Agenda for Health Care Reform (American Nurses Association, 1991) included in the President's Health Security Plan (1993). Economic, social, and demographic factors provide the input for future development and act as the major forces driving the evolution of healthcare organizations.

Economic Factors

The complexity of controlling costs is currently and will remain a major issue driving development of the healthcare system. Perhaps the most immediate change will be in the increasing direct involvement of industrial corporations as healthcare costs rise and as the financing of mandated employee benefit programs remains a major concern. This involvement is presently taking the form of initiating audits of employee healthcare use and designing benefits packages to control use. A form of a benefit package, previously referred to in the discussion of third-party insurers, is managed care, which uses specific standards for approving diagnostic testing, medical treatment, and technological interventions and duration of use of inpatient and community service. Another form of control of healthcare organization services is the development of local coalitions consisting of community health providers, consumers, and corporations, acting to unify business initiatives in healthcare cost containment and to provide consumers with input into health planning and policy development. Wellness programs designed to modify consumers' use of and demand for services such as health-promotion campaigns, ergonomic programs to reduce work-related injuries such as carpal tunnel syndrome, and fitness and exercise programs are other industrial corporate initiatives being introduced to reduce costs. Again, nurses are playing key roles in managed care and in organizing and directing wellness programs.

There are many implications for the economy related to nurses in healthcare organizations. Development of strategies that allow patients to become empowered controllers of their own health status is primary among these. Responsive structural changes in service delivery will be needed to maintain congruence with new missions and philosophies developed in response to changes. Continuous evaluation will be needed to assess cost and quality outcomes related to change. Continuous focus on quality care and access to care will be required so that bottom-line costs do not overshadow quality care provisions. Nurses have a major role to play in demonstrating that access to care and quality management are essential components of cost control. With the increasing involvement of industry, business management techniques will assume greater emphasis in healthcare organizations. Nurse leaders and managers will need to go beyond obtaining education in business techniques to gaining skill in adapting that knowledge to meet the specific needs of delivery of cost-effective, quality care.

Social Factors

Increasing consumer attention to disease prevention and promotion of healthful lifestyles is redefining relationships of healthcare organizations and their patients. Patients are becoming increasingly active in care planning, implementation, and evaluations and are seeking increased participation with their providers. Nursing's history of work with the development of patient-centered interactive strategies places nurses in a position to assume leadership roles in this area of organizational development.

Demands will be made of healthcare organizations for more personal, responsive, and coordinated care. Leadership will need to be taken by nurses to redesign roles and restructure healthcare organizations' departments.

Demographic Factors

Resources of geographic regions, such as regional employment status, incomes of the population, and age of the country's population, are chief among the demographic factors influencing the design of healthcare organizations.

Economic and demographic characteristics of many rural communities result in a larger number of uninsured and underinsured citizens in rural areas (President's Health Security Plan, 1993). Geographic isolation often limits access to necessary health services and impedes recruitment of healthcare personnel. Community-based rural health networks that provide primary care links to urban health centers for teaching, consultation, personnel sharing, and the provision of high-tech services are one solution to meeting needs in rural areas. Federal and state funding, which includes incentives for healthcare personnel to work in rural areas, is another approach. Strategic planning by nursing is critical to address community needs.

The largest influence exerted on healthcare organizations comes from the aging of the population. By the year 2025, more than 18% of the population is expected to be older than 65 years of age. The numbers of "the old-old," those older than 80, are increasing dramatically. Although this segment of the population does not necessarily have dependency needs, a need exists for more long-term beds, supportive housing, and community programs. To meet these emerging needs of el-

derly persons, new healthcare organizations will continue to evolve, be evaluated, and be restructured based on findings. New roles for nurses as leaders and managers of elderly care are evolving, such as the roles being played by advanced nurse practitioners in directing the care of patients who have become members of geriatric care organizations such as retirement centers.

Another major effect on the system will come from the increasing number of poor people who are able to afford care to meet only their most basic needs—if that. Without a broad array of basic healthcare services, failure to treat a minor problem, such as high blood pressure, results in a high-cost illness such as a cerebrovascular accident. This lack of healthcare provision is compounded by the number of people excluded from coverage due to preexisting health conditions and job loss. Means of financing care will change as partial solutions to these problems; those changes will affect existing healthcare organizations.

A SYSTEMS THEORETICAL PERSPECTIVE

Systems theory produces a model that explains the process of healthcare organization evolution (Figure 6-1). Systems theory presents an explanation of organizational evolution that is similar to biological evolution. This theory sees organizations as sets of interdependent parts that together form a whole (Thompson, 1967). The survival of the organization, as portrayed throughout this chapter, is dependent on its evolutionary response to changing environmental forces; it is seen as an open system. The response to environmental changes brings about internal changes (see Chapter 9), which produce changes that alter environmental conditions. The changes in the environment, in turn, act to bring about changes in the internal operating conditions of the organization.

A very simplified example of this can be seen by again studying the implementation of the prospective payment system that was caused by the economic driving force of escalating healthcare costs. Ambulatory surgery, same-day admissions, and hospital- and community-based home care organizations are some of the internal healthcare organization changes caused by this environmentally driven policy change, which put a cap on reimbursing

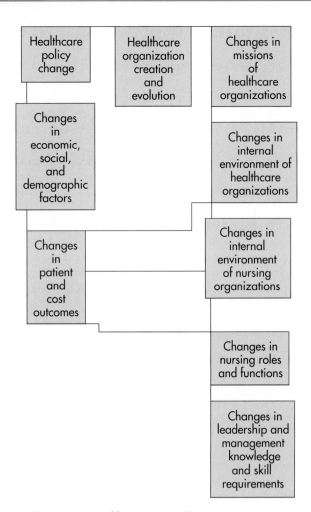

Figure 6-1   Healthcare organizations as open systems.

Exercise 6–5
Think about the changes you can quickly identify in your community. How will they influence healthcare organizations?

NURSING ROLE AND FUNCTION CHANGES

The implications for the increasing leadership and management skills and knowledge that nurses will need are clear in the evolving development of healthcare organizations. Nurses are responsible for providing a continuum of individualized care based on patient need, and they must make efforts to increase their economic viability and influence in designing and implementing healthcare policy. The decision by Ontario, Canada, to require a baccalaureate degree in nursing by 2005 will influence the preparation of the registered nurse population because of the expectation that leadership and management content will be required.

Leadership and management roles for nursing are proliferating in the changing healthcare organizations that are developing in response to environmental driving forces. The proportion of nursing jobs in the community is increasing. Nurses need new knowledge and skills to coordinate the care of patients with the many disciplines and organizational units that are providing the continuum of care. Nurses who can engage in the political process of policy development, coordinate care across disciplines and settings, use conflict management techniques to create win-win situations for patients and providers in resolving the healthcare system's delivery problems, and use business savvy to market and prepare financial plans for the delivery of cost-effective care are needed.

Because healthcare organizations function as open systems, nurses must be continuously alert to assessing both the internal and external environment for the forces that act as inputs to changes needed in healthcare organizations and for the effects of changes that are made. Awareness of the changing statuses of healthcare organizations and ability to play a leading role in creating and evaluating adaptation in response to changing forces will be a central function of nurse leaders and managers in healthcare organizations. Nurses will need to develop a foundation of leadership and management knowledge that they can build on through a planned program of continuing education.

expenses incurred by hospitalized patients. These internal organizational developments placed pressure on the external environment to create mechanisms to respond to increasing percentages of the population with self-care deficits who were returning to the community.

This open systems approach to organizational development and effectiveness emphasizes a continual process of adaptation of healthcare organizations to external driving forces and a response to the adaptations by the external environment, which generates continuing inputs for further healthcare organization development. This open system is in contrast to a closed system approach that views a system as being sufficient unto itself. The effects of external forces on internal structures of healthcare organizations are discussed in Chapter 9.

The Solution

I contacted the hospital case manager, who arranged for this patient to have access to special programs in the hospital to fund the medications and support the case management expenses. We arranged for the patient to be seen by a state agency that provides emergency funds for utilities and phone service and assisted him with a Medicaid application with a request for a retroactive initiation date. Finally, we contacted Hospice and the American Cancer Society to support the tube feeding expenses and worked with other agencies to delay billings until Medicaid was available. Clearly, today's nurse manager has to be connected with the extended resources in the community to ensure care for patients who require assistance.

— Beth A. Smith

 Would this be a suitable approach for you? Why?

CHAPTER CHECKLIST

Knowledge of types of healthcare organizations and characteristics used to differentiate healthcare organizations provides a foundation for examining the operation of the healthcare system. Understanding the economic, social, and demographic forces driving changes in healthcare organizations identifies needs that organizations must be designed to fit. A recognition that alterations in the environment and in healthcare organizations are mutually interactive is necessary to determine the effects of change and the steps that need to be taken in response to the constant changes. Changes in nursing roles and the settings in which nurses provide service are changing the leadership and management knowledge and skills that nurses need. These changes are part of a continual evolution that demands a foundation in leadership and management knowledge that serves as a basis for future development.

- Key characteristics that differentiate types of healthcare organizations are as follows:
  - For-profit or not-for-profit status
  - Public or private ownership
  - Teaching status
  - Geographic location
  - Clinical services provided
  - Number and types of units operated
  - Relationship with a healthcare network
- Major types of healthcare organizations are as follows:
  - Acute care facilities
  - Ambulatory-based facilities
  - Community-based facilities

- Third-party payers (insurers)
  - Regulatory and planning agencies
  - Pharmaceutical and medical equipment suppliers
  - Professional organizations
- Economic forces driving the development of healthcare organizations are numerous and are continually evolving, escalating the percentage of the GNP comprised of healthcare costs.
- Social forces driving development of healthcare organizations include the following:
  - A focus of society that is changing from illness to health (wellness)
  - An increasing demand by individuals that they participate in designing their own customized care plans
- Demographic forces driving development of healthcare organizations include the following:
  - The increasing percentage of society that is composed of elderly individuals
  - An increasing percentage of poor people who do not have the financial resources to have access to care
  - The inability of isolated rural areas to provide ready and economical access to needed health services
- Implications of healthcare organization evolution for leadership and management role functions of professional nurses include the following:
  - An increased ability to attune to the altered environmental driving forces that predict and direct necessary changes in healthcare organizations
  - An increased ability to attune to the healthcare organization's internal environment to predict and direct changes required in both the internal and external environment

Continued

CHAPTER CHECKLIST—cont'd

- Knowledge and skill both in influencing the development of and in developing healthcare policy at the federal, state, local, and organizational levels
- Knowledge and skill in coordinating and collaborating with peers and other disciplines providing services within a point of service and in networks created by the interconnection of many points of service
- Skill in using business knowledge in planning and evaluating delivery of healthcare in healthcare organizations that must market cost and outcome effectiveness to survive
- Knowledge and skill in planning and directing group work, which promotes optimal health statuses with minimal use of personnel and material resources

TIPS ON HEALTHCARE ORGANIZATIONS

- Knowledge of economic, social, and demographic changes is essential to redesigning healthcare organizations to meet society's needs.

- Consolidation of healthcare services into large networks that will provide all levels of care necessitates the development of communication systems that provide information on patients receiving services at the various points of care in the network.
- Diversified positions will be available for professional nurses in the various organizations that are developing to enhance the provision of care.
- New configurations of healthcare delivery will demand that professional nurses continually develop new knowledge in leadership and management.

TERMS TO KNOW

consolidated systems	private
fee-for-service	public
managed care	secondary care
networks	teaching institution
not for profit	tertiary care
primary care	third-party payers

REFERENCES

American Nurses Association. (1991). *Nursing's Agenda for Health Care Reform*. Washington, DC: Author.

Baker, C. M., Messmer, P. L., Gyurko, C. C., Domagala, S. E., Conly, F. M., Eads, T. S., Harshman, K. S., & Layne, M. K. (2000). Hospital ownership, performance, and outcomes: Assessing the state-of-the-science. *Journal of Nursing Administration, 30*(5), 227-240.

Barry-Walker, J. (2000). The impact of systems redesign on staff, patient, and financial outcomes. *Journal of Nursing Administration, 30,* 77-89.

Diania, N., Allen, M., Baker, K., Cartledge, T., Gwyer, D., Harris, S., et al. (1997). Merger motorway: Giving staff the tools to reengineer. *Nursing Management, 28*(3), 42-47.

Garry, R. J. (2000). Benchmarking: a prescription for healthcare. *Journal of Nursing Administration, 30,* 397-398.

Murphy, B. (Ed.). (1995). *Nursing centers: The time is now* (Pub. No. 41-2629). New York: National League For Nursing Press.

President's health security plan. (1993). New York: Random House.

Thompson, J. D. (1967). *Organization in action.* New York: McGraw-Hill.

SUGGESTED READINGS

Brzytwa, E., Copeland, L., & Hewson, M. (2000). Managed care education: A needs assessment of employers and educators of nurses. *Journal of Nursing Education, 39,* 197-204.

Cummings, K., & Abell, R. (1993). Losing sight of the shore: How a future integrated health care organization might look. *Health Care Management Review, 18*(2), 39-51.

Etheridge, P. (1997). The Carondelet experience. *Nursing Management, 28*(3), 26-28.

Glick, D., Hale, P., Kulbok, P., & Shettig, J. (1996). Community development theory: Planning a community nursing center. *Journal of Nursing Administration, 20*(7/8), 44-50.

Jeska, S., & Rounds, R. (1996). Addressing the human side of change: Career development and renewal. *Nursing Economics, 14*(6), 339-345.

Kast, F. E., & Rosenweiz, J. E. (1991). General systems theory: Applications for organizations and management. In M. J. Ward & S. A. Price (Eds.), *Issues in nursing administration: Selected readings* (pp. 60-73). St. Louis: Mosby.

Kellar, N., Martinez, J., Finis, N., Bolger, A., & VonGunter, C. F. (1996). Characteristics of an acute inpatient hospice palliative care unit in a U.S. teaching hospital. *Journal of Nursing Administration, 26*(3), 16-20.

Kerikes, J., Jenkins, M. L., & Torrisi, D. (1990). Nurse managed primary care. *Nursing Management, 28*(3), 44-48.

Mark, B. A., Sayler, J., & Smith, C. (1997). A theoretical model for nursing systems outcomes research. *Nursing Administration Quarterly, 20*(4), 12-27.

Nakamura, P. (1997, March 16). Parish nursing on the rise: A growing movement responds to the need of people for wellness. *The Living Church,* pp. 14-16.

Porter-O'Grady, T. (1996). The seven basic rules for successful redesign. *Journal of Nursing Administration, 26*(1), 46-55.

Shindul-Rothchild, J., & Duffy, M. (1996). The impact of restructuring and work design on nursing practice and patient care. *Best Practices and Benchmarking in Healthcare, 1,* 271-282.

Simms, L. M., Price, S. A., & Ervin, N. E. (2000). *Professional practice of nursing administration* (3rd ed.). Albany, NY: Delmar.

Stulginsky, M. M. (1993). Nurses' home health experiences. *Nursing and Health Care, 14,* 402-407.

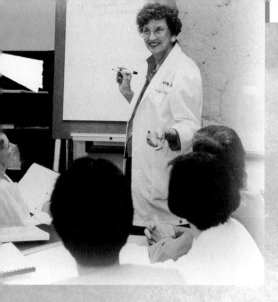

7

Strategic Planning, Goal Setting, and Marketing

Darlene Steven

his chapter discusses the application of several organizational elements of planning for the future, such as the strategic planning process, goal setting, management by objectives, and marketing. Examples of planning and marketing strategies used in the healthcare field are presented when appropriate.

Objectives

- Describe the importance of environmental assessment.
- Explain the planning process.
- Outline the purpose of a mission statement, a philosophy, goals, and objectives.
- Describe goal setting and strategic planning.

- Describe the process of strategic planning in establishing an entrepreneurial business in the healthcare field.

- Explain the importance of marketing plans in the healthcare field.

Questions to Consider

- *How is the strategic plan used to implement change in an organization?*
- *How do the mission statement, philosophy, goals, and objectives merge with the strategic plan of the facility?*
- *How can you influence the direction of your organization by effective planning?*
- *If you had a "vision" of where your facility should be directed in the future, how would you go about making your vision a reality?*

The Challenge

Tim Porter-O'Grady, RN, PhD, FAAN
Senior Partner, Tim Porter-O'Grady Associates, Inc., and Associate Professor, Emory University, Atlanta, Georgia

As the nurse manager on the medical surgical unit, I was dealing with an unmotivated and "burned out" staff. They could only complain about the workload and the increasing demands the organization was placing on their shoulders. They felt no one cared and that things were out of control. The staff believed that management was making decisions about their work and lives and they had no role to play in it. I had done everything I could to motivate them but found they still complained and exhibited no accountability for what was happening. I sensed the staff felt impotent and passive.

 What do you think you would do if you were this nurse?

INTRODUCTION

The present healthcare system is in a state of change. The pressure to contain costs in healthcare has resulted in major reforms. Restructuring of our healthcare system includes patient empowerment; comprehensive and coordinated service delivery; efficient and effective use of resources, manpower, and technology; and emphasis on health promotion and prevention. The demographics of our society are also in a state of change and include a dramatic increase in the elderly population.

Nurses have the opportunity to make a difference by planning new strategies for the future and by influencing the direction of healthcare. As nurses, our new paradigm shift is about embracing technology. We must be proactive in our use of it so that we may become active in its development. Only by fearlessly adopting and using new technologies can we garner the expertise and earn the credibility to serve as advisors, directors, and influencers of technology. Only by influencing technology can we ensure that it will be used to meet nursing's information needs, advance nursing practice, and realistically ensure nursing's continued viability. In short, where twenty-first century technology is concerned, it is embraced or replaced (Simpson, 1999).

Proactive simply means "aggressive planning," which provides direction for one's efforts and toward which others must then react. Thus greater control is possible so that the preferred future becomes a probability, not just a possibility. The importance of proactive, thoughtful, deliberate planning in the face of uncertainties cannot be overstated. Wilkinson (1988) offers this insight: "An employee in an organization, manager, supervisor or an [employee] who

has no clearly defined, benefit-oriented, attainable, measurable objectives is like a ship without a compass or a chart. Such people do not know where they are going, where they should be going, at what rate, at what cost, in what control. They are not managing their working lives or helping others to manage theirs" (p. 6).

In this chapter the strategic planning process is described. Planning is followed by an introduction to goal setting and management by objectives. The key concepts of marketing as it relates to the healthcare industry are discussed. When appropriate and feasible, examples of planning and marketing strategies used in the healthcare field are presented as case studies.

STRATEGIC PLANNING

Definition

Strategic planning is a process that is designed to encompass the organization's emphasis on mission statements, strategic action plans, changes in policies and procedures, environmental factors affecting the organization, and the development of new services.

The strategic planning process shown in Figure 7-1 consists of the following series of steps:

- Search of the environment to determine those forces or changes that may affect the work of the organization or that may be crucial to its survival
- Appraisal of the organization's strengths and weaknesses and its potential for dealing with change

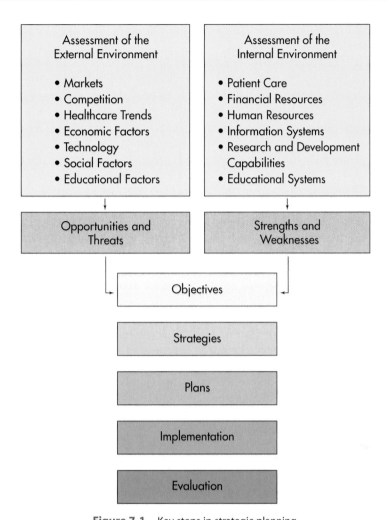

Figure 7-1   Key steps in strategic planning.

- Appraisal of the major opportunities and threats in the environment
- Identification and evaluation of the various strategies available to the organization to meet these opportunities and threats
- Selection of the best option that balances the organization's potential with the challenges of changing conditions, taking into account the values of its management and its social responsibilities
- Preparation of the strategy
- Implementation and evaluation of the strategy

Reasons for Planning

To survive the ongoing change and restructuring of the healthcare system, thoughtful and deliberate planning becomes a necessity. This process leads to success in the achievement of goals and objectives, gives meaning to work life, and provides direction for operational activities of the organization.

Furthermore, planning may result in efficient and effective use of resources and may assist in the formulation of visionary activities and the future direction of the agency. There are numerous reasons why nursing administrators should plan in a systematic manner: Knowledge regarding philosophy, goals, and external and internal operations of the organization are necessary; an understanding of the planning process is essential; and time must be divided on day-to-day operations rather than on short- and long-range plans.

Phases of the Strategic Planning Process

The strategic planning process is proactive, vision-directed, action-oriented, creative, innovative, and oriented toward change. "Healthcare providers increasingly are relying on strategic planning to guide the allocation of capital and other resources. Strategic planning helps identify and prioritize opportunities for financial improvement, particularly revenue-generating initiatives, which offer the greatest opportunities for significant long-term benefits" (Zuckerman, 2000, p. 54).

The term *strategic planning process* usually entails the development of a plan of action covering 3 to 5 years. The initial phase is the most difficult.

Phase 1: Assessment of the External and Internal Environment

External Environmental Assessment. Assessment of the external environment is the initial phase in the strategic planning process. The economic, demographic, technological, social, educational, and political factors are assessed in terms of their impact on opportunities and threats within the environment. Healthcare managers can assess the effect of competitors on their environment and thus plan and monitor their own operations and develop other creative and visionary programs. An example follows.

A rural northern community is undertaking a study to examine accessibility, availability, quality, and effectiveness of primary, secondary, and tertiary cardiac and cancer services provided to patients. One of the initial steps is to conduct an environmental scan. The factors taken into consideration include the following:

- Economic forces and the escalating rates of healthcare costs
- The numbers and types of health professionals, including shortages of adequately trained cardiologists, radiologists, physicists, internists, and family physicians
- Shortages of nurse practitioners, nurses, radiation therapists, and technicians
- The social, political, and regulatory forces, including strategic priorities of the government in health promotion and disease prevention
- The diagnostic services available, including magnetic resonance imaging (MRI) and nuclear diagnostic imaging
- Therapeutic capabilities (gene therapy, chemotherapy, radiation therapy, chelation, and laser therapy)
- Patient trends
- Demographic and population trends (population, employment, socioeconomic indicators, education, ethnicity, and lifestyle issues, with particular emphasis on minority groups)
- Trends in healthcare (increased emphasis on wellness programs and enhanced technologies)

Through a process of participatory research, the investigators plan to undertake "town hall" meetings so that residents can give thoughtful deliberation to the services that exist and provide visionary ideas for services in the future.

Exercise 7–1

What is your opinion about the economic situation in the city in which you live? What are the demographics of the area? What are the educational resources?

Internal Environmental Assessment. The internal assessment of the environment includes a review of the effectiveness of the structure, size, programs, financial resources, human resources, information systems, and research and development capabilities of the organization. The management team involves all levels of staff in this process and focuses on the purpose of the organization; the mission; the capabilities, skills, and relationships of various professional and related staff; and the weaknesses and strength of staff in such areas as leadership, planning, coordination, research, and staff development.

Phase 2: Review of Mission Statement, Philosophy, Goals, and Objectives

Mission Statement. A mission statement reflects the purpose and direction of the healthcare agency or a department within it. A statement of philosophy provides direction for the agency and/or department within it. The content usually specifies beliefs regarding the rights of individuals, beliefs regarding health and nursing, expectations of practitioners, and commitment of the organization to professionalism, education, evaluation, and research. The importance of the mission statement cannot be overstated, yet it is questionable how many individuals in an organization, when questioned directly, could enunciate the key points in the mission statement or the philosophy of a healthcare setting.

Covey (1990) relates that the mission statement is vital to the success of an organization. He believes that everyone should participate in the development of the mission statement: "The involvement process is as important as the written product and is the key to its use" (p. 139).

Covey relates the belief system of IBM: the dignity of the individual, excellence, and service. Everyone in IBM is committed to these values. This illustration of a mission statement is worthy of further consideration by healthcare agencies. "An organizational mission statement, one that truly reflects the deep shared vision and values of everyone within that organization, creates a unity and tremendous commitment" (p. 143).

Exercise 7-2

Select a clinical organization with which you have been affiliated. How effective is the structure? (Does the organization operate effectively and efficiently?) What overall human resources are present (e.g., various titles and numbers of people)? What information systems are used? Now apply these questions to the nursing component only.

An example of a mission statement of a newly developed community congestive heart failure program is to provide quality, patient-centered, and integrated care, utilizing the primary healthcare model, to people with congestive heart failure.

Goal Setting. Goal setting is the process of developing, negotiating, and formalizing the targets or objectives of an organization.

The community congestive heart failure program has six goals:

1. Provide comprehensive patient/family education through inpatient and outpatient programs.
2. Develop protocols for standardized patient care programs in terms of diet, exercise, smoking cessation, and other aspects of prevention and control.
3. Provide a multidisciplinary approach to patient care through the use of physicians, nurse practitioners, nurses, social workers, psychologists, physical and occupational therapists, dietitians, home care personnel, and pastoral care.
4. Enhance community support programs.
5. Develop telemetry and telemedicine programs in northern and remote communities.
6. Ensure that current information and services are available to patients on websites.

Exercise 7-3

Review a healthcare organization's mission statement. Tell a colleague in your own words what the statement means in general; then give specific examples of how it translates to nursing.

Practical insights from these studies that are important to nurse administrators are that specific goals are more likely to lead to higher performance than are vague or very general goals, such as "do your best." Feedback, or knowledge of results, is likely to motivate individuals toward higher performance levels and commitment to the achievement of goals.

Three key steps in implementing a goal-setting program are as follows:

1. Set goals that are specific and adhere to a deadline.
2. Promote goal commitment by providing instructions and support to employees and managers.
3. Support the achievement of goals with appropriate feedback as soon as possible.

Objectives. The ability to write clear and concise objectives is an important aspect of nursing administration. Characteristics of well-written objectives include the following:

1. The objective statement is properly constructed.
   - It begins with the word *to* followed by an action verb.
   - It specifies a single result to be achieved.
   - It specifies a target date for its attainment.
2. The objective is measurable.
3. The objective can be easily understood by those required to attain it.
4. The objective conforms to SMART criteria: *s*pecific, *m*easurable, *a*chievable, *r*esult-oriented, and *t*ime bound (Bowen, 2000).

Phase 3: Identification of Strategies

The third phase of the strategic planning process involves identifying major issues, establishing goals, and developing strategies to meet the goals. Strategy "is a broad plan of action by which an organization intends to reach its objectives" (Sommers & Barnes, 2001, p. 59). All departmental managers are involved in this process and are responsible for preparing a detailed plan of action, which may include the following: development of short- and long-term objectives, formulation of annual department objectives, resource allocation, and preparation of the budget.

Phase 4: Implementation

In the fourth phase of the strategic plan, the specific plans for action are implemented in order of priority. This entails open communication with staff in regard to the priorities for the next year and subsequent periods, formulation of revised policies and procedures in regard to the changes, and formulation of area and individual objectives related to the plan. The specific plans to be focused on include market plans, program plans, operating plans and budget, and human resource plans.

Phase 5: Evaluation

At regular intervals the strategic plan is reviewed at all levels to determine whether the goals, objectives, and activities are on target. As stated previously, it is important to consider that objectives may change as a result of legislation, budget cutbacks, and change in structure or other environmental factors. Therefore optional activities may need to be adapted to the situation. For example, one agency was informed that there had to be a decrease in the budget of $500,000 over the next 6 months. The staff were involved in the development of creative methods for ensuring that the necessary changes occurred. Savings were realized with organizational restructuring, the elimination of nursing supervisor positions, and changes in medication administration to a unit dose system.

Exercise 7-4

You are a staff nurse at a public health department in a small rural town. The director of nursing has assigned you to work on a planning committee. The purpose of the committee is to devise long- and short-term departmental goals.

The population of the town is 25,000, and the chief industry is agriculture. It is estimated that 8000 more people will move there in the next 5 years; a majority will be immigrants from Asia and Mexico.

The health department currently has four full-time baccalaureate nurses, and the state has not approved additional funding for this year.

Considering the concepts of strategic planning you have just read, in what direction should this department consider moving over the next 5 years? Does the department have an adequate number and mix of staff to accommodate this growth? How will you determine between long-term and short-term plans? What additional information will your committee need to realistically plan for the next 5 months and the next 5 years?

An example of a strategic plan of action for the development of a community congestive heart failure program is available at the website for this text.

MARKETING

Marketing may be defined as the "activities designed to generate and facilitate exchanges intended to sat-

isfy human wants and needs" (Sommers & Barnes, 2001, p. 4). Social marketing emphasizes "nontangible products such as ideas, attitudes, and lifestyle changes, as opposed to the more tangible products and services that are the focus of business marketing" (Blair, 1995, p. 528). Social marketing is used in a number of health-promotion activities undertaken by nurses. The benefits of marketing include increased consumer satisfaction, improved resource attraction, and improved organizational efficiency. The underlying assumption is that marketing helps manage the exchange of goods and services in a more efficient manner (Hoffman, 1997, p. 67). Marketing principles have been used successfully in a number of community programs designed to decrease the risks of heart disease (diet, exercise, antismoking campaigns, and alcohol and drug use awareness). One particular program that has generated a great deal of interest from adolescents is the campaign addressing date rape and date rape drugs. A group of high school students wrote a play and presented it to students in their community. This was followed by a town hall session whereby the audience could have questions answered by a panel of experts on the subject. In addition, the health unit prepared posters and forwarded them to all schools in the area, and advertisements were posted in bus shelters and underground transit stations. A follow-up study is being conducted by the health unit to determine the effectiveness of the program in decreasing the incidence of date rape.

An example of a survey designed to assess the knowledge, attitudes, and beliefs and practices regarding breast and cervical cancer screening of selected ethnocultural groups is presented in the Research Perspective box.

Strategic Marketing Planning Process

The strategic marketing planning process is similar in nature to the strategic planning process and the nursing process. Figure 7-2 offers a comparative chart outlining the steps in the process.

The steps of the strategic marketing planning are as follows:

- Analyze the organizationwide mission, objectives, goals, and culture to which the marketing strategy must contribute.
- Assess organizational strengths and weaknesses to respond to threats and challenges presented by the external environment.
- Analyze the future environment the marketer is likely to face with respect to public served; com-

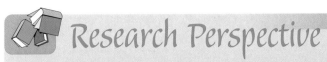
Research Perspective

Steven, D., Dhaliwal, H., Fitch, M., Choudhry, U., Clarke, E., Kirk-Gardner, R., Jamieson, J., Sevean, P., Stafford, J., Sellick, S., Woodbeck, H., & McPherson, D. (2002). Breast and cervical cancer screening: Knowledge, attitudes, beliefs and practices in selected ethno cultural groups in northwestern Ontario. Manuscript submitted for publication.

THE CONCEPTS OF RESEARCH

The objective of the project was to examine the knowledge, attitudes, beliefs, and practices regarding breast and cervical cancer screening of selected ethnocultural groups in a northern region.

SAMPLE SIZE

A convenience sample of 125 women aged 40 years and older who were of Italian, Ukrainian, Finnish, Ojibwa, and Oji-Cree descent was selected.

METHODOLOGY

An interview guide was designed specifically for this study. The interview guide contained information related to knowledge, attitudes, beliefs, and practices about breast self-examination (BSE), clinical breast examination (CBE), mammography, and cervical cancer screening procedures. A demographic data sheet was used to assess age, marital status, educational level, number of dependent children, and town of residence. A pilot study consisting of 25 women was conducted to determine the appropriateness of the tool.

FINDINGS

A comparison of groups regarding health-related behaviors was conducted. Aboriginal women were more likely to have ever smoked (77% compared with 40% or less in other groups). Most women exercised two times a week, and the exercise of choice was walking. The aboriginal women related that they consumed foods higher in fat and were more likely to add salt to food and had more

than four drinks per day. First Nations Women (aboriginal women in northwest Ontario, including those who live on and off reserves) were more likely than any other group to have not performed a BSE, have refused a BSE or mammogram, have not been told how to do a breast examination, have not received written information about BSE, and state they were uncomfortable and fearful about cervical cancer screening procedures (33% refused an internal examination compared with 0% to 8% in other ethnic groups).

IMPLICATIONS FOR PRACTICE

This study has tremendous implications for designing marketing strategies that are culturally sensitive and that take into consideration the literacy level of participants in any screening program. The researchers offer the following recommendations regarding education.

- Develop culturally sensitive health education programs and resources (pamphlets, videos, television, and media programs).
- Develop culturally appropriate written materials with consideration for literacy and visual appeal.
- Develop educational programs in the school system regarding the importance of screening, prevention, and early detection of breast and cervical cancer.
- Develop educational programs for healthcare professionals on cultural sensitivity regarding breast and cervical cancer screening for specific populations.

petition; and the social, political, technological, and economic environment.
- Determine the marketing mission, objectives, and specific goals for the relevant planning period.
- Formulate the core marketing strategy to achieve the specified goals.
- Implement the necessary organizational structure and the systems within the marketing function to

ensure proper follow-through of the designed strategy.
- Establish detailed programs and tactics to carry out the core strategy for the planning period, including a timetable of activities and the assignment of specific responsibilities.
- Establish benchmarks to measure interim and final achievements of the program.

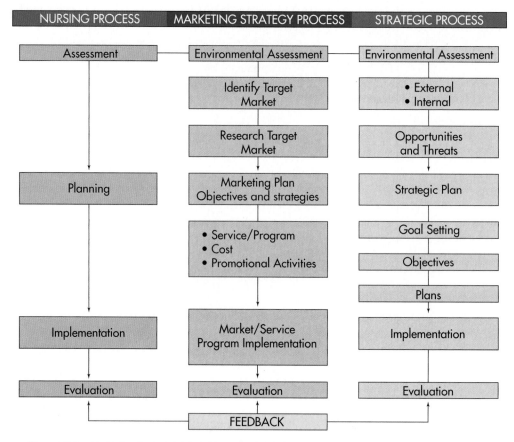

Figure 7-2 Marketing framework as compared with using the nursing process and strategic planning.

- Implement the planned program.
- Measure performance and adjust the core strategy, tactical details, or both as needed.

Assessment

Determining Organization-Level Missions, Objectives, and Goals

A marketing plan is developed by the top-level managers and advisory board to do the following:

1. Determine the organization-level long-term culture, mission, objectives, and goals.
2. Assess the organization's likely future external environment.
3. Assess the organization's present and potential strengths and weaknesses.

Analyzing Organizational Strengths and Weakness

During the marketing process an environmental assessment is conducted to identify and research the target market. An example of this is conducting a needs assessment of the services presently provided by an agency to develop new services or promotional activities to meet the needs of the population being served.

An audit may consist of interviews with key staff; review of documents; observation of staff; visits to competitors; and overview of advertisements, brochures, and other documents as deemed appropriate.

Analyzing External Threats and Opportunities

The three components of the external environment are (1) the public environment, which consists of groups and organizations that affect the organization (e.g., public, media, regulatory agencies); (2) the competitive environment, which consists of other organizations that vie for the attention and loyalty of clientele; and (3) the macroenvironment, consisting of demographic, economic, technological, political, and social forces to which the organization must adapt.

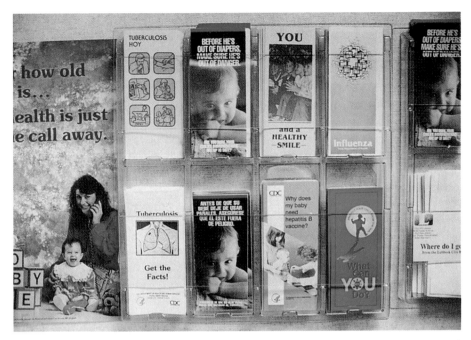

Pamphlets and brochures are promotional materials that inform clients about the benefits of a healthcare agency's programs and services.

Setting Marketing Mission, Objectives, and Goals

Kotler and Andreasen (1991) compared the essence of the development of a mission, objectives, and goals to financial management. The person who is managing an investment portfolio must decide whether to sell stocks or change from stocks to real estate. The same holds true for the marketing manager who "is constantly evaluating the portfolio against changing market conditions and changing performances of individual units" (p. 109).

Planning

The environmental assessment is followed by the development of a marketing plan. This plan outlines the service or program to be provided, includes a detailed budget-cost analysis, and describes the promotional activities designed to promote the program. "Predicting the future" is difficult in turbulent times. Forecasting allows the manager to plan for future and anticipated problems (Urban, Weinberg, & Hauser, 1996). The process requires several components:

- Assessment of the present situation
- Identification of strengths and weaknesses
- Outline of the driving forces in the environment
- Development of optional scenarios
- Identification of the preferred action
- Development of a plan of action
- Implementation of the plan of action
- Evaluation

In their article "Is Forecasting a Waste of Time?" Morrison and Metcalfe (1996) state that concerns about the usefulness of forecasts usually relate to concerns about accuracy. Forecasts should be estimates of how accurately a situation can be predicted, provide optional futures, be considered for their influence in convincing managers of the need for change, be a learning experience, be cost effective, and be used for their ritualistic purpose. Rather than using the "shooting at a target" metaphor, it may be more appropriate to consider forecasters as being like art teachers, helping line (and clinical) managers to paint updated pictures of their future. For example, in forecasting the number of patients who will need cardiac services in a community, a manager needs to consider an environmental scan, including factors related to mortality and morbidity; the fact that individuals are living longer as a result of medical, technological, and pharmaceutical interventions; and the effect of lifestyle and comorbidity. In the rural community described in the Research Perspective, diabetes is becoming more common among aboriginal people

BOX 7-1

Mission Statement, Goals, and Objectives of the Northwestern Ontario Breast Cancer Screening Program

Mission Statement

To reduce the leading cause of cancer deaths in women by delivering a comprehensive, organized, and evaluated breast cancer screening program for women between the ages of 50 and 69 years. In accordance with Ontario's health goals, the Cancer Care Ontario is committed to deliver a program that is sensitive to women's needs, builds on health-promoting behaviors, and fosters partnerships with interest groups in the community.

Overall Goal

To integrate health promotion strategies and medical practice to reduce mortality from breast cancer by 40% using breast screening of women aged 50 to 69 years.

Objectives

- To detect breast cancer earlier than would occur if organized screening were not available
- To develop and implement a community mobilization plan for the program
- To develop and implement a social marketing plan, including a health education component for the program
- To establish protocols and standards for healthcare professionals associated with the program
- To establish protocols for the interaction of the target population with the program
- To develop and implement training and technical assistance for those associated with the delivery of the program
- To develop a partnership with healthcare professionals that will facilitate program delivery
- To establish a regional breast screening service so that all women in the target population have equal access to breast screening
- To ensure that a minimum of 70% of women in the target population participate in screening every 2 years
- To document the follow-up of all women in whom an abnormality has been detected
- To provide screening that is sensitive and acceptable to the target population
- To evaluate the program on a continual basis, including needs assessment and measurement of process, economic, and outcome variables

because of hereditary and lifestyle changes; these changes could lead to an increased incidence of heart disease in the future. The community is developing culturally sensitive preventive programs for this population.

Implementation

The implementation phase includes the establishment of the program and promotional activities designed to communicate benefits of the service or program to patients. Forms of promotion may include media releases, brochures, pamphlets, newsletters, and "word-of-mouth" advertising.

Evaluation

The evaluation may incorporate satisfaction surveys, interviews with clients, and further research studies designed to assess reasons why clients are using or not using the service, program, or product. Feedback is an essential component of the marketing process.

Box 7-1 and Table 7-1 present steps in the strategic marketing planning process in relation to the delivery of breast cancer screening services to women in a widespread rural area of Ontario, Canada.

Nurses in all roles have rights and responsibilities relating to planning, goal setting, and marketing. Each of us has some sense of what is important today and sustainable for tomorrow in the context of our cultural perspective. Most of us sense the difference between fads and trends and how each affects us personally and professionally. Leaders are accountable for setting goals, including followers in those activities, and aligning tasks with the goals. Finally, each of us, as we represent our profession, organization, or community, are marketing each of those elements. We can contribute to formal marketing strategies through activities such as focus groups, or we can evaluate responses to marketing materials. Always, however, the focus should be on how what we are doing contributes to future quality.

Table 7-1   STRATEGIC PLAN OF ACTION FOR THE DEVELOPMENT, IMPLEMENTATION, AND EVALUATION OF A WOMAN'S HEALTH CENTER

Objective	Activities	Responsible Council	Time Frame
1. To develop a women's health center in a remote rural community	1.1 To conduct a needs assessment	Nurse practitioners	January 2004
	1.2 To conduct a literature review related to each of these topics: Women's health Entrepreneurship Programs related to women's health	Nurse practitioners and students	January 2004
	1.3 To form an advisory committee comprising community representatives to oversee the development and implementation of the center	Nurse practitioners	February 2004
	1.4 To develop the organizational structure, mission statement, philosophy, and objectives and revise accordingly	Nurse practitioners and advisory committee	February 2004
	1.5 To develop policy and procedure manuals for staff	Nurse practitioners	Ongoing
	1.6 To determine the business structure of the organization (i.e., legalities regarding partnerships, corporations, and proprietorship)	Nurse practitioners	Ongoing
	1.7 To develop a budget	Nurse practitioners	January 2004-ongoing
	1.8 To develop a business site for the organization: All renovations Office equipment Supplies Special healthcare equipment Filing and billing systems	Consultants and nurse practitioners	February 2004
	1.9 To develop a marketing program (newspapers, telephone, radio messages, signs, and direct mailings)	Nurse practitioners	February 2004-ongoing
2. To implement and evaluate the effectiveness and efficiency of these programs	2.1 To develop patient questionnaires related to satisfaction regarding care provided	Nurse practitioners	March 2004-ongoing
	2.2 To develop cost-effective analysis studies to evaluate each of the programs being provided	Nurse practitioners	Ongoing
	2.3 To collect and collate data related to utilization of services by clientele	Nurse practitioners	Ongoing

The Solution

I had read an article by a staff nurse from a large health center about forming a unit staff council that would be empowered to make decisions and solve problems. This council was totally led by the staff and its consultant/advisor.

I decided to get something like this started on my unit and undertook the following plan:

1. I copied the article for the staff, and I talked to the informal leaders about their interest in it. I had my staff talk with the staff at the successful health center about their experiences, which got this core staff excited about the possibilities.

2. I talked with the staff about what decisions they wanted to control and found that they were interested in self-scheduling, time and job sharing, clinical problem solving, and better time management. I set up a charter of authority with them and a process for getting together regularly to deal with their issues.

3. The staff set up a mechanism for getting everyone involved by rotating their tasks, processes, and decision-making responsibilities among the staff members. They determined that everyone on the staff would have to participate or move to another unit. They decided that this was the way they intended to "do their business."

4. I made sure that beginning issues were easy and resolvable, with measures of success built in. I cele-

brated the staff's successes with them no matter how small. As the staff got more confident and proficient, I introduced them to issues with more critical value and supported them with information, skill development, and good process.

5. As the staff became stronger and felt a higher level of ownership, I backed off and let them take more control and authority, and the council became an integral part of the unit's way of working. The staff had more authority, felt more autonomy, and had more control.

The result of this approach was a stronger investment of the staff in their own issues, a mechanism for managing their own issues, and a way to directly address problems they previously thought they had no control over. Energy and enthusiasm returned, a growing sense of maturity and accountability emerged, and other units and staff became intrigued enough with what was happening that they too wanted to establish similar approaches on their units. In many cases the staff became mentors and consultants to the efforts of other units in the system.

— Tim Porter-O'Grady

 Would this be a suitable approach for you? Why?

CHAPTER CHECKLIST

The effectiveness of any organization depends on its strategic planning. Nurse leaders/managers must be aware of the critical elements to facilitate the process. Setting goals and defining marketing strategies for product lines are part of the role professional nurses must perform to achieve effective organizational results in creating a niche in healthcare services.

- The planning process leads to success in the achievement of goals and objectives, gives meaning to work life, and provides direction for the organizational activities of the organization.
- Strategic planning is similar in nature to the nursing process and involves the following:
  - Assessment of the environment (internal and external)

  - Appraisal of the organization's strengths and weaknesses
  - Identification of the major opportunities and threats
  - Development of strategies to meet these opportunities
  - Implementation and evaluation of the strategy
- Marketing strategies will continue to play a vital role in healthcare settings as competition increases to provide services and programs to the public. Steps in the strategic marketing planning process are as follows:
  - Assessment
  - Planning
  - Implementation
  - Evaluation

- Nurses can play a pivotal role in the development of visionary programs and services that meet the needs of the population.

- Be clear about your role in the organization and its success.
- Think about what messages others need to hear about you and your services.

TIPS FOR PLANNING, GOAL SETTING, AND MARKETING

- Be clear about the organization's mission and vision.
- Read and listen to wide sources of data to determine what is happening and what trends could affect you and your organization.

TERMS TO KNOW

marketing
strategic planning

REFERENCES

Blair, J. (1995). Social marketing: Consumer focused health promotion. *AAOHN Journal, 43*(10), 527-531.

Bowen, J. (2000). The 4 P's of marketing. *Advisor's Edge, 3*(6), 38-40.

Covey, S. (1990). *The seven habits of highly effective people.* Toronto: Simon & Schuster.

Hoffman, S. (1997). Marketing professional services. *Journal of Professional Nursing, 13*(2), 67.

Kotler, P., & Andreasen, A. (1991). *Strategic marketing for nonprofit organizations.* Englewood Cliffs, NJ: Prentice Hall.

Morrison, M., & Metcalfe, M. (1996). Is forecasting a waste of time? *Journal of General Management, 22*(1), 28-34.

Simpson, R. (1999). Toward a new millennium: Outlook and obligations for 21st century health care technology. *Nursing Administration Quarterly, 24*(1), 94-97.

Sommers, M., & Barnes, J. (2001). *Fundamentals of marketing.* Boston: McGraw-Hill Ryerson.

Steven, D., Dhaliwal, H., Fitch, M., Choudhry, U., Clarke, E., Kirk-Gardner, R., Jamieson, J., Sevean, P., Stafford, J., Sellick, S., Woodbeck, H., & McPherson, D. (2002). Breast and cervical cancer screening: Knowledge, attitudes, beliefs and practices in selected ethno cultural groups in northwestern Ontario. Manuscript submitted for publication.

Urban, G., Weinberg, B., & Hauser, J. (1996). Premarket forecasting for really-new products. *Journal of Marketing, 60,* 47-60.

Wilkinson, R. (1988). Whether your face fits or not...it's the results that matter. *Supervision, 49*(12), 6-8.

Zuckerman, A. (2000). Leveraging strategic planning for improved financial performance. *Healthcare Financial Management, 54*(12), 54-57.

SUGGESTED READINGS

Achrol, R., & Kotler, P. (1999). Marketing in the network economy. *Journal of Marketing, 63*(Special Issue), 146-163.

American Organization of Nurse Executives. (1999). *Market-driven nursing: Developing and marketing patient care services.* San Francisco: Jossey-Bass.

Anderson, T. (2000) Strategic planning, autonomous actions and corporate performance. *Long Range Planning, 33,* 184-200.

Bagozzi, R., & Dholakia, U. (2000). Goal setting and goal striving in consumer behavior. *Journal of Marketing, 63*(Special Issue), 19-32.

Belt, J., & Bashore, E. (2000). Managed care strategic planning: The reality of uncertainty. *Healthcare Financial Management, 54*(5), 38-42.

Buzzell, R. (1999). Market functions and market evolution. *Journal of Marketing, 63*(Special Issue), 61-63.

Campbell-Hunt, C. (2000). What have we learned about generic competitive strategy? A meta-analysis. *Strategic Management Journal, 21,* 127-154.

Christensen, C., Bohmer, R., & Kenagy, J. (2000). Will disruptive innovations cure health care? *Harvard Business Review, 78*(5), 102-112.

Curtis, K. (1994). *From management goal setting to organizational results: Transforming strategies into action.* Westport, CT: Quorum Books.

Day, G. (1999). Creating a market driven organization. *Sloan Management Review, 41*(1), 11-22.

Day, G., & Montgomery, D. (1999). Charting new directions for marketing. *Journal of Marketing, 63*(Special issue), 3-13.

Durig, R. (2000). Strategic imperatives that will drive healthcare in a networked world. *Hospital Quarterly, 4*(1), 71-76.

Harris, I., & Ruefli, T. (2000). The strategy/structure debate: An examination of the performance implications. *Journal of Management Studies, 37*(4), 587-603.

Hendry, J. (2000). Strategic decision making, discourse, and strategy as social practice. *Journal of Management Studies, 37*(7), 955-977.

Kaplan, R., & Norton, D. (2000). Having trouble with your strategy? Then map it. *Harvard Business Review, 78*(5), 167-176.

Kenny, D., & Marshall, J. (2000). Contextual marketing. *Harvard Business Review, 78,* 119-125.

Liedtla, K. (2000). Strategic planning as a contributor to strategic change: A generative model. *European Management Model, 18*(2), 195-206.

McCarthy, K. (2000). Harmonizing health information initiatives: Review of INFOcus 2000. *HCIM & C 3rd Quarter, 14*(3), 36-37, 39.

Mullem, C., Burke, L., Dohmeyer, K., Farrell, M., Harvey, S., John, L., et al. (1999). Strategic planning for research use in nursing practice. *Journal of Nursing Administration, 29*(12), 38-45.

Oliver, R. (2000). A thousand year strategic plan. *Journal of Business Strategy, 21*(2), 7-9.

Pascal, W. (2000). Health care of the future: Vision 2020. Part II. *HCIM & C 3rd Quarter, 14*(3), 22-24.

Snyder-Halpern, R., & Chervany, N. (2000). A clinical information system strategic planning model for integrated health care delivery. *Journal of Nursing Administration, 30*(12), 583-591.

Sullivan, M., & Parisi, R. (1999). Strategic decision making on shifting sands. *Nursing Administration Quarterly, 23*(4), 75-80.

Vahey, D., Corser, W., & Brennan, P. (2001). Publicly available databases for administrative strategic planning. *Journal of Nursing Administration, 31*(1), 9-15.

Vitell, S., & Ho, F. (1997). Ethical decision making in marketing: A synthesis and evaluation of scales measuring the various components of decision-making in ethical situations. *Journal of Business Ethics, 16,* 699-717.

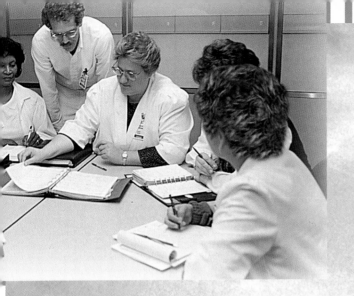

Chapter

8

Leading Change

Kristi D. Menix

This chapter describes the general nature of change in healthcare organizations. The theories and models, processes, responses, principles, and strategies typically involved in creating and leading change are discussed. The manager's primary role is that of change agent. This role includes responsibilities to anticipate, create, and manage the dynamic forces of change for desired outcomes and goal achievement. How to react to imposed change is part of that responsibility, but leading proactively to create change offers opportunities to better control outcomes. The effective change agent ensures staff empowerment to achieve change outcomes. The term change agent is used in this chapter to describe the nurse responsible and accountable for achieving a defined set of work outcomes through the efforts of an employee group. Change refers to an alteration in the work environment that is new or different from what existed previously. Change management refers to the overall processes and strategies used to moderate and manage the preparation for, effect of, responses to, and outcomes for conditions that are new and different from those that existed previously.

Objectives

- Analyze the general characteristics of change in open-system organizations.
- Relate the models of planned change to the process of low-level change.
- Relate nonlinear theories for managing high-level change.
- Evaluate the use of select functions, principles, and strategies for initiating and managing change.
- Formulate desirable qualities of effective change agents.

Questions to Consider

- *What are your beliefs about the benefits and disadvantages of change?*
- *What is your usual response to unexpected change? to deliberate, planned change? to sustained ambiguity in a change situation?*
- *Do you actively seek change to improve practice and management outcomes?*
- *What kinds of expertise and values do you possess that could facilitate change in a work setting?*
- *What strategies do you propose to support continuous learning?*

The Challenge

Joel Graeter, RN, BSN
Clinical Manager, East Texas Medical Center Specialty Hospital, Tyler, Texas

As a specialty hospital clinical manager accountable for the safe, quality care of acutely ill patients with multiple, complex, and long-term care needs and average lengths of stay of 30 to 32 days, I must simultaneously respond to constant administrative pressures to reduce operational costs. Recently, pay schedules for nurses changed hospitalwide. New pay incentives made it more appealing for nurses to work as much or as little (prn) as they wish with no benefits but at a higher hourly wage or as nurses contracted to the hospital through an agency at a high hourly wage. Full-time nurses, employees of the hospital, have benefits, but they earn less per hour than agency and prn nurses. Their services are available and more cost effective, so they are asked to work overtime and engage in other unit responsibilities. The challenge is to maintain appropriate staffing levels and mixes, as well as continuity of care, in the face of managing the dynamics of a nursing staff with varying commitment, values, and aptitudes. How could I manage this change and its forces effectively?

 What do you think you would do if you were this nurse?

INTRODUCTION

Change is a natural social process of individuals, groups, organizations, and society. The forces of change originate inside and outside healthcare organizations. Change today is constant, inevitable, pervasive, and unpredictable and varies in rate and intensity, which unavoidably influences individuals, technology, and systems at all levels of the organization.

Because most healthcare organizations operate as open systems, they are receptive to external and internal influences originating from a rapidly changing healthcare delivery system. Organization-wide change depends on the organization's stage of development, degree of flexibility, and history of response to change, as well as the maturity of its systems. The role of **change agents** is to lead change efforts through thinking that is systems and theory based, tolerant of ambiguity, and mindful of the whole picture. Thus the management of change in organizations requires moving from an emphasis on long-range planning and established goals to a greater focus on managing the dynamic forces in the **change situations** while moving toward a set of achievable outcomes. Balancing change in the long and short view is a key challenge today.

CONTEXT OF THE CHANGE ENVIRONMENT

The transformation of healthcare delivery is occurring rapidly, creating contextual alterations in change situations in such factors as time, information, decision making, and planning (Begun & White, 1995; Porter-O'Grady, 1997). Increased uncertainty challenges change agents to communicate differently and more extensively than is required with less complex change (DiFonzo & Bordia, 1998; Freeman, 1999; Geddes, Salyer, & Mark, 1999; McDaniel, 1998). Nursing entities, as open systems, need to begin viewing their work in less bureaucratic, inflexible ways and open themselves up to responding with flexibility and creativity to today's dynamic environment (Begun & White, 1995). The use of planned, linear change approaches for highly complex, accelerated, and unpredictable change situations may not be as effective as they are for low-level, **low-complexity change** in more stable environments (Nutt, 1992).

Nursing is a key component of healthcare delivery, a partner with multiple care providers, and a pivotal player in open systems organizations. "In order for the nursing profession to strategically adapt in a rapidly changing environment, it

BOX 8-1

Guidelines for Altering the Dominant Logic

DECREASE	INCREASE
Long-term forecasting	Short-term forecasting
Preplanned strategies	Emergent strategies
Emphasis on past successes	Search for new opportunities
One future vision	Multiple scenarios
Rigid, permanent structures	Self-organizing, temporary structures
Structural isolation in the workplace	Structural interdependence in the workplace
Stability of leadership	Leadership turnover
Standardization	Innovation, experimentation, diversity
Insulation from other professions and marketplace	Cooperation and competition
Marketplace "passivity"	Marketplace "aggression"
Expectation of job security	Self-learning

From Begun, J. W., & White, K. R. (1995). Altering nursing's dominant logic: Guidelines from complex adaptive systems theory. *Complexity and Chaos in Nursing, 2*(1), 10.

is important to consider its current 'dominant logic' as a source of structural inertia. A system's dominant logic is a screen that filters information deemed relevant by historical antecedents and by those analyzing the data" (Begun & White, 1995, p. 5). Using **chaos theory** components, Begun and White (1995) suggest that nursing in various areas is too stable and thus too unresponsive and unable to adapt to the influences of rapid change. They believe that nursing must change its entrenched, inflexible thinking and acting and its typical bureaucratic structures. Box 8-1 shows guidelines for altering the dominant logic. For example, because of environmental uncertainty and the need to be responsive, nursing leaders should avoid setting rigid goals. Instead they should envision several outcome scenarios to move toward within the context of the possibilities of changing circumstances (J.W. Begun, personal communication, July 8, 1997).

Planned change models, or linear approaches, can guide directional, more incremental, low-level, less complex changes, such as those needed to systematically reorganize the storage of unit supplies or to recommend a series of inservice offerings for nursing staff. High-level change, on the other hand, is characteristically more fluid and complex because of the interactions and activities of multiple players and influences across the organization. **Nonlinear** approaches are found in complexity/chaos and

learning organization theories. They offer helpful approaches for understanding dynamic, open-system healthcare organizations and for guiding change agents in managing accelerated, increasingly uncertain change environments (Menix, 2000, 2001). Change agents must primarily manage the forces of the change situation while considering several desired outcomes, potentially leading to more creative results (Begun & White, 1995; Wheatley, 1992).

PLANNED CHANGE USING LINEAR APPROACHES

Most **planned change** models—linear models—advocate that change can occur in a sequential and directional fashion when guided by effective change agents. Planned change models, such as those of Lewin (1947); Lippitt, Watson, and Westley (1958); and Havelock (1973), explain the nature of **change processes** and offer systematic problem-solving methods designed to achieve change. Rogers' (1995) innovation-decision model highlights individual change. The use of planned change can be useful for low-level change in more stable environments. Flexibility in implementing the plan and moderating the situational factors, as is advocated by nonlinear approaches, can improve the overall outcomes.

Lewin (1947) suggested that an analysis of change situations, which he termed *force field analysis,* includes early and ongoing assessment of **barriers** and **facilitators.** Barriers in change situations are factors that can hinder the change process; facilitators are factors that can expedite the process. These elements may originate with people, technology, structure, or values. For change to be effective, the force of facilitators must exceed the force of barriers; thus the work of change agents is to reduce the barriers in the situation and support the facilitators.

Lewin (1947) describes change as having three stages:

- Unfreezing
- Experiencing the change
- Refreezing

Unfreezing refers to the awareness of an opportunity, need, or problem for which some action is necessary; it also requires subsequent mental readiness to approach the issue. This phase may occur naturally as a progressive development, or it may result from a deliberate activity as a first step in planning a change. For example, when the current way of giving shift reports is ineffective, as evidenced by errors occurring in care delivery, the staff become aware of a problem and the need for change. As in The Challenge presented earlier, changes in nurses' pay schedules and their effects on staffing and scheduling brought about unfreezing for hospital leadership and all staff.

Exercise 8-1

Identify the facilitators and barriers in the following situation. Rate the potential strength of each in hindering or expediting attainment of the change. Use +5 for the highest positive strength toward change occurring and −5 for the greatest negative strength against the change:

Nursing administration wants the pediatric neurology unit to merge with the pediatric cardiac unit for improved care delivery and cost-effectiveness. Staff nurses and managers from both units—some enthusiastic, some reluctant—participate on the merger planning committee. The appointed chair is the organization's powerful personnel director. Administration wants a new facility to house the merged unit.

"Experiencing" the change or solution leads to incorporation of what is new or different into work and interpersonal processes (Lewin, 1947). Deciding to begin to use the change or being thrust into the change can result in potential integration of the new way of thinking or doing.

"Refreezing" occurs when the participants in the change situation accept and use the new attitude or behavior (Lewin, 1947). Acceptance is assumed once most staff integrate the change into their work processes. Surveys, structured or unstructured observations, or other data collection methods can be conducted at various points after the implementation of a designated change. Analysis of these data can help evaluate the degree of implementation and identify additional alterations needed to ensure an effective **change outcome.**

Although Havelock's (1973) six-stage model for planning change had particular application to educational entities (see Theory box), it shows similarities in the elements of the directional phases recommended by other planned change models. Two adjuncts to Havelock's model advocate development of the effective change agent and use of his model as a rational problem-solving process. The rational problem-solving process is "how change agents can organize their work so that successful innovation will take place" (p. 3).

Lippitt, Watson, and Westley's (1958) model suggests seven sequential phases to use to plan change (see Theory box). Inherent in this model is the change agent's appraisal of the "change and resistance forces which are present in the client system at the beginning of the change process as well as others which may be revealed as the process advances. Being continuously sensitive to the constellation of change forces and resistance forces is one of the most creative parts of the change agent's job" (p. 92).

The innovation-decision process (Rogers, 1995) describes the choice of an individual, over time, to accept or reject a new idea for use in practice (see Theory box). According to Rogers' work, the individual's decision-making actions pass through five sequential stages. The decision to not accept the new idea may occur at any stage. However, the change agent can facilitate movement by others through these stages by encouraging the use of the idea and providing information about its benefits and disadvantages.

Theory Box

THEORIES FOR PLANNED CHANGE

KEY CONTRIBUTORS	KEY IDEA	APPLICATION TO PRACTICE
Six Phases of Planned Change Havelock (1973) is credited with this planned change model.	Change can be planned, implemented, and evaluated in six sequential stages. The model is advocated for the development of effective change agents and use as a rational problem-solving process. The six stages* are as follows: 1. Building a relationship 2. Diagnosing the problem 3. Acquiring relevant resources 4. Choosing the solution 5. Gaining acceptance 6. Stabilizing the innovation and generating self-renewal	Useful for low-level, low-complexity change.
Seven Phases of Planned Change Lippitt, Watson, and Westley (1958) are credited with this planned change model.	Change can be planned, implemented, and evaluated in seven sequential phases. Ongoing sensitivity to forces in the change process is essential. The seven phases† are as follows: 1. The client system becomes aware of the need for change. 2. The relationship is developed between the client system and change agent. 3. The change problem is defined. 4. The change goals are set and options for achievement are explored. 5. The plan for change is implemented. 6. The change is accepted and stabilized. 7. The change entities redefine their relationships.	Useful for low-level, low-complexity change.
Innovation-Decision Process Rogers (1995) is credited with formulating this process.	Change for an individual occurs over five phases when choosing to accept or reject an innovation/idea. Decisions to not accept the new idea may occur at any of the five stages. The change agent can promote acceptance by providing information about benefits and disadvantages and encouragement. The five stages‡ are as follows: 1. Knowledge 2. Persuasion 3. Decision 4. Implementation 5. Confirmation	Useful for individual change.

*Modified from Havelock, R. G. (1973). *The change agent's guide to innovation in education.* Englewood Cliffs, NJ: Educational Technology Publications.

†Modified from Lippitt, R., Watson, J., & Westley, B. (1958). *The dynamics of planned change.* New York: Harcourt Brace.

‡Modified from Rogers, E. M. (1995). *Diffusion of innovations* (4th ed.). New York: The Free Press.

NONLINEAR CHANGE: CHAOS AND LEARNING ORGANIZATION THEORIES

Chaos Theory

Organizations can no longer rely on rules, policies, and hierarchies to get work accomplished in inflexible ways. Healthcare organizations are unable to control long-term outcomes (McDaniel, 1998), according to chaos theory perspectives, because of the rapidly changing nature of human and world factors. Organizations are open systems operating in complex, fast-changing environments. One important concept of chaos theory is that "organizations are potentially chaotic" (Thietart & Forgues, 1995, p. 19). Non–human-induced responses are characterized by random-appearing yet self-organizing patterns. "The richness of interactions among parts and between the system and its environment allows the system as a whole to undergo spontaneous self-organization" (McDaniel, 1998, p. 356). Typically, organizations will experience periods of stability interrupted with periods of intense transformation. Although not predictable in the long run, small changes in the internal or external environment can result in significant consequences to organizational work processes and outcomes. Chaos theory further explains that the conditions present in a particular organizational change will not occur again in the same form (McDaniel, 1998; Thietart & Forgues, 1995; Vicenzi, White, & Begun, 1997).

Wheatley (1992) and CRM Films (1997a, 1997b) propose that organizations have always been self-organizing systems with the potential for self-renewal. From Wheatley's perspective, employees and leaders/managers have exercised bureaucratic premises, such as control, prediction, and emphasis on structure and elements of the whole, rather than on the relationship of the parts in forming a whole. She encourages leaders to act, think, and lead in terms of nonlinear perspectives, particularly in three major interrelated, interacting domains: information as "currency" or vital "air," relationships as pathways to building teams and generating new information, and vision as a "field of vision" within which all members of the organization share values and beliefs in the development of organizational direction. Continuous learning by personnel as a matter of organizational philosophy further promotes adaptation to accelerated change.

Learning Organization Theory

Learning organizations are organizations that place emphasis on flexibility and responsiveness (Senge, 1990). Specifically, complex organizations responsive to internal and external influences are trying to survive in an unpredictable healthcare environment. They can best respond and adapt when members of the organization complete their work with others using a learning approach. Enactment of Senge's five disciplines is essential to achieving learning organization status. *Disciplines* refers to the critical and interrelated elements that comprise a grouping that can function effectively only when all elements are present, linked, and interacting. For example, a car with a working engine and other essential operational features but no tires could not be driven as designed. Without the knowledge of the interrelatedness of the car's operational features, one might not be able to take the right action to use this form of transportation.

Senge's (1990) five disciplines of learning organizations include the following:

- Systems thinking
- Personal mastery
- Mental models
- Shared vision
- Team learning

Dialogue (two-way discussion) promotes the individual, group, and organizational learning process. *Systems thinking* refers to the need for the organization to view the world as a set of multiple visible and invisible parts that interact constantly. When the organization values and facilitates development of the deeper aspirations of its members in addition to professional proficiency, it successfully matches organizational learning and personal growth or *personal mastery*. Each individual and each organization bases its activities on a set of assumptions, beliefs, and mental pictures about the way the world should work. When these invisible *mental models* are uncovered and consciously evaluated, it is possible to begin to determine, in a "learningful" (Senge, 1990, p. 9) way, their influence on work accomplishment. The *building of shared vision* occurs when leaders involve all members in moving personal visions of the future into a consolidated yet ongoing vision common to members and leaders. *Team learning* refers to the need for a cohesive group to learn together to benefit from the abilities of each member, thereby enhancing the overall outcomes of the team's efforts. Organizations value employees who can learn continuously, interact and communicate effectively as team members, and seek to meet their potential as team members.

Staff resilience and hardiness are other qualities needed by organizations and change agents to respond quickly and continuously to a dynamic organization and environment (Deevy, 1995). A hardy, resilient person is typically flexible, focused, positive, organized, and proactive.

Most organizational change is dynamic, is extensive, and affects all components of the organization—its employees, technology, structure, processes, and outcomes. McDaniel (1998) suggests 12 recommendations for the change agent to apply that integrate many chaos and learning theory concepts in dealing with change:

1. Dispense with controlling and planning.
2. Operate on the margin between order and disorder.
3. Develop new organizations with the help of everyone.
4. Promote internal interaction to develop organizational pride.
5. Encourage information sharing among staff.
6. Promote staff's knowledge of others' work.
7. Stimulate open learning through discussions generating "creative tension" (p. 360).
8. Consider the organization's structure as dynamic.
9. Help staff discover their goals.
10. Encourage cooperation, not competition.
11. Approach work from a smarter, not harder, view.
12. Uncover values continuously to form organizationwide visions.

An example of the application of chaos and learning organization theories is a community hospital that has been sensitive to and adapted to external and internal environmental influences, such as the need to make changes in reimbursement and accreditation policies. The process of adaptation involved times of fluctuation interrupted with times of stability. The implications of managed care induced by major insurance players may not have been predictable, but they have had significant consequences for the financial survival of the community hospital. New reimbursement strategies have forced the community hospital and other area hospitals to interact to seek consolidation for all to survive. Accelerated change of such magnitude has created change that appears chaotic. However, all hospitals are becoming transformed, and some order exists in the middle of perceived general chaos. It is likely that these exact conditions will not occur again for these hospitals. Hospital administrators and other personnel have shown resilience and assumed a "learning" philosophy to seek overall organizational adaptation.

MAJOR CHANGE MANAGEMENT FUNCTIONS

Change agents selectively use **change management** functions and activities to assist in the creation and management of change to reach specific outcomes. They may or may not be used sequentially; they may be applied simultaneously, based on the nature of the change process. Flexibility and appropriateness of use are essential. The five functions are as follows:

- Planning (includes assessment)
- Organizing
- Implementing
- Evaluating
- Seeking feedback

Feedback functions in conjunction with the first four management functions as a way to assess the ongoing status of the change process and movement toward desired change outcomes.

Planning is simply the activity of looking ahead to decide how to achieve some result, goal, or outcome. For any plan to be effective, both those who will implement the plan and those who will be affected by the changes must participate in the change-planning process from the beginning. Planning ideally occurs before implementation. Part of the initial and ongoing planning activity includes assessing the who, what, why, when, and how of the situation needing change and the factors desired to achieve the change. It is important to carefully assess factors in the change situation that predictably will support or interfere with the progress of a change (Lewin, 1947). This information clarifies the conditions and direction of the advancing plan. Putting general plans for change in writing can establish a visual method to communicate ideas, decisions, and responsibilities to others.

Organizing entails making decisions about reaching outcomes in terms of time, personnel, materials, communication, or other activities and resources. For reasons of efficiency, it is important to weigh the costs and benefits of options to reach several possible change outcomes. Organizing builds clarity into the plan by formalizing the desired sequence and means of accomplishing the change.

Exercise 8-2

From the perspective of a manager applying these functions to a change process, consider the manager's responsibility to orient a new staffing coordinator for a large surgicenter and identify the appropriate management function for each number. Ideally, the manager, the new staffing coordinator, and the assistant nurse manager will map out in writing (1) the goals of the orientation, (2) the activities for meeting goals, and (3) a schedule for accomplishing them. The assistant nurse manager and staffing coordinator agree to (4) meet as needed, as well as to (5) meet weekly to review progress and to (6) address informational or confidence needs. Part of this plan includes the option to (7) alter the plan based on unexpected changes. The staffing coordinator will (8) begin the position in 2 weeks and (9) put the prearranged outline of activities into (10) action. The assistant nurse manager's responsibility will be to (11) guide and support the education of the new staffing coordinator. Unexpected occurrences, such as the staff coordinator being absent for a few days, will create the need to (12) modify the goal, activities, or time frame of the orientation plan (dynamic quality of process). New information (feedback) guides the overall process.

Implementing ideally occurs after a plan is established. However, unexpected change may sometimes require immediate action. Plans made quickly after the change can facilitate handling the effects of the change. Successful implementation, or putting the plan into action, depends on the appropriateness of the change and the involvement of those involved in the change. An important aspect of change is that change in one part of a system can affect the function in other, related systems.

Evaluating entails continually judging the degree to which the change process is moving acceptably toward desired outcomes or goals and whether or when outcomes are met. Monitoring, or ongoing data collection, assists the change agent to recognize and correct process problems early. Judging whether or not an outcome has been fully or partially met occurs in the final stage of the change process.

Effective change agents obtain feedback by continuously gathering accurate, comprehensive, timely information about the progress of the change

process through a variety of sources. Classic references (Ashby, 1957; Cadwallader, 1959) describe that **cybernetic theory** purports that access to what the theory terms *negative feedback* can be accomplished by establishing communication networks that act as monitors of specific types of information. Analysis of this negative feedback, or information indicating a correction is needed in the system, informs the change agent where problems exist: whether the course of the accelerated change process has veered away from its progress toward desired outcomes or some action is needed to facilitate continued progress. Although some typical organizational feedback mechanisms include computerized data findings, staff meeting discussions, and informal or formal observations, negative feedback sources are found specifically in the reports of exceptions, such as incident reports, variances in budget expenditures, or new reimbursement policies. Multiple sources of unexceptional feedback produce information to build a picture of success for the change process.

RESPONSES TO CHANGE

Change, whether proactively initiated at the point of change or imposed from external sources, affects people, technology, and systems. Change can be mandated by higher administration, or it can originate within any department or unit or at the level of care delivery. Often, higher administration creates a change for managerial staff to integrate into their work areas. Thus it follows that the responses that arise across the organization will depend on how change is perceived. Effective change agents anticipate possible responses and apply strategies to deal with them for the best possible change outcomes.

Organizational culture and staff readiness influence responses to change. Knowledge of the values and beliefs of work groups and their managers and administrators—all part of organizational culture—are critical to identifying responses to change (Simms, Price, & Ervin, 2000). Readiness can be viewed as individuals' current attitudes or willingness, as well as their nursing abilities. Assessment of organizational culture and the readiness of staff and others to engage in making or participating in a change, whether minor or extensive, set the stage for the selection and use of strategies. For example, in Exercise 8-2, the willingness of the nursing and administrative managerial staff to successfully merge is interdependent with the different nursing

Table 8-1 **SELF-ASSESSMENT: HOW RECEPTIVE TO CHANGE AND INNOVATION ARE YOU?**			

Read the following items. Circle the answer that most closely matches your attitude toward creating and accepting new or different ways.

	Yes	Depends	No
1. I enjoy learning about new ideas and approaches.	Yes	Depends	No
2. Once I learn about a new idea or approach, I begin to try it right away.	Yes	Depends	No
3. I like to discuss different ways of accomplishing a goal or end result.	Yes	Depends	No
4. I continually seek better ways to improve what I do.	Yes	Depends	No
5. I commonly recognize improved ways of doing things.	Yes	Depends	No
6. I talk over my ideas for change with my peers.	Yes	Depends	No
7. I communicate my ideas for change with my manager.	Yes	Depends	No
8. I discuss my ideas for change with my family.	Yes	Depends	No
9. I volunteer to be at meetings when changes are being discussed.	Yes	Depends	No
10. I encourage others to try new ideas and approaches.	Yes	Depends	No

If you answered "yes" to 8 to 10 of the items, you are probably receptive to creating and experiencing new and different ways of doing things. If you answered "depends" to 5 to 10 of the items, you are probably receptive to change conditionally based on the fit of the change with your preferred ways of doing things. If you answered "no" to 4 to 10 of the items, you are probably not receptive, at least initially, to new ways of doing things. If you answered "yes," "no," and "depends" an approximately equal number of times, you are probably mixed in your receptivity to change based on individual situations.

and organizational skills required by the new unit. Answering the self-assessment questions in Table 8-1 can help determine how receptive one is to change and innovation.

Human Side of Change

The *human side* of managing change refers to staff responses to change that either facilitate or interfere with change processes. Responses to all or part of the change process by individuals and groups may vary from full acceptance and willing participation to open rejection. Responses may be categorized behaviorally (Rogers, 1983) or emotionally (Perlman & Takacs, 1990). Some nurses may manifest their dissatisfactions visibly; others may quietly accommodate the change. Some individuals consistently reject any new thinking or ways of doing things.

The initial response to change may be, but is not always, reluctance and resistance. Resistance and reluctance are common when the change threatens personal security. For example, changes in the structure of an agency can result in changes of position for personnel. Changing the position of a nurse from critical care nurse to home health nurse can result in the nurse feeling temporarily incompetent and isolated.

The change agent's recognition of the ideal and common patterns of individuals' behavioral responses to change can facilitate an effective change process (Rogers, 1983). These responses and brief descriptions are as follows:

- *Innovators* thrive on change, which may be disruptive to the unit stability.
- *Early adopters* are respected by their peers and thus are sought out for advice and information about innovations/changes.
- *Early majority* prefer doing what has been done in the past but eventually will accept new ideas.
- *Late majority* are openly negative and agree to the change only after most others have accepted the change.
- *Laggards* prefer keeping traditions and openly express their resistance to new ideas.
- *Rejectors* oppose change actively, even use sabotage, which can interfere with the overall success of a change process.

The change agent's challenge is to deal with these behavioral patterns of individuals by providing opportunities to channel their responses into those supportive of the change process.

Individuals moving through change may also experience an emotional grieving of 10 possible stages resulting from the loss of their former employment situation (Perlman & Takacs, 1990). These 10 phases are equilibrium, denial, anger, bargaining, chaos, depression, resignation, openness, readiness, and reemergence. Each phase is characterized by varying energy levels, attitudes, and willingness to engage in new change activities. The change agent's challenges are to be sensitive to employees' stages of loss and to promote transition by responding with appropriate interventions, such as active listening, informing, and problem solving (Lancaster, 1999).

Jost (2000) reported her development of an assessment tool using concepts from Levine's conservation model. The tool's purpose was to systematically assess and address staff members' issues. Discovering the nature of their concerns, the nurse manager intervened appropriately to support staff during times of change and transition, which ultimately had positive outcomes for productivity, job satisfaction, and employment longevity.

Systems and Technological Side of Change

The *systems and technological side of managing change* refers to responses that influence the efficiency and effectiveness of work processes and outcomes. The change agent's challenge is to monitor, recognize, and apply appropriate strategies to minimize responses that are destructive and maximize those that support the dynamics of an ongoing change.

Organizational systems and technology can both influence and be influenced by change. System responses to change may emerge as signs of more or less efficiency or effectiveness. Changes in the type of staff or technology used to deliver care may lead to initial responses of confusion, then to a period of adaptation by the staff and other systems. The quality of care and the morale of staff may change. Productivity and safety outcomes may be different. Reparation of the breakdowns in the affected work processes can restore efficient and effective functioning. Managing uncertainty is critical (see Research Perspective).

STRATEGIES

The change agent uses various strategies to facilitate both planned and nonlinear change processes (Figure 8-1). **Strategies** are approaches designed to achieve a particular purpose based on anticipation and consideration of myriad human, technological, and system responses. The intent of the change agent and those supporting the change is to promote the continued movement toward integrating the change and achieving outcomes and to decrease

 Research Perspective

Geddes, N., Salyer, J., & Mark, B. A. (1999). Nursing in the nineties: Managing the uncertainty. *The Journal of Nursing Administration, 29,* 40-48.

The report of this qualitative research study was part of the research conducted by the Outcomes Research in Nursing Administration Project (ORNA) funded by the National Institutes of Health (NIH). The researchers requested that individual informants in 53 hospitals submit journals monthly for 6 months. Entries in the journals followed a specific content outline to include critical incidents and implications. Findings described life at work in relation to perceived events that influenced their hospitals, units, the functioning of their patients, and select outcomes of patient care. From 40 topics, one recurring theme emerged: "environmental uncertainty" (p. 43) stemming from the turbulence in their acute care settings. Informants primarily expressed how events shaped their workload, altered their identity (loss of identities) associated with mergers, and formed

their responses to reengineering efforts resulting in changes in roles and responsibilities.

IMPLICATIONS FOR PRACTICE
Nurse administrators and nurse managers who function as change agents can validate the existence of similar critical events, then selectively apply appropriate strategies to reduce the sources of uncertainty in work settings experienced by nurses practicing in acute care settings. The qualitative data point to the need to reduce the fluctuations and effects of changes. Several strategies suggested are to support collaborative problem solving among disciplines, to build trust between staff and top administration, and to provide opportunities for education to prepare nurses for different roles and responsibilities as the result of changes in work structure and processes.

and eliminate, if possible, any harmful resistance to the change (Wheeler, 1995). The key to using the various strategies effectively is to learn to match the appropriate strategies with the demonstrated response as it relates to the change situation.

Strategies, such as education and communication; participation and involvement; facilitation and support; negotiation and agreement; and manipulation, cooptation, and coercion, can be used individually or in combination with each other (Kotter & Schlesinger, 1979). As supported by chaos and learning organization theory, the change agent also uses vision development, relationship building, and information management strategies.

Communication and *education* refer to interchanges among the change agent, the change participants, and others for the purpose of integrating the elements of the change process. Staff meetings, focus groups (Carney, 2000), and informal discussions inform staff and clarify change activities. Active and empathetic listening are essential. Early explanation and education, especially of informal leaders, can facilitate change.

MATCHING STRATEGIES TO SITUATIONS

Situation	Education	Support	Facilitation	Communication	Participation	Negotiation	Manipulation	Cooptation	Coercion	Learning	Visioning	Relationships	Information
Staff not sure of next best step in change process	√	√	√	√						√	√	√	√
Two staff members reluctantly try change	√	√	√	√	√	√				√		√	√
Staff has heard rumors about new program	√			√						√	√		√
Several staff members propose a different method		√	√		√					√	√	√	√
One nurse consistently lags behind in accepting a change	√		√		√					√	√	√	√
A group of staff expresses loss of previous roles		√	√	√						√		√	√
Three staff members challenge the need for a change	√		√	√	√	√				√	√		√
Staff member avoids change task force membership				√		√			√	√		√	√
Four staff members have become change agents with manager	√	√	√	√	√					√	√	√	√
A group of staff verbalizes satisfaction with status quo	√			√	√	√	√	√		√	√	√	√
One nurse disrupts the change process with other ideas	√			√	√	√	√	√		√	√	√	√
Two nurses try to get others to oppose change	√			√		√	√	√	√				

Figure 8-1   Matching strategies to situations.

Empowerment of staff through *participation* and *involvement* promotes ownership of both the process and the decisions made during the process. It is important to incorporate staff at all levels at the beginning or as early as possible and then throughout the change process.

Facilitation and *support* strategies typically are used to reassure and assist those in the change situation who do not accept a change because of anxiety and fear. When personal security is threatened or when loss and grief are experienced, people tend to want to continue doing what they have always done. A staff member with financial problems may believe that a new benefit plan will result in less take-home pay. The change agent can reassure that person by providing the actual calculation to show that the fear is unfounded.

Individuals or groups in the change situation may have the power or resources to adversely affect the success of a particular change. *Negotiation* and *agreement* strategies can revise these terms of the change to accommodate the involved parties.

Cooptation usually entails manipulated involvement through an appointed or assigned role. An example of this strategy is appointing a highly resistant individual to a change task force that necessitates more active involvement in the change process. *Manipulation* appeals to the motivational needs of others and influences them to participate in change when they might not do so on their own initiative. Expecting staff to be cooperative by participating in a pilot project of the proposed change on a 3-month basis can reduce barriers.

Coercion involves the use of power to force others to make a change, particularly when time is critical to implementation. An example of coercion would be offering to retain a staff member's position during staff reductions if that individual accepts certain conditions.

The ongoing creation of goals and visions (*visioning*) by all the change participants or change teams shows overt responsiveness to the dynamic nature of change (McDaniel, 1998; Senge, 1990; Wheeler, 1995). This required dialogue continually redefines the future, whether for the organization or for a project. Development of a set of possible outcomes rather than rigid pursuit of one outcome opens the possibilities to respond to unpredictable environmental influences (Begun & White, 1995). Change agents build work environments that support the time needed to create a shared vision and accept varied beliefs of staff (Senge, 1990; Wheatley, 1992).

Information management by the change agent focuses on delivery of the right information to the right place at the right time. Sound assessment of environmental influences and decision making depend on accurate and current information (Wheatley, 1992).

Managing *relationships* involves how individual capabilities and potential can facilitate creative solutions to projected organizational outcomes and is essential to change management. Formal position titles become irrelevant. Matching a staff member who has the needed abilities and attitudes with the demands of an appropriate project, for example, can lead to more creative outcomes. Peers can become coaches and teachers to help develop others' competencies.

The strategies discussed are useful when used appropriately. It is important to recognize cognitive responses or concerns, for example, that can be met with education, information, or other forms of communication. Participation, facilitation, and support can be choices to address the emotional components of accepting change, such as fear, anxiety, or grief. When the issue is sustained lack of motivation or unwillingness to cooperate, the more effective strategies to use may be manipulation, cooptation, or coercion. Effective change agents develop work environments that support continuous individual and group learning. Because of the dynamic nature of accelerated change environments, effective change agents stay focused on the dynamics of change by consistently managing information, relationships, and vision.

Typically, combinations of strategies are applied simultaneously, rather than one at a time. Figure 8-1 captures the deliberate selection of appropriate strategies to fit the ongoing needs and responses associated with leading change.

ROLES AND FUNCTIONS OF CHANGE AGENTS AND FOLLOWERS

Initiating change and managing its dynamics using linear and nonlinear approaches are key roles of change agents, with shared responsibilities by followers. Appropriate application of related functions, principles, and strategies can assist in meeting the challenges of any kind of change on the change continuum from **low-complexity change** to **high-complexity change**. The ultimate goal is a unified movement toward the adoption of something new or different.

Effective followership requires that followers communicate constructively with the formal or **informal change agent** to offer information, suggestions, or concerns. Followers also benefit by actively seeking participation in change, staying flexible, tolerating ambiguity, and thoughtfully supporting change efforts (Menix, 2001). Respect and trust between followers and change agents benefit both groups emotionally (Smith & Flarey, 1999).

Change agents, usually staff within healthcare organizations (insiders) or members of the community (outsiders), use their personal, professional, and managerial knowledge and skills to lead or influence change (Lancaster, 1999). Staff members who are not officially in charge—possessing only informal power—can also play important change agent functions. Through their early interest and expertise (early majority), informal leaders can model the new way of doing or thinking for others to simulate. Their positive attitudes toward integrating the change can positively influence staff participation and unity. The informal leader's close interaction with the formal change agent can lead to reinforcement with other staff about changes in direction.

Being an effective change agent, whether in charge or not, requires specific qualifications. Lancaster (1999) describes some key qualities of effective change agents: excellent communication skills, use of observational skills to monitor change, knowledge of group dynamics, perceptive nature about political issues, supportive attitude toward change participants, and the ability to establish trusting relationships.

Knowing how to build relationships, interact with others, and empower change participants is also critical to the achievement of change outcomes (Menix, 2001). Staff who share the creation of change that affects them directly and who trust the change agent usually are more receptive to change and integrate change more willingly. Giving and receiving information that includes clear explanations also encourage receptivity. Assertive communication projects self-confidence. Persistence and persuasion can communicate the change agent's commitment to the change outcome.

Because the human, systems, and technological responses to change are unpredictable, flexibility, timing, and conflict management by the change agent can keep the change on course (Menix, 2001). It is important to deal with potential or real conflict in effective ways. Understanding the interrelatedness of change and group dynamics assists the change agent in selecting appropriate strategies.

Change participants are members of unique work cultures, so the change agent's selection of strategies to manage responses considers the culture's dominant values and beliefs. Managing a change to fit the preferences of a group's culture can facilitate acceptance of a particular change (O'Connell, 1999).

Having credibility, often as a result of their expertise and legitimate power, allows change agents to sometimes make independent decisions without negative responses. Change agents can role model the change by actively participating in the change situation, which can translate into expectations for others to follow. For example, a manager who uses the new computerized medication dispenser may be more likely to earn the respect of the change participants.

Exercise 8-3

Recall a work or personal situation in which a particular individual tried to get you or a group to do something. What rationale supported the decision to cooperate or not? Was the idea worthwhile from your perception? Was the person making the suggestions known, understood, and trusted? Was the person making the suggestions aware of the real situation, an essential part of carrying out the idea, or had he or she not received official sanctioning to influence activities? Can you see that change agents need specific qualities and abilities to be trusted by others?

PRINCIPLES

Principles are assumptions and general rules that guide behavior and processes. Principles are useful for creating and leading change. Classic principles that characterize effective change implementation are provided in Box 8-2 (Harper, 1993).

Exercise 8-4

Prepare an actual or hypothetical change that is meaningful to you in your personal, work, or school life. Select a change that provides an opportunity to apply the linear (planned) and nonlinear principles of change. Draft a hypothetical or actual plan for change, drawing on the chapter content and paying particular attention to the array of change principles discussed. Share your plan and the rationale used with peers or a small group of other healthcare providers. Ask for their comments and suggestions. (If you need a hypothetical change to work with, consider this one: You are the assistant manager for a home health agency. The agency administrator just informed you by memorandum that in 1 month, because of new reimbursement rules, the agency will begin caring for patients receiving chemotherapy. How will you prepare for this change?)

BOX 8-2

Classic Principles Characterizing Effective Change Implementation

- Change agents within healthcare organizations use personal, professional, and managerial knowledge and skills to lead change.
- The recipients of change believe they own the change.
- Administrators and other key personnel support the proposed change.
- The recipients of change anticipate benefit from the change.
- The recipients of change participate in identifying the problem warranting a change.
- The change holds interest for the change recipients and other participants.
- Agreement exists within the work group about the benefit of the change.
- The change agent(s) and recipients of change perceive a compatibility of values.
- Trust and empathy exist among the participants of the change process.
- Revision of the change goal and process is negotiable.
- The change process is designed to provide regular feedback to its participants.

Modified from Harper, C. L. (1993). *Exploring social change* (2nd ed.). Englewood Cliffs, NJ: Prentice Hall.

The Solution

The changes in nurses' pay schedules essentially rearranged both the tangible and less tangible incentives of employment. Some nurses decided to stay in full-time positions; some became prn nurses. I continue to use prn and agency nurses, despite their higher costs. My goal in managing this change was to maintain the standards and continuity of care by providing the right number and type of competent staff around the clock. The hospital has clinical coordinators, too, who offer the added expertise and support for all staff and patients, regardless of their pay schedule classification. Most of my change management strategies had to do with keeping frequent contact with staff, being approachable, and addressing individual issues of concern before they became unit issues. Building trust, keeping their confidence, and always seeking to know their opinions and needs work toward retention of full-time nurses and hopefully making this place a quality place to work for all. My philosophy is to keep employees happy, not to just keep them! Besides staying informed about what is going on in this hospital and outside about the supply of nurses and other related issues, I do a variety of things to attract and interest future nursing staff. I talk with nursing students and serve as a preceptor for them. I talk to high school students as well. I support the informal learning and continuing education of my current staff. I try to help them meet their goals and the unit's needs. I observe for tiredness and burnout and try to act in their interest. I never discourage staff from leaving the unit; many times they return because they had positive experiences.

— Joel Graeter

 Would this be a suitable approach for you? Why?

CHAPTER CHECKLIST

Change is an unavoidable constant in the rapidly transforming healthcare delivery system. As a result, uncertainty is an element in most healthcare institutions. Creating and leading change rather than merely reacting can promote overall organizational effectiveness.

The nature of accelerated change demands flexibility and prompt response to sometimes unpredictable environmental pressures as opposed to inflexible thinking and acting. Planned change as a linear approach to managing change can be useful for dealing with low-level, less complex change. Nonlinear approaches offered by chaos and learning organization theories focus more on managing the dynamic elements of more complex, high-level change situations.

- Characteristics of change include the following:
  - Is a natural social process
  - Involves individuals, groups, organizations, and society
  - Is constant and accelerates at various rates and intensities
  - Is inevitable and unpredictable
  - Varies from high complexity to low complexity
- Planned change occurs in sequential stages, according to planned change theorists:
  - Lewin:
    - Awareness of need for change
    - Experience of change
    - Integration of change
  - Havelock:
    - Building a relationship
    - Diagnosing the problem
    - Acquiring relevant resources
    - Choosing the solution
    - Gaining acceptance
    - Stabilizing the innovation and generating self-renewal
  - Lippitt, Watson, and Westley:
    - The client system becomes aware of the need for change.
    - The relationship is developed between the client system and change agent.
    - The change problem is defined.
    - The change goals are set and options for achievement are explored.
    - The plan for change is implemented.
    - The change is accepted and stabilized.
    - The change entities redefine their relationship.
  - Rogers:
    - Knowledge
    - Persuasion
    - Decision
    - Implementation
    - Confirmation
- Nonlinear change occurs in a different manner according to nonlinear change theorists:
  - Chaos theory:
    - Organizations as open systems
    - Non–human-induced self-organizing patterns
    - Periods of stability interrupted with intense transformation

- Small changes resulting in significant consequences
- Conditions in one situation not recurring in the same pattern
  - Learning organization theory:
    - Emphasis on flexibility, responsiveness, and learning
    - Five disciplines interrelated by dialogue:
      Systems thinking
      Personal mastery
      Mental models
      Shared vision
      Team learning
  - Resilience
    - Manifested by beliefs, skills, behaviors, and knowledge
    - Personal qualities:
      Flexible
      Focused
      Positive
      Organized
      Proactive
  - Major change management functions:
    - Planning
    - Organizing
    - Implementing
    - Evaluating
    - Providing feedback/cybernetic theory
- The human responses to change manifest in various behavioral patterns that may help or hinder movement toward achievement of the change outcome:
  - Innovators
  - Early adopters
  - Early majority
  - Late majority
  - Laggards
  - Rejectors
- Multiple strategies are used selectively to promote involvement by the participants of change and to facilitate the overall change process:
  - Education and communication
  - Participation and involvement
  - Facilitation and support
  - Negotiation and agreement
  - Manipulation and cooptation
  - Coercion
  - Information management
  - Relationship facilitation
  - Ongoing vision development
  - Continuous learning

Continued

CHAPTER CHECKLIST—cont'd

- Effective change agents, both formal and informal (those not in charge), exhibit the following characteristics in the change situation:
  - Display leadership
  - Possess excellent communication skills
  - Use observation skills
  - Know how groups work
  - Are perceptive about political issues
  - Are trusted by others
  - Establish positive relationships
  - Empower others
  - Are flexible
  - Manage conflict
  - Participate actively in change
  - Are respected, credible members of organization or community
  - Possess expert and legitimate power
  - Understand change process
  - Display appropriate timing
- Principles guide change:
  - Ownership of change
  - Anticipated benefits as change consequence
  - Negotiability between change agent and participants
  - Benefits of feedback to change process

- Expect people to respond differently to change, which may either keep movement toward the outcome on course or slow it down.
- People cope and adapt better when they assume the role of continuous learner during accelerated change.
- People involved in change may assume the roles of followers or leaders and may emerge from both informal and formal, or internal and external sources.
- Creating a detailed plan and rigidly adhering to it reduces opportunities to moderate the inevitable and changing aspects of a change process, especially in an accelerated change environment. Building ambiguity and flexibility into a plan and how it's managed promotes responsiveness and movement toward desired outcomes.

TERMS TO KNOW

barriers	facilitators
change agents	high-complexity change
change management	informal change agent
change outcome	learning organization
change process	low-complexity change
change situations	nonlinear change
chaos theory	planned change
cybernetic theory	strategies

TIPS IN LEADING CHANGE

- Whether involved in planned (low-complexity) or nonlinear (high-complexity) change, create a group of outcome/goal scenarios with prospective actions to achieve.

REFERENCES

Ashby, W. R. (1957). *An introduction to cybernetics.* New York: John Wiley & Sons.

Begun, J. W., & White, K. R. (1995). Altering nursing's dominant logic: Guidelines from complex adaptive systems theory. *Complexity and Chaos in Nursing, 2*(1), 5-15.

Cadwallader, M. L. (1959). The cybernetic analysis of change in complex social organizations. *The American Journal of Sociology, 65,* 154-157.

Carney, M. (2000). The development of a model to manage change: Reflection on a critical incident in a focus group setting. An innovative approach. *Journal of Nursing Management, 8,* 265-272.

CRM Films. (1997a). *Leadership and the new science* [Review of the video program]. (Available from Best Sellers Series, 2215 Faraday Avenue, Carlsbad, CA, 92008).

CRM Films. (1997b). *Lessons from the new workplace* [Review of the video program]. (Available from Best Sellers Series, 2215 Faraday Avenue, Carlsbad, CA, 92008).

Deevy, E. (1995). *Creating the resilient organization.* Englewood Cliffs, NJ: Prentice Hall.

DiFonzo, N., & Bordia, P. (1998). A tale of two corporations: Managing uncertainty during organizational change. *Human Resource Management, 37*(3 & 4), 295-303.

Freeman, S. J. (1999). The gestalt of organizational down-sizing: Downsizing strategies as packages of change. *Human Relations, 52*(12), 1505-1541.

Geddes, N., Salyer, J., & Mark, B. M. (1999). Nursing in the nineties: Managing the uncertainty. *The Journal of Nursing Administration, 29*(5), 40-48.

Harper, C. L. (1993). *Exploring social change* (2nd ed.). Englewood Cliffs, NJ: Prentice Hall.

Havelock, R. G. (1973). *The change agent's guide to innovation in education.* Englewood Cliffs, NJ: Educational Technology Publications.

Jost, S. J. (2000). An assessment and intervention strategy for managing staff needs during change. *The Journal of Nursing Administration, 30*(1), 34-40.

Kotter, J., & Schlesinger, L. (1979, March/April). Choosing strategies for change. *Harvard Business Review, 57,* 106-114.

Lancaster, J. (1999). *Nursing issues in leading and managing change.* St. Louis: Mosby.

Lewin, K. (1947). Frontiers in group dynamics: Concept, method, and reality in social science, social equilibria and social change. *Human Relations, 1*(1), 5-41.

Lippitt, R., Watson, J., & Westley, B. (1958). *The dynamics of planned change.* New York: Harcourt Brace.

McDaniel, R. R. (1998). Strategic leadership: A view from quantum and chaos theories. In W. J. Duncan, P. Ginter, & L. Swayne (Eds.), *Handbook of health care management* (pp. 339-367). Oxford, England: Basil Blackwell Publishing.

Menix, K. D. (2000). Educating to manage the accelerated change environment. Part 1. *Journal for Nurses in Staff Development, 16,* 282-288.

Menix, K. D. (2001). Educating to manage the accelerated change environment. Part 2. *Journal For Nurses in Staff Development, 17,* 44-53.

Nutt, P. C. (1992). *Managing planned change.* New York: Macmillan.

O'Connell, C. (1999). A culture of change or a change of culture? *Nurse Administrator Quarterly, 23*(2), 65-68.

Perlman, D., & Takacs, G. J. (1990). The 10 stages of change. *Nursing Management, 21*(4), 33-38.

Porter-O'Grady, T. (1997). Quantum mechanics and the future of healthcare leadership. *The Journal of Nursing Administration, 27*(1), 15-20.

Rogers, E. M. (1983). *Diffusion of innovations* (3rd ed.). New York: The Free Press.

Rogers, E. M. (1995). *Diffusion of innovations* (4th ed.). New York: The Free Press.

Senge, P. M. (1990). *The fifth discipline.* New York: Doubleday.

Simms, L. M., Price, S. A., & Ervin, N. E. (2000). *Professional practice of nursing administration* (3rd ed.). Albany, NY: Delmar of Thomson Learning.

Smith, S. P., & Flarey, D. L. (1999). *Process-centered health care organizations.* Gaithersburg, MD: Aspen Publishers.

Thietart, R. A., & Forgues, B. (1995). Chaos theory and organization. *Organization Science, 6*(1), 19-31.

Vicenzi, A. E., White, K. R., & Begun, J. W. (1997). Chaos in nursing: Make it work for you. *American Journal of Nursing, 97*(10), 26-31.

Wheatley, M. J. (1992). *Leadership and the new science.* San Francisco: Berrett-Koehler.

Wheeler, M. M. (1995, January/February). The human side of change. *Canadian Journal of Nursing Administration, 8*(1), 26-32.

SUGGESTED READINGS

Asselin, M. (2001). Time to wear a third hat? *Nursing Management, 32*(3), 25-28.

Bennis, W. G., Benne, K. D., & Chin, R. (1984). *The planning of change* (4th ed.). Fort Worth: Holt, Rinehart & Winston.

Dianis, N. L., Allen, M., Baker, K., Cartledge, T., Gwyer, D., Harris, S., McNemar, A., Swayze, R., Wilson, M., & Walker, P. H. (1997). Merger motorway: Giving staff the tools to reengineer. *Nursing Management, 28*(3), 42-47.

Havelock, R. G., & Zlotolow, S. (1995). *The change agent's guide* (2nd ed.). Englewood Cliffs, NJ: Educational Technology Publications.

McCrea, M. A. (1998). Personal reflections on early learning in shared leadership. *Seminars for Nurse Managers, 6*(2), 83-88.

Perra, B. M. (2000). Leadership: The key to quality outcomes. *Nurse Administrator Quarterly, 24*(2), 56-61.

Salmond, S. W. (1998, September/October). Managing the human side of change. *Orthopaedic Nursing, 17*(5), 38-51.

Tiffany, C. R., & Lutjens, L. R. (1998). *Planned change theories for nursing.* Thousand Oaks, CA: Sage Publications.

Witkin, B. R., & Altschuld, J. W. (2000). *From needs assessments to action.* Thousand Oaks, CA: Sage Publications.

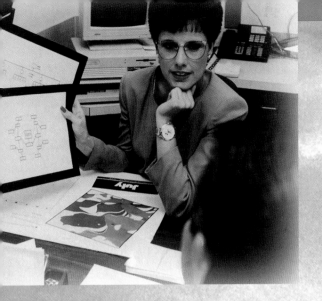

Chapter

9

Understanding and Designing Organizational Structures

Carol Alvater Brooks

T his chapter explains key concepts related to organizational structures and provides information on designing effective structures. This information can be used to help new managers function in an organization and to design structures that support work processes. An underlying theme is designing organizational structures that will respond to changes taking place in the current healthcare environment.

Objectives

- Analyze the relationships among vision, mission, and philosophy statements and organizational structure.
- Analyze factors that influence the design of an organizational structure.

- Relate types of organizational structures with three distinguishing characteristics of each.

- Evaluate the forces that are necessitating reengineering of organizational systems.

Questions to Consider

- *What is the nursing organization's reason for being?*
- *What are the beliefs and values regarding patients, patient care, and the employees?*
- *What characteristics of the nursing organization's structure would best serve patients' and employees' needs and support work processes? At what level are decisions about each made?*
- *What would a futuristic organizational chart look like? What management strategies would be prevalent for this organization?*

The Challenge

Rebecca M. Patton, RN, MSN, CNOR
Director of Nursing , University Hospitals Health System, Richmond Heights Hospital, Cleveland, Ohio

This is a newly acquired hospital in my health system. The hospital went through three different owners during the last 5 years. As a result, there were at least three sets of operating policies directing care. When I was appointed Director of Nursing, there was an organizational plan in place, but several of the head nurse positions and supervisor positions were vacant.

The standard of care, as a result, was driven by three different sets of policies, and sometimes there was no nursing administrator available to clarify which practice to follow or even to be aware of the fact that there was a major clinical conflict.

What do you think you would do if you were this nurse?

INTRODUCTION

Professional nurses work mostly in organizations. Learning to determine how an organization accomplishes its work, how to operate productively within an organization, and how to influence organizational processes is essential to survival.

Organization as it is used here refers to the structure that is designed to support organizational processes. A vision statement conveys some dramatic view of how to describe the organization at some future time. It suggests how far to strive in all endeavors. The **mission,** or reason for the organization's existence, influences the design of the structure, for example, to meet healthcare information needs of a designated population, to prepare patients for a peaceful death, or to provide supportive and stabilizing care to an acute care population. Another key factor influencing structure is the **philosophy,** which expresses the values and beliefs members of the organization hold about the nature of their work, about the people to whom they provide service, and about themselves and

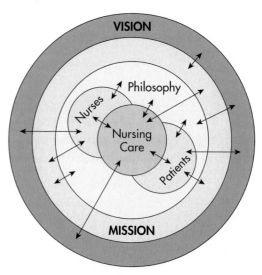

Figure 9-1 The interrelationship of vision, mission, and philosophy.

others providing the services. Figure 9-1 reflects how these elements interrelate.

Exercise 9–1

Consider how you might use the information in the Introduction (1) to analyze an organization that you are considering joining to determine whether it fits your professional development plans, (2) to assess the functioning of an organization that you are already a member of, or (3) to make a plan to reengineer the structure or philosophy to better accomplish the mission of an organization you are considering joining or are already a member of. Use Figure 9-1 as a test for interrelatedness.

VISION

Vision statements are future-oriented, purposeful statements designed to identify the desired future of an organization. They serve to unify all subsequent statements toward the view of the future. Typically, vision statements are brief, consisting of only one or two phrases or sentences. Mission and philosophy statements are crafted within the context of the vi-

BOX 9-1

Mission and Philosophy for a Neurosurgical Unit

Mission Statement

This unit's purpose is to provide quality nursing care for neurosurgical patients during the acute phase of their illness that facilitates their progression to the rehabilitation phase, to cultivate a multidisciplinary approach to the care of the neurosurgical patient, and to provide multiple educational opportunities for the professional development of neurosurgical nurses.

Philosophy

The philosophy is based on Roy's Adaptation Model and on the American Association of Neurosurgical Nursing Conceptual framework.

Patients

We believe

- It is the right of the patients to make informed choices concerning their treatment.
- Patients have a right to high-quality nursing care and opportunities for improving their quality of life regardless of the potential outcomes of their illness.
- The patient/family/significant other has a right to exercise personal options to participate in care to the extent of individual abilities and needs.

Nursing

We believe

- Neuroscience nursing is a unique area of nursing practice because neurosurgical interventions and/or neurological dysfunction affects all levels of human existence.
- The goal of the neuroscience nurse is to engage in a therapeutic relationship with his or her patients to facilitate adaptation to changes in physiological, self-concept, role performance, and interdependent modes.

- The ultimate goal for the neuroscience nurse is to foster internal and external unity of patients to achieve optimal health potentials.

Nurse

We believe

- The nurse is the integral element who coordinates nursing care for the neurosurgical patient using valuable input from all members of the patient care team.
- The nurse has an obligation to assume accountability for maintaining excellence in practice.
- The nurse has three basic rights: human rights, legal rights, and professional rights.
- The nurse has a right to autonomy in providing nursing care based on sound nursing judgment.

Nursing Practice

We believe

- Nursing practice must support and be supported by activities in practice, education, research, and management.
- Insofar as possible, patients must be assigned one nurse who is responsible and accountable for their care throughout their stay on the neurosurgical unit.
- The primary nurse is responsible for consulting and collaborating with other healthcare professionals in planning and delivering patient care.
- The contributions of all members of the nursing team are valuable, and an environment must be created that allows each member to participate fully in the delivery of care in accord with his or her abilities and qualifications.
- The nursing process is the vehicle used by nurses to operationalize nursing practice.
- Data generated in nursing practices must be continually and consistently collected and analyzed for the purpose of managing the quality of nursing practice.

Courtesy Upstate Medical University, University Hospital, Syracuse, NY (W. Painter, J. Van Nest-Kinne).

---

sion statement. A vision statement appropriate to Box 9-1, for example, might be as follows: To be the exemplar of neurosurgical nursing in the state.

▰ MISSION

The mission statement defines the organization's reason for being. This statement is the foundational

assertion from which subsequent statements flow. The mission identifies the organization's customers and the types of services offered, such as education, supportive nursing care, rehabilitation, acute care, and home care. It enacts the vision statement (see Box 9-1).

The mission statement sets the stage by defining the services to be offered, which, in turn, identify the kinds of technologies and human resources to be employed. Hospitals' missions are primarily treatment-oriented; the missions of ambulatory care group practices combine treatment, prevention, and diagnosis-oriented services; long-term care facilities' missions are primarily maintenance- and social support–oriented; and the missions of nursing centers are oriented toward promoting optimal health statuses for a defined group of people. The definition of services to be provided and its implications for technologies and human resources greatly influence the design of the **organizational structure.**

Nursing, as a profession providing a service within a healthcare agency, formulates its own mission statement that describes its contributions to achieve the agency's mission. A purpose of the nursing profession is to provide nursing care to clients. The statement should define nursing based on theories that form the basis for the model of nursing to be used in guiding the process of nursing care delivery. Nursing's mission statement tells why nursing exists (see Box 9-1). It is written so that others within the organization can know and understand nursing's role in achieving the agency's mission. The mission should be reviewed for accuracy and updated routinely by professional nurses providing care. It should be known and understood by other healthcare professionals, by clients and their families, and by the community. It indicates the relationships among nursing and patients, agency personnel, the community, and health and illness. This statement provides direction for the evolving statement of philosophy and the organizational structure.

Units that provide specific services such as intensive care, cardiac services, or maternity services also formulate mission statements that detail their specific contributions to the overall mission.

PHILOSOPHY

The philosophy states the values and beliefs held about the nature of the work required to accomplish the mission and the nature and rights of both the people being served and those providing the service. It states the nurse managers' and practitioners' vision of what they believe nursing management and practice are and sets the stage for developing goals to make that vision a reality. It states the beliefs of nurse managers and staff as to how the mission or purpose will be achieved. For example, the mission statement may incorporate the provision of individualized care as a purpose, and the philosophy would support this purpose through expression of a belief in the respon-

sibility of nursing staff to act as patient advocates and to provide quality care according to the wishes of the patient, family, and significant others. Philosophy both shapes and reflects the organizational culture; organizational culture is exemplified by behaviors that illustrate values and beliefs. Examples include rituals and customary forms of practice, such as celebrations of promotions, publications, degree attainment, professional performance, weddings, and retirements. Another example is the characteristics of the people who are recognized as heroes by the organizational members.

Philosophies are evolutionary in that they are shaped both by the social environment and by the stage of development of professionals delivering the service. The nursing staff reflects the values of the times and the values acquired through their education in their statements of philosophy. **Technology** development such as that of information systems also shapes the philosophy. For example, information systems can provide people with data that allow them greater control over their work; workers are consequently able to make more decisions and take more autonomous action. Philosophies require updating to reflect the extension of rights brought about by such changes.

Exercise 9–2

Obtain a copy of the philosophy of a nursing department and identify behaviors that you observe on a unit of the department that relate or do not relate to the beliefs and values expressed in the document.

Developing a philosophy can be an activity used for **reengineering** a nursing care delivery system. A group process of development provides a method of stating a believed-in ideal and envisioning methods to make that ideal a reality. Box 9-1 shows an example of a philosophy developed for a neurosurgical unit with the leadership of a nurse manager and clinical instructor.

FACTORS INFLUENCING ORGANIZATIONAL DEVELOPMENT

Organizational structure defines how work is organized, where decisions are made, and the authority and responsibility of workers. Structure is a map for communication and decision-making paths. As organizations change through acquisitions, mergers, and focusing, it is essential that structures change to accomplish revised missions.

Probably the best theory to explain today's nursing organizational development is chaos (complexity, nonlinear, quantum) theory. The Theory Box identifies key concepts associated with complexity theory. In essence, this theory suggests that life (and organizations) are really weblike. Pulling on one small segment rearranges the web; a new pattern emerges, yet the whole remains. This theory, applied to nursing organizations, suggests that differences logically exist between and among various organizations and that the constant environmental forces continue to affect the structure, its functioning, and the services. Wheatley suggests that understanding chaos as a life process releases our creative power (Wheatley, 1999).

The issues in healthcare delivery, with their concomitant changes, such as reimbursement regulation and the development of networks for delivery of healthcare, have profound effects on organizational structure designs. Consumerism, the demand by consumers of care that the care be customized to meet their individual needs, necessitates that decision making be done where the care is delivered. Change is ongoing as efforts are made to reduce cost and improve outcomes of healthcare. Increased consumer knowledge and greater responsibility for selecting healthcare providers and options have resulted in consumers who demand customized care. Competition for clients is another factor influencing structure design. These three factors—change, consumerism, and competition—necessitate reengineering healthcare structures. Reengineering involves a total overhaul of an organizational structure. An example is technological change, particularly in information services, that provides a means of customizing care. Its potential for making all informa-

tion concerning a client immediately accessible to direct caregivers has profound implications for altering decision-making points.

■ Exercise 9-3

Arrange to interview a nurse employed in a healthcare agency or use your own experience to identify examples of changes taking place that necessitate reengineering, such as implementation of capitation, development of policies to carry out legislative regulations related to the right to die, or development of labor/delivery/recovery rooms for marketing. Identify examples of how previous systems of communication and decision making were inadequate to cope with these changes.

CHARACTERISTICS OF ORGANIZATIONAL STRUCTURES

The characteristics of different types of organizational structures and the theories on which designs are based provide a catalog of options to consider in designing structures that fit specific situations. Knowledge of these characteristics and theories also assists managers in understanding the structures in which they currently function.

An organization is a group of people working together to achieve a purpose. Organizational theory is based largely on the systematic investigation of the effectiveness of specific organizational designs in achieving their purpose. Organizational theory development is a process of creating knowledge to understand the effect of identified factors, such as organizational culture; organizational technology, which is defined as all the work being carried out; and organizational structure or organizational development. A purpose of such work is to determine how organizational effectiveness might

Theory Box

COMPLEXITY (CHAOS/NONLINEAR/QUANTUM) THEORY

KEY CONTRIBUTORS	KEY IDEA	APPLICATION TO PRACTICE
Computer development allowed us to understand this theory described by Wheatley (1999).	Structures should encourage flexibility so that they remain relevant to changing needs.	Nurses should be well prepared to expect the unexpected and never assume predicted outcomes will occur. Organizations that would be described as "learning" should be created.

be predicted or controlled through the design of the organizational structure. Although many relationships among the variables just mentioned have been hypothesized, there is a need for research studies that test these relationships. This is especially important during acquisitions (George, Burke, & Rodgers, 1997).

Organizational designs are often classified by their characteristics of complexity, formalization,

and centralization. Figure 9-2 illustrates specialization, centralization, authority, and responsibility.

Complexity concerns the division of labor in an organization, the specialization of that labor, the number of hierarchical levels, and the geographic dispersion of organizational units. *Division of labor* and *specialization* refer to the separation of processes into tasks that are performed by designated people. The horizontal dimension of an **organizational chart**

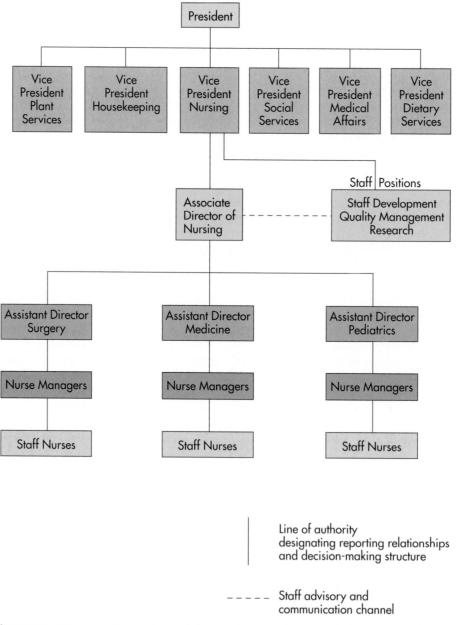

Figure 9-2　A bureaucratic organizational chart depicting specialization of labor, centralization, hierarchical authority, and line and staff responsibilities.

relates to the division and specialization of labor functions attended by specialists. **Hierarchy** connotes lines of authority and responsibility. **Chain of command** is a term used to refer to the hierarchy and is depicted in **vertical** dimensions of organizational charts. Hierarchy vests authority in positions on an ascending line away from where work is performed and allows for control of work. Staff are often placed on a bottom line of the organization, and authority, which provides for control, is placed in higher levels.

Geographic dispersion refers to the physical location of units. Units of work may be in one building; in several buildings in one location; spread throughout a city; or in different counties, states, or countries. The more dispersed an organization is, the greater are the demands for creative designs that place decision making related to client care close to the patient and consequently far from corporate headquarters. A similar type of complexity exists in organizations that deliver care at multiple sites in the community, such as school health programs in which care delivery sites are located in schools that usually are at great distances from the corporate office, which has overall responsibility for the school health program.

Formalization is the degree to which an organization has rules, stated in policy, that define a member's function. The amount of formalization varies among institutions.

■ *Exercise 9–4*

Review a copy of a nursing department's organizational chart and identify the divisions of labor, the hierarchy of authority, and the degree of formalization.

Centralization refers to the location where a decision is made. Decisions are made at the top of a centralized organization. In a decentralized organization, decisions are made at or close to the patient-care level. Highly centralized organizations delegate responsibility without the authority necessary to carry out the responsibility. For example, some hospitals have vested the charge nurse with admission decisions (decentralized), whereas others require the nurse supervisor or chief nurse executive to make such decisions (centralization).

■ *Exercise 9–5*

Review nursing policies in a city health department, a school health office, a home health agency, and a hospital.

Are there common policies? Does one of the organizations have more detailed policies than others? Is this formalization consistent with the structural complexity?

TYPES OF ORGANIZATIONAL STRUCTURES

Three types of organizational structures exist: **bureaucratic, matrix,** and **flat.** Nursing organizations often combine characteristics from the three types, forming a structure that is a **hybrid. Shared governance** is a term often used to describe the flat types of structures presently being designed to meet the changing needs of nursing organizations.

Bureaucracy

Bureaucracy evolved from early theories on organizing work. It arose at a time of societal development when services were in short supply, workers' and clients' knowledge bases were limited, and technologies for sharing information were undeveloped. Characteristics of bureaucracy arose out of a need to control workers and were centered around division of processes into discrete tasks. Bureaucratic structures are formal, centralized, and hierarchical and consist of divisions of labor and specialists. Rules, standards, and protocols ensure uniform actions and limit individualization of services and variance in workers' performance. As shown in Figure 9-2, communication and decisions flow from top to bottom, limiting employees' autonomy.

■ *Exercise 9–6*

Develop a list of decisions that you as a staff nurse would like to make to optimize care for your patients. Determine where those decisions are made in a nursing organization with which you are familiar. Consider issues such as (1) deciding on visiting schedules that meet your own, your clients', and their significant others' needs and (2) determining a personal work schedule that meets your personal needs and your clients' needs. An example of the latter is talking to the children of a confused elderly client during the evening because they work during the day shift, when you are on duty.

At the time that bureaucracies were developed, these characteristics promoted efficiency and production. As the knowledge base of the general population and employees grew and technologies developed, the bureaucratic structure no longer fit the evolving situation. Increasingly, employees and consumers functioning in bureaucratic situations complain of red tape, procedural delays, and general frustration.

Applying the characteristics of bureaucracy to an organization illustrates that the characteristics can be present in varying degrees. An organization can demonstrate bureaucratic characteristics in some areas and not in others. For example, nursing staff in intensive care units may be granted autonomy in making and carrying out direct client care decisions, but they may be granted no voice in determining work schedules or financial reimbursement systems for hours worked. A method of determining the extent to which bureaucratic tendencies exist in organizations is to assess the organizational characteristics of labor specialization (the degree to which client care is divided into highly specialized tasks), centralization (at what level of the organization decisions regarding carrying out work and remuneration for work are made), and formalization (what percentage of actions required to deliver patient care is governed by written policy and procedures).

Bureaucratic structures are commonly called *line structures*. Line structures usually have a staff component. Line structures have a vertical line, designating reporting and decision-making responsibility, that connects all positions to a centralized authority (see Figure 9-2).

Exercise 9-7

Analyze the decisions identified in Exercise 9-6 from a manager's perspective. Is that perspective similar to or different from the original perspective you identified?

Line functions are those that involve direct responsibility for accomplishing the objectives of a nursing department, service, or unit. Staff functions are those that assist the line in accomplishing the primary objectives. Line positions may include registered nurses, licensed practical/vocational nurses, and unlicensed assistive personnel who have the responsibility for carrying out all aspects of direct care. Staff positions may include staff development personnel, researchers, and special clinical consultants who are responsible for supporting line positions through activities of consultation, education, role modeling, and knowledge development, with no authority for decision making. Line personnel have authority for decision making, whereas staff provide support, advice, and counsel. Organizational charts

usually indicate line positions through the use of solid lines and staff positions through broken lines (see Figure 9-2).

To make line and staff functions effective, the authority for decision making is clearly spelled out in position descriptions. Effectiveness is further ensured by delineating competencies required for the responsibilities, providing methods of determining whether personnel possess these competencies, and providing means of maintaining and developing the competencies.

Matrix Structures

Matrix structures are designed to focus on both product and function. *Function* is defined as all the tasks required to produce a product that is designated as the end result of the function. In an acute care organization, the desired product may be a satisfactory outcome to the client's problem that necessitated treatment, and the function may be all the actions required to produce the product. In a matrix organization the manager of a unit responsible for a service reports both to a functional manager and to a product manager. For example, a director of pediatric nursing could report both to a chief executive officer (product manager) and to a vice president of nursing (functional manager) (Figure 9-3).

Matrix structures have been effective in the current healthcare environment. The matrix design enables timely response to the forces in the external environment that demand continual programming, and it facilitates internal efficiency and effectiveness through the promotion of cooperation among disciplines.

A matrix structure is a hybrid structure that combines both a bureaucratic structure and a flat structure; teams are used to carry out specific programs or projects. A matrix structure superimposes a horizontal program management over the traditional vertical hierarchy. Personnel from various functional departments are assigned to a specific program or project and become responsible to two bosses—their functional department head and a program manager. This creates an interdisciplinary team.

A line manager and a project manager function collaboratively. For example, in nursing, there may be a chief nursing executive, nurse managers, and staff nurses in the line of authority to accomplish nursing care. In the matrix structure, some of the nurse's time is allocated to project or committee

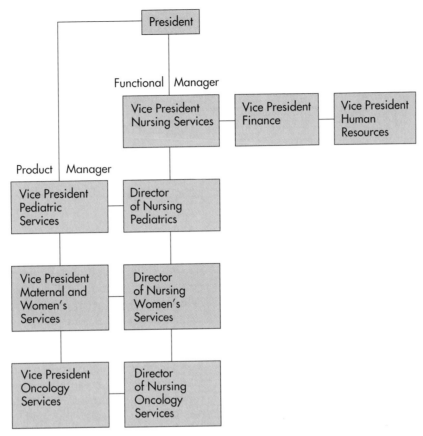

Figure 9-3   Matrix organizational structure.

work. Nursing care is delivered in a teamwork setting or within a collaborative model. The nurse is responsible to a nurse manager for nursing care and to a program or project manager when working within the matrix overlay. Well-developed collaboration and coordination skills are essential to effective functioning in a matrix structure. The nature of a matrix with its complex interrelationships requires workers with knowledge and skill in interpersonal relationships and teamwork.

One example of the matrix structure is the patient-focused care delivery model that is being implemented in some facilities. Another example is the program focused on specialty services such as geriatric services, women's services, and cardiovascular services. A matrix model can be designed to cover both a patient-focused care delivery model and a specialty service. Other examples are special healthcare facility programs such as discharge planning, total quality management, and cardiopulmonary resuscitation. Sometimes these elements are referred to as *product lines* or *service lines*.

Flat Structures

Delegation of decision making to the professionals doing the work, referred to as *participatory management*, is the primary characteristic of flat organizational structures. The term *flat* signifies the removal of hierarchical layers, thereby granting authority to act and placing authority at the action level (Figure 9-4). Decisions regarding work methods, nursing care of individual patients, and conditions under which employees work are made where the work is carried out. Decentralization replaces the centralization of decision making at the top of the organization. Providing staff with authority to make decisions at the place of interaction with clients reflects a flat structure.

Flat organizational structures are less formalized than hierarchical organizations. A decrease in rules and policies allows for individualized decisions that fit specific situations and meet current needs created by consumerism, change, and competition.

The degree of flattening varies from organization to organization. Organizations that are decen-

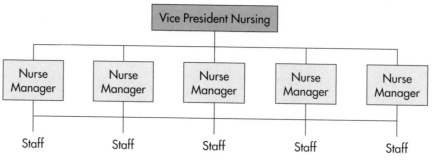

Figure 9-4   Flat organizational structure.

tralizing often retain bureaucratic characteristics. They may at the same time have units that are operating as matrix structures. *Hybrid* is a term applied to organizational structures that operate with characteristics of different types of structures.

■ *Exercise 9–8*

Organizational structures vary in the extent to which they have bureaucratic characteristics. Using observations from your current situations, place a check mark (✓) in the "Present" column beside the bureaucratic characteristics that you believe apply to the agency. What does this analysis indicate about the bureaucratic tendency of the agency? Do the environment and technologies fit the identified bureaucratic tendency? (Consider the state of development of information systems, method of care delivery, clients' characteristics, workers' characteristics, regulatory status, and competition.)

CHARACTERISTIC	PRESENT
Hierarchy of authority	___
Division of labor	___
Written procedures for work	___
Limited authority for workers	___
Emphasis on written communication related to work performance and workers' behaviors	___
Impersonality of personal contact	___

Problems with letting go of centralized control and of top managers changing from boss roles to facilitator roles are partially responsible for the development of hybrid structures. Managers are unsure of what needs to be controlled, how much control is needed, and which mechanisms can replace control. Fear of chaos without control predominates. Education that prepares managers to employ leadership techniques that empower nursing staff to take responsibility for their work is one method of eliminating managers' fears. These fears stem from

loss of centralized control, as authority with its concomitant responsibilities moves to the place of interaction. The evolutionary development of self-governance structures in nursing departments demonstrates a type of flat structure being used to replace hierarchical control.

Self-Governance

Self-governance goes beyond participatory management through the creation of organizational structures that allow nursing staff to govern themselves. Accountability forms the foundation for designing self-governance models. To be accountable, authority to make decisions concerning all aspects of responsibilities is essential. This need for authority and accountability is particularly important for nurses who treat the wide range of human responses to wellness states and illnesses. The major cause of nurses' dissatisfaction with their work revolves around the absence of this accountability. The early Magnet hospital study (McClure et al., 1983), which identified characteristics of hospitals successful in recruiting and retaining nurses, found that nursing departments with structures that provided nurses the opportunity to be accountable for their own practice were the major contributing characteristic to success. The Research Perspective box provides more recent findings.

Shared governance or self-governance structure designs, sometimes referred to as *professional practice models,* go beyond decentralizing and diminishing hierarchies. Accountability is determined by needs arising from the services provided to clients. Authority, control, and autonomy are placed in specifically defined areas of accountability. For example, all issues related to nursing practices are dealt with by nursing staff.

All organizations require a foundation for operation. In a shared governance organization, the

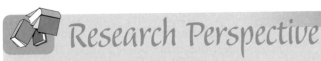

Research Perspective

Aiken, L. H., Havens, D. S., & Sloane, D. M. (2000). The Magnet Nursing Services Recognition Program: A comparison of two groups of Magnet hospitals. *American Journal of Nursing, 100,* 26-36.

This study compared seven current American Nurses Credentialing Center (ANCC) Magnet hospitals with the 13 original Magnet hospitals. Nurses on medical-surgical units responded to a 15-page survey. Factors such as job characteristics and outlook, organizational attributes, and job attitude were evaluated. Results included the following:

- Both sets of Magnet facilities had registered nurses with significantly higher education than non-Magnet facilities.
- The current ANCC Magnet hospitals had a significantly higher ratio of registered nurses (RNs) to patients than original Magnet hospitals.

- Nurses in current ANCC Magnet hospitals reported they had adequate support services and enough RNs to provide high quality care more often than nurses in original Magnet hospitals.
- Nurses in current ANCC Magnet hospitals reported significantly less burnout than those in the original Magnet hospitals.
- Nurses rated the quality of care as excellent more often in current ANCC Magnet hospitals than nurses in the original Magnet hospitals.

IMPLICATIONS FOR PRACTICE

Creating organizational structures and cultures reflective of Magnet facilities can enhance quality of care and nurse satisfaction.

---

structure's foundation is the workplace rather than the hierarchy. Authority, responsibility, and accountability for all aspects of the work are vested in the nurses delivering care. The management/administrative level serves to coordinate and facilitate the work of the practicing nurses. Areas of accountability, such as quality management, are points of final authority for their designated accountability and are not subject to other sources for approval and mandated performance. Mechanisms are designed outside of the traditional hierarchy to provide for the functional areas needed to support professional practice. These functions include areas such as quality management, competency definition and evaluation, and continuing education. Structures of shared governance organizations vary. Box 9-2 shows three self-governance structures in progressive stages of evolution. As shown, evolution is moving structure beyond committees imposed on hierarchical structures to governance structures at the unit level.

Shared governance structures require new behaviors of all staff, not just new assignments of accountability. Behaviors required are in the areas of interpersonal relationship development, conflict resolution, and personal acceptance of responsibility for action. Education and experience in group work and conflict management are essential for successful transitions.

Changing nurses' positions from dependent employees to independent, accountable professionals is a prerequisite for the radical redesign of healthcare organizations that is required to create value for clients and to abandon basic notions regarding the necessity of the division of labor. Structures providing nurses with accountability will meet needs for change while also meeting consumers' demands and remaining competitive. Fitting nursing process and function with the governance process and determining that organizational structure characteristics fit the technology is an ongoing process.

ANALYZING ORGANIZATIONS

When an organization is analyzed, it is important to scrutinize the various systems that exist to accomplish the work of the enterprise. This includes delineating the processes or procedures that have been developed to coordinate the work to be done. To conceptualize how the organization functions, it is imperative to know the recruitment procedures, the method of selecting individuals for positions, the reporting relationships, and the information network. A positive organization reflects a fit of the vision, mission, and philosophy with the structure and practices. Understanding the criteria for Magnet facilities (American Nurses Credentialing Center,

2000), irrespective of structure, could form the basis for evaluating nursing services.

EMERGING FLUID RELATIONSHIPS

As the continuum of care moves health services outside of institutional parameters, different skill sets, relationships, and behavioral patterns will be required. Boundaryless organizations are the emerging organizations. Old boundaries of hierarchy, function, and geography are disappearing. Vertical integration aligns dissimilar but related entities such as hospital, home care agency, rehabilitation center, long-term care facility, insurance provider, and medical office/clinic. The **virtual organization** is an-

---

BOX 9-2

Self-Governance Structure Evolution

Phase One

Representative staff nurses are members of clinical forums, which have authority for designated practice issues and some authority for determining roles, functions, and processes. Managers are members of the management forums, which are responsible for the facilitation of practice through resource management and location. Recommendations for action go to the executive committee, which has administrative and staff membership that may or may not be in equal proportion. The nurse executive retains decision-making authority.

Phase Two

Representative staff nurses belong to nursing committees that are designated for specific management and/or clinical functions. These committees are chaired by staff nurses or administrators appointed by the vice president of nursing. The nursing committee chairs and nurse administrators make up the nursing cabinet, which makes the final decision on recommendations from the committees.

Phase Three

Representative staff nurses belong to councils with authority for specific functions. Council chairs make up the management committee charged with making all final operational organizational decisions.

 Literature Perspective

Fitzpatrick, M. J., McElroy, M. J., & DeWoody, S. (2001). Building a strong nursing organization in a merged service line structure. *Journal of Nursing Administration, 31*(1), 24-32.

In an increasingly complex healthcare environment, the discipline of nursing is difficult to define. Although a "designated" department of nursing may be absent on the organizational chart, the functional elements of the discipline remain. The authors offer a five-phase methodology to enable the creation of a strong nursing organization in the face of mergers, service lines, and complex reporting structures.

Identifying the foundation of nursing, agreeing on a common philosophy, and identifying elements thought to contribute to a sound nursing organization are done in the first phase. The second phase of identifying where nursing is practiced and organizing nursing into like areas of practice enhanced the development of documentation tools and orientation plans for new staff, among other things. Standardization of job descriptions in the third phase provided for articulation of the orientation and training content for various jobs. Designing a nursing language system in the fourth phase led to identifying competencies and time for validation. Review, revision, and preparation for automation became the fifth phase.

IMPLICATIONS FOR PRACTICE

A methodology for maintaining a unified nursing presence in new organizations is necessary. Using the five-phase approach provides nursing leaders and staff with a methodology for keeping nursing's value known, its presence felt, and its unity intact.

other model that brings together various entities in providing continuity of care for a limited period to reach a specific goal. New technologies, fast-changing markets, and global competition are revolutionizing relationships in healthcare, and the roles that people play and the tasks that they perform have become blurred and ambiguous.

Nurses no longer practice in settings, but rather in systems of care that have extended boundaries. Nurses need to be able to work with other members of society to design organizational models for care delivery that meet patient/customer needs and priorities. It is essential to take a new look at the nature of the work of nursing and propose innovative models for nursing practice that take into account emerging labor-saving assistive technologies and rapidly changing healthcare needs. Employee participation and learning environments go hand in hand, and work redesign needs to be regarded as a continuous process. It is essential that nurses value their own and others' autonomy to deal successfully in these new structures. As the Literature Perspective illustrates, no matter what the structure is, it is important to have a strong nursing organization.

Reframing or changing an organization is a four-dimensional process (human, structural, political, and symbolic). In future organizations, healthcare delivery businesses will be knowledge-based organizations comprised largely of specialists who direct their performance through organized feedback from colleagues, customers, and headquarters.

The Solution

Immediately, I established what the management structure would be. For example, I changed the scope of responsibility for the individual managers. I then actively recruited for those positions and put in place specific retention strategies to ensure that those who were already a part of the team were engaged in the new direction. I also created a staff development position to fulfill my strategy of clinical management.

After I created the management team, I created core competencies for the clinical staff. Obviously, staff representatives participated in the establishment and design of the initial set of competencies. Now we are working on the design and implementation of the second set of competencies. It really is exciting to see how the nurses here have focused their energy in meeting this challenge. I am very fortunate also that the staff development educator has had experience in a university, so she has connections for recruitment, and she is acutely aware of standards and consistency.

— Rebecca M. Patton

 Would this approach be suitable for you? Why?

CHAPTER CHECKLIST

Nursing care delivered in healthcare organizations is determined by the vision and mission of the organization in which the care is delivered. Changes occurring in missions affect both the culture of the workplace and the philosophies regarding the work required to accomplish the mission. Actualizing new missions and philosophies requires reengineered organizational structures that place decision-making authority and responsibility where care is delivered. Decision-making responsibility requires staff to understand the organization's mission and to participate in the development of mission and philosophy statements.

- Five factors influencing design of an organization structure are as follows:
  - The types of service performed or the product produced
  - The characteristics of the employees performing the service or producing the product
  - The beliefs and values held by the people responsible for delivering the service concerning the work, the people receiving the services, and the employees
  - The technologies used to perform the service and produce the product
  - The needs, desires, and characteristics of the consumers using the product or service

Continued

CHAPTER CHECKLIST—cont'd

- Reengineering, the complete overhaul of an organization's structures, is driven by forces of the following:
  - Change
  - Consumerism
  - Competition
- Bureaucratic structures are characterized by the following:
  - A high degree of formalization
  - Centralization of decision making at the top of the organization
  - A hierarchy of authority
- Matrix structures are characterized by the following:
  - Dual authority for product and function
  - Mechanisms such as committees to coordinate actions of product and function managers
  - Success that is dependent on recognition and appreciation of each others' missions and philosophies and commitment to the organization's mission and philosophy
- Flat organizations are characterized by the following:
  - Decision making concerning work performed, decentralized to the level where the work is done
  - Authority, accountability, and autonomy, as well as responsibility, provided to staff performing care
  - Low level of formalization in relation to rules, with processes tailored to meet individual consumer's needs
- Vision, mission, and philosophy determine the characteristics of the organizational structure by doing the following:
  - Creating an ultimate state of existence (vision)
  - Describing the consumers and services as a prescription for the technologies and human resources needed to accomplish the defined purpose (mission)
  - Citing values and beliefs that shape and are shaped by the nature of the work and the rights and responsibilities of workers and consumers (philosophy)
  - Designing characteristics that support the service implementation to fulfill the mission and philosophy (structure)

TIPS ON UNDERSTANDING ORGANIZATIONAL STRUCTURES

- The mission of the organization and the mission for the specific unit where a professional nurse is employed or is seeking employment provide knowledge concerning the major focus for the work to be accomplished.
- Understanding the philosophy of the organization and/or unit where work occurs provides knowledge of the behaviors that are valued in the delivery of client care and in interactions with persons employed by the organization.
- Organizational structures describe channels of communication and decision making.
- Matrix organizations usually have two persons responsible for the work, so it is important to know to whom you are responsible for what.
- For a self-governance structure to function effectively, mechanisms must be put in place to promote decision making about client care by persons providing the care.
- Professional nurses in staff or followership positions need to understand the vision, mission, philosophy, and organizational structure to maximize their contributions to patient care.

TERMS TO KNOW

bureaucratic organization	organizational chart
chain of command	organizational structure
fit	philosophy
flat organization	reengineering
hierarchy	shared governance
hybrid organization	technology
matrix organization	vertical organization
mission	virtual organization

REFERENCES

Aiken, L. H., Havens, D. S., & Sloane, D. M. (2000). The Magnet Nursing Services Recognition Program: A comparison of two groups of Magnet hospitals. *American Journal of Nursing, 100,* 26-36.

American Nurse Credentialing Center. (2000). *Health care organization instructions and application process manual.* Washington, DC: Author.

Fitzpatrick, M. J., McElroy, M. J., & De Woody, S. (2001). Building a strong nursing organization in a merged service line structure. *Journal of Nursing Administration, 31*(1), 24-32.

George, V., Burke, L., & Rodgers, B. (1997). Research and planning for change. Assessing nurses' attitudes toward governance and professional practice autonomy after hospital acquisition. *Journal of Nursing Administration, 27*(6), 53-61.

McClure, M. L., Poulin, M. A., Sovie, M. D., & Wandelth, M. A. (1983). *Magnet hospitals, attrition and retention of professional nurses.* Kansas City, MO: American Nurses Association.

Wheatley, M. J. (1999). *Leadership and the new science.* San Francisco: Berrett-Koehler.

SUGGESTED READINGS

Aiken, L. H., Clarke, S. P., & Sloane, D. M. (2000). Hospital restructuring: Does it adversely affect care and outcomes? *Journal of Nursing Administration, 30,* 457-465.

Aiken, L. H., & Patrician, P. A. (2000). Measuring organizational traits of hospitals: The revised nursing work index. *Nursing Research, 49,* 146-153.

Begun, J. W., & White, K. R. (1995) Altering nursing's dominant logic: Guidelines from complex adaptive systems theory. *Complexity and Chaos in Nursing, 2*(1), 5-15.

Brzytwa, E., Copeland, L., & Hewson, M. (2001). Managed care education: A needs assessment of employers and educators of nurses. *Journal of Nursing Education, 39*(5), 197-204.

Garrett, D. K., & McDaniel, A. M. (2001). A new look at nurse burnout: The effects of environmental uncertainty and social climate. *Journal of Nursing Administration, 31,* 91-96.

Graham, P., Constantine, S., Balik, B., Bedore, B., Hoake, M. C. M., Papin, D., Quamme, M., & Rivaid, R. (1987). Operationalizing a nursing philosophy. *Journal of Nursing Administration, 17*(3), 14-18.

Kennedy, S. H. (1996). Effects of shared governance on perceptions of work and work environment. *Nursing Economics, 14*(2), 111-116.

Markus, M. L., Manville, B., & Agres, E. (2000). What makes a virtual organization work? *Sloan Management Review, 42*(1), 13-26.

McGuire, E. (1999). Chaos theory: Learning a new science. *Journal of Nursing Administration, 29*(2), 8-9.

Miller, J., Galloway, M., Coughlin, C., & Brennan, E. (2001). Care-centered organizations. Part 1: Nursing governance. *Journal of Nursing Administration, 31*(2), 67-73.

Netting, F. E., & Williams, F. G. (2000). Expanding the boundaries of primary care for elderly people. *Health & Social Work, 25*(4), 233-242.

Porter-O'Grady, T. (1996). The seven basic rules for redesign. *Journal of Nursing Administration, 26*(1), 46-53.

Poteet, G., & Hill, A. (1988). Identifying the components of a nursing service philosophy. *Journal of Nursing Administration, 18*(10), 29-35.

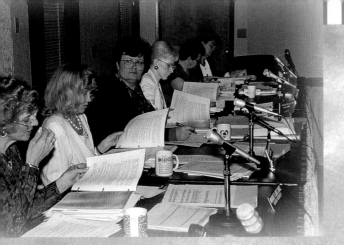

10

Collective Action

Fran Hicks

As society has moved toward a more egalitarian environment, employees are expecting and, in many situations demanding a greater voice in decisions involving their work life. These decisions involve both the context and the content of their work. Policy, education, and experience influence healthcare professionals to engage the consumer in healthcare decisions. These professionals see merit in being part of the decision-making process. Participation in decisions regarding practice is an appropriate expectation of a professional nurse. Collective action is one mechanism available to achieve that participation. The manager can capitalize on this strategy to accomplish positive outcomes.

Objectives

- Relate the participation of staff nurses in decision making to job satisfaction.
- Analyze the influence of culture on the selection of a governance model.
- Identify key characteristics of selected collective action strategies: shared governance, workplace advocacy, and collective bargaining.
- Distinguish between the rights of individuals included in collective bargaining contracts and the rights of at-will employees.
- Compare the factors that contribute to nurses' decisions to

be represented for the purpose of collective bargaining and the decision for no representation.

- Evaluate strategies for their effectiveness in diverse workplace environments.

Questions to Consider

- *How does nurse participation in decision making influence job satisfaction?*
- *What strategies can you use to participate in decision making?*
- *How can you transfer your knowledge of advocacy to workplace advocacy?*
- *What would influence you to practice in an organization in which nurses are organized for the purpose of collective bargaining?*
- *Within the context of labor law, how do the responsibilities of nurses who are supervisors differ from the responsibilities of nurses who are nonsupervisory?*

155

The Challenge

Peggy Reiley, RN, MSN, ScM
Vice President, Scottsdale Memorial Hospital—Osborn, Scottsdale, Arizona

I was a new vice president for patient services. After several months of assessing the new organization, I determined that I would like to redesign how care was delivered on the patient care unit. Specifically, I wanted to reevaluate vari-ous roles and possibly redesign certain roles to better meet the need of patients and their families.

 What do you think you would do if you were this nurse?

INTRODUCTION

The excitement of beginning a career in nursing or assuming the position of a manager is balanced by events taking place in healthcare and the effect of these events on nursing and nurses. The knowledge gained about healthcare provides a background for considering issues within healthcare and factors that promote or inhibit the achievement of professional practice.

Nurses are deeply involved in the complex clinical problems of individuals, families, and communities. Nursing practice requires an acquisition, synthesis, and retrieval of knowledge to provide competent nursing care. Having the time and resources to engage in this level of preparation for each situation may be viewed as the "high hard ground"; the current environment in which nursing practice occurs may be more akin to "the messy swamps and the pathways between" (Streets, 1990, p. 22).

COLLECTIVE ACTION

Collective action is a benign phrase; it refers to many aspects of daily life, including work. Inpatient health care has historically been delivered through the collective action of shifts of nurses. This pattern requires a level of independence during the shift and interdependence between shifts and other healthcare professionals. Nurses learn quickly to rely on their colleagues. "In a climate of job insecurity, it is easy to lose sight of our personal power as individuals and our collective power as professionals" (Harris, Ryan, & Belmont, 1997, p. 39). Nurses have been less comfortable with formal collectives. Their discomfort may be attributed to a number of factors.

Nursing is a female-dominated profession, and women have had less experience in working and playing within a team structure. Before Title IX, few women participated in competitive team sports. Women have demonstrated less interest in the structure of rules. Many women, including nurses, view employment as a job rather than a career. For these individuals the time to work with others to achieve common goals deprives them of personal time. Women have not perceived themselves to be powerful. The "good" nurse was considered obedient. (The Nightingale Pledge reinforced obedience: "With loyalty will I endeavor to aid the physician in *his work* . . ." [Kalisch & Kalisch, 1975].) This obedience or acquiescence to authority appears to have been transferred to other authority figures, including but not limited to, hospital administrators.

Minarik and Catramabone (1998) described four main purposes of collective participation for nurses: (1) to promote the practice of professional nursing, (2) to establish and maintain standards of care, (3) to allocate resources effectively and efficiently, and (4) to create satisfaction and support in the practice environment. Collective action helps define and sustain individuals in achieving their purposes. In the absence of collective action the average individual has limited influence in achieving his or her purpose. Perhaps you learned the strength and value of collective action early in life as you and your siblings banded together to make a request to your parents. The same strategy has probably served you in an organization as you brought together a group of peers to make a point or to plead your case. In nursing practice you may have observed nurses as they identified a practice concern and joined together to bring about change.

Developing networks, developing a collective voice, and cultivating a collective are strategies for building collectives (Mason, Talbott, & Leavitt, 1998).

■ *Exercise 10–1*

Identify three collectives to which you belong. List the purposes of each. How do you feel as a member of these groups?

The strategies of developing networks, developing a collective voice, and cultivating a collective require strong leaders and a broad **followership.** Matusak (1997) suggested that the relationship between leaders and followers is symbiotic; that is, two or more very dissimilar organisms form a relationship that is interdependent. Followers and leaders share many characteristics. Successful people move easily between the roles of follower and leader. The knowledge and skills of followers may differ from those of the leader; they are not less. Leaders and followers are knowledgeable of the context and content of their practice. Followers are active, involved participants committed to an agreed-upon agenda. They are loyal and supportive to the individual who is setting the pace and the agenda. The nurse who becomes a leader finds that the absence of followers is personally painful.

The change in an initiative or an agenda may result in today's leader being tomorrow's follower. The opposite is also applicable: Today's follower may be tomorrow's leader. The change may result from the context of the situation. In the operating room the surgeon is the acknowledged leader and the anesthesiologist follows that lead with respect to the extent of the anesthesia. If the patient's condition changes, the anesthesiologist becomes the leader and the surgeon may simply step away from the table, an overt act that demonstrates a change in leadership. As healthcare consumers and participants, we salute the clarity.

■ *Exercise 10–2*

Identify two groups in which you have been a leader (e.g., school, church, sports). Was your specific role the result of a group decision? How did your role as a leader differ from your role as a follower? List the skills you used in each role.

Followers are not submissive partisans blindly following a cultist personality. They are effective group members, not "groupies." They are skilled in group dynamics and accountable for their actions. They are willing and able to question, debate, compromise, collaborate, and act. Consider potential differences between being a subordinate in a hierarchical organization and being a follower committed to one's practice.

Collective action provides a mechanism for achieving professional practice through greater participation in decision making. The governance structure provides the framework for participation. Participation in decision making regarding one's practice is an appropriate expectation for professionals, provides for greater autonomy and authority over practice decisions, contributes to empowering the professional nurse, and is a major component of job satisfaction. The privilege and the obligation to participate are inherent in the discipline. Consistent with the Code of Ethics for Nurses (American Nurses Association [ANA], 2001), members of the discipline participate based on their competence. Although nurses are expected to be informed, active participants, not all nurses wish to participate in decisions. For these nurses, going to work and doing their assigned job may fulfill their expectations. They may not perceive themselves as being in a subordinate position, or if they do, it is not a concern for them. Their orientation is to serve the care recipient and to be loyal to the organization. For these individuals, asserting the right and responsibility to participate in decisions may be considered disrespectful to the organization's policies and to the physician. However, participation in practice-related decisions is critical to quality patient care, expected by society, and essential to autonomy for nursing. Lewis and Batey (1982) defined four key concepts: responsibility, authority, autonomy, and accountability; today's healthcare environment demands that nurses exercise each.

Responsibility

The history of nursing provides evidence of nurses accepting responsibility or the "charge to act." In the past this charge took the form of meticulously and unquestioningly following the "physician's orders" and "hospital procedures." The "good" nurse rendered disclosure at the convenience of the physician and management. Progressive healthcare organizations recognize "the rightful power of the nurse to act." The recognition of credentialing, especially certification, has contributed to the exercise of expert power by nurses.

Authority

Authority based on preparation and experience suggests a departure from the tradition of delegating authority to individual nurses based on the physician's knowledge of the nurse—a knowledge that too often was based on personal characteristics, not clinical competence. That statement does not denigrate the collegial relationship between nurse and physician, relationships that are based on mutual respect and trust. There is evidence that patient care improves when these relationships exist.

Autonomy

Autonomy, the freedom to decide and act, has come about more slowly. Dempster (1990) conceptualized four dimensions of autonomy: empowerment, readiness, application, and valuation. In today's cost-containment environment, the effort of all individuals must be maximized. To maximize the clinical effectiveness of registered nurses (RNs), they must have autonomy consistent with their scope of practice. It is unfortunate that autonomy for nurses is often based on management's trust of the individual nurse instead of the profession. Multiple studies demonstrate that a healthcare organization that provides a climate in which nurses have authority and autonomy retains nurses at a higher rate, is more cost effective, and has evidence of greater patient satisfaction than an organization in which such a climate does not exist. Based on her work, Kennerly (2000) posited that the future depends on designing and implementing freedom in decision making to create and sustain positive work environments in nursing. The study by Aiken, Clarke, and Sloane (2000) acknowledged the influence of organizational restructuring on job satisfaction and the important influence of nurse staffing, especially the RN-to-patient ratios, on patient care outcomes. Furthermore, they ". . . showed that nurse control over the practice setting explains almost all of the variation in patient satisfaction that is associated with different organizational forms of AIDS care" (p. 462). Nurse involvement in decision making contributes to higher levels of job satisfaction for the nurse and higher satisfaction with care for the patient and positively influences health outcomes.

Recruitment and retention are affected by participation. The "failure on the part of health care delivery organizations, physicians, and policy making bodies to fully recognize the decision making abilities of RNs has contributed to problems in recruiting and retaining nurses, hindered the develop-

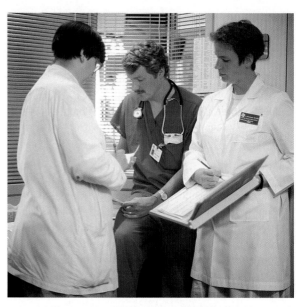

Decision making is at the core of nursing practice.

ment of a career orientation in professional nursing, and limited the efficiency and effectiveness of patient care delivery" (U.S. Department of Health and Human Services, 1988, p. vii). This statement was accurate when written and has become more important as the delivery of and payment for healthcare evolve.

Autonomy encourages innovation and increases productivity. Although automobile manufacturing is a highly mechanized process, management has learned that it is cost effective to give the employee on the shop floor the autonomy to "stop the line" when the potential for error is detected. Stopping errors before they occur is more efficient than recalling items and retrofitting and is more humane than causing injury and perhaps death. Unlocking minds by providing greater autonomy and diversifying tasks decreases fear, specifically fear of ridicule, fear of punishment, fear of loss of job, and even fear of favors.

Accountability

Accountability focuses the organization and all its members on the purposes and the outcomes of their collective activities. Accountability requires ownership. Porter-O'Grady and Wilson (1995) assert, "It is not possible to be accountable for what one does not own" (p. 30). These researchers identified five accountability basics: (1) Accountability is about outcomes, not processes; (2) accountability is individually defined; (3) accountability is inherent in the role—it is not delegated; (4) accountability must be clear to all those in related roles; and (5) accountability is the foundation for evaluation.

The value of process is determined by the extent to which individuals observe a particular protocol while accomplishing a goal. Accountability focuses on the achievement of the specified outcome. This shift in thinking has had a tremendous effect on healthcare reimbursement. An example of the shift is evident in patient education. Initialing a form to indicate that patient teaching has occurred is no longer acceptable. The criterion now expects that the patient's behavior has changed. "Accountability is all about outcomes" (Porter-O'Grady & Wilson, 1995, p. 29).

GOVERNANCE

Nursing governance is the methodology or system by which a department of nursing controls and directs the formulation and the administration of nursing policy. Organizational structure provides a framework for fulfilling the organization's mission. Organizational charts show the relationship among and between roles. The structure of the organization and the relationship among the components of the structure are influenced by the individuals selected to interpret and implement the organization's philosophy. A particular form of governance evolves from the mission and values of the organization and the relationships among and between its components. Although nurses must be knowledgeable of the structure, relationships, and influential individuals to achieve collective action, evidence suggests that organizational structure is not a significant influence on the leadership behaviors of nurse managers (Drayton-Hargrove, 1996). To paraphrase an adage, behavior speaks louder and has more clout than organizational charts.

Nurses have at their disposal multiple strategies to achieve collective action; three prevalent ones are **shared governance, workplace advocacy,** and collective bargaining. These strategies are not mutually exclusive. As noted, governance is influenced by the context within which the organizational culture is embedded.

The culture of the geographic area influences the organizational culture and the selected governance structure. For example, in right-to-work states, collective bargaining may be tolerated more

BOX 10-1

Right-to-Work Legislation

Right-to-work legislation prevents unions from mandating membership by workers in a given organization. In states with right-to-work laws, unions are not allowed to mandate membership of employees in a bargaining unit. Therefore unionization is less prevalent. Nurses working in these states are less likely to choose unionization as a strategy to achieve collective action in part because they may see fewer examples in society at large.

than supported by nurses and administration. Box 10-1 summarizes some key factors about these states. The "purity" of geographic cultures has been diluted because of mobility and the mass media. However, it is prudent to acknowledge how deeply embedded these cultural influences are within the fabric of American society.

When the respective subcultures are clearly rooted in the mission of the organization (delivery of quality care in a cost-effective environment), the possibility of genuine negotiation or problem solving is enhanced. The presence of congruent subcultures supports healthy relationships. Healthy relationships are an important variable in the development of a strong internal governance structure capable of supporting a professional practice environment that works well for everyone involved.

Exercise 10-3

Is your state a right-to-work state? If it is not, what is the nearest state that is a right-to-work state? Are any workers in the right-to-work state organized for the purpose of collective bargaining? How would you describe these workers (e.g., laborer, professional)?

Subcultures form within organizations as "distinct clusters of ideologies, cultural forms, and other practices that identifiable groups of people in an organization exhibit" (Trice & Beyer, 1992, p. 5-1). Nurses and administrators are often members of separate subcultures. This phenomenon should not be given a negative connotation. Several factors may increase the distinct ideologies of the two groups, including the presence of a union and the existence of a distant corporate structure. Both factors may be considered external tensions. By

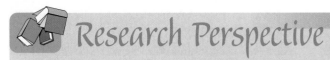

Research Perspective

Moss, R., & Rowles, C. (1997, January). Staff nurse job satisfaction and management style. *Nursing Management, 29,* 32-33.

Job satisfaction for staff nurses is related directly to the perceived management style of managers. In a study of 623 staff nurses from three Midwestern hospitals, researchers found that the greater the perceived level of participatory style was, the greater the level of job satisfaction of staff nurses was. Job satisfaction was higher when the manager's style incorporated characteristics of the participatory style, including loyalty, trust, group problem solving, and high levels of consideration.

IMPLICATIONS FOR PRACTICE
The staff nurse's perception of the style is key. As managers begin a process of changing practice and perception, nurses must be kept informed of proposed changes and changes must be implemented slowly. Individuals who expect certain behaviors experience unnecessary job stress with a rapid change in style.

---

tradition, decision making in the United States has been centralized at the top administrative level. There is a tendency to increase the concentration of decision making during economic downturns. Actions are taken to avoid risk. However, history shows that broader input, not less, is important during these times.

When efforts have been made to address nurses' perceptions about job satisfaction, there has been a resulting effect on the relationship between nursing and the top administration of a hospital. Job satisfaction and the perceived level of care are greater when organizations provide for interaction between staff and management and when decision making is at the point of service (Parker & Gadbois, 2000). The relationship is damaged when organizations do not address job satisfaction. The Research Perspective identifies the important role of managers.

Exercise 10-4

Identify four factors in your practice (experience) that contribute to job satisfaction. Compare your responses to those of three practicing nurses who are not supervisors and three practicing nurses who are supervisors. Are your factors common in the responses of others? Are you surprised by the responses?

In the past, nurses experienced practice environments and working conditions controlled by the medical profession and hospital administration. Increasingly, nurses expect a motivating, satisfying work environment that includes a role in decision making. Many nurses today are unwilling

to remain outside of the decision-making loop. However, restructuring efforts to increase productivity and lower costs contribute to increased tension regarding the role of nursing and nurses in decision making. Evolving or creating a system that incorporates others in the decision-making process may be difficult for many individuals in upper management positions. Organizations that provide quality healthcare create climates that provide for participation by all stakeholders. Each group shares responsibility and risk that requires optimism and trust.

Contractual models provide for nurses to form an organization and contract with the healthcare organization to provide nursing services. A contractual model can be characterized as a self-governance model as opposed to shared governance. Nurses become contract providers instead of employees. Although direct contracting has been discussed as the "wave of the future" for subacute healthcare organizations (Stahl, 1997), a limited number of nurses have selected this strategy.

Shared Governance

Shared governance is a democratic, egalitarian concept. Shared governance builds a structure that supports the point of care and sustains ownership and accountability at the point of care (Porter-O'Grady, Hawkins, & Parker, 1997). According to Porter-O'Grady, Hawkins, and Parker, basic principles of shared governance include partnerships, equity, accountability, and ownership. It is more accurate to say that shared governance *demands* participation in decision making rather than *provides* for partici-

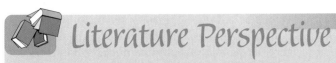

Literature Perspective

Allen, D., Calkin, J., & Peterson, M. (1988). Making shared governance work: A conceptual model. *Journal of Nursing Administration, 17*(1), 37-43.

A significant increase in decisional participation can be expected to produce a number of positive outcomes for the employees and the overall organization. They can be expected to become more involved in their practice, their practice becomes more important to them, and they will be more internally motivated and more committed to the organization. These relationships will be stronger for those with strong desires for achievement, responsibility, and autonomy; for those who perceive themselves as decisionally deprived; and for those whose work is difficult and varied. One can anticipate that people may come to value autonomy and responsibility more highly and to find their jobs more challenging. Nurses must understand the relationship between performance and reward, as well as how their role contributes to the organization and its services. Nurse participation in those decisions that they perceive as being most important to them is essential.

IMPLICATIONS FOR PRACTICE

Nurses and managers can use participative decision making to create a true win-win situation while enhancing professional practice. A participative program can increase that challenge if it affects an employees' autonomy. If the intervention promotes variety, taps more of the nurses' abilities, and helps them develop new skills, it can also make their work more challenging and hence more satisfying. Staff nurses who perceive support for their input will be more likely to risk input. The potential to improve the cost-effectiveness of care is increased by increasing the input of staff nurses into decisions and the issues around which decisions need to be made.

pation. Shared governance creates a framework for ensuring that the processes of empowerment operate effectively throughout a system at every point where work and relationship intersect (Porter-O'Grady & Wilson, 1995).

When asked to rate five consensus-building activities in terms of how they relate to their job satisfaction, staff nurses demonstrated a preference for shared governance models (American Hospital Association [AHA], 1990). In addition to shared governance, the activities included interdisciplinary conferences, interdisciplinary team-building activities, physician-nurse collaborative practice committees, and joint practice. It is ironic that although shared governance received the highest score, it was planned for implementation by only about 18% of the hospitals that did not have it in place. The Literature Perspective illustrates the value of shared governance.

Some organizations mislabel their governance structures. Although structures may be labeled "shared governance," they possess few of the characteristics outlined by those who are recognized as experts on the topic. In addition, many organizations have developed thinly veiled mechanisms designed to preclude nurses from participating in collective bargaining. Evidence suggests that organizations design the systems for that purpose. In 1994 a "National Labor Relations Board administrative law judge ruled that a labor-management cooperative effort at a hospital was illegal. The hospital had established a core group of six employees and supervisors to look into staffing issues. The committee was formed with the purpose of establishing new and innovative ideas including the drafting for a newly created position" (ANA, 1995, p. 11). Such a mechanism would have diminished the role of the union by "setting up a pattern and practice of dealing with the union on a variety of mandatory subjects" (ANA, p. 11). In today's competitive environment, being informed of potential implications of approaches and not rushing to judgment prematurely are important.

Professional-practice climates recognize individual performance. The ability to find organizations that provide professional-practice climates often influences a nurse's decision on where to practice (Jones, 1994). Planning to interview nurses within the organization before finalizing employment decisions is a wise strategy.

Workplace Advocacy

Workplace advocacy is an umbrella term encompassing activities within the practice setting. The choice of advocacy to reflect the framework in which nurses control the practice of nursing is consistent with the goals of the profession. Workplace advocacy includes an array of activities undertaken to address the challenges faced by nurses in their practice settings. The focus of these activities is on career development, employment opportunities, terms and conditions of employment, employment rights and protections, control of practice, labor-management relations, occupational health and safety, and employee assistance. The objective of workplace advocacy is to equip nurses to practice in a rapidly changing environment. Advocacy occurs within a framework of mutuality, facilitation, protection, and coordination.

The manifestations of advocacy include (1) ensuring relevant information, (2) enabling the selection of information, (3) disclosing a personal view, (4) providing support for making and implementing decisions, and (5) helping determine personal values (Gadow, 1990).

■ *Exercise 10-5*

Contact nurses who are not represented by contract. Discuss the strategies they use to influence practice decisions (e.g., staffing, skill mix, responsibilities) and economic decisions (e.g., wages, benefits, time off, retirement).

Ensuring Relevant Information

Within the practice setting, nurses must have relevant information to support their practice. Access to information is the basis for initiatives, full participation, and sharing information. Clinical nursing practice demands that nurses begin with patient information. The use of clinical data is necessary for patient well-being. However, patient information is the beginning of data gathering, not the end. It is equally important for nurses to have information related to occupational health and safety issues, equal employment opportunity information, professional liability, and labor law.

Enabling the Selection of Information

Just as healthcare patients must have relevant information to make good decisions, nurses must be able to select information that is relevant to their practice. Nurses have an obligation to know about a workplace. Begin by learning the mission of the organization and becoming knowledgeable of the culture. Acquaint yourself with nurses who practice in the organization. Although you will need to devote some time and effort to this activity, you will find that it is time and effort well spent. Many nurses and other individuals spend more time making decisions about the cars that they drive than a potential employment site. Think about a time when you were deciding about a car. You probably checked various makes and models and determined price; you may have visited a website or visited the dealership; you may have visited the service department and talked with those who had purchased a car from the dealership; you may have, literally or figuratively, kicked the tires. A similar process should be used to select a place of employment. Data regarding the workplace inform nurses of the history of the workplace. These data are available through the organization's Occupational Safety and Health Administration (**OSHA**) 200 logs (www.OSHA.gov) (Shogren, Calkins, & Wilburn, 1996).

Disclosing a Personal View

Nurses and managers disclose their views on issues related to the work environment. Disclosure of management's perspective is important. The failure to build a trusting relationship jeopardizes the achievement of outcomes.

Healthcare organizations constitute one of the most unsafe work environments in the United States. This environment is characterized by "speed-ups," fewer personnel, fewer full-time personnel, and a propensity to underemploy. An increasingly cynical public holds the "face" of the organization accountable for their pain and frustration. Often, a nurse is the organizational face.

Violence toward healthcare personnel continues to increase. Risk is greater in emergency departments and psychiatric settings. Evidence reveals that many incidents are not reported. The identified toxins in the workplace are also increased. Latex is a particular problem. Disinfectants, sterilants, antineoplasticine agents, radiation, and noise are constants. The organization has a responsibility to ensure a safe environment for staff and patients. Nurses need to be involved in addressing workplace safety. Occupational health nurses provide expert consultation in the identification of potential hazards and suggestions for change. Although back injuries are the most common and most expensive injury in today's nursing care environment, hospitals have been

BOX 10-2

Safety in the Workplace

The Occupational Safety and Health Act of 1970 requires employers to provide a safe and healthy environment. Fire protection, construction and maintenance of equipment, worker training, machine guarding, and protective equipment are specified. Employers are required to familiarize themselves with applicable standards. The **Centers for Disease Control and Prevention (CDC)** guidelines assume that all patients are infectious for human immunodeficiency virus (HIV) and other bloodborne pathogens. Although the CDC is not an enforcement agency, its guidelines are adopted as professional practice standards.

slow to seek these experts to reduce injury (Rogers, 1996). Box 10-2 describes two key sources of environmental support.

Providing Support for Making and Implementing Decisions

The support needed to make and implement decisions is achieved through **role models, mentors,** and empowerment. Role models may include the nurse who has exquisite clinical skills in assessment. Perhaps you have had the opportunity to observe nurses who seem to "absorb" information when they enter a patient's environment. This is a rare and coveted skill. Similarly, observing someone skillful in assertive communications transform an explosive situation into a positive interaction is impressive. The implementation of a primary mentorship program may contribute to the development of these and other skills. It is clear that a brief program with an external expert will not achieve the goal. A mentoring relationship is an ongoing, "hands-on" process. Those who are products of a successful mentorship have identified positive, frequently occurring behaviors that characterized their mentor. The most striking of these learned behaviors may be the encouragement of independent decision making (Holloran,

Exercise 10–6

List the characteristics that you would want your mentor to possess. If you have identified a person you would want as a mentor, ask if he or she is willing to mentor you. Identify any factors that may be a barrier to your seeking a mentorship relationship with the individual. Consider ways that you can address the factor(s).

1993). The value to the individual is professional growth. The value to the organization is in the outcome: The individual will make good decisions.

Today's healthcare environment requires nurses to make many difficult decisions. One painful decision for the beginning nurse and the long-time employee is the act of documenting an unsafe assignment. Accepting an unsafe assignment or refusing an assignment is difficult for nurses—both those at the beginning of their careers and those who are experienced. The ANA (1997) developed a form that documents the acceptance of an assignment despite objections. The completed form may be useful to nurse managers as a source of necessary data to support the preparation of their budgets. Experience shows that many assignments are classified as unsafe because of a lack of personnel and a lack of training of the existing personnel. Nurses need to prepare themselves to respond when an assignment is inappropriate. During an employment interview, ask about the criteria for classifying an assignment as unsafe and the procedure for documenting an unsafe assignment. It is important for your patients and for your practice to become informed about the procedures for refusing an assignment in practice settings and for accepting an assignment despite objection.

Consider the consequences of accepting an assignment that is beyond your scope of practice and skills. These consequences have the potential to affect a patient, the organization, your colleagues, and yourself. One consequence may be conflict. The Alternative Dispute Resolution (ADR) model provides assistance to nurses and is particularly useful in noncontract facilities. ADR uses techniques other than litigation. These techniques include negotiation, facilitation, mediation, and arbitration (Bachman, 2001).

Helping Determine Personal Values

As you enter the profession, your personal values will be internalized. Your professional values have evolved through your education in classroom settings and in your clinical assignments. "Professional values are beliefs and ideologies that are generally held in common by members of the profession and are used to guide professional practice" (Chinn & Kramer, 1999, p. 42). You will have an opportunity to solidify your own values as skillful mentors guide your practice and assist you to engage in value clarification. Ethical codes, standards of practice, standards for protecting participants, willingness to challenge social traditions, priorities for allocating resources, cultural mores, and priorities for allocating resources are examples of specific factors inherent in professional values (Chinn & Kramer, 1999).

Individuals' value to an organization is increased when the individuals are empowered to make decisions within their scope of practice. This situation is both that simple and that complex. Empowerment requires redefining the managerial role and a change in behavior by nurses and administrators. The behavior changes to one in which trust replaces distrust and respect replaces disrespect. How will the beginning nurse determine individual values within various types of decisions if there are inadequate, guided opportunities to practice decision making?

Organizational models that follow a traditional pattern tend to segment the responsibility for the provision of care and management of resources for that care. It is in the best interest of healthcare consumers for nurses to participate in decisions regarding the provision of care and resources. The involvement of nurses can vary from none whatsoever to a high degree of input by nurses in virtually every decision affecting the conditions of employment and their practice. Nurses must be prepared and willing to participate.

▇ *Exercise 10–7*

Identify four factors that you consider most empowering in a governance model. Would the presence of one or more of these factors influence you to practice in this environment? Identify four factors that you would consider least empowering in a governance model. Would the presence of one or more of these factors influence you to avoid practicing in this environment?

Collective Bargaining

Collective bargaining is "the performance of the mutual obligation of the employer and the representatives of the employees to meet at reasonable times and confer in good faith with respect to wages, hours, and other terms and conditions of employment or the negotiation of any agreement or any question arising thereunder . . ." (Labor Management Reporting Act, 1947, section 8). The purpose of collective bargaining by nurses (Box 10-3) is to secure reasonable and satisfactory conditions of employment, including the right to participate in decisions regarding their practice. These conditions are not self-serving; they are directly correlated with the quality of care (Flanagan, 1995).

Union activity in the healthcare sector has become more aggressive in the recent past in part because of changes in labor law. The federal role in labor relations is a dynamic, evolving one. The 1935 Wagner Act (National Labor Relations Act) established election procedures for employees to be able to freely choose their collective bargaining representatives. Two years later, the ANA included provisions for improving nurses' work and professional lives. The 1947 Taft-Hartley Act placed curbs on

BOX 10-3

Unionization

In nonhealthcare industries, unionization is acknowledged as a usual and expected business practice. Improved communication and good will cannot eliminate the gap between labor and management. Cooperation between management and labor will remain an illusion unless or until there is sharing of responsibility, power, and profits (Levitan & Johnson, 1983). If cooperation and trust exist between the union and the company, the members of the union will understand when the company is experiencing financial difficulties. Mills (1983) cites examples of companies in which employees voluntarily accepted wage reductions to help the company decrease expenses. By the same token, management will understand when members of the union experience difficulties. In 1996 the Malden Mills continued to assist employees from company funds when the company was unable to produce popular Polartec items because of a fire. In 2001 unions representing 1200 workers voted to accept a reduction in pay and benefits in an effort to keep Freightliner in Portland, Oregon (Columbian, 2001).

Some individuals (Reisman & Compa, 1985) see no benefit to employees for management and the union to have a positive relationship. Heckscher (1989) suggests that the union model is outdated because of trends that have made the public policy framework of unionization less useful. Porter-O'Grady (2001) suggests there can be a partnering and that the formal requirements of the union contract "advances the practice of managing well and maintains the foundation of good management" (p. 32).

some union activity and excluded from coverage employees of not-for-profit hospitals. The Labor Management Reporting and Disclosure Act of 1959, the Landrum-Griffin Act, provides for greater internal democracy within unions. The 1974 amendments to the Taft-Hartley Act removed the exemption of not-for-profit hospitals, and employees of these types of organizations have the same rights as industrial workers to join together and form labor unions. The removal of the exemption for not-for-profit hospitals created a frenzy of activity as traditional industrial unions targeted healthcare facilities. The National Labor Relations Board (NLRB) administers the National Labor Relations Act. In addition, state laws further define labor law.

Why is there an increase in organizing nurses and other healthcare professionals? Healthcare is a "hot" topic at the state and federal levels. The morning newspaper, nightly news, and a continuous parade of "news magazines" have featured countless articles related to health and illness. One may paraphrase Willie Sutton when he was asked why he robbed banks: "That is where the money is." Why organize nurses and other healthcare workers? That is where potential members are.

As technology replaces unskilled workers, a smaller pool of workers is available for trade-union organizing. Declining union membership has been the catalyst for unions to explore other membership bases (U.S. Department of Labor, 2001). NLRB data confirm that organizing campaigns are more successful in healthcare than in other industries. In 1993 the win rate for all industries was 48%, whereas the win rate in healthcare was 58.3% ("Keep Employees Involved," 1994). Nurses seeking collective bargaining should carefully consider

the representing agent. (See Box 10-4 for suggested screening criteria.)

Traditional industrial unions are increasingly seeking opportunities to represent nurses for the purpose of collective bargaining and to speak for nursing with boards of nursing, regulatory agencies, and legislatures. Organizing nurses and other healthcare workers for the purpose of collective bargaining is very attractive because of the large numbers of people involved and the decrease in organizing in other sectors. The share of wage and salary workers who are union members decreased from 20.1% in 1983 to 13.5% in 2000. Other highlights of the 2000 data include the following: Government workers have a higher rate of unionization than the private sector; within the public sector, local government workers, including school teachers, police, and firefighters, had the highest rate of unionization, 43.2% (U.S. Bureau of Labor Statistics, 2001). Nurses have a low rate of unionization: 19.1% of the 2,074,741 employed nurses. The United American Nurses (UAN) of the ANA represents 32.9% of nurses covered by a union contract (U.S. Department of Labor, 2001).

Historically, nurses were reluctant to be identified with unions; however, that view is changing. In the words of one nurse, "As a staff nurse presently working in health care, I know that nurses need as much help as possible when decisions can affect quality patient are made" (Brengman, 2000). The relationship between management and unions may be adversarial; however, moving from an adversarial relationship to one of cooperation contributes to the institution's flexibility in responding to the demands of consumers and in decreasing patient care costs (Preuss, 1998).

Nurses have a legal right to bargain. The AHA has spent millions of dollars challenging the appropriateness of all-RN bargaining units or a unit separate from other organized employees. In a 1991 unanimous opinion, the U.S. Supreme Court upheld the NLRB's ruling that provides for RN-only units. This decision was critical for nursing. At stake was the ability of nurses to control nursing practice and the quality of patient care. Employees, including nurses, must be accorded workplace rights and the protection that allows them to practice. Nurses must have the freedom to do what the profession and their license require them to do.

Some healthcare organizations have the role of the state nurses' associations as a collective bargaining representative based on the presence of statutory

---

BOX 10-4

Suggested Criteria for Selecting a Bargaining Agent

- A strong commitment to nursing practice, legislation, regulation, and education
- A well-prepared practice, policy, and labor staff: a minimum of a bachelor's degree in nursing
- Representative of those they represent in both gender and ethnic makeup
- National in scope and local in implementation
- Control by individual members over bargaining unit activities

supervisors on the board of directors. The establishment of a separate labor arm, UAN, has addressed these issues. A third challenge has been labeling all RNs as supervisors. RNs monitor and assess patients as a part of their professional practice, not as a statutory supervisor within the definition of the National Labor Relations Act (ANA, 1997). A 1996 NLRB ruling held that RNs were not statutory supervisors and were protected by federal labor law; the decision was upheld in 1997 by the U.S. Court of Appeals for the Ninth Circuit (Nguyen, 1997). However, a 2001 Supreme Court decision (*National Labor Relations Board v. Kentucky River Community Care, Inc.*, 2001) upheld a lower court's decision to classify RNs as supervisors. Costly, time-consuming challenges have the effect of denying timely representation to nurses.

Nurses as Knowledge Workers

The change from producing a product to providing a service has many implications for management and labor. In the past employees in manufacturing were treated like interchangeable cogs: When a cog was broken, it was replaced. A large pool of unskilled workers was available to step forward in the steel mill, the coal mine, and the shop floor. The increased number of technical workers in healthcare seems to be replacing the technical workers in other industries who were displaced as a result of technology. The move from an industrial model requires "knowledge workers." One such trend is the shift to replace blue-collar workers with knowledge workers. The unskilled worker of yesterday did not have a high school diploma. Today, knowledge workers may have multiple college degrees and certifications. When knowledge workers unionize, they develop organizations that are more similar to associations than traditional industrial unions. They become involved in activities such as lobbying and coalition building. Today's nurses are knowledge workers. The tools of knowledge workers differ. As the knowledge content of the work increases, the practice of the worker (nurse) becomes more individualized.

There was a time when union leaders negotiated contracts for thousands of workers and instructed them how to vote. Nurses in Canada demonstrated that solidarity between the union and its leadership does not exist as it did in the past. The leaders of the union approved an agreement only to have the membership repudiate it. Although an agreement was reached, the anger toward the union leaders endured (Kerr & MacPhail, 1991).

For many nurses the question may be, "Why be represented for collective bargaining?" A collective bargaining contract requires management to bargain, a requirement not present in noncontract organizations. Multiple factors, such as discontent with working conditions, the negotiation of contract provisions addressing professional concerns, and the successes that have been achieved by others, influence nurses to seek collective bargaining.

"Patients' current concerns about their hospital experiences derive from what they see as an absence of nursing care in the hospital" (Fagin, 2001, p. 5). Nurses have observed a decline in the quality of care, attributable in large measure to decreased professional nurse staffing; they have observed that dividends to stockholders and plan officers have escalated. The increase in the number of conglomerates has been accompanied by a decreased concern with humanistic factors (Shindul-Rothschild, Berry, & Long-Middleton, 1996). The victims are the public and the providers. As healthcare has become a commodity traded on the stock market, allegiance appears to have shifted from the patient to the stockholder. Healthcare is a labor-intensive industry that manifests many of the ills of other labor-intensive industries: impersonal management, discrimination, favoritism, and arbitrary termination. Nursing as a profession and nurses as individuals have a distinguished record of "going beyond the call of duty" in emergency situations. However, when extraordinary effort is demanded as ordinary effort, nurses resist the expectation and resent a system that takes advantage of the legacy.

Union or At-Will

Nurses are seeking assistance from external sources in an effort to balance the assistance available to the organization's administrative personnel. The fear of arbitrary discipline and dismissal may be the catalyst for nurses to seek ways to protect themselves from what are perceived to be arbitrary actions. A collective bargaining contract has the potential to contribute to a balance of power. The discipline structure provided by contract treats all employees in the same manner and may decrease the manager's flexibility in designing or selecting discipline. Although there is **whistleblower** legislation (Box 10-5), the current environment in healthcare places the **at-will employee** who voices concern about the quality of care in a vulnerable position. Managers of at-will employees have greater latitude in selecting disciplinary measures for specific infractions.

BOX 10-5

Whistleblower Protection

Whistleblowing "refers to a warning issued by a current or former employee of an organization to the public about a serious wrongdoing or danger created or concealed within the organization" (Hunt, 1995, p. 155). The 1989 Whistle Blower Protection Act protects federal workers. The law does not cover the private sector. Some states have specific laws. It is imperative that the whistleblower understand the consequences of action and inaction. The underlying premise of the work by Fletcher, Sorrell, Silva (1998) is that whistleblowing often is a result and symptom of organizational failure.

State and federal laws do provide a level of protection; however, an at-will employee may be terminated at any time for any reason except discrimination. At-will employees, in essence, work at the will of the employer.

Contract language requires management to follow "due process" for represented employees. That is, management must provide a written statement outlining disciplinary charges, the penalty, and the reasons for the penalty. Management is required to maintain a record of attempts to counsel the employee. Employees have the right to defend themselves against charges and the opportunity to settle disagreements in a formal grievance hearing. They have the right to have their representative with them during the process. Management must prove that the employee is wrong or in error. In a nonunion environment, the burden of proof is on the employee. However, Carson and Franklin (2001, p. 56) cited changes in the interpretation of the law: "The ability to avail oneself of protection does not depend on whether the employees are represented by a union to the interpretation of the law."

Nurse managers maintain the record of counseling. The commitment to nursing requires the manager to be clear about the charge. Although all disciplinary charges are important, those directly related to patient care have a more critical dimension. Clarity in describing the situation is important because it affects patient care, the individual nurse, and nurse colleagues.

Many nurses continue to be intimidated by the charge that "unions are unprofessional." Nurse colleagues, hospital management, and physicians have made these charges. However, many physicians now have collective bargaining contracts. Why? They want to have greater control of their practice, improve working conditions, and influence their remuneration, and contracts fit in the cultures where they have unionized. Contracts are a usual part of our present-day environment.

A labor contract, a collective bargaining agreement, is unrelated to being professional. Sociologists characterize the responsibilities of the professional as a respect for the duty to perform, respect for the duty to learn, respect for the public interest, and preservation and enhancement of the image (Moore, 1970). There are many adages in our language that characterize the relationship between parties; they include "a man's word is his bond," "let's shake on it," and "I am as good as my word." These expressions convey a trust between the two parties. In today's marketplace, one rarely "shakes on it." The purchase of a house or a car results in a written contract between individuals and financial institutions that details the responsibilities of the parties involved. It is ironic that a contract between an employer and employee is considered unusual. Replacing the adversarial system should be the goal of efforts to redesign the workplace. A new social order in the workplace must be based on a spirit of genuine cooperation between management and nurses.

Selecting a Bargaining Agent

Leaders in nursing have maintained that the ANA is the only organization that can speak authoritatively for nursing and nurses. As a professional society, ANA maintains that all RNs and only RNs may hold membership in the constituent member association (states and others). The Constituent Member Associations (CMA) and ANA represent the interests of the profession, nurses, and healthcare at the state, federal, and international levels. In 1999 the House of Delegates of the ANA created the UAN to ensure that nurses have a meaningful access to collective bargaining through the ANA. The collective bargaining program of the UAN is designed to implement strategies that maintain or attain improvement in nursing practice in addition to addressing the economic issues. The UAN has "won significant gains in patient care, health and safety, and compensation" (Bronder, 2001). Lucille Joel, a former president of the ANA, provided eloquent support for ANA's involvement. "As long as professionals (nurses) look to collective action to assure public access to quality service, this professional association must offer workplace representation to its members. Where collective bargaining is the model of choice for work place representation, our appeal must lie in something above and beyond what competing unions offer" (Joel, 1990, p. 7).

Exercise 10-8

If you work in a setting with a collective bargaining agreement, secure a copy. Identify the articles of this contract. Are they practice issues or economic issues? What is the relationship between the two? If you work in a setting that does not have a collective bargaining agreement, secure dispute resolution policies. Identify the areas that may be disputed. Are they practice issues or economic issues? What is the relationship between the two?

Not all nurses are eligible to participate in collective bargaining. The nurse who is a statutory supervisor is excluded. Statutory supervisors are those nurses who have the authority to act in the interest of the employer, including the power to hire, terminate, reward, and discipline. These functions are stipulated in the statute (the law). These acts differ from those of nonsupervisory nurses, who act in the interest of the patient. Supervisory nurses share a concern for working conditions, practice standards, and the care delivery environment with nonsupervisory nurses. Many supervisory nurses may think that they are unnecessarily placed in an adversarial relationship with nonsupervisory nurses in the hospital who are represented by the union. Unfortunately, there are healthcare organizations that, as a condition of employment terms, prevent supervisory nurses from maintaining membership in the CMA that represents nurses employed by the hospital.

Canadian nurses have two separate organizations: a professional association and a union. In the province of British Columbia, the Registered Nurses Association of British Columbia is the professional association and the British Columbia Nurses Union is the union. The professional association focuses on maintaining appropriate standards of nursing care and serving the public interest. The union focuses on the socioeconomic needs of members and is not legally bound to protect the public interest. Strategies that allow the separate organizations to cooperate differ from province to province (Kerr & MacPhail, 1991). "Where collective bargaining is controlled by nurses and where professional values predominate, the greater the likelihood of cooperation between the professional body and the negotiating body" (Conroy & Hibberd, 1983). This statement continues to be a valid descriptor of the practice environment.

FRAMEWORKS FOR COLLECTIVE ACTION

Nurses practice in multiple settings; some have collective bargaining contracts, and others do not. Collective bargaining and noncollective bargaining environments espouse safe, quality care. Both environments exist within the context of state and federal laws. Professional practice models may exist in both environments. Nurses may feel valued in both environments. The noncollective bargaining environment *may* be supportive of nursing practice and provide opportunities for nurses to give input into decisions regarding the care that is provided and the environment in which care occurs. There is a critical difference. A contract *requires* the employer to negotiate within a legally binding framework. Noncollective bargaining environments do not provide that assurance.

The future may hold new relationships, and public policy may continue to include provisions that were formally negotiated through contracts. Nurses practice in highly competitive environments. Decision making is at the core of nursing practice. Nurse involvement in decision making contributes to higher levels of job satisfaction for the nurse and higher satisfaction with care for the patient, and it also has a positive influence on health outcomes. Nurses, and those they serve, benefit from collective action that uses a wide range of strategies.

The Solution

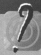

In any redesign effort, involving the staff is critical. I began by meeting with the staff and telling them why I wanted to begin a redesign process and what I hoped to accomplish from such efforts. I then set up redesign teams that have a great deal of staff involvement.

Involving the staff is critical for several reasons. First, the individuals who are actually taking care of patients most of the time think of the most creative solutions for redesign. Second, staff are more likely to embrace redesign activities if they feel that they have been actively involved in the process. Finally, staff can often anticipate issues or problems with these efforts and help develop solutions before the implementation of redesign.

If I worked in a unionized environment, my approach would not differ, except I would meet with the union representatives before initiating the redesign efforts. Again, I would explain what I hoped to accomplish through these efforts, answer any questions or concerns, and ask for their support of the project.

— Peggy Reiley

 Would this be a suitable approach for you? Why?

CHAPTER CHECKLIST

Collectively, nurses possess the knowledge, skills, abilities, and numbers to influence decisions. Collective action may take many forms. Geographic and organizational contexts influence the formal and informal structures in which nurses participate. An organization's structure establishes the parameters for participation in decision making. Managers establish the context for participation. The decision to organize for the purpose of collective bargaining represents an important decision for nurses and for the organization in which they practice. A level of tension exists when an external group becomes a part of an organization's decision-making processes. External groups may enter as a new management consultant, as a part of a merger, as a new owner, or as a union representing registered nurses. The acceptance and appreciation of the external group are influenced by understanding the rationale for the group's entry and by the respect between the constituencies.

- The purposes of collective participation by nurses are to do the following:
  - Promote the practice of professional nursing
  - Establish and maintain standards of care
  - Allocate resources effectively and efficiently
  - Create satisfaction and support in the practice environment (Minarik & Catramabone, 1993)

- Increased autonomy and diversification decrease the following:
  - Fear of ridicule
  - Fear of punishment
  - Fear of loss of job
  - Fear of favors
- Governance strategies dictate levels of participation. The level of participation in decision making influences job satisfaction.
- Shared governance is characterized by partnerships, equity, accountability, and ownership.
- The framework for advocacy includes mutuality, facilitation, protection, and coordination. The manifestations of advocacy are as follows:
  - Ensuring relevant information
  - Enabling the selection of information
  - Disclosing a personal view
  - Providing support for making and implementing decisions
  - Helping determine personal values
- The goal of workplace advocacy is to equip nurses to practice in a rapidly changing environment.
- Collective bargaining is an effective mechanism used by nurses to obtain the right to participate in decisions regarding their practice.
- Represented nurses must be proven wrong or in error. Unrepresented nurses bear the burden of proving themselves to be correct.

Continued

CHAPTER CHECKLIST—cont'd

- Representation for the purpose of collective bargaining, or belonging to a union, is neither professional nor unprofessional.
- Nurses who are statutory supervisors are excluded from representation.

TIPS FOR COLLECTIVE ACTION

- Managers and staff should understand the culture and the organization's approach to any collective action strategy.
- Some states have laws that are more supportive of whistleblowing than others.
- Where collective bargaining is the appropriate strategy, develop criteria for the selection of the appropriate collective bargaining agent.

TERMS TO KNOW

at-will employee
Centers for Disease Control and Prevention (CDC)
collective action
collective bargaining
culture
empowerment
followership
governance
labor law
mentor
OSHA
role model
shared governance
whistleblowing
workplace advocacy

REFERENCES

Aiken, L., Clarke, S., & Sloane, D. (2000, October). Hospital restructuring: Does it adversely affect care and outcomes? *Journal of Nursing Administration, 30*(10), 457-465.

Allen, D., Calkin, J., & Peterson, M. (1988). Making shared governance work: A conceptual model. *Journal of Nursing Administration, 18*(1), 37-43.

American Hospital Association. (1990). *Survey of the hospital nursing strategies pretest.* Chicago: Author.

American Nurses Association. (1995, March 10). Legal developments. *ANA's Labor & Employment Newsletter,* 11.

American Nurses Association. (1997). *What you need to know about today's workplace: An independent study continuing education module.* Washington, DC: Author.

American Nurses Association. (2001). *The code of ethics for nurses with interpretive statements.* Washington, DC: Author.

Bachman, J. (2001). *Alternative dispute resolution.* Washington, DC: ANA.

Brengman, S. (2000). Do unions promote quality nursing care? *MCN, 25*(5), 232.

Bronder, E. (2001). Collective bargaining agreements. *American Journal of Nursing, 101*(8), 59–61.

Carson, W., & Franklin, P. (2001, February). Workplace advocacy: How can it help you? *American Journal of Nursing, 101*(2), 55–57.

Chinn, P., & Kramer, M. (1999). *Theory and nursing: Integrated knowledge development* (5th ed.). St. Louis: Mosby.

The Columbian. (2001, October 6).

Conroy, M., & Hibberd, J. (1983). Areas for cooperation and conflict between nursing associations and negotiating bodies. In S. Quinn (Ed.), *Cooperation and conflict: Caring for the carers.* Geneva: International Council of Nurses.

Dempster, J. (1990). Autonomy in practice: Conceptualization, construction, and psychometric evaluation of an empirical instrument. *Dissertation Abstracts International, 51*(7), 3320B.

Drayton-Hargrove, S. (1996, May). Leadership behaviors of nurse managers in traditional and participatory settings. *Journal of Nursing Science, 1*(3/4): 77-87.

Fagin, C. (2001). *When care becomes a burden: Diminishing access to adequate nursing.* New York: Milbank Memorial Fund.

Flanagan, L. (1995). *What you need to know about today's workplace: A survival guide for nurses.* Washington, DC: American Nurses Publishing.

Fletcher, J., Sorrell, J., & Silva, M. (1998). Whistleblowing as a failure of organizational ethics. *Online Journal of Issues in Nursing,* December 31, 1998.

Gadow, S. (1990). Existential advocacy: Philosophic foundations of nursing. In T. Pence & J. Cantrell (Eds.), *Ethics in nursing: An anthology.* New York: NLN.

Harris, A., Ryan, M., & Belmont, M. (1997, May). More than a friend: The special bond between nurses. *American Journal of Nursing, 97,* 37-39.

Heckscher, D. (1989). *The new unionism: Employee involvement in the changing corporation.* New York: Basic Books.

Holloran, S. (1993, February). Mentoring: The experience of nursing service executives. *Journal of Nursing Administration, 22,* 49–54.

Hunt, G. (1995). *Whistleblowing in the health service: Accountability, law and professional practice.* London: Edward Arnold.

Joel, L. (1990, March). Workplace representation: Continuing commitment, new choices. *The American Nurse, 22*(3), 7.

Jones, P. (1994). Developing a collaborative professional role for the staff nurse in a shared governance model. *Holistic Nurse Practitioner, 8,* 32-37.

Kalisch, B., and Kalisch, P. (1975). Slaves, servants, or saints: An analysis of the system of nurses training in the United States, 1873–1948. *Nurse Forum 14*(3), 114.

Keep employees involved in decision-making process. (1994). *Modern Healthcare, 24*(26), 86.

Kennerly, S. (2000). Perceived worker autonomy: The foundation for shared governance. *Journal of Nursing Administration, 30*(12), 611–617.

Kerr, J., & MacPhail, J. (1991). *Canadian nursing: Issues and perspectives.* St. Louis: Mosby.

Levitan, S., & Johnson, C. (1983, September/October). Labor and management: The illusion of cooperation. *Harvard Business Review, 61,* 8-16.

Lewis, F., & Batey, M. (1982, October). Clarifying autonomy and accountability in nursing service: Part 2. *Journal of Nursing Administration, 12*(10), 10-15.

Mason, D., Talbot, D., & Leavitt, J. (1998). *Policy and politics for nurses: Action and change in the workplace, government, organizations and community* (3rd ed.). Philadelphia: Saunders.

Matusak, L. (1997). *Finding your voice: Learning to lead . . . Anywhere you want to make a difference.* San Francisco: Jossey-Bass.

Mills, D. (1983, May/June). When employees make concessions. *Harvard Business Review, 61,* 103-113.

Minarik, P., & Catramabone, C. (1998). Collective participation in workforce decision-making. In D. Mason, D. Talbot, & J. Leavitt (Eds.), Policy and politics for nurses: Action and change in the workplace, government, organizations and community (3rd ed.). Philadelphia: Saunders.

Moore, W. (1970). *The professions: Roles and rules.* New York: Russell Sage Foundation.

Moss, R., & Rowles, C. (1997, January). Staff nurse job satisfaction and management style. *Nursing Management, 29,* 32-34.

National Labor Relations Act (NLRA) Sec. 8(5), 29 U.S.C.A. § 158 (5).

National Labor Relations Board v. Kentucky River Community Care, Inc., 121 S. Ct. 1861; No. 99-1815 (Argued February 21, 2001; decided May 29, 2001).

Nguyen, B. (1997, September/October). Long-awaited Providence ruling upholds right of charge nurses to bargain. *The American Nurse, 29,* 1, 14.

Parker, M., & Gadbois, S. (2000). Building community in the healthcare workplace, Part 3. *Journal of Nursing Administration, 30*(10), 466–473.

Porter-O'Grady, T. (2001, June). Collective bargaining: The union as partner. *Nursing Management, 32,* 30-32.

Porter-O'Grady, T., Hawkins, M., & Parker, M. (1997). *Whole systems shared governance: Architecture for integration.* Gaithersburg, MD: Aspen Publishers.

Porter-O'Grady, T., & Wilson, C. (1995). *The leadership revolution in health care: Altering systems, changing behaviors.* Gaithersburg, MD: Aspen Publishers.

Preuss, G. (1998). *Sharing care: The changing nature of nursing in hospitals.* Washington, DC: Economic Policy Institute.

Reisman, B., & Compa, L. (1985, May/June). The case for adversarial unions. *Harvard Business Review, 63,* 22-36.

Rogers, B. (1996). Nursing injury, stress, and nursing care. In *Nursing staff in hospitals and nursing homes: Is it adequate?* Washington, DC: IOM.

Shindul-Rothschild, J., Berry, D., & Long-Middleton, E. (1996, November). Where have all the nurses gone? Final results of our patient care survey. *American Journal of Nursing, 96,* 25-39.

Shogren, E., Calkins, A., & Wilburn, S. (1996). Restructuring may be hazardous to your health. *American Journal of Nursing, 96,* 64-66.

Stahl, D. (1997, May). Direct contracting: A new wave for subacute care. *Nursing Management, 28,* 22-23.

Streets, A. (1990). *Nursing practice—High, hard, ground, messy swamps and the pathways in between.* Geelong, Australia: Deskin University Press.

Trice, H., & Beyer, J. (1992). *The cultures of work organizations.* Englewood Cliffs, NJ: Prentice Hall.

U.S. Bureau of Labor Statistics. (2001). *Union members in 2000.* Retrieved January 21, 2001, from http://stats.bls.gov/newsrels.htm

U.S. Department of Health and Human Services. (1988). *Secretary's commission on nursing: Final report.* Washington, DC: U.S. Government Printing Office.

U.S. Department of Labor. (2001, January 18). *Union members in 2000. Current Population Survey.* Washington, DC: U.S. Government Printing Office.

SUGGESTED READINGS

Fisher, R., Ury, W., & Patton, B. (1991). *Getting to yes: Negotiating agreement without giving in.* New York: Penguin Books.

Mohr, W. K. (1997). Outcomes of corporate greed. *Image: Journal of Nursing Scholarship, 29*(1), 39-45.

Powers, J. (1993, September). Accepting and refusing assignments. *Nursing Management, 24*(9), 64-66, 68.

Slaikeu, K. A., & Hasson, R. H. (1998). *Controlling the costs of conflict: How to design a system for your organization.* San Francisco: Jossey-Bass

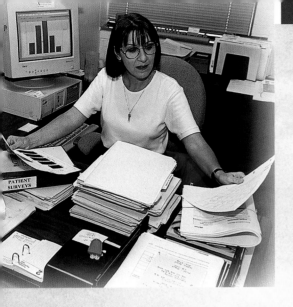

11

Managing Quality and Risk

Deborah A. Wendt

Darla J. Vale

T his chapter explains key concepts and strategies related to quality and risk management. All healthcare professionals must be knowledgeable about, and involved in, the continuous improvement of patient care.

Objectives

- Apply quality management principles to clinical examples.
- Use the six steps of the quality improvement process.
- Practice using selected quality improvement strategies to do the following:
  - Identify customer expectations.
  - Diagram clinical procedures.
  - Develop standards and outcomes.
  - Evaluate outcomes statistically.
- Demonstrate the importance of planning in quality management.

- Differentiate between *quality management* and *risk management*.

- Employ the "five-why" technique and triangulation method to obtain data about a situation or problem.

Questions to Consider

- *How can a staff nurse make effective suggestions to improve nursing practice?*
- *If a colleague makes a mistake, what can you do to prevent future errors while protecting your colleague's self-esteem?*
- *How can patients' expectations be used to improve nursing care?*

The Challenge

Deborah Anderson, RN, MPA
Assistant Health Commissioner, Cincinnati, Ohio

The Cincinnati Health Department applies the philosophy of total quality management to all its programs and services. Within the community health nursing programs, committees meet regularly to plan, implement, and evaluate quality improvement ideas. These committees are composed of both managers and staff workers, and each focuses on a specific area of nursing service. We have standards, audit, documentation, and staff development committees. This approach to quality improvement has been very successful in the past and has resulted in the implementation of changes and innovations in nursing care. However, at a recent staff meeting, nursing supervisors expressed the concern that several quality improvement committees were working on similar projects. This duplication of effort was a waste of the committee members' time and the health department's scarce resources.

 What do you think you would do if you were this nurse?

INTRODUCTION

Healthcare agencies and health professionals want to provide the highest quality of care with minimal risk to patients. But what is quality care? How can it be measured? As healthcare costs continue to rise, third-party payers and healthcare consumers, as well as health professionals, increasingly ask these questions. The philosophy of quality management and the process of quality improvement strive to answer such questions by redesigning the corporate culture and teaching all employees specific skills for assessment, measurement, and evaluation of patient care. Quality management stresses the prevention of patient care problems, but if problems occur, risk management activities focus on reducing the negative impact of such problems.

QUALITY MANAGEMENT IN HEALTHCARE

The path to quality in healthcare has become crowded in the last few years as providers recognize that survival and competitiveness are built on improved patient outcomes. Shortcuts to quality have been tried, but success depends on a philosophy that permeates the organization and values a continuous process of improvement. The quality management philosophy differs from other evaluation techniques because it focuses on the customer instead of the provider, prevention instead of inspection, and the process instead of the person.

The terms **quality management (QM)** and **quality improvement (QI)** have evolved from the business philosophy known as **total quality management,** which is discussed later in this chapter. Many healthcare organizations prefer to use the term *quality management* or **continuous quality improvement** because total quality management can never be achieved. The term **performance improvement (PI)** is sometimes used interchangeably with *quality improvement,* but usually emphasizes improving the activities of individuals or groups, not the systems. Quality-related terminology or jargon continues to evolve. Table 11-1 lists past, present, and evolving quality terms. These terms are defined in the glossary.

In this chapter *quality management* refers to a philosophy that defines a corporate culture emphasizing customer satisfaction, innovation, and employee involvement. *Quality improvement* refers to an ongoing process of innovation, prevention of error, and staff development that is used by corporations and institutions that adopt the quality management philosophy.

BENEFITS OF QUALITY MANAGEMENT

Healthcare systems can benefit in a number of ways from QM. First, the current financial environment with prospective payments has constrained budgets, which has caused a decrease in staff. Greater efficiency and proactive planning while maintaining

Table 11-1 PAST, PRESENT, AND EVOLVING QUALITY TERMS

Past Quality Terms	Present Quality Terms	Evolving Quality Terms
Quality control	Total quality management	Quality management
Quality assurance	Continuous quality improvement	Quality improvement Performance improvement

quality may overcome some of the problems with prospective payments. Second, the abundance of legal malpractice suits emphasizes the need for quality of care. QM is based on the philosophy that things should be done right the first time and that improvement is always possible. Third, QM involves everyone on the improvement team and encourages everyone to make contributions. This style of participative management enhances job satisfaction. Employees feel valued as team members who can really make a difference.

PLANNING FOR QUALITY IMPROVEMENT

Multidisciplinary planning is integral to the quest for quality. Issues are examined from various perspectives using a systematic process. Planning takes time and money; however, quality managers say, "We don't have time not to plan." The price of poor planning can be very expensive. Poor planning costs might involve redoing what was originally done poorly, increasing the risk of liability, making costly accidents and errors, risking a negative public image, and increasing employee frustration and turnover. The costs of errors and ineffective nursing actions are considered avoidable costs.

EVOLUTION OF QUALITY MANAGEMENT

W. Edwards Deming lectured about building quality into every product and service during a tour of postwar Japan. Using Deming's 14 points of QM as a guide, Japan recovered from the devastation of World War II and rapidly gained a reputation for efficient production and excellent products (Hansen, 2000). A summary of Deming's 14 management points appears in Box 11-1.

BOX 11-1

Deming's 14 Points

1. Create constancy of purpose for improvement of product and service.
2. Adopt the new philosophy.
3. Cease dependence on inspection to achieve quality.
4. End the practice of awarding business on the basis of price tag.
5. Improve constantly and forever the systems of production and service.
6. Institute training on the job.
7. Institute leadership.
8. Drive out fear.
9. Break down barriers between departments.
10. Eliminate slogans, exhortations, and targets for the workforce.
11. Eliminate numerical quotas for the workforce and numerical goals for management.
12. Remove barriers that rob people of pride and workmanship.
13. Institute a vigorous program of education and self-improvement for everyone.
14. Put everyone in the company to work to accomplish the transformation.

From Deming, W. E. (1986). *Out of the crisis.* Cambridge, MA: Massachusetts Institute of Technology.

During the 1980s the United States faced increased competition for products in a global market. Deming's philosophy was rediscovered by Americans, who enthusiastically began applying QM to business, industrial, educational, and healthcare systems (Stahl, 1999).

Deming's original management philosophy has been expanded and modified by various management theorists. Crosby stressed conformance to standards and zero defects. According to Crosby,

QI is not a program but a permanent process of prevention (Stahl, 1999). Juran developed a structured process for QI and encouraged the use of self-directed QI teams comprised of workers (Juran & Godfrey, 1999). The quality control circle, a team of workers who meet regularly to detect and correct quality problems, was the idea of Kaoru Ishikawa. He valued the use of statistical measurements and believed that all workers should be able to use basic statistics to improve the quality of products (Stahl, 1999).

Within healthcare systems, QI has traditionally stressed assessment of structure, process, and outcomes (Donabedian, 1966). These three factors are usually considered interrelated, so research has been conducted to determine characteristics of effective structures and processes that would result in better outcomes.

Magnet hospital research has demonstrated the relationship of these factors. *Magnet hospital* is a term that was first used in the early 1980s to describe a hospital that attracted and retained nurses even in times of nursing shortages. Currently, Magnet status is obtained through an accreditation process with the American Nurses Credentialing Center (ANCC) (Aiken & Havens, 2000).

Magnet hospital research has examined the characteristics of hospital systems that impede or facilitate professional practice in nursing and also promote outcomes. Common organizational characteristics of Magnet hospitals include structural factors (decentralized organizational structure, participative management style, and influential nurse executives) and process factors (professional autonomy and professional development/education) (McClure, Poulin, Sovie, & Wandelt, 1983). The

findings show a direct correlation between the control nurses reported having in the practice setting and the patients' rating of the quality of care. Subsequent analyses show that Magnet hospitals have a lower mortality rate for Medicare patients (Aiken & Havens, 2000).

This combination of QI ideas from theorists and research is sometimes referred to as *total quality management* or, more simply, *quality management*. The basic principles of QM are summarized in Box 11-2 and are developed further in the next section of this chapter.

QUALITY MANAGEMENT AND QUALITY IMPROVEMENT

QM operates most effectively within a flat, democratic organizational structure. Healthcare agencies in the past have often adopted a traditional bureaucratic organizational structure. Within a bureaucratic structure, workers usually specialize in one function or skill and decisions related to that skill are made at the management level above the worker (Marriner-Tomey, 2000). This type of structure tends to be quite rigid, with limited communication across levels of the organization.

Many healthcare organizations have shifted to a different type of corporate structure. This democratic structure, flatter in style with decentralized authority, encourages teamwork and shared leadership among all levels of employees (Heckman, 1996). In a democratic structure, workers can perform more than one function and are involved in decisions related to their areas of expertise (Heckman, 1996). Figure 11-1 shows the difference in organizational design between the traditional bureaucratic model and the democratic model.

Involvement

Managers and workers must be committed to QI. Top-level managers retain the ultimate responsibility for QM but must involve the entire organization in the QI process. Although some healthcare organizations have achieved significant QI results without systemwide support, total organizational involvement is necessary for a cultural transformation (Hansen, 2000). If all members of the healthcare team are to be actively involved in QI, a nonthreatening environment must be established. Deming believed that fear was not an effective motivator of employees and even advocated eliminating annual

---

BOX 11-2

Principles of Quality Management and Quality Improvement

1. Quality management operates most effectively within a flat, democratic organizational structure.
2. Managers and workers must be committed to quality improvement.
3. The goal of quality management is to improve systems and processes, not to assign blame.
4. Customers define quality.
5. Quality improvement focuses on outcomes.
6. Decisions must be based on data.

performance reviews because they inhibit creativity (Deming, 1986).

To work effectively in a democratic, quality-focused corporate environment, nurses and other healthcare workers must accept QI as an integral part of their role. When a separate department controls quality activities, healthcare managers and workers often relinquish responsibility and commitment for quality control to these quality specialists. Employees working in an organizational culture that values quality freely make suggestions for improvement and innovation in patient care. Exercise 11-1 may help nurses make QI suggestions.

Exercise 11–1

Think of a problem or potential problem that exists in the agency where you practice. Describe the problem, using as many specific facts as possible. List the advantages to the staff, patients, and agency of correcting this problem. Describe several possible solutions to the problem. Decide whom you would contact about this suggestion.

Goal

The goal of QM is to improve the system, not to assign blame. Managers strive to provide a system in which workers can function effectively. To encour-

age commitment to QI, nurse managers must clearly articulate the organization's mission and goals. All levels of employees, from nursing assistants to hospital administrators, must be educated about QI strategies.

Communication should flow freely within the organizational structure. To enhance communication, the nurse manager uses a participative or transformational management style. The nurse manager does not micromanage by concentrating on details but rather leads by demonstrating knowledge, integrity, and commitment to quality care (Fiscel, 1999). Because QM stresses improving the system, detection of employees' errors is not stressed, and if errors occur, reeducation of staff is emphasized rather than imposition of punitive measures.

Customers

Customers define quality. Successful organizations measure the factors that are most important to their customers and focus their energies on enhancing quality in these areas. As patients become more sophisticated and view themselves as "consumers" who can take their business elsewhere, they want input into treatment decisions. Although typical patients may not be knowledgeable about a specific

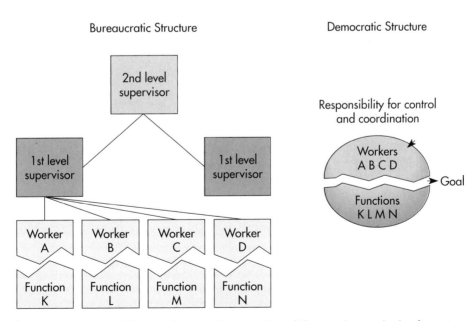

Figure 11-1   Design differences between bureaucratic and democratic organizational structures. (Modified from Heckman, F. [1996]. The participative design approach. *Journal of Quality and Participation, 2*[3], 48-51.)

treatment, they know if they were satisfied with their experience with the healthcare provider.

Every nurse and healthcare agency has internal and external customers. Internal customers are people or units within an organization who receive products or services. A nurse working on a hospital unit could describe patients, nurses on the other shifts, other hospital departments, and nursing managers as internal customers. Staff members working with a manager are that person's internal customers. External customers are people or groups outside the organization who receive products or services. For nurses, these external customers may include patients' families, physicians, managed care organizations, and the community at large. Managers and staff nurses can use Exercise 11-2 to identify their internal and external customers.

Exercise 11-2

For 1 week, list every person with whom you interact as a nurse. Which of these people work for, or receive care in, your organization? These are the internal customers. Which of these people come from outside the organization? These are the external customers.

Consumer satisfaction with healthcare can be assessed through the use of questionnaires, interviews, focus group discussions, or observation. However, patients cannot always adequately assess the competence of clinical performance. Healthcare providers may use additional tools to assess the safety, effectiveness, and timeliness of patient care (Krulish, 2001).

Focus

QI focuses on outcomes. Patient outcomes are statements that describe the results of healthcare (Plotkin & Roche, 2000). They are specific and measurable and describe patients' behavior. Outcome statements may be based on patients' needs, ethical and legal standards of practice, or other standardized data systems. Sources for outcome statements are described further in the next section of this chapter.

Decisions

Decisions must be based on data. The use of statistical tools enables nurse managers to make objective decisions about QI. However, Ishikawa (1985) warned against collecting data merely to support a preconceived idea. In Japan this was one of the most common reasons for poor decision making. Quality information must be gathered and analyzed without bias before improvement suggestions and recommendations are made.

THE QUALITY IMPROVEMENT PROCESS

QI involves continual analysis and evaluation of products and services to prevent errors and to achieve customer satisfaction. The work of continuous QI never stops because products and services can always be improved. The adage "If it ain't broke, don't fix it" conflicts with the main assumption of QI. Improvement is always possible.

The QI process is a structured series of steps designed to plan, implement, and evaluate changes in healthcare activities. Many models of the QI process exist, but all contain steps similar to those listed in Box 11-3.

The six steps in Box 11-3 can easily be applied to clinical situations. In the following example, a community clinic staff uses the QI process to handle patient complaints about waiting for appointments.

A community clinic receives a number of complaints from patients about waiting up to 2 hours for scheduled appointments. The clinic secretary and staff nurses suggest to the clinic manager that scheduling clinic appointments be investigated by the QI committee, which is composed of the clinic secretary, two clinic nurses, one physician, and one nurse practitioner. The clinic manager agrees to the staff's sug-

---

BOX 11-3

Steps in the Quality Improvement Process

1. Identify needs most important to the consumer of healthcare services.
2. Assemble a multidisciplinary team to review the identified consumer needs and services.
3. Collect data to measure the current status of these services.
4. Establish measurable outcomes and quality indicators.
5. Select and implement a plan to meet the outcomes.
6. Collect data to evaluate the implementation of the plan and the achievement of outcomes.

gestion and assigns the problem to the QI committee. At their next meeting, the QI committee uses a flow-chart to describe the scheduling process from the time a patient calls to make an appointment until the patient sees a physician or nurse practitioner in the examining room. Next, the committee members decide to gather and analyze data about the important parts of the process: the number of calls for appointments, the number of patients seen in a day, the number of canceled or missed appointments, and the average time each patient spends in the waiting room. The committee discovers that too many appointments are scheduled because many patients miss appointments. This overbooking often results in long waiting times for the patients who do arrive on time. The QI committee also gathers information on clinic waiting times from the literature and through interviews with patients and colleagues. A measurable outcome is written: "Patients will wait no longer than 30 minutes for an appointment." After a discussion of options, the team recommends that appointments be scheduled at more reasonable intervals, that patients receive notification of appointments by mail and by phone, and that all clinic patients be educated about the importance of keeping scheduled appointments. The committee communicates its suggestions for improvement to the manager and staff and monitors the results of the implementation of their improvement suggestions. Within 3 months the average waiting room time per patient decreases by 30 minutes and the number of missed patient appointments decreases by 20%.

Identify Consumers' Needs

The QI process begins with the selection of a clinical activity for review. Theoretically, any and all aspects of clinical care could be improved through the QI process. However, QI efforts should be concentrated on changes to patient care that will have the greatest effect. The Pareto principle applies here: 80% of positive improvement in clinical care will come by focusing quality improvement activities on 20% of essential patient care tasks and processes (Juran & Godfrey, 1999).

To determine which 20% of clinical activities are most important, nurse managers or staff nurses may interview or survey patients about their healthcare experiences. What would have helped them at a particular time? Although many QI activities focus on physical tasks, studies show that interpersonal care is just as important. The results of the research study (Stichler & Weiss, 2001) highlighted in this chapter's Research Perspective box identify the aspects of quality as defined by patients, nurses, payers, and physicians.

Assemble a Team

Once an activity is selected for possible improvement, a multidisciplinary team implements the QI process. QI team members should represent a cross

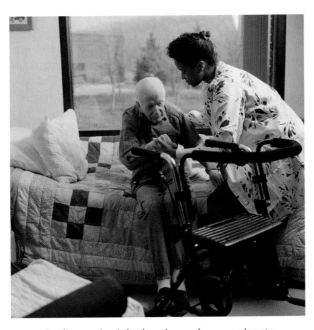

Quality nursing is both caring and compassionate.

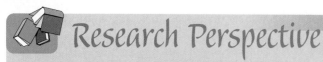

Research Perspective

Stichler, J., & Weiss, M. (2001). Through the eye of the beholder: Multiple perspectives on quality in women's health care. *Quality Management in Health Care, 8*(4), 1-13.

This qualitative study used semistructured interviews to examine the definitions of quality from different perspectives. A sample of 108 physicians, nurses, payer representatives, and female patients from a woman's hospital in the western United States were asked questions about what quality in women's healthcare meant to them. Although each group identified dimensions from their own unique perspective, there were eight common themes that emerged across groups: outcomes, caring, competence, timeliness, professional relationships, scope of services, environment, and support systems.

IMPLICATIONS FOR PRACTICE

Quality improvement activities often focus on tasks of nursing, but this study reveals that quality is a multidimensional concept. Because satisfaction of consumers is an important quality indicator, nurses and healthcare agencies may need to assess and support the interpersonal aspects of patient care, as well as system effectiveness, to improve patient satisfaction.

section of workers who are involved with the problem. Team members may need to be educated about their roles before starting the QI process.

To develop effective QI teams, the workplace environment must promote teamwork. Some healthcare facilities are more open to teamwork than others. Nurse managers can use Exercise 11-3 to decide whether their clinical facility is ready for QI teams.

Exercise 11-3

Ask yourself the following questions about your system:
1. Is communication between nurses and other professionals promoted? If so, how?
2. Could the communication process be improved in any way?
3. Does your system encourage nurses to act as a team?
4. Are other disciplines/departments included in team activities?
5. Can the team focus be improved in any way?

Collect Data

After the multidisciplinary team forms, the group collects data to measure the current status of the activity, service, or procedure under review. Various data tools may be used to analyze and present this information. These data tools include flowcharts, line graphs, histograms, Pareto charts, and fishbone diagrams. The use of empirical tools to organize QI data is an essential part of the QI process (Juran & Godfrey, 1999).

A detailed flowchart is used to describe complex tasks. The flowchart is a data tool that uses boxes and directional arrows to diagram a process or procedure. Sometimes just diagramming a patient care process in detail reveals opportunities for improvement. The flowchart in Figure 11-2 depicts the process of a home health agency receiving a new patient referral.

Line graphs present data by showing the connection among variables. The dependent variable is usually plotted on the vertical scale, and the independent variable is usually plotted on the horizontal scale. In QI this technique is often used to show the trend of a particular activity over time, and the result may be called a *trend chart*. The line graph in Figure 11-3 illustrates the number of referrals a home health agency receives during a year.

The histogram in Figure 11-4 illustrates the number of home health referrals that come from five different referral sources during 1 year. A histogram is a bar chart that shows the frequency of events.

A bar chart that identifies the major causes or components of a particular quality control problem is called a *Pareto chart*. Used often in QI, the Pareto chart helps the QI team determine priorities. The Pareto chart in Figure 11-5 demonstrates that on a medical-surgical unit over a 1-month period, omission of vital signs was the most common type of documentation error.

The fishbone diagram, also called the *cause-effect diagram,* was developed by Ishikawa as a

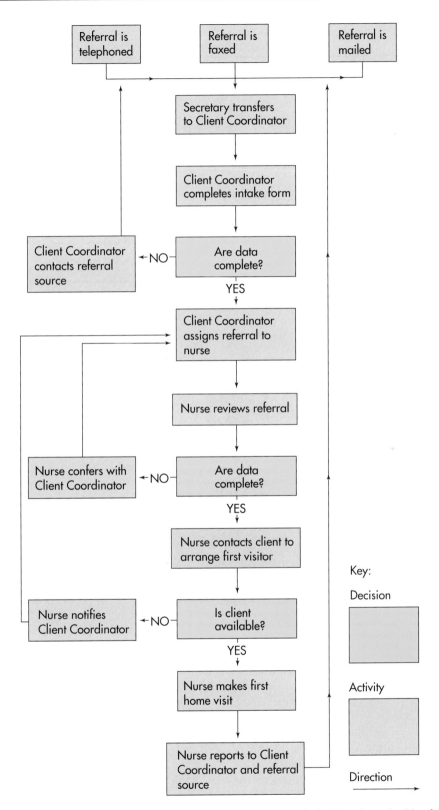

Figure 11-2   Steps in a flowchart diagramming process starting with the time a home health referral is made and ending with the first home visit.

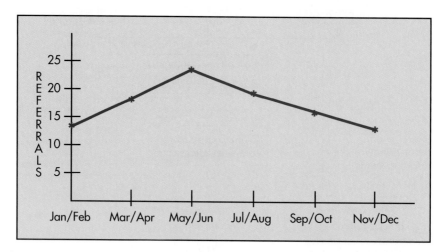

Figure 11-3   Line graph depicting the number of home health referrals received during 1 year.

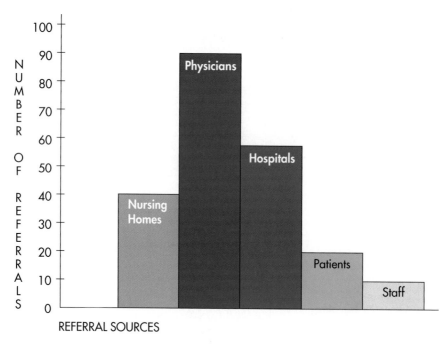

REFERRAL SOURCES

Figure 11-4   Histogram depicting the number of home health referrals received from five sources during 1 year.

quality control tool (Juran & Godfrey, 1999). A specific problem or outcome is written on the horizontal line. All possible causes of the problem or strategies to meet the outcome are written in a fishbone pattern. This tool is an effective method of summarizing a brainstorming session. Figure 11-6 uses a fishbone diagram to present possible causes of patients' complaints about extended waits for clinic appointments.

Although QI teams should be able to use these basic statistical tools, more complex analysis is sometimes necessary. In this situation a statistical expert could be included on the QI team, or the team may use a statistician as a consultant.

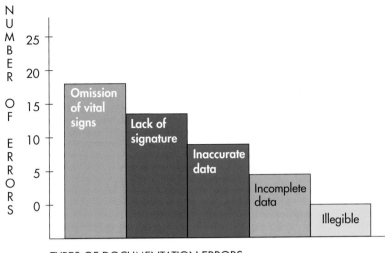

Figure 11-5 Pareto chart presenting major types of documentation error that occurred on a medical/surgical unit over a 1-month period.

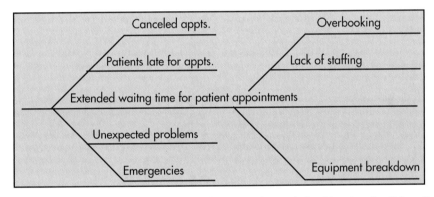

Figure 11-6 Fishbone diagram showing possible causes of extended waiting time for clinic patients.

Establish Outcomes

After analyzing the data, the team next sets a goal for improvement. This goal can be established in a number of ways but always involves a standard of practice and a measurable **patient care outcome.** The multidisciplinary team should use accepted standards of care and practice whenever possible. Evidence-based practice emphasizes the integration of the best research evidence along with other sources of knowledge (Glanville, Schirm, & Wineman, 2000). Sources that establish these standards include the following:

1. State nurse practice acts
2. Accrediting bodies such as the Joint Commission on Accreditation of Healthcare Organizations

(JCAHO) and the Community Health Accreditation Program (CHAP)
3. Nationally recognized professional organizations
4. Nursing research
5. Internal policies and procedures
6. Governmental bodies such as the Agency for Healthcare Research and Quality (AHRQ)

Although individual healthcare organizations may have unique patient needs related to their specific population or environment, many patients and outcomes are similar. One way to evaluate the quality of outcomes is to compare one agency's performance against that of similar organizations. In a process called **benchmarking,** a widespread search is conducted to identify the best performance against which to measure others. Through this process of comparing the best practices against your practice and process, your organization learns more about itself. For example, documentation of discharge teaching can be compared with that of other institutions and with readmission rates. Unfortunately, the usefulness of the information from other institutions continues to be hampered by differences in terminology. A consistent information system would provide a vast database regarding outcomes of care and resource allocation.

Documentation on computers has greatly increased the amount of data available for QI. Information technology plays a vital role in QI by increasing the efficiency of data entry and analysis, thereby enhancing informed decision making. This increased access to data identifies high-risk procedures and systematic errors, which can then be the focus for QI (Ang, Davies, & Finlay, 2001).

Nursing has been a leader in the information system field by developing standardized nursing classification systems. The availability of standardized nursing data enables the study of health problems across populations, settings, and caregivers. Consistent use of standardized language enhances the process of QI and also demonstrates the contributions of nursing to lawmakers, healthcare policy makers, and the public. Three leading nursing classification systems have been identified: the North American Nursing Diagnosis Association's (NANDA) nomenclature, the Nursing Intervention Classification (NIC) System, and the Nursing Outcomes Classification (NOC) system (Aquilino & Keenan, 2000).

Each classification system focuses on one component of the nursing process. Nursing diagnoses can be labeled using NANDA. These diagnosis labels represent clinical judgments about actual or potential health problems. Each diagnosis contains a definition, major and minor defining characteristics, and related factors (NANDA, 2001).

The NIC System consists of interventions that represent both general and specialty nursing practice. Each intervention includes a label, definition, and a set of activities that nurses perform to carry it out. For example, pain management is defined and more than 36 specific activities are listed to alleviate pain or reduce the pain to a level that is acceptable to the patient (McCloskey & Bulechek, 2000).

The NOC system consists of outcomes that focus on the patient and include patient states, behavior, and perceptions that are sensitive to nursing

interventions. Each outcome includes a definition, a 5-point scale for rating outcome status over time, a set of specific indicators to be used in rating the outcomes, and a list of background readings (Johnson, Maas, & Moorhead, 2000). Clinical testing for validation and refinement has occurred in various settings, and the standardization of terms continues to develop to reflect current knowledge and changes in nurses' roles and the structure of healthcare systems. The consistency of terms is essential in providing a large database across healthcare settings to predict resource requirements and establish outcomes of care.

Discuss Plans

The team discusses various strategies and plans to meet the new outcome. One plan is selected for implementation, and the process of change begins. Because QM stresses improving the system rather than assigning blame to employees, change strategies emphasize open communication and education of workers affected by the new standard and outcome. QI is impossible without continual education of all managers and workers. Even in a cost-conscious environment, staff education is not a luxury but a necessity.

Policies and procedures may need to be written or rewritten during the QI process. Policies should be reviewed frequently and updated so that they do not become barriers to innovation. Communication about the change or improvement to the team members at large is essential.

Evaluate

As the plan is implemented, the team continues to gather and evaluate data to document that the new outcomes are being met. If an outcome is not met, revisions in the implementation plan are needed. Sometimes improvement in one part of a system presents new problems. For example, a school nurse wanted to improve the psychosocial assessment of children with possible family problems. A result of this improvement in care was a greatly increased number of referrals for counseling, which overwhelmed the two school psychologists. The interdisciplinary team may need to reassemble periodically to handle the inevitable obstacles that develop with the implementation of any new process or procedure. The example that follows illustrates this idea.

A hospital is implementing a pneumatic tube system to dispense medications. A multidisciplinary team is assembled to discuss the process from various viewpoints: pharmacy, nursing, pneumatic tube operation managers, aides who take the medications from the pneumatic tube to the patient medication drawers, administrators, and physicians. The tube system is implemented. A nurse on one unit realizes that several patients do not have their morning medications in their med boxes. The nurse borrows medications from another patient's drawer and orders the rest of the medications stat from pharmacy. Other nurses on that unit and other units have the same problem and are doing the same or similar things. Several problems are occurring—some of the medications are being given late, nurses waste precious time by searching other med boxes, the pharmacy charges extra for the stat medications and is overwhelmed with stat requests, and the situation increases the nurses' frustration level. QM principles would encourage the nurses to report the problems to the nurse manager or appropriate team member. The pneumatic tube team could compile data such as frequency of missing medications, timing of medication orders, and nursing units involved. The problems are analyzed with a system perspective to effectively solve the late medication problem.

When the change is implemented successfully, the QI team disbands after celebrating their success. One of the crucial tasks of the nurse manager is to publicize and reward the success of each QI team. The nurse manager must also evaluate the work of the team and the ability of individual team members to work together effectively.

Some organizations that have used the QM philosophy for several years establish permanent QI teams or committees. These QI teams do not disband after implementing one project or idea but rather may meet regularly to focus on improvements in one specific area of patient care. In this chapter's Challenge and Solution, the assistant health commissioner in a Midwest health department describes the use of permanent QI teams and how she prevented duplication of efforts within the quality teams.

QM organizations stress system-level change and the evaluation of outcomes; however, in recent years the need for process/performance improvement, including individual performance appraisal, has reemerged within healthcare organizations (Crane & Crane, 2000). Peer review, multidimensional appraisal, and self-evaluation are performance assessment methods that fit within the QM philosophy (Crane & Crane, 2000; DiMauro, 2000; Johnstone, Rohde, May, Peng, & Hulick, 1999).

Any nurse can use the six steps of the QI process to self-evaluate and improve individual performance. For example, a nurse on a medical unit who wants to improve documentation skills might study past entries on patient records; review current institution policies, professional standards, and literature related to documentation; set specific performance improvement goals after consultation with the nurse manager and expert colleagues; devise strategies and a timeline for achieving performance goals; and after implementing the strategies, review documentation entries to see whether self-improvement goals have been met.

QUALITY ASSURANCE

Although QI is a comprehensive process to prevent problems, it is naive to suggest the total abandonment of periodic inspection. One method of monitoring of healthcare is done with **quality assurance (QA)** programs. QA focuses on clinical aspects of the provider's care, often in response to an identified problem. The focus may differ from that of QI, asking questions such as, "Did the nurse document the response to the pain medication within the required time period?" instead of, "Did the patient receive adequate pain relief postoperatively?" The similarities and differences between QI and QA are summarized in Table 11-2.

One of the methods most often used in QA is chart review or chart auditing. Chart audits may be conducted using the records of active or discharged patients. Charts are selected randomly and reviewed by qualified healthcare professionals. In an internal audit, staff members from the same hospital or agency that generated the records examine the data. External auditors are qualified professionals from outside the organization who conduct the review. An audit tool containing specific criteria based on standards of care is applied to each chart under review. For example, auditors might compare documentation related to use of restraints with the criterion, "Physician order is obtained for physical restraints within 8 hours of application." Auditors note compliance or lack of compliance with each audit criterion and report a summary of these findings to the appropriate manager or committee for corrective action (Marriner-Tomey, 2000).

QA staff usually conduct or supervise the chart audits within an agency. Although these nurses are internal auditors, they may not be directly involved

Table 11-2 COMPARISON OF QUALITY ASSURANCE AND QUALITY IMPROVEMENT PROCESS

	Quality Assurance (QA) Process	Quality Improvement (QI) Process
Goal	To improve quality	To improve quality
Focus	Discovery and correction of errors	Prevention of errors
Major tasks	Inspection of nursing activities Chart audits	Review of nursing activities Innovation Staff development
Quality team	QA personnel or department personnel	Multidisciplinary team
Outcomes	Set by QA team with input from staff	Set by QI team with input from staff and patients/customers

with the staff nurses whose charting is under review. Because the focus of the chart audit is on detecting errors and determining the person responsible for them, many staff members tend to view QA as a nuisance or a threat.

RISK MANAGEMENT

Although QM and **risk management** are related concepts, QM emphasizes the prevention of patient care problems, whereas risk management attempts to analyze problems and minimize losses after a patient care error occurs. These losses include incurring financial loss as a result of malpractice or absorbing the cost of an extended length of stay for the patient. They can also include negative public relations and employee dissatisfaction. If QM were 100% effective, there would be no need for risk management. In the current healthcare environment, however, risk management departments are needed and used.

Risk management has blossomed since the malpractice crisis in the 1970s. Before that time, healthcare was assumed to be safe and of high quality, with few exceptions. Healthcare professionals were revered, and medical treatment was not questioned. The abundance of liability suits in the 1970s caused people to doubt the validity of their faith in quality healthcare. The inclusion of risk management standards in the 1990 JCAHO guidelines further emphasized the importance of risk management (Marriner-Tomey, 2000).

The risk management department has several functions. These include the following:

- Defining situations that place the system at some financial risk, such as medication errors or patient falls

- Determining the frequency of occurrence of those situations
- Intervening and investigating identified events
- Identifying potential risks or opportunities to improve care

Each individual nurse is a risk manager. Each nurse has the responsibility to identify and report unusual occurrences and potential risks to the proper authority. One method of communicating risks is through incident reporting. Incident reports should be a nonpunitive means of communicating an incident that did cause or could have caused harm to patients, family members, visitors, or employees. These reports should be used to improve quality of care and decrease risk.

Nurses should also be able to recognize **sentinel events** and participate with nurse managers in the **root-cause analysis.** A sentinel event is a serious unexpected occurrence involving death or physical or psychological harm such as suicide, infant abduction, or surgery on the wrong body part (Anderson, 1998). JCAHO calls for voluntary self-reporting of sentinel events by both inpatient institutions and home health agencies. After a sentinel event is identified, a root-cause analysis is performed by a team that includes those directly involved in the event and those in leadership positions. A root-cause analysis is very similar to the QI process described in this chapter except that the root-cause analysis emphasizes getting to the major cause or root of the problem. The root-cause analysis leads to the development of specific risk-reduction strategies (Friedman, 1998).

Evaluating Risks

In gathering data about unusual occurrences, the risk manager may use the **"five-why" technique.** This technique involves asking "Why" several times to help discover underlying problems that a cursory overview might miss.

Risk managers also use a technique called **triangulation.** This technique involves using multiple data sources, data collection techniques, and perspectives to collect and interpret the data. Triangulation is used to enhance credibility of the findings and create a more accurate representation of the truth (Polit, Beck, & Hungler, 2001). Quantitative methods such as a yes/no questionnaire or records of medication administration are merged with qualitative methods such as open-ended question interviews. For example, a survey of patients conducted at discharge showed a lack of satisfaction with discharge instructions. Follow-up telephone interviews were conducted with the same

patients to ask open-ended questions. The interviews revealed that the patients were satisfied with the written and verbal instructions given by the nurse but were dissatisfied because they felt overwhelmed by what they did not know. Without the qualitative information, the problem may appear to be the teaching technique rather than the timing and volume of information.

Triangulation is also used in nursing research as a means to gain a broader perspective on nursing questions. Triangulation gives researchers, nurse managers, and risk managers additional information that might have been missed by using only one method. Triangulation takes more time to conduct and evaluate than just reading an incident report, so it should be used for significant issues.

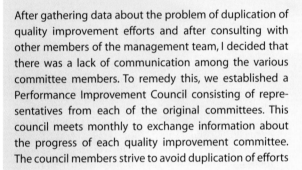

The Solution

After gathering data about the problem of duplication of quality improvement efforts and after consulting with other members of the management team, I decided that there was a lack of communication among the various committee members. To remedy this, we established a Performance Improvement Council consisting of representatives from each of the original committees. This council meets monthly to exchange information about the progress of each quality improvement committee. The council members strive to avoid duplication of efforts

and to encourage collaboration and coordination among the teams. This adjustment in our quality improvement process has allowed us to save time and to maximize the use of our resources.

— Deborah Anderson

 Would this be a suitable approach for you? Why?

CHAPTER CHECKLIST

Many healthcare organizations are in the process of transforming their system to QM. Greater efficiency with improved quality is the goal of this approach. Effective QI includes identifying consumer expectations, planning, using a multidisciplinary approach, evaluating outcomes, and changing the system to provide an environment where employees can perform their best.

- The main principles of QM and QI are as follows:
  - QM operates most effectively within a flat, democratic organizational structure.
  - Managers and workers must be committed to QI.
  - The goal of QM is to improve systems and processes—not to assign blame.

  - Customers define quality.
  - QI focuses on outcomes.
  - Decisions must be based on facts.
- QM strives to prevent errors. It requires effective planning. Initially, planning requires both time and money, but QM saves money in the long run. The QM philosophy originated with Deming and is being modified by contemporary management theorists.
- The major steps in the continuous QI process to evaluate and improve patient care are as follows:
  - Identify needs most important to the consumer of healthcare services.
  - Assemble a multidisciplinary team to review the identified consumer needs and services.
  - Collect data to measure the current status of these services.

Continued

CHAPTER CHECKLIST—cont'd

- • Establish measurable outcomes and quality indicators.
- • Select and implement a plan to meet the outcomes.
- • Collect data to evaluate the implementation of the plan and the achievement of outcomes.
- ■ Any process can be improved. Risk management focuses on minimizing loss after a patient care error occurs. Techniques to obtain data include the "five-why" technique and triangulation.

TIPS ON QUALITY MANAGEMENT

- ■ QM is based on data—what gets measured and recorded can be improved.
- ■ Concentrate QI energies on factors that are most important to your customers.
- ■ Working together to prevent problems is more effective than fixing problems after they occur.

TERMS TO KNOW

benchmarking
continuous quality improvement
"five-why" technique
patient-care outcome
performance improvement (PI)
quality assurance (QA)
quality improvement (QI)
quality management (QM)
risk management
sentinel event
root-cause analysis
total quality management
triangulation

REFERENCES

Aiken, L., & Havens, D. (2000). The Magnet nursing services recognition program: A comparison of two groups of Magnet hospitals. *American Journal of Nursing,* *100*(3), 26-35.

Anderson, M. (1998, October). Sentinel events: Policy & preparation. *CARING Magazine,* 26-30.

Ang, C., Davies, M., & Finlay, P. (2001). An empirical study of the use of information technology to support total quality management. *Total Quality Management, 12*(2), 145-163.

Aquilino, M., & Keenan, G. (2000). Having our say: Nursing's standardized nomenclatures. *American Journal of Nursing, 100*(7), 33-38.

Crane, J. S., & Crane, N. K. (2000). A multi-level performance appraisal tool: Transition from the traditional to a CQI approach. *Health Care Management Review, 25*(1), 64-73.

Deming, W. E. (1986). *Out of the crisis.* Cambridge, MA: Massachusetts Institute of Technology.

DiMauro, N. M. (2000). Continuous professional development. *The Journal of Continuing Education in Nursing, 31*(2), 59-62.

Donabedian, A. (1966). Evaluating the quality of medical care. *Millbank Memorial Fund Quarterly, 44*(3), 166-206.

Fiscel, M. R. (1999). Home care organizational leadership and structure in a changing environment. *Home Health Care Management Practice, 11*(6), 49-60.

Friedman, M. M. (1998). To tell the truth: The Joint Commission's sentinel event policy. *Home Healthcare Nurse, 16*(10), 659-664.

Glanville, I., Schirm, V., & Wineman, N. (2000). Using evidence-based practice for managing clinical outcomes in advanced practice nursing. *Journal of Nursing Care Quality, 15*(1), 1-11.

Hansen, C. (2000). Continuous quality improvement. *Arkansas Nursing News, 17*(2), 31-34.

Heckman, F. (1996). The participative design approach. *Journal of Quality and Participation, 2*(3), 48-51.

Ishikawa, K. (1985). *What is total quality control? The Japanese way.* Englewood Cliffs, NJ: Prentice Hall.

Johnson, M., Maas, M., & Moorhead, S. (Eds.). (2000). *Nursing outcomes classification (NOC)* (2nd ed.). St. Louis: Mosby.

Johnstone, P. A. S., Rohde, D. C., May, B. C., Peng, Y. P., & Hulick, P. R. (1999). Peer review and performance improvement in a radiation oncology clinic. *Quality Management in Health Care, 8*(1), 22-28.

Juran, J. M., & Godfrey, A. B. (1999). *Juran's quality handbook.* New York: McGraw-Hill.

Krulish, L. H. (2001). Using OBQI to improve assessment and management of pain. *Home Healthcare Nurse, 19*(3), 165-174.

Marriner-Tomey, A. (2000). *Guide to nursing management and leadership* (6th ed.). St. Louis: Mosby.

McCloskey, J., & Bulechek, G. (2000). *Nursing interventions classification (NIC): Iowa intervention project* (3rd ed.). St. Louis: Mosby.

McClure, M. L., Poulin, M. A., Sovie, M. D., & Wandelt, M. A. (1983). *Magnet hospitals: Attraction and retention of professional nurses.* Kansas City, MO: American Academy of Nursing.

North American Nursing Diagnosis Association. (2001). *Nursing Diagnoses: Definitions and classification 2001-2002* (4th ed.). Philadelphia: Author.

Plotkin, K., & Roche, J. (2000). Linking interventions to outcomes. *Home Healthcare Nurse, 18*(7), 443-448.

Polit, D., Beck, C., & Hungler, B. (2001). *Essentials of nursing research: Methods, appraisal and utilization* (5th ed.). Philadelphia: Lippincott.

Stahl, M. J. (1999). *Perspectives in total quality.* Milwaukee: Blackwell.

Stichler, J., & Weiss, M. (2000). Through the eye of the beholder: Multiple perspectives on quality in women's health care. *Quality Management in Health Care, 8*(4), 1-13.

SUGGESTED READINGS

Blegen, M. A., Vaughn, T. E., & Goode, C. J. (2001). Nurse experience and education. *AORN, 31*(1), 33-39.

Coeling, H. V., & Cukr, P. L. (2000). Communication styles that promote perceptions of collaboration, quality, and nurse satisfaction. *Journal of Nursing Care Quality, 14*(2), 63-74.

Cohen, J., Saylor, C., Holzemer, W., & Gorenber, B. (2000). Linking nursing care interventions with client outcomes: A community outcomes model. *Journal of Nursing Care Quality, 15*(1), 22-31.

Edick, V. W., & Whipple, T. W. (2001). Managing patient care with clinical pathways: A practical application. *Journal of Nursing Care Quality, 15*(3), 16-31.

Gingerich, B. (1999). Compliance concerns: Risk management and management of employee risk. *Home Health Care Management Practice, 11*(4), 65-66.

Horbar, J. D., Rogowski, J., Plsek, P. E., Delmore, P., Edwards, W. H., Hocker, J., Kantak, A. D., Lewallen, P., Lewis, W., Lewit, E., McCarroll, C. J., Mujsce, D., Payne, N. R., Shiono, P., Soll, R. F., Leahy, K., & Carpenter, J. H. (2001). Collaborative quality improvement for neonatal intensive care. *Pediatrics, 107*(1), 14-22.

Jones, J. (2000). Performance improvement through clinical research utilization: The linkage model. *Journal of Nursing Care Quality, 15*(1), 49-54.

Lee, T., & Mills, M. E. (2000). Analysis of patient profile in predicting home care resource utilization and outcomes. *AORN, 30*(2), 67-75.

Leff, E. W., & Lambert, P. (2001). Improving the performance of continuous care hospice nurses. *Home Healthcare Nurse, 19*(2), 95-102.

Murray, M. E. (2001). Outcomes of concurrent utilization review. *Nursing Economics, 19*(1), 17-23.

Pratt, J. R. (2000). Customer service. *Home Health Care Management Practice, 12*(6), 64-66.

Rakich, J. S. (2000). Strategic quality planning. *Hospital Topics: Research and Perspectives on Healthcare, 78*(2), 5-11.

Resick, L. K. (1999). Challenges in measuring outcomes in two community-based nurse-managed wellness clinics: The development of a chart auditing tool. *Home Healthcare Management Practice, 11*(4), 52-59.

Richard, A. A., Crisler, K. S., & Stearns, P. M. (2000). Using OASIS for outcome-based quality improvement. *Home Healthcare Nurse, 18*(4), 232-237.

Turner, J. T., Lee, V., Fletcher, K., Hudson, K., & Barton, D. (2001). Measuring quality of care with an inpatient elderly population: The geriatric resource nurse model. *Journal of Gerontological Nursing, 27*(3), 8-18.

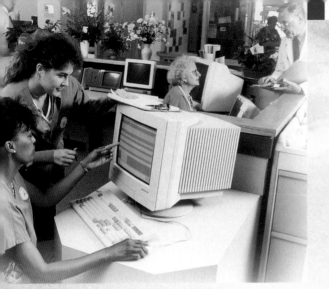

Chapter

12

Managing Information and Technology: Caring and Communicating With Computers

Christine R. Curran

This chapter describes current uses of information and information technology that allow nurses to use the data gathered at the point of care most effectively and efficiently. It discusses nurses as knowledge workers, the science of informatics, evidence-based practice, informatics competencies, various types of information technologies, standardized nursing terminologies, and future trends. Nurses need to build knowledge from practice by comparing and contrasting not only current patient data with previous data for the same patient but also data across patients with the same diagnosis. Information tools and skills are essential for these decision-making processes now and in the future.

Objectives

- Analyze the core components of informatics: data, information, and knowledge.
- Describe a model to change accepted practice into evidence-based practice.
- Evaluate three types of computerized information technologies used in nursing.
- Apply one structured nursing language to a nursing situation.
- Analyze three types of technology for capturing data at the point of care.
- Discuss knowledge systems and their uses for patient care.

- Explore the issues of nurse ethics and patient confidentiality in information technology.

- Understand the use of the Internet for healthcare information.

Questions to Consider

- *What types of technology are needed for effective patient care?*
- *How do you convert data gathered during patient care into information and then knowledge for future use?*
- *How can technology enhance efficiency and effectiveness?*
- *What competencies do you need to develop to take advantage of information processes and new technology?*
- *How can you be instrumental in promoting the use of informatics and technology skills and knowledge to keep nursing current?*

The Challenge

Michelle DeStefano, MPA, RN
Administrator, Women's Health Department, Milton S. Hershey Medical Center, Hershey, Pennsylvania

How can I, as a nurse leader and hospital administrator, take advantage of the new point-of-care technology, such as the PDA (personal digital assistant), to enhance productivity of my nurses? Because I oversee patients across the continuum of care, I have nurses who work in both inpatient and outpatient settings, as well as nurses who run community outreach programs. We are in the process of implementing a longitudinal and integrated clinical information system. Can one point-of-care device be used for nurses regardless of their practice setting, or would different technologies be needed? What about software applications on these devices?

 What do you think you would do if you were this nurse?

INTRODUCTION

Technology surrounds us! Computers are being used at the bank, at the grocery checkout, in our cars, and in almost every other aspect of daily living, including the provision of healthcare. Healthcare is an information-intensive business; therefore how the nurse gathers, manages, and uses information and the supporting information technologies will determine his or her success.

Nurses are **knowledge workers.** Knowledge workers need **data** and **information** to do their jobs effectively. Knowledge work is nonrepetitive, nonroutine work that requires considerable levels of cognitive activity (Drucker, 1993). The core activity of knowledge work is critical thinking, and the outcome is shared expertise.

Nurse knowledge workers need support from information technologies. Data and information must be accurate, reliable, and presented in an actionable form. Information technologies should facilitate and extend the nurses' decision-making abilities. They should support nurses in the following areas: (1) storing clinical data, (2) translating clinical data into information, (3) linking clinical data and domain knowledge, and (4) aggregating clinical data (Snyder-Halpern, Corcoran-Perry, & Narayan, 2001).

INFORMATICS

Informatics is "a science that combines a domain science, computer science, information science, and cognitive science" (Hunter, 2001, p. 180). In this case the domain science is nursing. In 1989 Graves and Corcoran published a classic work that describes the study of nursing informatics. Their initial model has subsequently been expanded and is depicted in Figure 12-1 (Graves, Amos, Huether, Lange, & Thompson, 1995).

The core of this model is the transformation of data into information and then into **knowledge.** This transformation occurs to facilitate decision making, new discoveries, and the creation of designs. Information and computer literacy, as well as the informatics infrastructure, influence this transformation of data into knowledge.

Data are discrete entities that describe or measure something without interpreting it. Numbers are data; for example, the number 30, without interpretation, means nothing. Information consists of interpreted, organized, or structured data. The number 30 interpreted as milliliters or as a length of time in minutes or hours has meaning. *Knowledge* refers to information that is combined or synthesized so that interrelationships are identified. For example, the number 30, when included in the statement "all patients who had indwelling catheters for longer than 30 days developed infections" becomes knowledge, something that is known.

The progression from data to information to knowledge can occur quickly in practice as data are interpreted and compared with previous information about the patient to provide knowledge. Much of the value is lost, however, if these data are not stored where others might retrieve and use them to synthesize new knowledge. Box 12-1 provides an

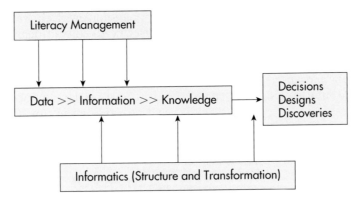

Figure 12-1 Nursing informatics conceptual model. (From Graves, J. R., Amos, L. K., Huether, S., Lange, L. L., & Thompson, C. B. [1995]. Description of a graduate program in clinical nursing informatics. *Computers in Nursing, 13*[2], 60-70.)

BOX 12-1

Using the Information Triad

Several patients in the coronary care unit had fallen at night over the last 3 weeks. This was very unusual because patients with heart conditions do not usually become disoriented at night. The nurse manager became concerned about this and began to look for commonalities among the patients who had fallen. She found that they were all taking the same sleeping medication. She mentioned this at a meeting and found that several other nurse managers had noticed the same situation. Together they contacted the pharmacist, who contacted the pharmaceutical representative. He found that the medication dosage had been tested on college students and that the dose was too high for older, less healthy patients. This is an example of combining data to provide information that, when aggregated and processed, becomes new knowledge.

Exercise 12-1

Think about the data that you gather every day: vital signs, intake and output, and the symptoms that you communicate during shift report. What data did you automatically combine or reorganize to help you make a decision regarding patient care? How did you use this information to improve your patient's outcome?

For example, you are charting vital signs and notice that the patient's blood pressure is lower than it was the day before. He is also complaining of nausea and light-headedness. You check his medications and see that he is receiving hydralazine (Apresoline). Based on your processing of the data that you have collected, you make a note to check his blood pressure and other symptoms again and notify the physician if the situation has not changed.

example that illustrates combining and interpreting data to provide information, which, when synthesized, provides new knowledge.

EVIDENCE-BASED PRACTICE

Nurses need to stay on the cutting edge of new knowledge. Therefore both the building of knowledge from practice and the application of clinical

evidence into practice are needed to advance nursing practice. **Evidence-based practice** is the integration of "individual clinical expertise with the best available external clinical evidence from systematic research" (Sackett, Rosenberg, Gray, Haynes, & Richardson, 1996, p. 71).

Rosswurm and Larrabee (1999) have proposed a model for evidence-based practice. Their model involves six steps: (1) assessing the need for change, (2) linking the problem with the interventions and outcomes, (3) synthesizing the best evidence, (4) designing a change in practice, (5) implementing and evaluating the practice change, and (6) integrating and maintaining the practice change. Nurses can use this framework to take existing heuristic practices and change them to evidence-based practices.

Informatics forms the infrastructure upon which evidence-based practice exists. Five building blocks form this informatics infrastructure: standardized terminologies and structures, digital sources of evidence, data exchange standards, informatics processes, and **informatics competencies** (Bakken, 2001).

Standardized terminologies are needed to uniformly "code" data within and between **databases.** Using consistent terms and concepts facilitates retrieval of comprehensive, accurate, and reliable information when a database is queried. Because no one source of data can meet all patient care needs, a common vocabulary allows links between databases to be effective.

Digital sources of evidence, such as the *Cochrane Database Library* and the *Online Journal of Knowledge Synthesis for Nursing,* provide access to evidence for practice. These databases are composed of systematic reviews of research intended to convey information on "best practices." Although meta-analyses and randomized clinical trials are viewed as the gold standards of evidence for practice, evidence is also built up from practice. Thus data collected from individual patients and across patient populations and then entered into clinical databases should be aggregated to generate knowledge.

Data exchange standards allow for communication of data between electronic systems. These protocols specify how data must be formatted to be sent and received between computer systems (i.e., at the interface of the systems). HL7 (health level seven) is perhaps the most widely known standard for the transmission of healthcare data.

Informatics processes, such as making clinical decisions or providing reminders to clinicians, affect the quality of care provided. A fundamental skill for nurses to build evidence from practice is systematic inquiry. Systematic inquiry includes asking an answerable question, tracking down reliable and relevant data (i.e., data based on research and expertise), weighing the evidence for validity and usefulness, and integrating conclusions into practice.

All nurses need informatics competencies. These competencies encompass computer skills, informatics knowledge, and information skills (Staggers, Gassert, & Curran, 2001). All nurses need to know how to identify, collect, record, analyze, and interpret pertinent patient and nursing data and information; use computer applications designed for delivery of patient care; and manage the privacy, confidentiality, and security of data and

information (American Nurses Association, 2001). Nurses need skills in quantifying data and aggregating information from multiple patients to gain knowledge of patient populations. Nurse leaders, in addition to possessing these competencies themselves, must assess for these competencies in staff and provide a means for staff to acquire those that are absent.

TYPES OF TECHNOLOGIES

As nurses we commonly use and manage three types of technologies: biomedical technology, information technology, and knowledge technology. **Biomedical technology** involves the use of equipment in the clinical setting for diagnosis, physiological monitoring, testing, or administering therapies to patients. **Information technology** entails recording, processing, and using data and information, in this case, for the purpose of delivering patient care. **Knowledge technology** is the use of expert and decision-support systems to assist nurses in making decisions about patient care. These systems are designed to mimic the reasoning of nurse experts in making such decisions.

Biomedical Technology

Biomedical technology is used for (1) physiological monitoring, (2) diagnostic testing, (3) drug administration, and (4) therapeutic treatments. Physiological monitoring systems measure heart rate, blood pressure, and other vital signs. They also monitor arrhythmias, record pressures such as central venous pressure or pulmonary wedge pressure, and analyze oxygen and carbon dioxide levels in the blood.

Continuous arrhythmia monitors and electrocardiograms (ECGs) are used to provide visual representation of electrical activity in the heart. Two types of arrhythmia systems are detection surveillance and diagnostic, or interpretive, systems. In the detection system the criteria for a normal cardiac rhythm are programmed into the computer, which then continuously surveys the patient's cardiac rhythm for normal and abnormal waveforms. The detection systems also monitor rhythm, rate, and pacemaker artifacts. The computer can audibly and visually alert the nurse when a preset number of abnormal waveforms is reached or when deviations from any other preset limit occurs. These data are stored so that the patient's history can be retrieved.

These systems can also be diagnostic. The computer, after processing the ECG, generates an analysis report. The ECG tracings may be transmitted over telephone lines from remote sites, such as the patient's home, to the physician's office or clinic. Patients with implantable pacemakers can have their cardiac activity monitored without leaving home.

Many hospitals are using oximetry to continuously monitor arterial oxygenation. This is a simple noninvasive procedure that can detect any trend in the patient's oxygenation status within seconds. The oximeter can measure oxygenation through ear, pulse, or nasal septal oximetry. Ear oximetry measures the arterial oxygen saturation by monitoring the transmission of light waves through the vascular bed of the earlobe. If low cardiac output causes insufficient arterial perfusion in the earlobe, a pulse oximeter may be used to measure the wavelengths of light transmitted through a pulsating vascular bed such as a fingertip. As the pulsating bed expands and relaxes, the light path length changes, producing a waveform. Because the waveform is produced from arterial blood, the pulse oximeter calculates the arterial oxygen saturation for every heartbeat without interference from surrounding tissues. If the patient has reduced peripheral vascular pulsations or is taking vasoactive drugs, a nasal probe may be used. This device fits around the septal anterior ethmoidal artery to detect vascular pulsations.

Systems for diagnostic testing include blood gas analyzers, pulmonary function systems, and intracranial pressure monitors. Blood gas analyzers use arterial blood to sense and calculate arterial blood gases, saturation curves, and buffer curves from normal data. These analyzers measure the partial pressures of oxygen and carbon dioxide and the pH of the arterial blood used in the test, enter primary results as soon as they are available, communicate the results quickly, and generate trend analysis for patients throughout their hospitalization.

Pulmonary function systems automate and simplify routine lung mechanics, lung volume, and diffusion capacity measurements. They can store data, calculate results, generate a numeric report, and display volumes graphically.

Intracranial pressure (ICP) monitoring systems monitor the cranial pressure in patients with closed head injuries or postoperative craniotomy patients. The ICP, along with the mean arterial blood pressure, can be used to calculate perfusion pressure. This allows for assessment and early therapy as changes occur. When the ICP exceeds a set pressure, some systems allow ventricular drainage. These systems supplement rather than replace nursing observations of the patient.

Drug administration systems are often used with implantable infusion pumps that administer medications. This equipment can be programmed to deliver medication at a predetermined rate for a defined period. These pumps are commonly used for hormone regulation; treatment of hypertension, chronic intractable pain, diabetes, and thrombosis; and cancer chemotherapy.

Therapeutic systems may be used to regulate intake and output, regulate breathing, and assist with the care of the newborn. Intake and output systems are linked to infusion pumps that control arterial pressure, drug therapy, fluid resuscitation, and serum glucose levels. These systems calculate and regulate the intravenous drip rate.

Ventilators are used to deliver a prescribed percentage of oxygen and volume of air to the patient's lungs and to provide a set flow rate, inspiratory-to-expiratory time ratio, and various other complex functions. Ventilators also provide sophisticated, sensitive alarm systems for patient safety. Some computer-assisted ventilators are electromechanically controlled by a closed-loop feedback system to analyze and control lung volumes and alveolar gases by a preset inspiratory pressure.

In the newborn nursery, computers monitor the heart and respiratory rates of the babies. In addition, these newborn nursery systems can regulate the temperature of the isolette by sensing the infant's temperature and the air of the isolette. Alarms can be set to notify the nurse when preset physiological parameters are exceeded. Newer systems are used to monitor fetal activity before delivery; these systems monitor the ECGs of the mother and baby and the pulse oximetry, blood pressure, and respirations of the mother.

Developments in biomedical technology include the use of implantable devices such as automated defibrillators, artificial organ transplants, gene therapy, and the use of robot servants for people who are disabled. Biomedical technology affects nursing care because nurses assume responsibility for monitoring the data generated by these devices and assessing their effectiveness.

Nurse leaders must be aware of how these technologies fit into the delivery of patient care and the strategic plan of the institution or corporation for which they work. They must have a vision for the future and be ready to suggest solutions that will assist nurses across specialties and settings.

■ *Exercise 12–2*

List the types of biomedical technology available for patient care in your organization. List ways that you currently use the information gathered by these systems. How does this information help you care for patients? Can you think of other ways to use the technology? the information? For example, patients with respiratory problems often have frequent arterial blood gases drawn to assess the effectiveness of treatment. Are there instances when the noninvasive pulse oximetry might be used? Nurses spend many hours learning to use the devices and to interpret the information gained from them. Have we come to rely on technology rather than on our own judgment?

Nurse managers must be aware of the latest technologies for the monitoring of patients' physiological status, diagnostic testing, drug administration, and therapeutic treatments. It is important to identify the data to be collected, the information that might be gained, and the many ways that these data might be used to provide new knowledge. More important, nurses must remember that these systems are tools for our use and do not replace our responsibility for assessing and monitoring the patient. Box 12-2 describes the development of informatics skills from novice to expert.

BOX 12-2

Development of Informatics Skills From Novice to Expert Practice

Novice nurses focus on learning what data to collect and how to use this information. They learn what clinical applications are available for use and how to use them. Computer and informatics skills focus on applying concrete concepts.

As nurses grow in expertise, they look for patterns in the data and information. They aggregate data across patient populations to look for similarities and differences in responses to therapies. Expert nurses integrate theoretical knowledge with practical knowledge gained from experience.

Expert nurses know the value of reflection on knowledge gained and synthesis and evaluation of information for discovery and decision making.

Information Technology

Computers offer the advantage of storing, organizing, retrieving, and communicating digital data with accuracy and speed. Patient care data can be entered once, stored in a database called a *central data repository,* and then quickly and accurately retrieved many times and in many combinations by healthcare providers and others. A database is a collection of data elements organized and stored together. Data processing is the structuring, organizing, and presenting of data for interpretation as information. For example, vital signs for one patient can be entered into the computer and communicated on a graph; the vital signs of several patients can be compared with the number of doses of antiarrhythmic medication. Vital signs for male patients between the ages of 40 and 50 years can be correlated and used to show a relationship between blood pressures and use of hypertensive medications.

Nurses process data continuously, but in an analog form. Computers process data in a digital form, process data faster and more accurately than humans, and provide a method of storage so that the data can be retrieved as needed. The Theory Box provides key ideas about information processing.

Structured Nursing Terminologies

The **nursing minimum data set (NMDS)** was defined to establish uniform standards for the collection of comparable essential patient data. Collecting a set of basic data from every healthcare encounter makes sense because comparisons can be made among many patients, institutions, or countries, almost in any combination imaginable, as well as across time. The NMDS is based on the concept of the uniform minimum health data set (UMHDS), a minimum set of items of information with uniform definitions and categories that meets the needs of multiple data users. UMHDSs have been developed for long-term care, hospital discharge, and ambulatory care.

Werley and Lang (1988) developed the NMDS, which represents nursing's first attempt to standardize the collection of nursing data. It follows UMHDS criteria in that (1) data items included in the set must be useful to healthcare professionals and administrators and to local, state, and federal planning, regulatory, and legislative bodies; (2) data items must be readily collectible and with reasonable accuracy; (3) data items should not duplicate data available from other sources; and (4) confidentiality must be protected.

Theory Box

INFORMATION THEORY

KEY CONTRIBUTORS	KEY IDEAS	APPLICATION TO PRACTICE
Tan (1995) describes the elements of information theory as source, transmitter, channel, receiver, and destination.	The information source selects the message or information to be transmitted. An underlying code or set of characters represents the message to be processed by the computer. The transmitter has an encoding function that converts the message to be sent. The communication channel (cable, air waves) provides the medium necessary for the information to be transmitted over distance. The receiver converts the information from its transmitted form, and the destination is the final stage of reception, in which the message is decoded to be understandable.	The physician enters an order for laboratory tests *(source, message)*. The computer program converts the message *(transmitter)*. The converted order is sent over the computer network *(communication channel)* to the laboratory *(receiver)*, where it is converted and read by the computer system in the laboratory *(destination)*.

The purposes of the NMDS are to (1) establish the comparability of patient care data across clinical populations, settings, geographic areas, and time; (2) describe the care of patients and families in various settings; (3) provide a means to mark the trends in the care provided and the allocation of nursing resources based on health problems or nursing diagnosis; (4) stimulate nursing research through links to existing data; and (5) provide data about nursing care to influence and facilitate healthcare policy decision making. Box 12-3 lists the elements of the nursing minimum data set.

Some NMDS elements (e.g., interventions and outcomes) are not collected as easily as the demographic and service elements, many of which are captured at patient registration or discharge, because of the lack of a uniform or unified **structured nursing language**. Significant efforts have been made to bridge this gap. Currently, 12 classification systems have been recognized by the American Nurses Association (Elfrink, Bakken, Coenen, McNeil, & Bickford, 2001) based on the following criteria (Bakken, Button, Konicek, Matney, McCormick, Ozbolt, Saba, Warren, & Westra, 2001):

- Support for nursing practice by providing clinically useful terminology (e.g., nursing diagnoses, nursing interventions) and rationale for development
- A level of development beyond an application, adaptation, or synthesis of currently recognized

BOX 12-3

Elements of the NMDS

Nursing Care Elements
1. Nursing diagnosis
2. Nursing intervention
3. Nursing outcome
4. Intensity of nursing care

Patient Demographic Elements
5. Personal identification*
6. Date of birth*
7. Sex*
8. Race and ethnicity*
9. Residency*

Service Elements
10. Unique facility or service agency number*
11. Unique health record number of the patient
12. Unique number of the principal registered nurse provider
13. Episode, admission, or encounter date*
14. Discharge or termination date*
15. Disposition of patient or client*
16. Expected payer for most of the bill

From Werley, H. H., & Lang, N. M. (1988). The consensually derived nursing minimum data set: elements and definitions. In H. H. Werley & N. M. Lang (Eds.), *Identification of the nursing minimum data set* (pp. 402-411). New York: Springer.
*Elements comparable to those in the UMHDS.

American Nurses Association vocabulary/classification schemes or presentation of an explicit rationale for seeking recognition for synthesis, application, or adaptation of existing schemes

- Clear and unambiguous terms
- Documented testing of reliability, validity, and utility in practice
- A systematic method of development
- A named entity responsible for a formal process of documenting evolving development and maintenance, including tracking of deleted terms and version control
- A coding scheme that provides a unique identifier for each term
- Identification of pertinent data elements as the variables of interest to whom and within what context
- Definition of the set of possible values for each variable
- A clear description of a defined structure or architecture with explicit principles of division

- Terms that can be combined to represent more complex concepts
- A classification structure that supports multiple parents and multiple children as relevant
- Preestablished rules for combining the terms

These recognized classification systems differ in specialty focus and included components. Some contain vocabularies for diagnosis, interventions, and outcomes, whereas others focus only on one or two of these groups. Some terminologies are specialty specific, such as the perioperative nursing data set. Table 12-1 lists the recognized standardized languages, with included components and a reference for each. An example of outcomes research being conducted using the NMDS and a structured nursing terminology can be found in the Research Perspective box.

Nurse managers must advocate for use of structured nursing terminologies so that data can be collected and aggregated within and across pa-

Table 12-1 ANA-RECOGNIZED STANDARDIZED LANGUAGES

Standardized Terminology	Problems/ Diagnoses	Interventions	Goals/ Outcomes	Reference
Complete Complementary Alternative Medicine Billing and Coding Reference		•		Gianinni (in press)
Home Health Care Classification	•	•	•	Saba (1990)
International Classification for Nursing Practice	•	•	•	International Council of Nurses (1999)
North American Nursing Diagnosis Association (NANDA) Taxonomy	•			NANDA (1999)
Nursing Interventions Classification		•		McCloskey & Bulechek (2000)
Nursing Management Minimum Data Set				Huber, Delaney, & Crossley (1992)
Nursing Minimum Data Set	•	•	•	Werley & Lang (1988)
Nursing Outcomes Classification			•	Johnson, Maas, & Moorehead (2000)
Omaha System	•	•	•	Martin & Scheet (1992)
Patient Care Data Set (1994)	•	•		Ozbolt, Fruchtnight, & Hayden
Perioperative Nursing Data Set	•	•	•	Kleinbeck (2000)
SNOMED RT	•	•	•	Spackman, Campbell, & Cote (1997)

tient populations to build evidence from practice and to use evidence in practice. These data are also needed to quantify and describe nursing practice and its effect on patient outcomes and the quality of care delivered.

Exercise 12–3

Examine the elements of the NMDS. Which of them would be collected by patient registration? Which information do you need to collect? For example, in an acute care setting, you have given pain medication several times today. The nursing diagnosis was alteration in comfort due to pain. You charted the medication given and the patient's quantitative rating of pain 30 minutes after medicating him. You have documented an intervention and an outcome, two nursing care elements of the NMDS. Can you locate the service elements in the medical record?

Information Systems

An information system may be manual or automated. Automated systems are needed to manage large volumes of data. They use computer hardware and software to process data into information needed to examine patterns and trends, solve prob-

lems, and answer questions. Data should be gathered at the point of care and information made available to healthcare providers when and where it is needed. This is accomplished by networking computers both within and between organizations to form larger systems. These networked systems might encompass several hospitals, clinics, hospice centers, home health agencies, and/or physician practices. Data from all patient encounters with the healthcare system are stored in a central data repository, where they are accessible to authorized users located anywhere in the world. These become the **computerized patient records,** which contain health data from birth to death.

Nursing leaders must influence and make choices that will benefit the staff and patients. Box 12-4 lists elements of the ideal hospital information system for consideration in choosing a system for an institution. These systems must make sense to the people who use them and not increase the workload. Nurse leaders and staff should be members of the selection team so that the systems chosen reflect the work being done. Remember: All nurse knowledge workers need information to deliver effective patient care.

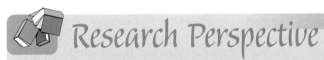

Research Perspective

Barton, A. J., Skiba, D. J., Baramee, J., & Erickson, V. I. (2000). Collecting the NMDS across multiple advanced practice nursing sites. *Proceedings from the 7th International Congress in Nursing Informatics,* Auckland, New Zealand.

The University of Colorado Health Sciences Center School of Nursing initiated collection of the nursing minimum data set (NMDS) at their faculty practice sites to demonstrate the value-added component of nurse practitioner care. For the nursing care elements of diagnosis, intervention, and outcome, they used the Omaha system as their structured nursing language. The current procedural terminology (CPT) was used as a proxy for the nursing intensity component of the NMDS.

Data were collected on 522 patient visits. Care was provided by eight different nurse practitioners. More than 1048 problems were identified. The majority of interventions involved health education (35%) and monitoring of a specific problem (32%). Outcomes indicated that the patients

had basic knowledge, displayed moderate signs and symptoms, and inconsistently demonstrated appropriate behavior.

IMPLICATIONS FOR PRACTICE
This study gave the faculty practice quantifiable insight into their patient population as a whole (i.e., the volume and types of patients seen, interventions chosen, and outcomes experienced as they related to interventions). They were able to understand the level of patient care workload through use of the CPT coding. The researchers believed that the amount of health education and monitoring were consistent with most nurse practitioner practices. Furthermore, the data supported that patients were understanding the education provided.

BOX 12-4

Elements of the Ideal Hospital Information System

1. The hardware is fail-safe.
2. The software requires minimal staff support.
3. The system is integrated wherever possible.
4. Data from the patient care process are gathered at the point of care.
5. The medical record is online and almost paperless, and the previous medical record is available on the system.
6. The database is complete, accurate, and easy to modify.
7. Physicians' offices, satellites, and future external sites are interfaced to the system.
8. Data are gathered by instrumentation whenever possible so that only minimal data entry is necessary.
9. The system has rapid response time (almost instantaneous).
10. Screen displays can be customized by the users.

Modified from McAlindon, M., Danz, S., & Theodoroff, R. C. (1987). Choosing the hospital information system: a nursing perspective. *Journal of Nursing Administration, 17*(19), 11-15.

Exercise 12-4

Select a hospital with which you are familiar. What information systems are used? Make a list of the names of these systems and the information that they provide. How do they help you in caring for patients? in making management decisions? Think about the communication of data and information between departments. Do the systems communicate with each other? If you do not have computerized systems, think about how data and information are communicated. How might a computer system help you be more efficient?

As an example, assume that a barium enema has been ordered. Handwritten requisitions are sent to nutritional services, the pharmacy, and the radiology department. With a computerized system, the barium enema is ordered, and the requests for dietary changes, bowel preparation medications, and the barium enema itself are automatically sent to the appropriate departments. Radiology will compare its schedule openings with the patient's schedule and automatically place the date and time for the barium enema on the patient's automated plan of care.

Nurse leaders have a responsibility to ensure that cost-effective, quality patient care is being delivered by the nursing staff under their supervision. Nursing databases that support decision making for this purpose are needed. Both clinical data and management data are required. Administrative databases assist in the development of the organization's information infrastructure, which ultimately allows for links between management and clinical outcomes. Table 12-2 lists the essential components of a nursing administration information system.

Once these data are available on the computer, nurse leaders can use this information to monitor staff performance, unit error rates (e.g., from incident reports), patient acuity levels, and staffing and scheduling patterns in relation to budget and census. Computerized personnel files could be used to generate reminders for license renewal and track position changes to produce reports for budgeting and forecasting purposes. Staffing levels and skill mix could be correlated with patient outcome data.

Quality management and the measurement of efficiency, effectiveness, and patient care outcomes have become necessary for the accreditation and licensing of healthcare organizations. This can be accomplished through documentation of the patient care processes and outcomes. The computerized plan of care outlines what patient care needs to occur, orders are executed to make the prescribed care happen, nursing documentation confirms that it was done, and then the computer can be used to aggregate the data and evaluate patient outcomes.

Beginning with the 1994 *Accreditation Manual*, the Joint Commission on Accreditation of Healthcare Organizations (JCAHO) provides a separate chapter that addresses the management of information. Within these standards the goals of information management are to obtain, manage, and use information to improve patient outcomes and individual and organizational performance in patient care, as well as to improve performance in other organizational processes. The standards address the identification, design, capture, analysis, communication, integration, and use of information. Four areas of management of information are reviewed: (1) patient-specific data and information, (2) aggregate data and information, (3) expert knowledge–based information, and (4) comparative performance data and information (JCAHO, 2001).

In 1997 JCAHO introduced the ORYX initiative, which integrated outcome and performance measurement data into the accreditation review process. Organization-specific performance data are used to guide the accreditation survey process and to monitor performance between surveys when indicated. In addition, core performance measures, categorized by type of institution, have been selected to

Table 12-2 ESSENTIAL COMPONENTS OF A NURSING ADMINISTRATION INFORMATION SYSTEM

Level	Administrative Data	Clinical Data
Interinstitution	Nursing management minimum data set (NMMDS)	Nursing minimum data set (NMDS)
Organization	Organizational productivity measures Referral patterns Cost per drug or procedure; profit calculations Case mix analysis Achievement of accrediting body standards Strategic planning data (e.g., forecasting market share, patient distribution by county of residence)	Site of care (e.g., inpatient, outpatient, skilled-care facility, home care, community-based site) Outcomes research findings Number of caregivers per patient Aggregate patient profile (e.g., volume, type, diagnosis by service, outcomes, utilization rates)
Department or discipline	Staffing profile (skill mix, educational mix, experience mix) Employee satisfaction Chief nurse executive profile Salary—total and distribution	Research studies with findings Clinical knowledge Number of caregivers per patient Standards of care Average patient intensity Patient satisfaction
Division or product line	Type of division/product line Staffing profile (skill mix, educational mix, experience mix) Salary—total and distribution Units of service (patient days, procedures, visits) Size of division (number of beds available, operational, and occupied) Budget Nursing resources (FTEs—total and by skill level) Activity levels (admission, discharge, and transfer) Costs—direct and indirect expenses Resources (equipment, supplies) Nursing turnover Employee satisfaction Profile of the director	Average intensity (e.g., HPPD or HPWI) Patient satisfaction Division profile (e.g., volume, type, diagnosis by service, outcomes, utilization rates) Standards of care
Unit or patient population/service	Type of unit Care delivery system (e.g., primary, team, functional, care partners) Nurse manager profile Staff mix Units of service (patient days, procedures, visits) Size of unit (number of beds available, operational, and occupied) Budget Nursing resources (FTEs—total and by skill level) Activity levels (admission, discharge, and transfer) Costs—direct and indirect expenses	Standards of care Patient educational information Aggregate patient profile (histories, diagnoses, interventions, outcomes, volume, patterns of care/day, educational needs, LOS, discharge disposition and summary) Modeling of preferred care Average intensity (e.g., HPPD or HPWI)

From Curran, C. R. (1995). *Data requirements of the nurse executive.* Unpublished paper.
DRG, Diagnosis-related group; *FT,* full-time; *FTE,* full-time equivalent; *HPPD,* hours per patient day; *HPWI,* hours per workload index; *LOA,* leave of absence; *LOS,* length of stay; *PT,* part time.

Continued

Table 12-2 ESSENTIAL COMPONENTS OF A NURSING ADMINISTRATION INFORMATION SYSTEM—cont'd

Level	Administrative Data	Clinical Data
Unit or patient population/ service—cont'd	Resources (equipment, supplies) Administrative standards Nursing turnover Nonfunctional positions by pay period (vacancy rate by job category, orientation time, unfilled positions because of LOAs or employees offered positions but not here yet)	
Individual	Salary (base, differentials, and bonuses) and salary plan (e.g., regular, Baylor, per diem) Skill level Credentials (license type, number, and expiration date; educational preparation; experience; work history—FT and PT; certification types, numbers, and expiration dates) Current work history (hire date, change in positions and salary, termination date) Clinical ladder appointment(s) Clinical privileges Performance evaluation Demographic data (SSN, name, position number, gender, date of birth, address, race, phone number) Continuing education programs and hours Cost center Position title Appointment fraction Schedule (include shift length) Nonproductive time (e.g., LOAs, sick, vacation) Employee satisfaction Audits of practice by nurse	Individual patient intensity score Individual nurse assignment Each patient medical record (patient history, diagnosis, plan of care, interventions, outcomes, primary nurse, demographic data, LOS, discharge disposition and summary) Patient satisfaction Incident reports by patient and by nurse Uniform billing information (cost per patient)

From Curran, C. R. (1995). *Data requirements of the nurse executive.* Unpublished paper.
DRG, Diagnosis-related group; *FT,* full-time; *FTE,* full-time equivalent; *HPPD,* hours per patient day; *HPWI,* hours per workload index; *LOA,* leave of absence; *LOS,* length of stay; *PT,* part time.

begin a process of comparing performance across organizations (JCAHO, 2001).

Communication networks are used to transmit information that is entered at one computer and received by another. These networks are usually part of the integrated system and reduce the clerical functions of nursing. They can provide patient census and locations, results from tests, and lists of medications. Nursing policies and procedures may be entered onto a communication network to be accessible to authorized personnel.

Discussion has focused on information systems for acute care institutions, but many patients are cared for in outpatient or community settings. Nursing focus in these settings involves health promotion, maintenance, and education, as well as coordinated continuity of care and monitoring of chronic diseases. Information systems also support nursing functions in these settings. They are used for financial management and billing, statistical reporting, and patient care information systems. These systems can be used within the agency or at the point of care to connect the nurse to an enterprise-integrated data network that allows access to the computerized patient record.

Links can be provided between the patient's home, hospital, and/or physician office with bedside computers, handheld technologies, voice-activated systems, or laptop computers. Day-to-day events can be recorded on these devices and downloaded into the patient record remotely or, in the case of portable devices, back at the office at the end of the day.

Nurses caring for patients in the home healthcare industry have many government and insurance requirements for form completion. Computers offer a means of reducing this paperwork burden by allowing direct entry of data in the required format. Portable and wireless computers have made recording of patient care information more efficient and have improved personnel productivity.

These portable computers are used to download files of the patients to be seen during the day from the main database. During each visit, the computer prompts the nurse for vital signs, assessments, diagnosis, interventions, long- and short-term goals, and medications based on previous entries in the medical record. The nurses then enter any new data, modifications, or nursing notes directly into the portable computer. Entries related to patient care can be transmitted by telephone to the main computer at the office or downloaded from the device at the end of the day. This automatically updates the patient record and any verbal order entry records, home visit reports, federally mandated treatment plans, productivity and quality improvement reports, and other documents for review and signature.

The elimination of the paper trail has been partially accomplished by the placement of computers at the bedside or through the use of handheld devices. In this way, information can be entered once at the point of care and accessed over and over again. Documentation of the patient assessment at the bedside saves time, gives others access to more timely data, and decreases the likelihood of forgetting to document vital information. Point-of-care systems that adapt to the nurse's workflow, personalize patient assessments, and simplify care planning are available. Patient care areas with point-of-care computers have improved the quality of

patient care by decreasing errors of omission, providing greater accuracy and completeness of documentation, reducing medication errors, providing more timely response to patient needs, and improving discharge planning and teaching. These systems shorten or eliminate shift-to-shift communication and eliminate redundant charting of data.

Wireless (WL) messaging is changing the way we work. WL communication is an extension of an existing wired network environment and uses radio-based systems to transmit data signals through the air without any physical connections. Nurses can communicate with offices/departments, other healthcare team members, and patients through the use of pagers, cellular phones, or personal digital assistants (PDAs). These devices can send and receive alphanumeric data. Nurses can send and receive **emails**, clinical data, and other textual messages. They can also access the **Internet** on these devices.

WL systems are being used by emergency medical personnel to request authorization for the treatments or drugs needed in emergency situations. Laboratories use WL technology to transmit laboratory results to physicians, patients awaiting organ transplants are being provided with WL pagers so that they can be notified if a donor is found, and parents of critically ill children carry them when they are away from a phone. A home monitoring system in use by visiting nurses uses WL technology to enter vital signs and other patient-related information. Inpatient nurses can send a message to the admissions department when a patient is being transferred to another unit without having to wait for someone to answer the telephone.

Voice technology will also enhance the use of computer systems when this technology is further developed. Voice technology is the ability to control a computer system through voice input by the user. The machine gathers, processes, interprets, and executes audible signals by comparing the spoken words with a template already resident in the system. If the patterns match, recognition occurs and a previously stored command is executed by the computer. This allows untrained personnel or those whose hands are busy to work in computer-based environments without touching the computer. Voice technology will also allow quadriplegic and other physically challenged individuals to function more efficiently when using the computer.

These systems recognize a large number of words but are still immature. The speaker must use staccato-like speech, pausing about one tenth of a second between each clearly spoken word, and these systems must be programmed for each user so that the system recognizes the user's voice patterns.

Technology has both advantages and disadvantages. The use of handheld devices is less expensive because each caregiver on a shift can be equipped with a device rather than placing a stationary computer in each patient room. They allow access to information at the point of care, both for retrieval of information and entry of patient data. Disadvantages of handheld technology stem from their size and portability; they can be put down and forgotten, or dropped and broken, and are a target for theft. There must also be a convenient and adequate place to store them when they are not in use and to charge their batteries if needed. These computers have a small display screen, which limits the amount of data available on the screen and the size of the text.

Bedside computers must be suited to patient rooms. They should have quiet fans, must be lighted to be viewed in the dark, and must be either mounted on the wall or placed on portable stands. In addition, automating the healthcare delivery process is not an easy task. Processes are not standardized across settings, and vendors cannot afford to customize applications for each organization. Some current versions of the computerized medical record have merely automated the existing schema of the chart rather than considering how computers could permit data to be viewed or used differently from the previous manual method.

Management of these technologies is important. Nurse leader and managers must make knowledgeable decisions about the type of technology to use, the education needed, and the proper care and maintenance of the equipment. Important questions to ask include the following: What data and information do we need to gather? When and where should it be gathered? How difficult is the equipment to use? Has the technology been tested sufficiently to ensure purchase of a dependable product?

■ Exercise 12-5

Think about the data you gather as you go through the day. How do you communicate the information and knowledge gleaned about your patient to others? Does the information system support the way you need this information organized, stored, retrieved, and presented to other healthcare providers? For example, if a patient's pain medication order is about to expire and you want to assess the patient's use and response to the pain medication over the last 24 hours, can the information system generate a graph for this patient comparing the time, dose, and pain score for this period? If your assessment is that the medication needs to be renewed, can you leave an electronic message for the physician to renew this medication—is there an "electronic sticky note" function?

Knowledge Technology

Knowledge technology consists of systems that generate or process knowledge. Knowledge technology involves **expert systems.** An expert system is a computer program that mimics the inductive or deductive reasoning of a human expert. These programs process knowledge to produce decisions by means of a knowledge base and a software application that controls the use of the knowledge (an inference engine). To automate this process, the necessary data elements must be identified and rules for combining the data established. The same data elements are always required, and the same formula or rule is applied in the same way to the same data. The knowledge base contains the knowledge (rules, heuristics) that an expert nurse would apply to the data and information to solve a problem. The inference engine controls the use of the knowledge by providing the logic for its use. Box 12-5 illustrates the use of an expert system for giving a maximum dose of pain medication. The knowledge base contains eight items that are to be considered when giving the maximum dose. The inference engine controls the use of the knowledge base by applying logic that an expert nurse would use in making the decision to give the maximum dose.

This decision frame states that *if* pain is severe (A) or a painful procedure is planned (B), and there is an order for pain medication (C) and the time since surgery is less than 48 hours (H) and the time since the last dose is greater than 3 hours (G), and there are no contraindications to the medication (D) or history of allergy (E) or contraindication to the maximum dose (F), then the "decision" would be to give the dose of pain medication. The rule, or heuristics, appearing in this logic are those that expert nurses would apply in making the decision to give pain medication. The inference engine controls the *if* logic or knowledge.

One of the benefits of computerized expert systems is that they outperform nonexpert human clinicians by assisting with the decision making for novices, nurses working outside their areas of expertise, and orientees. Because the systems obtain their information directly from patient care documentation, the computer never forgets when a pa-

BOX 12-5

Expert Decision Frame for "Give Maximum Dose of Pain Medication"

The Knowledge Base

A. Severe pain
B. Painful procedure planned
C. Pain medication order
D. Contraindications to the medication
E. History of allergic reaction to opiate analgesics
F. Contraindication to maximum dose of opiate analgesic
G. Time since last dose
H. Time since surgery

The Inference Engine:

Logic: Give the maximum dose of pain medication *if* (A or B) and (C and H <48 hours and G >3 hours) and not (D or E or F)

or:

(C and H <48 hours and G >4 hours) and not (D or E or F)

---

tient needs pain medication or the effectiveness of the last treatment. If the expert system is used in conjunction with an information system, the documentation of observations, care, and patient outcomes can be expected to increase significantly and improve the quality of care.

Nurse managers must be aware of the usefulness of expert systems for nursing. By helping to develop the logic used in the knowledge base through the use of critical-thinking skills, changes in current practice can be made for the improvement of patient care.

Exercise 12–6

Mr. Jones' heart rate is 58 beats per minute. Tony is about to give Mr. Jones his atenolol (Tenormin). When Tony enters Mr. Jones' identification number and the medication name, the computer warns him that atenolol should not be given for a heart rate less than 60 beats per minute. What should Tony do?

PROFESSIONAL ISSUES

Data Privacy and Confidentiality

Patients' rights to privacy of their data must be maintained whether in a manual or automated system. Converting the patient record to a computer-

generated document increases the likelihood that a breach in confidentiality will have broader implications. With manually generated documents, there is only one copy of the data, and caregivers access the chart individually and in a geographically limited place. With computerized data, any person with the proper permission anywhere in the world may access the information, and multiple people can do so simultaneously. Data can also be inadvertently sent to the wrong individual or site.

System users must never share the passwords that allow them access to information in the computerized database. Each password uniquely identifies a user to the system by name and title, gives approval to carry out certain functions, and provides access to data appropriate to the user. When a nurse signs on to a computer, all data and information that are entered or reviewed can be traced to that password. Thus you are accountable for all actions taken using your password.

A firewall protects the information in the central data repository from access by unauthorized users. It is a network security measure that keeps electronic intruders from accessing an organization's data on its private network while allowing members of the organization to reach the Internet. Organizational policies on the use, security, and accuracy of data must be written and enforced.

Ethics

Ethics is a form of thinking about morality, moral problems, and moral judgments. Principles are general action guides for judgment; an ethical principle might be to prevent harm and promote the highest level of health possible. Despite security measures available in computerized systems, the integrity and ethical principles of the users of these systems provide the only safeguard of patients' welfare, privacy, and confidentiality of data.

Because of the increasing ability to preserve and maintain human life via technological interventions, questions dealing with life become complex, both conceptually and ethically. Conceptually, it becomes more difficult to define extraordinary treatment and human life because technology has changed our concepts of living and dying. The ethics problem becomes one of precedence, such as the dilemma of how to relieve pain without hastening death.

A frequent source of ethical dilemmas is the use of invasive technological treatment to prolong life for patients with limited or no decision-making capabilities. Healthcare institutions that use technology strive for efficiency and cost-effectiveness with an ethical mandate of the greatest good for the greatest number. The nursing profession holds a holistic orientation and is concerned with individual patient welfare and effect of technological intervention as it affects the immediate and long-term quality of the patients and their families. Patient advocacy remains an important function of the professional nurse.

Nurse leaders must promote the existence and use of an ethics committee in their institutions and assign knowledgeable nurses to serve on these committees. Nurse managers must ensure that policies and procedures for the collection and entering of data and the use of security measures (e.g., passwords) are established to maintain confidentiality of patient data and information. Nurse managers must also be knowledgeable patient advocates in the use of technology for patient care by referring ethical questions to the organization's ethics committee. Staff nurses must be aware of their responsibilities for the confidentiality and security of the data they gather and for the security of their passwords.

FUTURE TRENDS

Because of escalating healthcare costs, insurance companies (third-party payers) and the federal government are supporting new technologies to reduce costs. Longitudinal computerized patient records, telecommunications, and WL devices that store health history data are technologies that will grow in the future. Use of the Internet and **World Wide Web** (WWW) will also provide new exciting options for healthcare. Use of robotics will be commonplace. Miniaturization of devices will occur, and wearable computers are in development.

Computerized Patient Records

Managed care is an effort by the insurance companies, the payers for healthcare, to manage healthcare costs by limiting the care provided for each diagnosis. In the hospital this means that the number of days a patient is permitted to stay is limited, depending on the diagnosis. If the patient remains longer than the permitted days, the health insurer will not reimburse the costs of the care for the unapproved days. The concept of managed care has resulted in the redesign of patient care plans to clinical pathways that detail the interventions needed day by day to achieve the outcome of discharge by the final approved day. Data from the clinical pathway form the basis of the episode of care in the **computerized patient record (CPR)**. The federal government has mandated use of a CPR.

Credit card–like devices called **smart cards** store a limited number of pages of data on a computer chip. The implementation of computer-based health information systems will lead to computer networks that will store health records across local, state, national, and international boundaries. The smart card serves as a bridge between the clinician terminal and the central repository, making patient information available to the caregiver quickly and cheaply at the point of service because the patients bring it with them. This will help coordinate care; improve quality-of-care decisions; and reduce risk, waste, and duplication of effort. Patients are mobile and consult many practitioners, thereby causing their records to be fragmented. With the electronic smart card, patients, providers, and notes can be brought together in any combination at any place. Box 12-6 provides examples of the kinds of data that are recorded on smart cards.

Telecommunications

Telecommunications and systems technology facilitate clinical oversight of healthcare via telephone or cable lines, remote monitoring, information links, and the Internet. **Telehealth** is the use of modern telecommunications and information technologies for the provision of healthcare to individuals at a distance and the transmission of information to provide that care. This is accomplished through the

---

BOX 12-6

Smart Card Information

1. Patient classification with a link to insurance plans
2. Emergency care information
3. Recent care encounter data, including medications
4. Past care encounter summaries
5. Record of locations and electronic address information for patient records

Modified from Elliott, J. (1996). The smart card: Wising up on plastic money. *Healthcare Informatics, 13*(5), 29-32.

use of two-way interactive video-conferencing and high-speed telephone lines, fiberoptic cable, and satellite transmissions. Patients sitting in front of the teleconferencing camera can be diagnosed, treated, monitored, and educated by nurses and physicians. ECGs and x-ray films can be viewed and transmitted. Sophisticated electronic stethoscopes and dermascopes allow nurses and physicians to hear heart, lung, and bowel sounds and to look closely at wounds, eyes, ears, and skin. Ready access to expert advice and patient information is available no matter where the patient or information is located. Patients in rural areas and prisons especially benefit from this technology.

Internet

Another vehicle for health information is the Internet. The Internet, which can provide health education and other health information, is a worldwide network of computers that fosters communication, collaboration, resource sharing, and information access. It is a multicultural library that is open all day, every day to ordinary computer users.

The main uses of the Internet are sending and receiving electronic mail (email) and browsing the WWW. Mail may be sent to individuals in any part of the world through email if they have an email address, or email of particular interest may be obtained by subscribing to a listserv. A *listserv* is a group of people who have similar interests. Subscribers to a listserv become part of the "conversation." All messages sent to the listserv are forwarded to all subscribers, who can then read and respond to them.

Email is rapidly becoming a preferred communication method between healthcare providers and patients. This asynchronous mode of communication allows for timely responses to nonemergent healthcare issues at the convenience of both the patient and provider. It prevents "telephone tag" and avoids the interruptions often encountered when paging healthcare providers. However, reimbursement for these "virtual office visits" is currently a problem. Third-party payers need to financially support this method of care delivery.

Email can be a very effective means of delivering health services to people. It provides documentation of the patient-provider communication and gives patient instructions in writing. Emails can have embedded links to information on the WWW. Box 12-7 presents guidelines for the use of email between patients and providers.

The WWW is a network of information in the form of text, pictures, video, and sound. Web pages contain text and "links" to other documents filled with information. Links are highlighted or underlined words that are clicked on with the mouse to activate another linked document. Web servers are located all over the world, so information can be retrieved from linked web pages without knowledge of whether the server is located in Australia, Europe, or California. A software program called a *browser* is needed to view web pages. Box 12-8 lists websites of interest to nurses.

Web users need to evaluate the quality of healthcare information found on the WWW. Websites can be created but may not be updated. Links are often "broken" when websites relocate to another address.

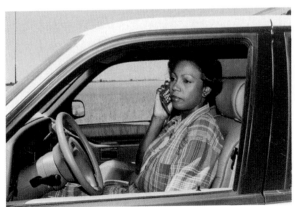
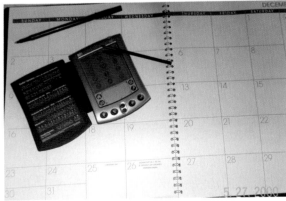

Nurses working in the community often use cellular phones and other technologies (e.g., personal digital assistants) to communicate and remain connected with their offices.

BOX 12-7

Guidelines for Use of Patient-Provider Email

Communication Issues

- Establish an expected response time for messages.
- Discuss who will see messages (i.e., how private is the email).
- Establish boundaries of acceptable and unacceptable types of email messages.
  1. Purpose
  2. Content
- Have the patient include his or her name in the body of the message.
- Suggest a list of categories the patient could use in the subject heading.
- Print all emails to document the information in the medical record.
- Send reply messages so that receipt of the message is confirmed.

Administrative Issues

- Obtain informed consent from the patient before using email.
- Do not share your password with anyone.
- Use an email package that encrypts messages.
- Perform routine backups of the email system.
- Do not forward any patient-identifiable information without the written consent of the patient.
- Have a written policy in place for the use of email in the practice setting.

Modified from Kane, B., & Sands, D. (1998). Guidelines for the clinical use of electronic mail with patients. *Journal of the American Medical Informatics Association, 5,* 104-111.

BOX 12-8

Health-Related Website Uniform Resource Locators (URLs)

Description	URL
American Heart Association	http://www.americanheart.org
Centers for Disease Control and Prevention	http://www.cdc.gov
Department of Health/Human Services	http://www.healthfinder.gov
Health on the Net	http://www.hon.ch/
World Health Organization	http://www.who.int/

Additional Sites	
Excellent links to health information	http://members.tripod.com/HealthCareWorld
Guide to Evidence Based Practice	http://www.nursingresearch.jgh.mcgill.ca/Cnr.htm
Nursing and healthcare resources	http://nmap.ac.uk/
Public mailing lists	http://www.paml.net
Resources for nurses and families	http://pegasus.cc.ucf.edu/%7Ewink

BOX 12-9

Criteria for Evaluation of Healthcare Websites

- Credibility
  - Source authority/credentials of the author
  - Context
  - Updated/current information
  - Utility of information
  - Editorial review process
- Content
  - Accuracy
  - Hierarchy of evidence
  - Original source stated
  - Disclaimer
  - Omissions
- Disclosure
  - Purpose of the site
  - Profiling

- Links
  - Selection
  - Architecture
  - Content
  - Back linkages and descriptions
- Design
  - Accessibility
  - Logical organization/navigation
  - Internal search engine
- Interactivity
  - Mechanism for feedback
  - Chat rooms and bulletin boards
  - Tailoring
- Caveats

Source: Health Information Technology Institute of Mitretek Systems, Inc., of Falls Church VA, and the Health Summit Working Group. (1997). *Criteria for assessing the quality of health information on the internet.* White paper accessed at http://hitiweb.mitretek. org/docs/criteria.html.

How does one evaluate the credentials of the author of the information or site? Several texts and articles suggest criteria for the evaluation of websites related to health (Goldsborough, 1999; Hollaway, Kripps, Koepke, & Skiba, 2000; Nicoll, 2001). Box 12-9 lists criteria for evaluation of these sites.

Search engines are often used to look up information on the WWW. Even the best search engines are currently not very effective; a recent study found that only about one third of all available information on a topic was typically retrieved (Lawrence & Giles, 1998). Thus the data retrieved should be considered a starting point and not an end point of possible information on the subject.

Exercise 12-7

Think about the use of the WWW in healthcare. How do you use it to look up healthcare information? How would you advise a patient to select appropriate sites? (Hint: See Box 12-9.)

 SUMMARY

We have discussed the advances of technology in a managed care environment that will stress wellness, health promotion, and illness management, as well as the linking of local and global communities. Care in this new era will focus on empowering patients and their families through information and education. Everyone (families, employers, insurers, and providers) will evaluate care based on outcomes. Healthcare in the future will emanate from wherever the client is located. Clinicians will move beyond the traditional walls of healthcare facilities to become as skilled with wellness maintenance activities and prevention methods as with direct care delivery. Technology has become the bond that links people and information together in a rapidly changing world of healthcare, and with technology comes the need for a new set of competencies. We need to prepare for this exciting future.

The Solution

This should not be a quick decision, nor one made alone, because it has broad implications for cost and quality of patient care delivery. In this age of information explosion, it is unlikely that any one person can have all the answers. Therefore I decided to form a project team consisting of key stakeholders to look at the options and select the best approach to implement point-of-care technology within my service line. A staff member from each setting, a member of the clinical information system application team from IT, our budget administrator, and the nurse manager of the inpatient unit formed the team. Options explored were bedside/office-based computers, hand-held devices, and portable laptop computers. Information needs were identified, and software applications to sup-port these information needs were researched and prioritized. Both the need to have electronic reference materials, such as an updated medication database to look up drug information, and the need to enter and retrieve patient data into and from the clinical information system were addressed. The advantages and disadvantages and the cost of implementation of each approach were discussed before one technology was selected.

— Michelle DeStefano

 Would this approach be suitable for you? Why?

CHAPTER CHECKLIST

Nurses are the key personnel in the healthcare system to mediate the interaction among science, technology, and the patient because of our unique holistic view-point and "24 by 7" role of vigilant healthcare providers who preserve the patients' humanity, optimal functioning, and promotion of health. The challenge for the profession is to continue to provide human and moral care that gives life, health, and death their meaning in a technological society that strives for efficiency and cost-effectiveness. Nurse leaders, managers, and staff must provide leadership in managing information and technology to meet the challenge.

- Nurses are knowledge workers.
- Informatics is the transformation of data into knowledge. It consists of three core components:
  - Data
  - Information
  - Knowledge
- Evidence-based practice involves both the application of evidence to practice and the building of evidence from practice.
- The five building blocks of an informatics infrastructure are as follows:
  - Standardized terminologies and structure
  - Digital sources of evidence
  - Data exchange standards
  - Informatics processes
  - Informatics competencies
- Nurses commonly manage three types of information technology:
  - Biomedical
  - Information
  - Knowledge
- Biomedical technology includes the use of the following:
  - Physiological monitoring
  - Diagnostic testing
  - Drug administration
  - Therapeutic interventions
- *Information technology* refers to computers and programs that are used to process data and information.
- Use of structured nursing languages provides standards for gathering data so that they can be retrieved and compared across time and place.
- Information systems for nursing administration provide information for the following:
  - Quality improvement
  - Personnel tracking
  - Summary reports
  - Budgeting and payroll
  - Skill mix and staffing levels
  - Forecasting and planning
- Point-of-care computer devices have improved communication by providing immediate access to information when and where it is needed.

- Knowledge technology is used to mimic the information processing of an expert nurse.
- The computerized patient record contains healthcare information for each individual from birth to death, allowing immediate and complete access to health information.
- Smart cards are credit card–like devices that store a limited amount of data. These cards and the information they provide help coordinate care across local, state, national, and international boundaries—wherever patients may need access to healthcare.
- Confidentiality issues have become important with increased access to, and therefore potential broad misuse of, patient care data.
- The Internet is a worldwide network of computers that fosters communication, collaboration, resource sharing, and information access. It is a multicultural library that is open all day, every day to ordinary computer users. The main uses of the Internet are sending and receiving electronic mail (email) and browsing the WWW.
- Telehealth is the process of using modern telecommunication and information technologies to provide healthcare remotely.
- In the future, computers will be smaller, wearable, faster, and smarter.

TIPS FOR MANAGING INFORMATION AND TECHNOLOGY

- Create a vision for the future.
- Tie your vision to the institution's strategic plan.
- Learn what you need to know to fulfill the vision.

- Join initiatives that are moving in the direction of your vision.
- Be prepared to initiate, implement, and support new technology.
- Never stop learning, or you will always be behind.

TERMS TO KNOW

biomedical technology
computerized patient record (CPR)
data
database
email
evidence-based practice
expert system
informatics
informatics competencies
information
information technology
Internet
knowledge
knowledge technology
knowledge worker
nursing minimum data set (NMDS)
smart card
structured nursing language
telehealth
voice technology
wireless (WL) messaging
World Wide Web

REFERENCES

American Nurses Association. (2001). *The scope of practice of nursing informatics and the standards of practice and professional performance for the informatics nurse specialist.* (Draft document dated December 7, 2001).

Bakken, S. (2001). An informatics infrastructure is essential for evidence based practice. *Journal of the American Medical Informatics Association, 8*(3), 199-201.

Bakken, S., Button, P., Konicek, D., Matney, S., McCormick, K., Ozbolt, J. G., Saba, V. K., Warren, J. J., & Westra, B. (2001). Standardized terminologies for nursing concepts: Collaborative activities in the United States. In NI 2000 Postconference Proceedings. Rotorua, New Zealand: Premier Press.

Barton, A. J., Skiba, D. J., Baramee, J., & Erickson, V. I. (2000). Collecting the NMDS across multiple advanced practice nursing sites. Proceedings from the 7th International Congress in Nursing Informatics. Auckland, New Zealand.

Curran, C. R. (1995). Data requirements of the nurse executive. Unpublished paper.

Drucker, P. (1993). *Post capitalist society.* New York: Harper Business Publishers.

Elfrink, V., Bakken, S., Coenen, A., McNeil, B., & Bickford, C. (2001). Standardized nursing vocabularies: A foundation for quality care. *Seminars in Oncology Nursing, 17*(1), 18-23.

Elliott, J. (1996). The smart card: Wising up on plastic money. *Healthcare Informatics, 13*(5), 29-32.

Gianinni, M. (in press). *The CAM and nursing coding manual*. Albany, NY: Delmar.

Goldsborough, R. (1999). Information on the net often needs checking. *RN, 62*(5), 22, 24.

Graves, J. R., & Corcoran, S. (1989). The study of nursing informatics. *Image: Journal of Nursing Scholarship, 21*(4), 227-231.

Graves, J. R., Amos, L. K., Huether, S., Lange, L. L., & Thompson, C. B. (1995). Description of a graduate program in clinical nursing informatics. *Computers in Nursing, 13*(2), 60-70.

Health Information Technology Institute of Mitretek. (1997). Criteria for assessing the quality of health information on the Internet. Retrieved June 12, 2001, from http://hitiweb.mitretek.org/docs/criteria.html.

Hollaway, N., Kripps, B., Koepke, K., & Skiba, D. J. (2000). Evaluating healthcare information on the internet. In J. Fitzpatrick & K. S. Montogomery (Eds.), *Internet resources for nurses*. New York: Springer.

Huber, D. G., Delaney, C., & Crossley, J. (1992). A nursing management minimum data set. *Journal of Nursing Administration, 22*(7/8), 35-40.

Hunter, K. M. (2001). Nursing informatics theory. In V. K. Saba & K. A. McCormick (Eds.), *Essentials of computers for nurses: Informatics for the new millennium* (pp. 179-190). New York: McGraw-Hill.

International Council of Nurses. (1999). *International classification for nursing practice—Beta version*. Geneva, Switzerland: Author.

Joint Commission on Accreditation of Healthcare Organizations. (2001). *JCAHO accreditation manual*. Chicago: Author.

Johnson, M., Maas, M., & Moorhead, S. (2000). *Nursing outcomes classification* (2nd ed.). St. Louis: Mosby.

Kane, B., & Sands, D. (1998). Guidelines for the clinical use of electronic mail with patients. *Journal of the American Medical Informatics Association, 5*(1), 104-111.

Kleinbeck, S. V. (2000). Dimensions of perioperative nursing for a national specialty nomenclature. *Journal of Advanced Nursing, 31*(3), 529-535.

Lawrence, S., & Giles, C. L. (1998). Searching the World Wide Web. *Science, 280*, 98-100.

McAlindon, M., Danz, S., & Theodoroff, R. C. (1987). Choosing the hospital information system: A nursing perspective. *Journal of Nursing Administration, 17*(19), 11-15.

McCloskey, J. C., & Bulechek, G. M. (Eds.). (2000). *Nursing intervention classification* (3rd ed.). St. Louis: Mosby.

Martin, K. S., & Scheet, N. J. (1992). *The Omaha system: Applications for community health nursing*. Philadelphia: WB Saunders.

North American Nursing Diagnosis Association. (1999). *Nursing diagnoses: Definitions and classification, 1999-2000*. Philadelphia: Author.

Nicoll, L. H. (2001). *Nurses' guide to the Internet* (3rd ed.). Philadelphia: Lippincott.

Ozbolt, J. B., Fruchtnight, J. N., & Hayden, J. R. (1994). Toward data standards for clinical nursing information. *Journal of the American Medical Informatics Association, 1*(2), 175-185.

Rosswurm, M. A., & Larrabee, J. H. (1999). A model for change to evidence based practice. *Image: Journal of Nursing Scholarship, 31*(4), 317-322.

Saba, V. K. (1990). Home health care classification (HHCC system) [online]. Retrieved May 31, 2001, from http://www.sabacare.com.

Sackett, D. I., Rosenberg, W. M., Gray, J. A., Haynes, R. B., & Richardson, W. S. (1996). Evidence based medicine: What it is and what it isn't. *British Medical Journal, 312*(7023), 71-72.

Snyder-Halpern, R., Corcoran-Perry, S., & Narayan, S. (2001). Developing clinical practice environments supporting the knowledge work of nurses. *Computers in Nursing, 19*(1), 17-23.

Spackman, K. A., Campbell, K. E., & Cote, R. A. (1997). SNOMED: A reference terminology for health care. In D. Masys (Ed.), *Proceedings of the American Medical Informatics Association Annual Symposium* (pp. 640-644). Philadelphia: Hanley & Belfus.

Staggers, N., Gassert, C., & Curran, C. R. (2001). Informatics competencies for nurses at four levels of practice. *Journal of Nursing Education, 40*(7), 303-316.

Tan, J. (1995). *Health management information systems: Theories, methods, applications*. Gaithersburg, MD: Aspen.

Werley, H. H., & Lang, N. M. (Eds.). (1988). *Identification of the nursing minimum data set*. New York: Springer.

SUGGESTED READINGS

American Nurses Association. (1999). *Core principles on telehealth*. Washington, DC: Author.

Averill, C. B., Marek, K. D., Zielstorff, R., Kneedler, J., Delaney, C., & Milholland, D. K. (1998). ANA standards for nursing data sets in information systems. *Computers in Nursing, 16*(3), 157-161.

Ball, M., Hannah, K., Newbold, S., & Douglas, J. (Eds.). (1995). *Where caring and technology meet*. New York: Springer-Verlag.

Gabrieli, E. R. (1997). Longitudinal electronic patient records: A challenge of our time. *Computers in Nursing, 15*(2), S48-S52.

Henry, S. B., Warren, J. J., Lange, L., & Button, P. (1998). A review of the major vocabularies and the extent to which they have the characteristics required for implementation in computer-based systems. *Journal of the American Medical Informatics Association, 5*(4), 321-328.

McCormick, K. A., & Jones, C. B. (1998). Is one taxonomy needed for health care vocabularies and classifications? *Online Journal of Issues in Nursing*. Retrieved May 21, 2001, from http://www.nursingworld.org/ojin/tpc7/tpc7_2.htm.

Saba, V. K., & McCormick, K. A. (2001). *Essentials of computers for nurses: Informatics for the new millennium* (3rd ed.). New York: McGraw-Hill.

Staggers, N., Thompson, C. B., & Synder-Halpern, R. (2001). History and trends in clinical information systems in the United States. *Journal of Nursing Scholarship, 33*(1), 75-81.

Stetler, C. B., Brunell, M., Giuliano, K. K., Morsi, D., Prince, L., & Newell-Stokes, V. (1998). Evidence-based practice and the role of nursing leadership. *Journal of Nursing Administration, 28*(7/8), 45-53.

Tallon, R. (1996). Oximetry: State of the art. *Nursing Management, 27*(11), 43-44.

Tallon, R. (1996). Infusion pumps. *Nursing Management, 27*(12), 44-46.

Vahey, D. C., Corser, W. D., & Brennan, P. F. (2001). Publicly available healthcare databases for administrative strategic planning. *Journal of Nursing Administration, 31*(1), 9-15.

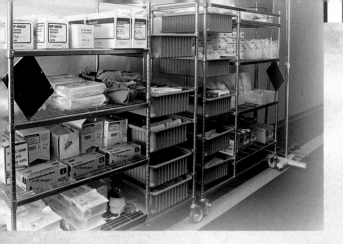

13

Managing Costs and Budgets

Donna Westmoreland

T his chapter focuses on methods of financing healthcare and specific strategies for managing costs and budgets in patient care settings. Factors that escalate healthcare costs, sources of healthcare financing, reimbursement methods, cost-containment and healthcare reform strategies, and implications for nursing practice are discussed. Various budgets and the budgeting process are explained. In addition to clinical competency and caring practices, understanding the cost issues in healthcare delivery and the ethical implications of financial decisions are essential for nurses to contribute fully to the health and healing of patients and populations.

Objectives

- Explain several major factors that are escalating the costs of healthcare.
- Compare and contrast different reimbursement methods and their incentives to control costs.
- Differentiate costs, charges, and revenue in relation to a specified unit of service, such as a visit, hospital stay, or procedure.
- Demonstrate why all healthcare organizations must make a profit.
- Give examples of cost considerations for nurses working in managed care environments.

- Discuss the purpose of and relationship among the operating, cash, and capital budgets.

- Explain the budgeting process.
- Identify variances on monthly expense reports.

Questions to Consider

- *How can you stay abreast of changes in the healthcare system and what they mean for the practice of nursing?*
- *What are the typical nursing care activities and supplies charges?*
- *Who are the major payers to your organizations? What is their method of payment or reimbursement?*
- *Does the organization recoup all of the charges? If not, what portion of the charges do they get for various patient groups?*
- *How is nursing reimbursed in your organization?*
- *How can you increase your cost-effectiveness as a nurse?*
- *Do the nursing practices in your organization add value for patients?*

The Challenge

Robin Stoupa, RN, MSN
Director of Ambulatory Services, University of Nebraska Medical Center, Omaha, Nebraska

The Internal Medicine Clinic (IMC) consists of one primary care section and eight specialty sections. The IMC is one of many clinics owned and managed by a physician group. Professional fees are the sole source of revenue for the IMC and are pooled into one fund. Professional fees are received for physician services provided in the hospital, in special procedure laboratories, and in the ambulatory clinic.

For the past 3 years, the IMC has experienced a 15% to 18% increase in ambulatory visit volume. At the same time, IMC revenues have declined. However, administrators want to stay budget neutral. As payers decrease payment in all areas, it is easy for administrators to assume that the areas of greatest activity are the areas losing money. The next logical step then is to require that vari-able expenses in that area be reduced. Because nursing personnel are the greatest variable expense in the clinic, such thinking often leads to demands to reduce nursing staff or to substitute lower-paid personnel. As nurse manager of the IMC, my goal is to maintain a high-quality, high-performance work team that adds value for patients. In this situation, what steps can be taken before reducing staff in the IMC ambulatory clinic? How can I justify that the amount spent currently for staff keeps the clinic functioning in the black?

 What do you think you would do if you were this nurse?

INTRODUCTION

Healthcare costs in the United States continue to rise at a rate greater than general inflation. In 1999 Americans spent $1.2 trillion for healthcare, approximately 13% of the gross domestic product (GDP) (Heffler, Levit, Smith, Smith, Cowan, Lazenby, & Freeman, 2001). This equals $4368 per person and surpasses the per capita expenditures of other Western nations by almost 50%. Yet millions of uninsured and underinsured Americans do not have access to basic healthcare services. With the exception of South Africa, the United States is the only industrialized nation where healthcare is a privilege rather than a right.

Despite our huge expenditures, major indicators reveal significant health problems in the United States, as well as large disparities in health status related to gender, race, and socioeconomic status (*Healthy People 2010*). Our infant mortality rate is among the highest of all industrialized nations, and black infants die at more than twice the rate of white infants. Average life expectancy is lower than in most developed countries, and men have a life expectancy that is 6 years less than that of women. One in eight women will develop breast cancer during their lifetime, with black and American Indian women experiencing a much higher death rate than white women.

Violence-related injuries are on the rise, and unintentional injuries, such as motor vehicle accidents, are a leading cause of death. Clearly, we are not getting a high value return for our healthcare dollar.

The large portion of the GDP that is spent on healthcare poses problems to the economy in other ways, too. Funds are diverted from needed social programs such as child care, housing, education, transportation, and the environment. The **price** of goods and services is increased, so the country's ability to compete in the international marketplace is compromised. One illustration is that up to 10% of the cost of a new American car is allocated to pay for the healthcare costs of automobile workers.

WHAT ESCALATES HEALTHCARE COSTS?

Total healthcare **costs** are a function of the prices and the **utilization** rates of healthcare services (Costs = Price × Utilization) (Table 13-1). *Price* is the rate that healthcare **providers** set for the services they deliver, such as the hospital rate or physician fee. *Utilization* refers to the quantity or volume of services provided, such as diagnostic tests provided or number of patient visits.

Table 13-1 RELATIONSHIP OF PRICE AND UTILIZATION RATES TO TOTAL HEALTHCARE COSTS

Price	×	Utilization Rate	=	Total Cost	% Change
$1.00		100		$100.00	0
$1.08*		100		$108.00	+8.0%
$1.08		105†		$113.40	+13.4%
$1.08		110‡		$118.80	+18.8%

*8% increase for inflation.
†5% more procedures done.
‡10% more procedures done.

Price inflation and administrative inefficiency are leading contributors to increasing prices for health services. In recent decades, rises in healthcare prices have significantly outpaced general inflation. Examples of factors that stimulate price inflation are physician incomes that rise faster than average worker earnings and the high prices of prescription drugs, which are often 50% higher than prices in other nations (Bodenheimer & Grumbach, 1998). Administrative inefficiency or waste is primarily a result of the large numbers of clerical personnel that organizations use to process reimbursement forms from multiple **payers.** U.S. hospitals spend an average of 20% of their **budgets** on billing administration alone.

Several interrelated factors contribute to increased utilization of medical services. These include unnecessary care, consumer attitudes, healthcare financing, pharmaceutical usage, and changing population demographics and disease patterns. Numerous studies show substantial amounts of unnecessary care that do not add health benefits for patients (Bodenheimer & Grumbach, 1998). Inappropriate or ineffective medical procedures are also prevalent and have led to national initiatives to demonstrate efficacy of interventions and to decrease variations in physician practice.

Our attitudes and behaviors as consumers of healthcare also contribute to rising costs. In general, we prefer to "be fixed" when something goes wrong rather than to practice prevention. When we need "fixing," expensive high-tech services typically are perceived as the best care. Many of us still believe that the physician knows best, so we do not seek much information related to costs and effectiveness of different healthcare options. When we do seek information, it is not readily available or understandable. Also, we are not accustomed to using other, less costly, healthcare providers, such as nurse practitioners.

The way healthcare is financed contributes to rising costs. When healthcare is reimbursed by third-party payers, consumers are somewhat insulated from personally experiencing the direct effects of high healthcare costs. For example, the huge rise in consumer demand for prescription drugs since 1995 was fueled by low copayments for drugs required by most insurance companies (Heffler et al., 2001). As consumer out-of-pocket expenses for drugs increase, consumer demand should decrease. In most instances, however, consumers do not have many incentives to consider costs when choosing among providers or using services. In addition, the various methods of reimbursement have implications for how providers price and use services.

Changing population demographics also are increasing the volume of health services needed. For example, chronic health problems increase with age, and the number of elderly Americans is rising. The fastest growing population is the group aged 85 or older, and Baby Boomers are beginning to move into their senior years. Infectious diseases such as acquired immunodeficiency syndrome (AIDS) and tuberculosis, as well as the growing societal problems of homelessness, drug addiction, and violence, increase demands for health services.

HOW IS HEALTHCARE FINANCED?

Healthcare is paid for by four sources: government (45%), private insurance companies (33%), individuals (16%), and other, primarily philanthropy (6%)

(Figure 13-1). Three fourths of the government funding is at the federal level. Federal programs include Medicare and health services for members of the military, veterans, Native Americans, and federal prisoners. Medicare, the largest federal program, was established in 1965 and pays for care provided to people 65 years and older and some disabled individuals. Medicare Part A is an insurance plan for hospital, hospice, home health, and skilled nursing care that is paid for through Social Security taxes. Nursing home care that is mainly custodial is not covered. Medicare Part B is an optional insurance that covers physician services, medical equipment, and diagnostic tests. Part B is funded through federal taxes and monthly premiums paid by the recipients. Medicare does not cover outpatient medications, eye or hearing examinations, or dental services.

Medicaid, a state-level program financed by federal and state funds, pays for services provided to persons who are medically indigent, blind, or disabled and to children with disabilities. The federal government pays between 50% and 83% of total Medicaid costs based on the per capita income of the state. Services funded by Medicaid vary from state to state but must include services provided by hospitals, physicians, laboratories, radiology departments; prenatal and preventive care; and nursing home and home healthcare services.

Private insurance is the second major source of financing for the healthcare system. Most Americans have private health insurance, which usually is provided by employers through group policies. Individuals can purchase health insurance, but typically the rates are very high and provide minimal coverage. Health insurance that is so intertwined with employment is problematic and contributes to the number of uninsured and underinsured Americans. Many of the uninsured work in small businesses that cannot afford to provide group insurance, or they have part-time, seasonal, or service positions.

Individuals also pay directly for health services when they do not have health insurance or when insurance does not cover the service. Costs paid by individuals are called out-of-pocket expenses and include deductibles, copays, and coinsurance. Health insurance benefits often do not cover preventive care or things such as eyeglasses, nonprescription medications, cosmetic surgeries, or alternative healthcare therapies.

REIMBURSEMENT METHODS

Four major payment methods are used for reimbursing healthcare providers: **charges, cost-based reimbursement,** flat-rate reimbursement, and capitated payments (Neuman, Suver, & Zelman, 1988). These methods are summarized in Box 13-1. Health-service researchers do not agree on the exact effects of these reimbursement methods on cost and quality. However, considering these effects is important because changes in payment systems have implications for how care is provided in healthcare organizations.

Charges consist of the cost of providing a service plus a markup for **profit.** Third-party payers often put limitations on what they will pay by establishing usual and customary charges by surveying all providers in a certain area. Usual and customary charges rise over time as providers continually increase their prices. In cost-based reimbursement, all allowable costs are calculated and used as the basis for payment. Each payer (government or insurance company) determines what the allowable costs are for each procedure, visit, or service. Charges and cost-based reimbursement are retrospective payment methods because the amount

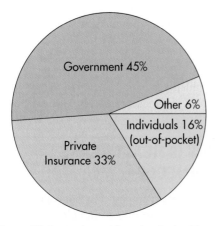

Figure 13-1   Sources of financing for healthcare.

BOX 13-1

Major Reimbursement Methods

- Charges
- Cost based (retrospective)
- Flat rate (prospective)
- Capitated

of payment is determined after services are delivered. When the reimbursed costs are less than the full charge for the service, a **contractual allowance** or discount exists. Charges and cost-based reimbursement were the predominant payment method in the 1960s and 1970s but have been largely supplanted by payer fee schedules determined before service delivery.

Flat-rate reimbursement is a method in which the third-party payer decides in advance what will be paid for a service or episode of care. This is a **prospective reimbursement** method. If the costs of care are greater than the payment, the provider absorbs the loss. If the costs are less than the payment, the provider makes a profit. In 1983 Medicare implemented a prospective payment system (PPS) for hospital care that uses diagnosis-related groups (DRGs) as the basis for payment.

■ *Exercise 13–1*

What is the contractual allowance when a hospital charges $800 per day to care for a ventilator-dependent patient and an insurance company reimburses the hospital $685 per day? What is the impact on hospital income (**revenue**) if this is the reimbursement for 2500 patient days?

DRGs, a classification system that groups patients into categories based on the average number of days of hospitalization for specific medical diagnoses, considers factors such as the patient's age, complications, and other illnesses. Payment includes the expected costs for diagnostic tests, various therapies, surgery, and length of stay (LOS). The cost of nursing services is not explicitly calculated. With a few exceptions, DRGs do not adequately reflect the variability of patient intensity or acuity within the DRG. This is problematic for nursing because the amount of resources (nurses and supplies) used to care for patients is directly related to the patient acuity. Thus many nurses believe that DRGs are not a good predictor of nursing care requirements. Recently, Medicare also began reimbursing home health agencies, nursing homes, and ambulatory care providers through a PPS.

In addition to Medicare, some state Medicaid programs and private insurance companies use a DRG payment system. Although DRGs are not currently used for specialty hospitals (pediatric, psychiatric, and oncology), they are a dominant force in hospital payment. Implementation of a PPS with DRGs resulted in increased patient acuity and de-

creased LOS in hospitals, along with a greater demand for home care. The need for hospital and community-based nurses also increased.

The resource-based relative value scale (RBRVS) is a flat-rate reimbursement method the federal government uses to pay physicians. Fees in this system are set by estimating the time, cognitive and technical skills, and physical effort required to provide the specific service. Another common flat-rate method is the discounted payments payers negotiate with providers in preferred provider organizations (PPOs).

Capitated payments are based on the provision of specified services to an individual over a set period such as 1 year. Providers are paid a per-person-per-year (or per-month) fee. If the services cost more than the payment, the provider absorbs the loss. Likewise, if the services cost less than the payment, the provider makes a profit. **Capitation** is the mode of payment characteristic of health maintenance organizations (HMOs) and other **managed care** systems.

■ *Exercise 13–2*

Medicare reimburses a hospice $70 for home visits. For one particular group of patients, it costs the hospice an average of $98 per day to provide care. What are the implications for the hospice? What options should the hospice nurse manager and nurses consider?

THE CHANGING HEALTHCARE ECONOMIC ENVIRONMENT

Healthcare is a major public concern, and rapid changes are occurring in an attempt to reduce costs and improve the health and wellness of the nation. As shown in Box 13-2, strategies shaping the evolving healthcare delivery system include managed care; **organized delivery systems (ODSs)**; and competition based on price, patient outcomes, and

BOX 13-2

Healthcare Delivery Reform Strategies

- Managed care
- Organized delivery systems
- Competition based on price, patient outcomes, and service quality

service quality. These strategies affect both the pricing and use of health services.

For each reimbursement method, think about the incentives for healthcare providers (individuals and organizations) regarding their practice patterns. Are there incentives to change the quantity of services used per patient or the number or types of patients served? Are there incentives to be efficient? List the incentives. How might each method affect overall healthcare costs? (Think in terms of effect on utilization and price.) What do you think the effect on quality of care might be with each payment method?

Managed care is a health plan that brings together the delivery and financing function into one entity, in contrast with a traditional fee-for-service plan, in which insurers pay providers based on costs (Chang, Price, & Pfoutz, 2001). A major goal of managed care is to decrease unnecessary services, thereby decreasing costs. Managed care also works to ensure timely and appropriate care. HMOs are a type of managed care system in which the primary physician serves as a gatekeeper who determines what services the patient uses. Because HMOs are paid on a capitated basis, it is to their advantage to practice prevention and use ambulatory care rather than more expensive hospital care. In other forms of managed care, a nonphysician case manager arranges and authorizes the services provided. Many insurance companies have used case managers for years. Nurses who work in home health and ambulatory settings often communicate with insurance company case managers to plan the care for specific patients. PPOs and point-of-service (POS) plans are other types of managed care plans that give the patient more options than traditional HMOs for selecting providers and services.

ODSs are composed of networks of healthcare organizations, providers, and payers. Typically, this means hospitals, physicians, and insurance companies. The aim of such joint ventures is to develop and market collectively a comprehensive package of healthcare services that will meet most needs of large numbers of consumers. Hospitals, physicians, and payers will share the financial risks of the enterprise. Although hospitals share some risk now with prospective payment, physicians have not generally shared the risk. This risk sharing is expected to provide incentives to eliminate unnecessary services, use resources more effectively, and improve quality of services.

Competition among healthcare providers increasingly is based on cost and quality outcomes. Decision making regarding price and utilization of services is shifting from physicians and hospitals to payers, who are demanding significant discounts or lower prices. Scientific data that demonstrate positive health outcomes and high-quality services are required. Providers who are unable to compete on the basis of price, patient outcomes, and service quality will find it difficult to survive as the system evolves.

WHAT DOES THIS MEAN FOR NURSING PRACTICE?

What does the healthcare economic environment mean for the practicing professional nurse? We must value ourselves as providers and think of our practice within a context of organizational viability and quality of care. To do this we must add "financial thinking" to our repertoire of nursing skills, and we must determine whether the services we provide add value for patients. Services that add value are of high quality, affect health outcomes positively, and minimize costs. The following sections help develop financial thinking skills and ways to consider how nursing practice adds value for patients by minimizing costs.

WHY IS PROFIT NECESSARY?

Private, nongovernmental healthcare organizations may be either for-profit (FP) or not-for-profit

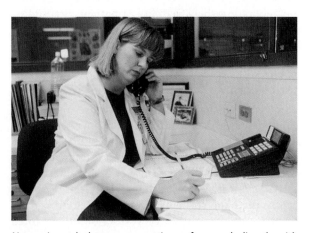

Nurses in ambulatory care settings often work directly with insurance companies to plan patient care.

(NFP). This designation refers to the tax status of the organization and designates how the profit can be used. Profit is the excess income left after all expenses have been paid (Revenues − Expenses = Profit). FP organizations pay taxes, and their profits can be distributed to investors and managers. NFP organizations, on the other hand, do not pay taxes and must reinvest all profits in the organization to better serve the public.

All private healthcare organizations must make a profit to survive. If expenses are greater than revenues, the organization experiences a loss. If revenues equal expenses, the organization breaks even. In both cases, nothing is left over to replace facilities and equipment, expand services, or pay for inflation costs. Some healthcare organizations are able to survive in the short run without making a profit because they use interest from investments to supplement revenues. The long-term viability of any private healthcare organization, however, is dependent on consistently making a profit. Box 13-3 presents an example of an income statement from a neighborhood nursing center.

Nurses and nurse managers directly affect an organization's ability to make a profit. Profits can be achieved or improved by decreasing costs or increasing revenues. In tight economic times, many managers think only in terms of cutting costs.

Although cost-cutting measures are important, especially to keep prices down so that the organization will be competitive, ways to increase revenues also need to be explored.

■ *Exercise 13–4*

Obtain a copy of an itemized patient bill from a healthcare organization and review the charges. What was the source and method of payment? How much of these charges was reimbursed? How much was charged for items you regularly use in clinical care?

▍COST-CONSCIOUS NURSING PRACTICES

Understanding What Is Required to Remain Financially Sound

Understanding what is required for a department or agency to remain financially sound requires that nurses move beyond thinking about costs for individual patients to thinking about income and expenses and numbers of patients needed to make a profit. In a fee-for-service environment, revenue is earned for every service provided. Therefore increasing the volume of services, such as diagnostic tests and patient visits, increases revenues. In a

BOX 13-3

An Income Statement
Neighborhood Nursing Center Statement of Revenues and Expenses
FYE December 31, 2002

Revenues		
Patient revenues	$115,700	
Grant income	60,000	
Other operating revenues	5,300	
TOTAL	$181,000	$181,000
Expenses		
Salary costs	$130,500	
Supplies	14,400	
Other operating expenses (rent, utilities, administrative services, etc.)	29,900	
TOTAL	$174,800	174,800
Excess of revenues over expenses [profit]*		$6,200

FYE, Fiscal year ending.
*Loss would be shown in parentheses ( ) or brackets < >.

capitated environment where one fee is paid for all services provided, increasing the overall number of patients served and decreasing the volume of services used is desirable. With capitation, nurses must strive to accomplish more with each visit to decrease return visits and complications. Many healthcare organizations function in a dual-reimbursement environment, part capitated and part fee-for-service. Nurses need to understand their organization's reimbursement environment and strategy for realizing a profit in its specific circumstances.

Knowing Costs and Reimbursement Practices

As direct caregivers and case managers, nurses are constantly involved in determining the type and quantity of resources used for patients. This includes supplies, personnel, and time. Nurses need to know what costs are generated by their decisions and actions. Nurses also need to know what things cost and how they are paid for in an organization so that they can make cost-effective decisions. For example, nurses need to know per-item costs for supplies so that they can appropriately evaluate lower-cost substitutes.

In ambulatory and home health settings, nurses must be familiar with the various insurance plans that reimburse the organization. Each plan has different contract rules regarding preauthorization, types of services covered, required vendors, and so on. Although nurses must develop and implement their plans of care with full knowledge of these reimbursement practices, the payer does not totally drive the care. Nurses still advocate for patients in important ways while also working within the cost and contractual constraints. Moreover, when nurses understand the reimbursement practices, they can help patients maximize the resources available to them.

In hospitals, the cost of nursing care usually is not calculated or billed separately to patients but is part of the general per-diem charge. One major problem with this method is the assumption that all patients consume the same amount of nursing care. Another problem with bundling the charges for nursing care with the room rate is that nursing as a clinical service is not perceived by management as generating revenue for the hospital. Rather, nursing is perceived predominantly as an expense to the organization. Although this perception may not matter in a capitated setting where all provider services are considered a cost, accurate nursing care cost data are needed to negotiate managed care contracts.

■ *Exercise 13–5*

How was nursing care charged on the bill you obtained? What are the implications for nursing in being perceived as an expense rather than being associated with the revenue stream? Why will this perception be less important in a capitated environment?

Capturing All Charges in a Timely Fashion

Nurses also help contain costs by making sure that all possible charges are captured. Several large hospitals report more than $1 million a year lost from supplies that were not charged. In hospitals, nurses must know which supplies are charged to patients and which ones are charged to the unit. In addition, the procedures and equipment used need to be accurately documented. In ambulatory and community settings, nurses often need to keep abreast of the codes that are used to bill services. These codes change yearly, and sometimes items are bundled together under one charge and sometimes they are broken down into different charges. Turning in charges in a timely manner is also important because delayed billing negatively affects cash flow by extending the time before an organization is paid for services provided. This is particularly considerable in smaller organizations.

In home health, hospice, and long-term care organizations, billing is closely integrated with the clinical information system. For example, to ensure reimbursement, the physician's plan of care and documentation that the patient meets the criteria for admission must be on the clinical record. Typically, nurses are responsible for documenting this information.

■ *Exercise 13–6*

You used three intravenous (IV) catheters to do a particularly difficult venipuncture. Do you charge the patient for all three catheters? What if you accidentally contaminated one by touching the sheet? How is the catheter paid for if not charged to the patient? Who benefits and who loses when patients are not charged for supplies?

Using Time Efficiently

The adage that time is money is fitting in healthcare and refers to both the nurse's time and the patient's time. When nurses are organized and efficient in their care delivery and in scheduling and coordinating patients' care, the organization will save money. With capitation, doing as much as possible during each episode of care is particularly important to decrease repeat visits and unnecessary service utilization. Because LOS is the most important predictor of hospital costs (Finkler & Kovner, 2000), patients who stay extra days cost the hospital a considerable amount. Decreasing LOS also makes room for other patients, thereby potentially increasing patient volume and hospital revenues. Nurses can become more efficient and effective by evaluating their major work processes and eliminating areas of redundancy and rework. Automated clinical information systems that support integrated practice at the point of care will also increase efficiency and improve patient outcomes.

■ *Exercise 13–7*

The Visiting Nurse Association (VNA) cannot file for reimbursement until all documentation of each visit has been completed. Typically, the paperwork is submitted a week after the visit. When the number of home visits increases rapidly, the paperwork often is not turned in for 2 weeks or more. What are the implications of this routine practice for the agency? Why would the VNA be very vulnerable financially during periods of heavy workload? What are some options for the nurse manager to consider to expedite the paperwork?

Discussing the Cost of Care With Patients

Talking with patients about the cost of care is important, although it may be uncomfortable. Discovering during a clinic visit that a patient cannot afford a specific medication or intervention is preferable to finding out several days later in a follow-up call that the patient has not taken the medication. Such information compels the clinical management team to explore optional treatment plans or to find resources to cover the costs. Talking with patients about costs is important in other ways, too. It involves the patients in the decision-making process and increases the likelihood that treatment plans will be followed. Patients also can make informed choices and better use the resources available to them if they have appropriate information about costs.

■ *Exercise 13–8*

A new patient visits the clinic and is given prescriptions for three medications that will cost about $120 per month. You check her chart and discover that she has Medicare and no supplemental insurance. How can you determine whether or not she has the resources to buy this medicine each month and if she is willing to buy it? If she cannot afford the medications, what are some options?

Meeting Patient Rather Than Provider Needs

Developing an awareness of how feelings about patients' needs influence decisions can help nurses better manage costs. A nurse administrator in a home health agency recently related the story of a nurse who continued to visit a patient for weeks after the patient's health problems had resolved. When questioned, the nurse said she was uncomfortable terminating the visits because the patient continued to tell her he needed her help. Later the patient revealed that he had not needed nursing care for some time, although he had continued telling the nurse he did because he thought she wanted to keep visiting him. This story illustrates how nurses need to verify whose needs are being met with nursing care.

Evaluating Cost-Effectiveness of New Technologies

The advent of new technologies is presenting dilemmas in managing costs. In the past, if a new piece of equipment was easier to use or benefited the patient in any way, nurses were apt to want to use it for everyone, no matter how much more it cost. Now they are forced to make decisions regarding which patients really need the new equipment and which ones will have good outcomes with the current equipment. Essentially, nurses are analyzing the cost-effectiveness of the new equipment with regard to different types of patients to allocate limited resources. This is a new and sometimes difficult way to think about patient care and at times may not feel like a caring way to make decisions regarding patient care. However, such decisions conserve resources without jeopardizing patients' health and thus create the possibility of providing additional healthcare services.

■ *Exercise 13–9*

Last year a new positive-pressure, needleless system for administering IV antibiotics was introduced. Because it was so easy and convenient for patients, the nurses in the home infusion company where you worked ordered them for everyone. Typically, patients get their IV antibiotics four times each day. The minibags and tubing for the regular procedure cost the agency $22 a day. The new system costs

$24 per medication administration, or $96 a day. The agency receives the same per-diem (daily) reimbursement for each patient. Discuss the financial implications for the agency if this practice is continued. Generate some optional courses of action for the nurses to consider. How should these options be evaluated? What secondary costs, such as the cost of treating fewer needlestick injuries, should be included?

Predicting and Using Nursing Resources Efficiently

Because healthcare organizations are service institutions, the largest part of their **operating budget** typically is for personnel. For hospitals in particular, nurses are the largest group of employees and often account for the majority of the personnel budget. Staffing is the major area nurse managers can affect with respect to managing costs, and supplies are the second area. To understand why this is so, it is helpful to understand the concepts of **fixed** and **variable costs.**

The total fixed costs in a unit are those costs that do not change as the volume of patients changes. In other words, with either a high or low patient census, expenses related to rent, loan payments, administrative salaries, and salaries of the minimum amount of staff to keep a unit open must be paid. Variable costs are costs that vary in direct proportion to patient volume or acuity. Examples include nursing personnel, supplies, and medications. Break-even analysis is a tool that uses fixed and variable costs for determining the volume of patients needed to just break even (revenue = expenses) or to realize a profit or loss.

In hospitals and community health agencies, patient classification systems are used to help managers predict nursing care requirements (see Chapter 16). These systems differentiate patients according to acuity of illness, functional status, and resource needs. Some nurses do not like these systems because they believe the essence of nursing is not captured. However, we need to remember that these are tools to help managers predict resource needs. Describing all nursing activities and judgments is not necessary for a tool to be a good predictor. Misguided efforts to sabotage classification systems with the hope for better staffing work primarily to prevent the development of tools to better manage practice. Used appropriately, patient classification systems can help evaluate changing practice patterns and patient acuity levels as well as provide information for **budgeting processes.**

Exercise 13-10

Given the definitions for fixed and variable costs, why do you think nurse managers have the greatest influence over costs through management of staffing and supplies?

Managing staffing and decreasing LOS can achieve the most immediate reductions in costs. Hospitals strive to lower costs so that they will attract new contracts and be attractive as partners in provider networks. Thus staffing methods and patient care delivery models are being closely scrutinized. Work redesign, a process for changing the way to think about and structure the work of patient care, is the predominant strategy for developing systems that better utilize high-cost professionals and improve service quality. Increased staff retention, patient safety, and positive patient outcomes result from effective work redesign processes.

Using Research to Evaluate Standard Nursing Practices

Another way nurses are restructuring their work to make sure they add value for patients is through research. For example, in the internal medicine clinics at the University of Nebraska Medical Center, nurses and physicians developed a rule to predict which patients are at risk for orthostatic hypotension. This is significant because the mortality rates are high in patients who have orthostatic hypotension. Yet performing the sitting and standing blood pressure readings on all patients is costly in terms of nursing resources. Full implementation of the rule, which was developed and validated through research, results in nurses taking orthostatic blood pressure readings on less than 25% of the clinic's patients. This chapter's Research Perspective illustrates cost savings from another practice alteration. Box 13-4 summarizes some cost-conscious strategies for nursing practice.

BUDGETS

The basic financial document in most healthcare organizations is the budget, a detailed financial plan for carrying out the activities an organization wants to accomplish for a certain period. An organizational budget is a formal plan that is stated in terms of dollars and includes proposed income and expenditures. The budgeting process is an ongoing activity in which plans are made and revenues and ex-

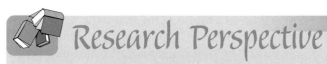
Research Perspective

Petryshen, P., Stevens, B., Hawkins, J., & Stewart, M. (1997). Comparing nursing costs for pre-term infants receiving conventional vs. developmental care. *Nursing Economics, 15*(3), 138-145, 150.

The purpose of this study was to compare the nursing costs of two different approaches for treating very-low-birth-weight (VLBW) infants. One group received conventional care, which included primary nursing, standardized care plans, and routine noise and lighting levels on the patient care unit. The other group received developmental care, which is a more individualized approach to caregiving that includes coordinating clinical interventions to prevent frequent interruption during infant sleep and reducing the lighting and noise levels. In addition, developmental care includes positioning and bundling infants in ways that prevent disorganization and promote self-regulation. Sixty infants were in each group.

Infants who received developmental care had improved physiological stability measures and fewer days in the neonatal intensive care unit (NICU) than infants receiving conventional care. The infants who received developmental care were moved from the NICU to a transitional care unit earlier, and their nursing intensity needs were lower. The average cost savings for infants in the developmental group was $4340 per infant during the first 35 days of life (or less if they were discharged).

IMPLICATIONS FOR PRACTICE
The findings from this economic evaluation support the implementation of developmental care for VLBW infants by demonstrating improved patient outcomes and lower costs.

BOX 13-4

Strategies for Cost-Conscious Nursing Practice

1. Understanding what is required to remain financially sound
2. Knowing costs and reimbursement practices
3. Capturing all possible charges in a timely fashion
4. Using time efficiently
5. Discussing the costs of care with patients
6. Meeting patient, rather than provider, needs
7. Evaluating cost-effectiveness of new technologies
8. Predicting and using nursing resources efficiently
9. Using research to evaluate standard nursing practices

penses are managed to meet or exceed the goals of the plan. The management functions of planning and control are tied together through the budgeting process.

A budget requires managers to plan ahead and to establish explicit program goals and expectations. Changes in medical practices, reimbursement methods, competition, technology, demographics, and regulatory factors must be forecast to anticipate their effects on the organization. Planning encourages evaluation of different options and assists in more cost-effective use of resources.

Exercise 13–11
A community nursing organization performs an average of 36 intermittent catheterizations each day. A prepackaged catheterization kit that costs the organization $17 is used. The four items in the kit, when purchased individually, cost the organization a total of $5. What factors should be considered in evaluating the cost-effectiveness of the two sources of supplies?

TYPES OF BUDGETS

Several types of interrelated budgets are used by well-managed organizations. Major budgets that are discussed in this chapter include the operating budget, the capital budget, and the **cash budget**. The way these budgets complement and support one another is depicted in Figure 13-2. Many organizations also use program, product line, or special purpose

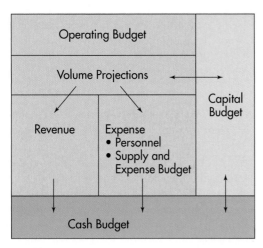

Figure 13-2   Interrelationships of the operating, capital, and cash budgets. (Modified from Ward, W. [1988]. *An introduction to health care financial management.* Ownings Mills, MD: National Health Publishing.)

budgets. Long-range budgets are used to help managers plan for the future. Often, these are referred to as *strategic plans* (Finkler & Kovner, 2000).

Operating Budget

The operating budget is the financial plan for the day-to-day activities of the organization. The expected revenues and expenses generated from daily operations, given a specified volume of patients, are stated. Preparing and monitoring the operating budget, particularly the expense portion, is often the most time-consuming financial function of nurse managers.

The expense part of the operating budget consists of a personnel budget and a supply and expense budget for each **cost center.** A cost center is an organizational unit for which costs can be identified and managed. The personnel budget is the largest part of the operating budget for most nursing units.

Before the personnel budget can be established, the volume of work predicted for the budget period must be calculated. A **unit of service** measure appropriate to the work of the unit is used. Units of service may be patient days, clinic or home visits, hours of service, admissions, deliveries, treatments, and so on. Another factor needed to calculate the workload is the patient acuity mix. The formula for calculating the workload or the required patient care hours for inpatient units is as follows: Workload volume = Hours of care per patient day × Number of patient days (Table 13-2).

In some organizations the workload is established by the financial office and given to the nurse manager. In other organizations nurse managers forecast the volume. In both situations nurse managers should inform administration about any factors that might affect the accuracy of the forecast, such as changes in physician practice patterns, new treatment modalities, or changes in inpatient versus outpatient treatment practices.

The next step in preparing the personnel budget is to determine how many staff members will be needed to provide the care. (This topic is discussed in more detail in Chapter 16.) Because some people work full-time and others work part-time, **full-time equivalents (FTEs)** are used in this step rather than positions. Generally, one FTE can be equated to working 40 hours per week, 52 weeks per year, for a total of 2080 hours of work paid per year. One half of an FTE (0.5 FTE) equates to 20 hours per week. The number of hours per FTE may vary within an organization in relation to staffing plans, so it is important to check.

The 2080 hours paid to an FTE in a year consist of both **productive** and **nonproductive hours.** Productive hours are paid time that is worked. Nonproductive hours are paid time that is not worked, such as vacation, holiday, orientation, education, and sick time. Before the number of FTEs needed for the workload can be calculated, the number of productive hours per FTE is determined by subtracting the total number of nonproductive hours per FTE from total paid hours. Alternatively, payroll reports can be reviewed to determine the percentage of paid hours that is productive for each FTE. Finally, the total number of FTEs needed to provide the care is calculated by dividing the total patient care hours required by the number of productive hours per FTE (Box 13-5).

The total number of FTEs calculated by this method represents the number needed to provide care each day of the year. It does not reflect the number of positions or the number of people working each day. In fact, the number of positions may be much higher, particularly if many part-time nurses are employed. On any given day, some nurses will be off, on vacation, or ill. Also, some positions that do not provide direct patient care, such as nurse managers or unit secretaries, may not be replaced during nonproductive time. Only one FTE is budgeted for any position that is not covered with other staff when the employee is off.

Table 13-2 WORKLOAD CALCULATION (TOTAL REQUIRED PATIENT CARE HOURS)

Patient Acuity Level*	Hours of Care Per Patient Day (HPPD)†	×	Patient Days‡	=	Workload§
1	3.0		900		2,700
2	5.2		3,100		16,120
3	8.8		4,000		35,200
4	13.0		1,600		20,800
5	19.0		400		7,600
TOTAL			10,000		82,420

*1, Low; 5, high.
†HPPD = number of hours of care on average for a given acuity level.
‡1 patient per 1 day = 1 patient day.
§Total number of hours of care needed based on acuity levels and numbers of patient days.

BOX 13-5

Productive Hours Calculation

Method 1:	Add all nonproductive hours/FTE and subtract from paid hours/FTE

Example:

Vacation	15 days
Holiday	7 days
Average sick time	4 days
TOTAL	26 days

26 × 8 hours = 208 nonproductive hours/FTE
2080 − 208 = 1872 productive hours/FTE

Method 2: Multiply paid hours/FTE by percentage of productive hours/FTE

Example: productive hours = 90%/FTE
(1872 productive hours of total 2080 = 90%)
2080 × 0.90 = 1872 productive hours/FTE

Total FTE Calculation

Required Patient Care Hours	÷	Productive Hours Per FTE	=	Total FTEs Needed
82,420	÷	1872	=	44 FTEs

■ *Exercise 13-12*

Change the number of patients at each acuity level listed in Table 13-2, but keep the total number of patients the same. Recalculate the required total workload. Discuss how changes in patient acuity affect nursing resource requirements.

The next step is to prepare a daily staffing plan and to establish positions (see Chapter 16). Once the positions are established, the labor costs that make up the personnel budget can be calculated. Factors that must be addressed include straight-time hours, overtime hours, differentials and premium pay, raises, and benefits (Finkler & Kovner, 2000). Differentials and premiums are extra pay for working specific times such as evening or night shifts and holidays. Benefits usually include health and life insurance, Social Security payments, and retirement plans. Benefits often cost an additional 20% to 25% of a full-time employee's salary.

Exercise 13-13

If the percentage of productive hours per FTE is 80%, how many worked or productive hours are there per FTE? If total patient care hours are 82,420, how many FTEs will be needed?

The supply and expense budget is often called the *other-than-personnel services* (OTPS) expense budget. This budget includes a variety of items used in daily unit activities such as medical and office supplies, minor equipment, books and journals, orientation and training, and travel. Although different methods are used to calculate the supply and expense budget, the prior year's expenses usually are used as a baseline. This baseline is adjusted for projected patient volume and specific circumstances known to affect expenses, such as predictable personnel turnover, which increases orientation and training expenses. A percentage factor is also added to adjust for inflation.

The final component of the operating budget is the revenue budget. The revenue budget projects the income the organization will receive for providing patient care. Historically, nurses have not been directly involved with developing the revenue budget, although this is beginning to change. In most hospitals the revenue budget is established by the financial office and given to nurse managers. The anticipated revenues are calculated according to the price per patient day. Data about the volume and types of patients and reimbursement sources, that is, the **case mix** and the **payer mix,** are necessary to project revenues in any healthcare organization. Even when nurse managers do not participate in developing the revenue budget, learning about the organization's revenue base is essential for good decision making.

Capital Expenditure Budget

The **capital expenditure budget** reflects expenses related to the purchase of major capital items such as equipment and physical plant. A capital expenditure must have a useful life of more than 1 year and must exceed a cost level specified by the organization. The minimum cost requirement for capital items in healthcare organizations is usually from $300 to $1000. Anything below that is considered a routine operating cost.

Capital expenses are kept separate from the operating budget because their high cost would make the costs of providing patient care appear too high during the year of purchase. To account for capital expenses, the costs of capital items are depreciated. This means that each year, over the useful life of the equipment, a portion of its cost is allocated to the operating budget as an expense. Therefore capital expenditures do get subtracted from revenues and in turn affect profits.

Organizations usually set aside a fixed amount of money for capital expenditures each year. Complete well-documented justifications are needed because the competition is stiff. Justifications should include projected amount of use; services duplicated or replaced; safety considerations; need for space, personnel, or building renovation; effect on operational revenues and expenses; and contribution to the strategic plan.

Cash Budget

The cash budget is the operating plan for monthly cash receipts and disbursements. Organizational survival depends on paying bills on time. Organizations can be making a profit and still run out of cash. In fact, a profitable trend, such as a rapidly growing census, can induce a cash shortage because of increased expenses in the short run. Major capital expenditures can also cause a temporary cash crisis. Because cash is the lifeblood of any organization, the cash budget is as important as the operating and capital budget (Finkler & Kovner, 2000).

The financial officer prepares the cash budget in large organizations. Understanding the cash budget helps nurse managers discern when constraints on spending are necessary even when the expenditures are budgeted and the importance of carefully predicting when budgeted items will be needed.

THE BUDGETING PROCESS

The steps in the budgeting process are similar in most healthcare organizations, although the budgeting period, budget timetable, and level of manager and employee participation vary. Budgeting is done annually and in relation to the organization's fiscal year. A fiscal year exists for financial purposes and can begin at any point on the calendar. In the title of some financial reports, a phrase similar to "FYE June 30, 2003," appears and means that this report is for the fiscal year ending on the date stated.

Major steps in the budgeting process include gathering information and planning, developing unit budgets, developing the cash budget, negotiating and revising, and using feedback to control budget results and improve future plans (Finkler &

Kovner, 2000). A timetable with specific dates for implementing the budgeting process is developed by each organization. The timetable may be anywhere from 3 to 9 months. The widespread use of computers for budgeting is reducing the time spread for budgeting in many organizations. Box 13-6 outlines the budgeting process.

The information-gathering and planning phase provides nurse managers with data essential for developing their individual budgets. This step begins with an environmental assessment that helps the organization understand its position in relation to the entire community. The assessment includes the changing healthcare needs of the population, influential economic factors such as inflation and unemployment, differences in reimbursement patterns, patient satisfaction, and so on.

Next, the organization's long-term goals and objectives are reassessed in light of the organization's mission and the environmental analysis. This helps all managers situate the budgeting process for their individual units in relation to the whole organization. At this point, programs are prioritized so that resources can be allocated to programs that best help the organization achieve its long-term goals.

Specific, measurable objectives are then established, and the budgets must meet these objectives. The financial objectives might include limiting ex-

penditure increases to 3% or making 4% reductions in personnel costs. Nurse managers also set operational objectives for their units that are in concert with the rest of the organization. This is where units or departments interpret what effect the changes in operational activities will have on them. For instance, how will using case managers and care maps for selected patients affect a particular unit? Establishing the unit-level objectives is also a good place for involving staff nurses in setting the future direction of the unit.

Along with the specific organization and unit-level operating objectives, managers need the organizationwide assumptions that underpin the budgeting process. Explicit assumptions regarding salary increases, inflation factors, and volume projections for the next fiscal year are essential. With this information in hand, nurse managers can develop the operating and capital budgets for their units. These are usually developed in tandem because each affects the other. For instance, purchasing a new monitoring system will have implications for the supplies used, staffing, and staff training.

The cash budget is developed after unit and department operating and capital budgets. Then the negotiation and revision process begins in earnest. This is a complex process because changes in one budget usually require changes in others. Learning to defend and negotiate budgets is an important skill for nurse managers. Nurse managers who successfully negotiate budgets know how costs are allocated and are comfortable speaking about what resources are contained in each budget category. They also can clearly and specifically depict what the effect of not having that resource will be on patient, nurse, or organizational outcomes.

BOX 13-6
Outline of Budgeting Process

1. Gathering information and planning
   - Environmental assessment
   - Mission, goals, and objectives
   - Program priorities
   - Financial objectives
   - Assumptions (employee raises, inflation, volume projections)
2. Developing unit and departmental budgets
   - Operating budgets
   - Capital budgets
3. Developing cash budgets
4. Negotiating and revising
5. Evaluating
   - Analysis of variance
   - Critical performance reports

Modified from Finkler, S., & Kovner, C. (2000). *Financial management for nurse managers and executives* (2nd ed.). Philadelphia: WB Saunders.

Exercise 13–14

If you can interview a nurse manager, ask to review the budgeting process. Ask specifically about the budget timetable, operating objectives, and organizational assumptions. What was the level of involvement for nurse managers and nurses in each step of budget preparation? Is there a budget manual?

The final and ongoing phase of the budgeting process relates to the control function of management. Feedback is obtained regularly so that organizational activities can be adjusted to maintain efficient operations. **Variance analysis** is the major control process used. A **variance** is the difference between the projected budget and the actual performance for a particular account. For expenses, a favorable, or positive, variance means that the budgeted amount was greater than the actual amount spent. An unfavorable, or negative, variance means that the budgeted amount was less than the actual amount spent. Positive and negative variances cannot be interpreted as good or bad without further investigation. For example, if fewer supplies were used than were budgeted, this would appear as a positive variance and the unit would save money. This would be good news if it means that supplies were used more efficiently and patient outcomes remained the same or improved. A problem might be suggested, however, if using fewer or cheaper supplies led to poorer patient outcomes. Or it might mean that exactly the right amount of supplies was used but that the patient census was less than budgeted. To help managers interpret and use variance information better, some institutions use flexible budgets that automatically account for census variances.

Exercise 13-15

Examine Table 13-3 and identify significant budget variances for the current month. Are they favorable or unfavorable? What additional information would help you explain the variances? What are some possible causes for each variance? Are the causes you identified controllable by the nurse manager? Why or why not? Is a favorable variance on expenses always desirable? Why or why not?

MANAGING THE UNIT-LEVEL BUDGET

How is a unit-based budget managed? At a minimum, nurse managers are responsible for meeting the fiscal goals related to the personnel and the supply and expense part of the operations budget. Typically, monthly reports of operations (see Table 13-3) are sent to nurse managers, who then investigate and explain the underlying cause of variances greater than 5%. Many factors can cause budget variances, including patient census, patient acuity, vacation and benefit time, illness, orientation, staff meetings, workshops, employee mix, salaries, and staffing levels. To accurately interpret budget variances, nurse managers need reliable data about patient census, acuity, and LOS; payroll reports; and unit **productivity** reports.

Nurse managers can control *some* of the factors that cause variances, but not all. After the causes are determined, and if they are controllable by the nurse manager, steps are taken to prevent the variance from occurring in the future. However, even uncontrollable variances that increase expenses might require actions of nurse managers. For example, if supply costs rise drastically because a new technology is being used, the nurse manager might have to look for other areas where the budget can be cut. Information learned from analyzing variances also is used in future budget preparations and management activities.

In addition, nurse managers monitor the productivity of their unit. Productivity is the ratio of outputs to inputs; that is, productivity = output/input. In nursing, outputs are nursing services and are measured by hours of care, number of home visits, and so forth. The inputs are the resources used to provide the services such as personnel hours and supplies. Only decreasing the inputs or increasing the outputs can increase productivity. Hospitals often use hours per patient day (HPPD) as one measure of productivity. For example, if the standard of care in a critical care unit is 12 HPPD, then 360 hours of care are required for 30 patients for 1 day. When 320 hours of care are provided, the productivity rating is 113% (360/320 = 1.13), meaning productivity was increased. In home health, the number of visits per day per registered nurse is one measure of productivity. If the standard is 5 visits per day but the weekly average was 4.8 visits per day, then productivity was decreased. Variances in productivity are not inherently favorable or unfavorable and thus require investigation and explanation before judgments can be made about them.

Although they do not have a direct accountability for the budget, staff nurses play an important role in meeting budget expectations. Many nurse managers find that routinely sharing the budget and budget-monitoring activities with the staff fosters an appreciation of the relationship between cost and the mission to deliver high-quality patient care. Providing staff with access to cost and utilization data allows them to identify patterns and participate in selecting appropriate, cost-effective practice options that work for the staff and patients. Managers and staff who work in partnership to understand that cost versus care is a dilemma to manage rather than a problem to solve will develop innovative, cost-conscious nursing practices that produce good outcomes for patients, nurses, and the organization (Johnson, 1996; Wesorick, Shiparski, Troseth, & Wyngarden, 1997).

Table 13-3 STATEMENT OF OPERATIONS
NEIGHBORHOOD NURSING CENTER PROFIT AND LOSS STATEMENT
MARCH 31, 2002

Current Month				Year-to-Date		
Budget	Actual	Variance	REVENUES	Budget	Actual	Variance
			Patient Revenues			
11,500	12,050	550	Insurance payment	34,500	35,750	1,250
1,500	1,550	50	Donations	4,500	4,750	250
13,000	13,600	600	Net Patient Revenues	39,000	40,500	1,500
			Nonpatient Revenues			
5,000	5,000	0	Grant income (#138-FG)	15,000	15,000	0
500	500	0	Rent income	1,500	1,500	0
5,500	5,500	0	Net Nonpatient Revenues	16,500	16,500	0
18,500	19,100	600	Net Revenues	55,500	57,000	1,500
			EXPENSES			
			Personnel			
7,750	8,500	(750)	Managerial/professional	23,250	24,400	(1,150)
2,000	1,800	200	Clerical/technical	6,000	5,800	200
9,750	10,300	(550)	Net salaries and wages	29,250	30,200	(950)
1,200	1,400	(200)	Benefits	3,600	4,000	(400)
10,950	11,700	(750)	Net Personnel	32,850	34,200	(1,350)
			Nonpersonnel			
2,500	2,500	0	Office operating expenses	7,500	7,500	0
1,000	1,100	(100)	Supplies and materials	3,000	3,050	(50)
300	450	(150)	Travel expenses	900	450	450
3,800	4,050	(250)	Net Nonpersonnel	11,400	11,000	400
14,750	15,750	(1,000)	Net Expenses	44,250	45,200	(850)
3,750	3,350	(400)	**REVENUES OVER/ UNDER EXPENSES**	11,250	11,800	550

The Solution

I began by investigating the assumption that the IMC ambulatory clinic was losing money. Because expenses were reported as a whole for the IMC, they had to be broken down by section and by location where services were provided. A spreadsheet was used, and expenses were determined either by the hours of utilization or by the percentage of visit volume for that section. Once the expenses were calculated, the revenue needed to break even was determined for each section.

Next, revenues were predicted. This was challenging because of the complexity of the payer mix. The Medicare Resource-Based Relative Value Scale (RBRVS) was used to calculate all predicted payments. In this system, each physician service is assigned a "relative value" based on the time, skill, and intensity it takes to provide the service. Relative values are then adjusted for geographic variations and multiplied by a national conversion factor to determine the dollar amount of payment. This system was selected because it was the minimum payment expected for all categories of payers, including managed care contracts. Thus using this system provided a conservative estimate of revenues. Once the payment for a specific service was calculated, it was multiplied by the number of times that service was provided in the ambulatory setting. The result was the potential revenue for that service in that section. The potential revenues for each service were added to provide a total predicted revenue for the section.

Predicted revenue for each section was compared with the revenue required to break even. In every instance the predicted revenue exceeded the break-even revenue. As a result of this work, the administrators changed their view of the IMC ambulatory service as a "loss leader" and staff reductions were not required. In addition, a performance strategy for physicians based on relative value units was developed, and some fees were increased because they were found to be lower than allowed by the RBRVS system.

— Robin Stoupa

 Would this be a suitable approach for you? Why?

CHAPTER CHECKLIST

Financial thinking skills are the cornerstone of cost-conscious nursing practice and are essential for all nurses. Nurses must also determine whether the services they provide add value for patients. Services that add value are of high quality, positively affect health outcomes, and minimize costs.

Understanding what constitutes profit and why organizations must make a profit to survive is basic to financial thinking. Knowing what is included in operating, capital, and cash budgets; how they interrelate; and how they are developed, monitored, and controlled is also important. Considering the ethical implications of financial decisions and collectively managing the cost-care dilemma is imperative for cost-conscious nursing practice.

- U.S. health indicators suggest that as a nation we are not getting a high value return on our healthcare dollar.
  - Infant mortality and breast cancer rates are two critical examples.
- Total healthcare costs are a function of price and utilization of services.
  - Administrative waste or inefficiency increases the price of healthcare services.
  - Our attitudes as consumers who want to be fixed, as well as healthcare insurance that buffers us from full healthcare costs, contribute to the high use of healthcare services.
- The government and insurance companies are the major payers for healthcare services. Individuals are the third major payer.
  - Payments may be based on cost reimbursement, flat rates, or capitated payments.
- Healthcare has moved toward managed care, organized delivery systems, and competition based on cost and quality outcomes.
- All private healthcare organizations must make a profit to survive.
- Nurse and nurse managers directly influence an organization's ability to make a profit.
- Cost-conscious nursing practices include the following:
  - Understanding what is required to remain financially sound

- Knowing costs and reimbursement practices
- Capturing all possible charges in a timely fashion
- Using time efficiently
- Discussing the costs of care with patients
- Meeting patient, rather than provider, needs
- Evaluating cost-effectiveness of new technologies
- Predicting and using nursing resources efficiently
- Using research to evaluate standard nursing practices
- Nurse managers have the most influence on costs in relation to managing personnel and supplies.
- Variance analysis is the major control process in relation to budgeting.

TIPS ON MANAGING COSTS AND BUDGETS

- Know the cost and charges (if applicable) of the 20 most frequently used supplies on your unit.
- Evaluate what each of your patients would find most helpful during the time you will be caring for them.
- Decide which of your actions create costs for the patient or the organization.
- Be aware of how changes in patient acuity and patient census affect staffing requirements and the unit budget.
- Know how charges are generated and how the documentation systems relate to billing.
- Consciously examine the upsides and downsides of the cost-care polarity.

TERMS TO KNOW

budget
budgeting process
capital expenditure budget
capitation
case mix
cash budget
charges
contractual allowance
cost
cost-based reimbursement
cost center
fixed costs
full-time equivalent (FTE)
managed care
nonproductive hours
operating budget
organized delivery systems (ODSs)
payer mix
payers
price
productive hours
productivity
profit
prospective reimbursement
providers
revenue
unit of service
utilization
variable costs
variance
variance analysis

REFERENCES

Bodenheimer, T., & Grumbach, K. (1998). *Understanding health policy: A clinical approach* (2nd ed.). Stamford, CT: Appleton & Lange.

Chang, C., Price, S., & Pfoutz, S. (2001). *Economics and nursing: Critical professional issues*. Philadelphia: F.A. Davis.

Finkler, S., & Kovner, C. (2000). *Financial management for nurse managers and executives* (2nd ed.). Philadelphia: WB Saunders.

Healthy People 2010. Retrieved December 12, 2001, from http://www.health.gov/HEALTHYPEOPLE/document/.

Heffler, S., Levit, K., Smith, S., Smith, C., Cowan, C., Lazenby, H., & Freeland, M. (2001). Health spending growth up in 1999: Faster growth expected in the future. *Health Affairs, 20*(2), 193-203.

Johnson, B. (1996). *Polarity management: Identifying and managing unsolvable problems*. Amherst, MA: HRD Press.

Neuman, B., Suver, J., & Zelman, W. (1988). *Financial management: Concepts and applications for health care providers* (2nd ed.). Ownings Mills, MD: National Health Publishing.

Petryshen, P., Stevens, B., Hawkins, J., & Stewart, M. (1997). Comparing nursing costs for pre-term infants receiving conventional US developmental care. *Nursing Economics, 15*(3), 138-145, 150.

Ward, W., (1998). *An introduction to healthcare financial management*. Ownings, MD: National Health Publishing.

Wesorick, B., Shiparski, L., Troseth, M., & Wyngarden, K. (1997). *Partnership council field book: Strategies and tools for co-creating a healthy work place.* Grand Rapids, MI: Practice Field Publishing.

SUGGESTED READINGS

Blumenthal, D. (2001). Controlling health care expenditures. *New England Journal of Medicine, 344*(10), 766-769.

Carruth, A., Carruth, P., & Noto, E. (2000). Financial management: Nurse managers flex their budgetary might. *Nursing Management, 31*(2), 16-17.

Cavouras, C., & McKinley, J. (1997). Variable budgeting for staffing: Analysis and evaluation. *Nursing Management, 28*(5), 34, 36, 38.

Goode, C., Tanaka, D., Krugman, M., O'Connor, P., Bailey, C., Deutchman, M., & Stolpman, N. M. (2000). Outcomes from use of an evidence-based practice guideline. *Nursing Economics, 18*(4), 202-207.

Gormley, K., & Verdejo, T. (2000). A systems approach—Budgeting for the 21st century: Turning challenges into triumphs. *Nursing Administration Quarterly, 24*(4), 51-59.

Hall, M., & Anderson, F. (1997). Maintaining quality care while decreasing hospice costs. *Nursing Economics, 15*(3), 157-159, 163.

Petryshen, P., Stevens, B., Hawkins, J., & Stewart, M. (1997). Comparing nursing costs for pre-term infants receiving conventional vs. developmental care. *Nursing Economics, 15*(3), 138-145, 150.

Shi, L., & Singh, D. (2001). *Delivering health care in America: A systems approach* (2nd ed.). Gaithersburg, MD: Aspen.

Sultz, H., & Young, K. (2001). *Healthcare USA: Understanding its organization* (3rd ed.). Gaithersburg, MD: Aspen.

Vincent, D., Oakley, D., Pohl, J., & Walker, D. (2000). Survival of nurse-managed centers: The importance of cost analysis. *Outcomes Management for Nursing Practice, 4*(3), 124-128.

Ward, W. (1988). *An introduction to health care financial management.* Ownings Mills, MD: National Health Publishing.

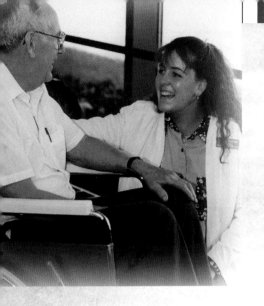

Chapter

14

Consumer Relationships

Brenda L. Cleary

T his chapter explores the changes that have altered consumer relationships with healthcare providers and looks specifically at the nurse's responsibilities to the consumer. Nurses set the tone for effective staff-patient interaction. Because nurses are the healthcare providers who spend the most time with the consumer, this chapter provides concepts and strategies to assist in developing effective nurse-consumer relationships.

Objectives

- Categorize health consumers' interactions into three relationship structures.
- Interpret the results of selected changes that have influenced consumer relationships in healthcare.
- Examine the importance of a service-oriented philosophy to the quality of the nurse-consumer relationship.
- Apply the four major responsibilities of nursing—service, advocacy, teaching, and leadership—to the promotion of successful nurse-consumer relationships.

Questions to Consider

- *Why is the consumer perspective so important to nursing leaders?*
- *What changes have taken place that have altered the relationships between consumers and providers of healthcare?*
- *What concepts must you apply to provide service-oriented nursing care to consumers?*
- *How do you take into consideration cultural diversity and individual differences when you practice nursing?*
- *What is consumer advocacy, and who is responsible for it?*

The Challenge

Suzanne Freeman, RN, MBA
President of Carolinas Medical Center, Charlotte, North Carolina

Customer satisfaction is the number one goal in our healthcare facilities. The hospital board officially acknowledged this goal, and systems were set in place to measure, monitor, and improve customer satisfaction. The staff ultimately defined principles to illustrate their commitment to this goal: teamwork, integrity, caring, commitment, and communication. Each individual would be treated with dignity and as a valued member of a "family."

The husband of a patient seen in the emergency room (ER) some time ago called the nurse manager a few days after her visit. When his wife arrived at the ER, her chief complaint was intermittent chest pain for 2 days. She had indicated that she did not have pain upon arrival to the ER and was ultimately admitted to the hospital with the diagnosis statement "Chest pain, rule out MI."

The husband complained that his wife had been required to "sign herself in," even though he had asked the nurse to have his wife seen immediately. He felt the nurse had not taken his wife's complaints seriously and the resulting delay had caused her condition to worsen. He attributed this issue to the fact that his wife required coronary artery bypass surgery the following day.

The nurse manager immediately met with the triage nurse involved. They talked through the encounter and examined the documentation. The triage nurse felt her assessment of "nonemergent" was valid. She noted that the patient was registered by the patient registration person-

nel and the physician saw her within 30 minutes of her arrival. The triage nurse's assessment indicated "Vital Signs stable, no history of heart disease, right-sided chest pain × 2 day." The pain scale records indicated "No pain now." The assessment made by the triage nurse appeared valid to the nurse manager. The nurse manager also noted that the nurse's competency in assessing patients for triage was historically reliable. The triage nurse did not recall the husband asking for his wife to be seen immediately.

The nurse manager visited the patient and her spouse in the coronary care unit. She apologized for their expectations not being met during the triage process. She assured the couple that their concerns were taken seriously and rendered her sincere apology. Her words seemed to be well received by the couple. Each thanked her for her concern and visit.

Apparently the couple was not satisfied, however, because the Vice President for Patient Services received a call from the husband that same day. He related the story, including the nurse manager's visit. He added that he had recently viewed a news report about how women were undertreated and misdiagnosed with regard to chest pain. The vice president listened carefully and promised to follow-up quickly with a response.

 What do you think you would do if you were this nurse?

INTRODUCTION

A Dilbert cartoon declared that there are two essential rules of management: (1) Customers are always right, and (2) they must be punished for their arrogance! The days of thinking that a patient or consumer who becomes actively engaged in healthcare decisions is stepping out of bounds, a mind-set often referred to as *paternalistic*, are fortunately coming to an end.

In the delivery of healthcare, the term *consumer relationships* refers to the multitude of encounters between the consumer (client/patient/customer) and the representatives of the healthcare system. Who are the consumers of healthcare, and what do they ex-

pect from providers? What are their likes and dislikes, and how do they evaluate the care they receive?

We all are consumers of healthcare—friends, neighbors, families, people like us, and people very different from us. Consumers are diverse culturally, ethnically, socially, physically, and psychologically. Consumers are indeed becoming better connoisseurs of healthcare than in the past. One sure sign of the healthcare industry's response to that fact is direct marketing of pharmaceuticals and other health-related products, a phenomenon for which the impact is not yet fully understood (Wilkes, Bell, & Kravitz, 2000). More than 40 million American adults report using the Internet specifically to obtain health information (Lewis & Pesut, 2001). Consumers today have access to a limitless amount of information regarding health, although such access varies to some degree by ethnicity and especially by socioeconomic status. Although not all of what they read, hear, or see is valid, **healthcare consumers** are, in general, better informed now than they ever have been. They question providers regarding the care they receive or do not receive, and they ask, "Why are you doing that?" "Where can I get the best care?" and "How do I make the right healthcare decisions?"

The Consumer Focus

Consumer relationships are constantly changing and thus affect the providers of health services: primary care and public health services, managed care organizations, hospitals, home health agencies, and nursing homes, as well as individual providers such as physicians and nurses. As inpatient services shrink, outpatient services grow, and competition for patients becomes fierce, the focus is moving from **healthcare providers** to healthcare consumers. As noted in The Challenge, the consumer will drive what goes on in our healthcare settings. The healthcare processes are being redefined with the consumer as the center. How consumers view and value the care they receive becomes important data. There are distinct relationships that consumers enter into in meeting their healthcare needs, including the relationships with the healthcare agency, the insurer or payer, the physician, the nurse, and allied health providers. Changes in physician practices, access to service, insurance coverage, and nurses' roles and responsibilities are a few of the significant factors that have influenced these relationships.

Physician-Consumer Relationships

Physician-consumer relationships changed as the physician's typical mode of practice moved from a single, private enterprise to multigroup practices. Some groups are even incorporated into health maintenance organizations, managed care programs, or physician-hospital organizations. When consumers visit a group practice, they may not have the option of selecting a specific physician. Patients no longer know their physicians as they did in the past, and physicians may be less familiar with their patients, resulting in decreased opportunity for the development of mutual respect and trust.

Rural consumers of healthcare have seen their local hospitals close and have had to seek care in regional health centers. They may not have a relationship with the physicians to whom they are directed to seek care, which often leads consumers to be more critical and less accepting of the care delivered. They often feel alienated and insecure in unfamiliar circumstances, even if they are receiving the best medical attention. The patient's perceptions are becoming an increasingly valued outcome of care.

Agency-Consumer Relationships

Consumers of health services are accustomed to receiving acute care in an inpatient setting. In many situations, this option is no longer available. Patients may be angry and frightened at the thought of being on their own or with service provided only periodically from home health agencies. When inpatient services are deemed appropriate, the specific hospital or health agency most likely will be dictated by the type of insurance coverage and the insurance carrier. Managed care options require that the consumer use particular and specific health facilities or be responsible for all or a larger portion of the bill.

No longer is a trip to the emergency room an option for a sore throat at midnight. The price tag for that service is prohibitive, although, sadly, the emergency room may provide the only access to care for the growing number of uninsured. Consumers' options for seeking care are shrinking and the costs are increasing. The insurance plans available to most people include a copayment or a deductible clause requiring the consumer to meet a certain dollar amount before the insurance companies will pay their 60% to 90% of the bill, resulting in a significant impact on the consumer. Medicare and Medicaid recipients also find themselves in the midst of changes in terms of how healthcare costs are managed.

Many healthcare organizations are still operating under an old paradigm, in which the needs of physicians and third-party payers drive the agency's priorities. In increasingly competitive current healthcare markets, executives need to focus on their patient customers who are becoming more knowledgeable and assertive (Ford & Fottler, 2000).

Nurse-Consumer Relationships

Nurses are the healthcare providers who spend the most time with the consumer. These encounters are generally personal and intensely meaningful. Therefore the nurse is in a unique position to influence and promote positive consumer relationships. The nurse manager sets the tone for effective staff-patient interactions, with exciting opportunities presented in patient-focused care.

Changes from hospital or nursing home care to outpatient and in-home care have particularly altered the nurse-consumer relationship. Nurses are taking leadership roles as primary providers (e.g., nurse practitioners, midwives), teachers and educators, and home healthcare managers and advocates, particularly in compensation and insurance arenas. Nurses may emerge as the **gatekeepers** of the healthcare system, the liaisons between the consumer and a complex healthcare market. The nurse in the role of gatekeeper can be an influential advocate for consumers who fall through the cracks of the complicated healthcare system. This group includes those who receive no care and need it most, such as those who are homeless, uninsured or underinsured persons, persons who abuse drugs or alcohol, children of poverty, migrant workers, and people with acquired immunodeficiency syndrome (AIDS).

Nurses are held in high regard by consumers. They view the nurse as knowledgeable, worthy of respect, concerned for others, honest, caring, confidential, friendly, hardworking, and especially trustworthy. In fact, according to a November 2000 Gallup poll, for the second year in a row, the public ranked nursing the number one occupation when it comes to honesty and ethics. In the 2000 Harris Poll, 92% of Americans reported that they trusted information that registered nurses provide about healthcare (American Nurses Association, 1999). Nurses, by virtue of this favorable status with the public, occupy positions of influence and can foster and promote successful consumer relationships across healthcare settings.

Henson (1997) presented an analysis of the concept of mutuality (i.e., mutual accountability) in relationships with patients. Mutuality balances power and respect and promotes productive communication.

Four major responsibilities of nurses in promoting successful consumer relationships are developed in this chapter:

1. Service
2. Advocacy
3. Teaching
4. Leadership

Exercise 14-1

List as many ways as you can think of that the nurse might carry out the four aforementioned responsibilities listed. Compare your list with those of your peers.

 # SERVICE

A **service** orientation responds to the needs of the customer. In The Challenge, activities were centered around the patient and family, including how nursing care and all other services were delivered so that patient care was a "whole" concept. As Box 14-1 illustrates, no matter where the services are delivered, the focus is the patient (**consumer focus**).

A service orientation is different from the concept of **service lines,** in which all related types of services are grouped into one functional unit of management. Some typical service line units are women's services, cardiac services, orthopedic services, emergency services, and oncology services (Fitzpatrick, McElroy, & DeWoody, 2001).

Even with an increasing emphasis on customer service, most healthcare facilities are not as "customer-friendly" as they could be; that is, they are built and organized in a manner that best serves the organization, not the consumer. They are departmentalized, with each department having specialized functions. Patients are transported from department to department to receive services. They risk loss of privacy, excessive exposure, and increased discomfort and fatigue during the transfer and waiting episodes. On an average day, a seriously ill hospitalized patient may to be exposed to up to 50 different personnel in the course of receiving treatment and care. This approach is not "service-oriented." A service mentality means delivering services in a manner that is least disruptive to the consumer. When possible, services should come to the patient and should be as easy, comfortable, pleasant, and effective as possible. In healthcare, components of customer service include areas such as technical competence, people skills, systems, and the environment (Leebov, Scott, & Olson, 1998).

Exercise 14-2

List the things that you think are not consumer-friendly in your nursing situation. (Example: Patients admitted to healthcare facilities are asked to repeat information several times to various people in the agency, such as admitting staff, nurses, and x-ray technicians.)

Providing satisfying and meaningful service is not easy. Every consumer is different, and every situation is different. How things are done and how needs are met vary in each situation. Service is not a prescribed set of rules and regulations and is not

BOX 14-1

Seven Primary Dimensions of Patient-Centered Care

- **Respect for patient's values, preferences, and expressed needs,** which includes attention to quality of life, involvement in decision making, preservation of a patient's dignity, and recognition of patients' needs and autonomy
- **Coordination and integration of care,** which involve clinical care, ancillary and support services, and "frontline" patient care
- **Information, communication, and education,** which include information on clinical status, progress, and prognosis; information on processes of care; and information and education to facilitate autonomy, self-care, and health promotion
- **Physical comfort,** which considers pain management, help with activities of daily living, and hospital environment

- **Emotional support and alleviation of fear and anxiety,** which demand attention to anxiety over clinical status, treatment, and prognosis; anxiety over the effect of the illness on self and family; and anxiety over the financial impact of the illness
- **Involvement of family and friends,** which recognizes the need to accommodate family and friends and involve family in decision making; to support the family as caregiver; and to recognize family needs
- **Transition and continuity,** which address patient anxieties and concerns about information on medication, treatment regimens, follow up, danger signals after leaving the hospital, recovery, health promotion, and prevention of recurrence; coordination and planning for continuing care and treatment; and access to continuity of care and assistance

From Gerteis, M., Edgman-Levitan, S., Daley, J., & Debanco, T. L. (1993). *Through the patient's eyes: Understanding and promoting patient-centered care.* San Francisco: Jossey-Bass.

BOX 14-2

Differentiating Characteristics Between a Service and a Product

Service	Product
• Intangible (without physical boundaries)	• Tangible (possesses physical properties)
• Unpredictable	• Predictable
• Spontaneous	• Produced and stored
• Created and consumed simultaneously	• Created/can be consumed at a later time
• Heterogeneous (no two items are alike)	• Homogeneous
• Personal, human interaction	• Impersonal

a unidimensional concept. Service means placing a premium on the design, development, and delivery of care. For example, a home care patient needs intravenous (IV) antibiotic therapy. Inserting the IV catheter is the task-oriented, production part of the care. The service aspect involves taking into consideration the special needs of the patient, such as placing the needle in the left arm so he can continue to use his cane with his right arm, or using some local anesthetic before inserting the needle to reduce discomfort. Several characteristics are used to differentiate a service from a product. Some of these are shown in Box 14-2.

In delivering nursing care, both service and product characteristics are present. Some of the ac-

tions in nursing require very prescribed rituals—the actual physical act of production, such as insertion of a Foley catheter. In performing this act, certain physical properties are apparent and the outcome predictable. At the same time, no two patients are alike; human interaction alters the situation, and unforeseen variables demand spontaneity. Caring, concern, and respect for the individual are intangible characteristics that affect the ultimate success or failure of the physical nursing act. Quality nursing care must be both clinically correct and satisfying to the customer. "Clinically correct" is the product aspect and "satisfying to the consumer" is the service orientation. An example of touching is highlighted in the Research Perspective.

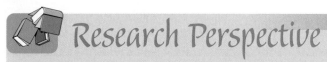

Research Perspective

Chang, S. O. (2001). The conceptual structure of physical touch in caring. *Journal of Advanced Nursing, 33*, 820-827.

This study of in-depth interviews of 39 adult subjects (healthcare professionals, inpatients, and healthy people) focused on the phenomenon of physical touch. This study found that physical touch in caring is a complex concept that focuses around five aspects of touch: promoting physical comfort, promoting emotional comfort, promoting mind-body comfort, performing social role, and sharing spirituality. The researcher concluded that physical touch could positively affect patients' well-being and comfort.

IMPLICATIONS FOR PRACTICE

Touching is an important part of nursing care. Because it has multiple meanings, it can promote positive consumer perceptions of their care.

Healthcare agencies, as service organizations, must be sensitive as to whether the agency milieu is indeed a healing environment that supports and reinforces the actual quality of clinical care. The challenge in the busy, unpredictable, cost-constrained world of healthcare is to provide settings of care that meet or exceed customer expectations. People are looking for an environment that meets their needs for safety and security, support, and psychological and physical comfort. Such needs are best addressed in healthcare organizations that deliver clinically competent care within a service orientation (Fottler, Ford, Roberts, & Ford, 2000).

A service orientation is consumer driven and consumer focused, and it places the emphasis on the quality of the nurse-patient relationship. The importance of relationships is reflected in current nursing theory in the caring philosophy. Caring has been described as the essence of nursing. It denotes a special concern, interest, or feeling capable of fostering a therapeutic nurse-patient relationship. Caring is important, but it is not enough to simply care. The ability to think and take appropriate, timely action must be a part of the therapeutic process. The nurse must do the right thing right at the right time.

The concept of nursing as a caring service is seen in the reality of "high tech–high touch." **High tech** denotes a mechanistic perspective, whereas **high touch** denotes a caring, humanistic perspective. Caring for patients can be described as challenging in an environment driven by technology. At the same time, patients depend on nurses to deliver high-tech care in a caring, humanistic manner. The more high technology is used in healthcare, the more the patient wants and needs high touch—

someone who is trusted and respected and who will add humanness to the experience. The quality of these human contacts becomes the measure by which the consumer forms perceptions and judgments about nursing and the health agency. Particularly in healthcare, consumers are frequently unable to judge or evaluate the quality of interventions, but they always have the ability to evaluate the quality of the relationship with the person delivering the service.

An essential component of a strong customer service program is a service recovery element, according to a 2001 study by Bendall-Lyon and Powers that was sponsored by the Agency for Healthcare Research and Quality. The authors identified six steps in using complaint management as an effective service recovery tool: (1) Encourage complaints as part of the quality improvement process, (2) establish a team to address the complaints, (3) resolve consumer issues quickly and effectively, (4) develop a database of complaints to analyze trends and generate information for management and staff, (5) commit to identifying failure points in the system, and (6) use information to improve service processes.

Exercise 14-3

Make a "what-if" list of things that would enhance services to the consumers of healthcare. (Example: What if nurses were referred to patients at the same time that physicians were referred to patients?)

Each individual nurse is responsible for providing quality patient care. The nurse manager is accountable for quality management. A consulting firm of organizational strategists (Booz-Allen) generated the term *patient-focused care.* However, there is no clearly explicated model or one widely accepted definition for this concept. A common thread across healthcare systems using patient-focused care strategies is refocusing on expected patient outcomes rather than on a multiplicity of tasks (O'Donnell et al., 1999; Geron, Smith, Tennstedt, Jette, Chassler, & Kasten, 2000).

ADVOCACY

Nurses today practice in a healthcare environment dominated by unrest and insecurity. Some of these forces are shown in Box 14-3.

Such forces bring about ethical and moral questions: Who gets care? Where do they get care? How much care? Who has the right to die? Who has the right to live? Who makes the decisions? Differing values and beliefs, along with economic constraints and limited resources, affect decisions that are made.

Consumers have some basic rights that need to be protected—the right to individualized care; the right to their own values, beliefs, and cultural ways; and the right to be informed and participate in care decisions. Within the healthcare system remains the unresolved issue of two levels of care that are rationally based on economics but tend to result in racial-cultural discrimination. Not only has care been on a two-tiered basis, but also minorities and women have been significantly underrepresented in health-related research, resulting in significant health disparities.

Who in the healthcare system is in a position to be the guardian of these rights for the consumer? The nurse is! The nurse acts as the primary person to be alert to circumstances that may prevent a successful outcome for the patient and to intervene on the patient's behalf. The nurse is in the position to address the issues of cultural, ethnic, and racial sensitivity.

Advocacy is a multidimensional concept and has many different meanings and applications. An advocate is one who (1) defends or promotes the rights of others; (2) changes systems to meet the needs of others; (3) empowers and promotes self-determination in others; (4) promotes autonomy of diverse cultures and social groups; (5) ensures respect, equality, and dignity for others; and (6) cares for the humanness of all.

Nurses practice in a healthcare system that is as culturally, economically, and socially diverse as con-

---

BOX 14-3

Forces of Unrest and Insecurity in Today's Healthcare Environment

1. Increased costs
2. Shift to outpatient services
3. Complex social problems (acquired immunodeficiency syndrome [AIDS], violence, poverty)
4. Decreased access to healthcare
5. Aging population (increasing life span)
6. Technological and genetic advances
7. Culturally and ethnically diverse work/consumer groups
8. Underrepresentation of women and ethnic groups in health-related research

---

sumers are. Nurses are responsible to consumers to assist them in successfully accessing and participating in the system. Some patients enter the healthcare system much like immigrants entering a foreign country. The result may be culture shock for such patients as they enter a system with a set of values, beliefs, behaviors, and language unlike their own. Nurses need to recognize the culture of their work setting, realizing that it may differ markedly from the culture of the consumer who enters the system, and move beyond ethnocentrism to provide culturally competent care. **Cultural competence** brings together attitudes, behaviors, and policies in an organization in such a way that allows people to work effectively in cross-cultural situations (National Alliance for Hispanic Health, 2000).

The advocate role requires the nurse to perceive and be comfortable with conflict and then mediate, negotiate, clarify, explain, and intervene. The nurse can advocate by being a liaison between the consumer and the system. The nurse's role is to interpret the rules and customs of the agency to the consumer. It is also to negotiate changes when the consumer and agency differ in values and beliefs. An example is shown in Box 14-4.

To provide culturally appropriate care, the nurse must possess knowledge about various culturally diverse groups (see Chapter 18). It takes time to develop cultural sensitivity and awareness. Some guidelines that are useful in learning to appreciate and value diversity are as follows:

1. Avoid stereotyping.
2. Avoid making assumptions.

BOX 14-4

Racial and Cultural Differences

SCENARIO: A young adult African-American male, shot while running from the police, had been hospitalized for more than 3 weeks. A psychiatric clinical nurse specialist made the following assessment:

PERSPECTIVE OF NURSING STAFF

1. No one wants to take care of this patient. Avoiding him is common. His call light goes unanswered.

2. The patient is loud, rude, and uses vulgar language.

3. Nursing staff suspects that sexual activity is occurring between the man and his girlfriend in the hospital.

4. Nurses feel physically and sexually threatened when trying to provide care.

PERSPECTIVE OF PATIENT OF COLOR

1. Patient feels isolated and forgotten. His room is at the end of the hall. He infrequently sees nurses and physicians, has little information about his gunshot wounds, and fears he's never going to walk again. He fears he will die in his room and no one will know.

2. Patient speaks loudly and uses vulgar talk to emphasize his concerns.

3. Patient makes comments with sexual overtones and spends hours with his girlfriend when she visits; he seeks comfort and affirmation through sexuality.

4. Patient's family only comes on weekends and then in large numbers.

Summary: Stereotypes about African-American males were operational on the unit. The staff members avoided the patient because of the sexual overtones, and they withheld information regarding his condition. Overt and covert battles of will with the patient resulted in further patient isolation.

Modified from Malone, B. L. (1993). Caring for culturally diverse racial groups: An administrative matter. *Nursing Administration Quarterly, 17*(2), 21-29.

3. Learn by observing ethnic groups interact.
4. Adjust expectations to be culturally sensitive.
5. Create a more level playing field—modify your behavior to accommodate diversity.

Powerlessness or an imbalance in power between the consumer and the system can result in value systems being forced on the recipient of care. Consumers who lack economic means by being either uninsured or underinsured often become powerless in the healthcare delivery system. They are at the mercy or will of those who control the power and the money. These consumers (described earlier) may be denied access to care, or if they achieve access, they may not receive equal care.

Less privileged consumers have a right to healthcare and a right to know what services or care they are entitled to. The nurse must be willing to ensure that economic constraints do not prevent them from receiving what they need. Some advocacy for the recipients of inequality in our healthcare system is done on the here-and-now level—initiating a referral to a social agency, appealing on behalf of the consumer to the ethics committee. On a broader scale advocacy means becoming involved professionally and politically to change the systems and policies to provide equality and access to healthcare.

Exercise 14-4

Using the scenario in Box 14-4, determine how the culturally competent nurse can mediate the cultural differences between the staff and the patient.

Race and ethnicity as a factor in health and healthcare has been the subject of concern, yet minority health is often erroneously assumed to be a unitary phenomenon when, in fact, there is extraordinary diversity. The interactions and relationships among race and ethnicity, social class, and health need further exploration (Geron et al., 2000).

Nursing can be described as a cultural phenomenon. Nursing as a profession has strived for greater diversity among its ranks with only very modest progress (National Sample Survey, 2001). In the meantime, cultural diversity training and sensitivity have never been greater in importance (Brooks, 2001). The U.S. Census of 2000 revealed remarkable increases in the diversity of our population. The Census Bureau predicts that by 2040, more than half the U.S. population will be composed of ethnic minorities. Currently, residents of the United States speak at least 329 languages! (Agency for Healthcare Research and Quality, 2001). It is most useful to define diversity broadly, to include not only race and ethnicity but also age, gender, class, religion, and sexual orientation. Persons with disabilities also should be considered in diversity programs.

Some of the keys to becoming a successful nurse advocate are (1) developing networking systems within work agencies and professional associations to assist in providing information and services to patients, (2) acquiring the knowledge needed to access systems, (3) learning about community resources and support networks, and (4) developing skill in referring and engaging patients.

A patient advocate's ultimate aim is to empower the patient (i.e., the consumer of healthcare). Patient empowerment is an emerging, fashionable trend in healthcare today. However, as VanderHenst (1997) points out, there is a lack of a clear, conceptual definition for the term. The nurse manager should keep in mind the most basic element of empowerment—helping people assert control. In the healthcare industry, control applies to factors that affect health. For example, the application of a "strengths" model of case management in a long-term care Medicaid waiver program helped people and communities identify and develop capacities, talents, skills, and interest and connect with necessary resources (Fast & Chapin, 1996). According to a 1996 analysis by Doty, Kasper, and Litvak, Medicaid patients in three states were more satisfied with program elements that gave them more choice and control. Kelly-Powell (1997) used a grounded theory research approach to explore how patients with life-threatening conditions choose to personalize treatment decisions and thus exercise control over their health and healthcare.

In health facilities, nurses can evaluate the quality of care the consumer is receiving by comparing it with the quality indicators or critical pathways in the quality review process. For example, if patient care standards cite that patients with a particular bronchial condition need chest x-ray examinations on day 2 and another on day 5, all patients should receive this same level of care. In agencies using critical paths to prescribe the plan of care, patients who cannot pay for services should not be denied treat-

ment, therapy, or tests if the critical path requires specific action. Nurse managers are in a unique position to ensure that all patients receive appropriate care. The tone set by the manager signals staff to report and document discrepancies and omissions. Nurse managers must acknowledge and respect the legal, ethical, and moral responsibilities of the staff to advocate for patients.

The savvy manager knows that the way in which consumers define quality may not always be in sync with the way "experts" define it. Research suggests that in the area of subacute care, for example, healthcare providers need to focus greater attention on (1) access to services, (2) communication and coordination, and (3) values (Stahl, 1997).

Quality medical care and quality nursing care are not dependent on the ability to pay or social acceptance. Good care is irrespective of the economic circumstance of the consumer. Nurses are the guardians of that right for consumers. Nurses have historically been the champions for the poor and the underserved. It is no different today.

TEACHING

Consumers of healthcare have a right to know and a need to know how to care for their own health needs. Nurses have an obligation to teach the consumer. This obligation is mandated in the states' nurse practice acts. Accrediting organizations such as the Joint Commission on Accreditation of Healthcare Organizations (JCAHO) also mandate patient teaching in their family and patient education standards. The American Nurses Association has advocated patient teaching since the publication of its Model Nurse Practice Act in 1975. More and more, consumers are demanding information about their health status and plan of care. Consumers are entitled to information regarding health concerns, to participate in caring for their health needs, and to contribute to finding solutions to their health problems. Education empowers consumers to exercise self-determination. It allows them to have greater control over what happens, to make informed decisions, and to choose wisely from options. An ancient proverb says that if you give a man a fish, you feed him for a day, but if you teach a man to fish, you feed him for a lifetime. Knowledge is power. Sharing knowledge means sharing power. Research supports the value of providing health-related education to consumers (Broom, 2001).

BOX 14-5

Three P's for a Successful Consumer Education Focus

1. Philosophy—Patient education is an investment with a significant positive return. Money invested in teaching is money well spent. Time and energy invested are time and energy well spent.
2. Priority—Education is important. Quality nursing care always has an educational component. Informed consumers want to participate and look to nurses to teach them.
3. Performance—Clinical teaching excellence is a required skill of nurses. They must possess a variety of techniques and methods to meet the needs of the diverse consumers served.

The changes in healthcare actively affect the way nurses teach consumers. Probably the most significant change is shorter hospital stays and thus more care in outpatient settings. This requires that patients be able to manage their own healthcare earlier and more independently. Hands-on, technical training is needed in many instances, such as self-catheterization. Research has shown that in patient teaching, nurses' perceptions of their patients' understanding of postdischarge treatment plans differ from the perception of patients themselves. Nurses often perceive patients to be much more knowledgeable than the patients themselves report. Teaching prevention and health promotion will increase the consumer's quality of life. Three *P*'s for a successful consumer education focus are shown in Box 14-5.

Teaching can be simple or complex. In teaching elemental, task-oriented behaviors, the nurse uses basic materials, simple relationships, guides, sequencing of steps, and cause-and-effect relationships. Teaching directed more broadly toward changing health behaviors actually seeks to modify beliefs and attitudes through persuasive communication (Stubblefield, 1997). The nurse manager needs to ensure that teaching resources exist and must validate that teaching is documented as part of the plan of care. Teaching behaviors should be addressed in performance evaluations.

In addition to being easy to read, written teaching materials need to reflect relevance, accuracy, and thoroughness and need to be updated regularly.

The tone needs be warm and personal and in an inviting format (Winslow, 2001).

EXAMPLE: Teaching insulin administration

1. Material	Demonstrate the use of the equipment. Have trainee do a return demonstration.
2. Simple relationships	Interpret the significance of the blood sugar level to the amount and type of insulin given.
3. Guides	Illustrate the rotation of injection sites with a chart.
4. Sequencing	Apply a step-by-step procedure to follow to encompass the task from start to finish.
5. Cause and effect	Explain the relationship of sterile technique to infection prevention— "If you contaminate the needle, infection can result."

As a step-by-step process, teaching can be adapted to the problem-solving process model shown in Figure 14-1.

The following example uses the nursing process model in teaching a patient about diabetes.

Assess	Patient is a 16-year-old, Hispanic boy with no prior knowledge of diabetes or skill in drug administration. English is a second language. He needs to administer his own insulin, using sterile technique, by the time he is discharged from the hospital.
Plan	Begin with a demonstration and return demonstration of basic subcutaneous injection. Progress step by step to basic understanding of diabetes, blood sugar, and insulin dosage by the time of discharge. Home health agency to continue training.
Implement	Set times, twice a day, to spend 1 hour in instruction with patient. Begin with a demonstration, a return demonstration, and repeat instructions. Adjust learning materials to accommodate language barrier.
Evaluate	Patient has met minimal skill level of subcutaneous technique. He can administer insulin safely but has limited disease and cause-and-effect understanding. To be followed per home health with continued teaching.

As a conceptual process, teaching fits into the general systems theory model as shown in Figure 14-2. The following example uses the gen-

ASSESSING

Analyze the learner
Assess knowledge
 and skills
Analyze the task
Assess performance level
 needed

DIAGNOSING
AND
PLANNING

Set the strategy
Plan the content
Develop the time frame
Assess readiness to
 learn
Establish expectations

IMPLEMENTING

Initiate planned strategies
Test for readiness
Sequence the tasks
Vary the learning aids
Adjust for cultural diversity

EVALUATING

Analyze achievements
Examine consumer
 skill level
Compare progress to
 plan strategy
Validate success
 or revise

Figure 14-1   Teaching model adapted to the nursing process.

eral systems theory model in teaching a patient with diabetes:

Input	Present information about the disease, the procedures to be learned, the skills necessary for successful achievement, and the cause-and-effect relationships. Have materials in Spanish at a high school reading level. Demonstrate the drug administration technique.
Throughput	Language barrier eased with materials printed in Spanish. Fear threat to macho image typical of 16-year-old boy. Allow time to practice techniques demonstrated.
Output	Return demonstration successful. Give posttest to assess knowledge (in Spanish).
Feedback	Praise for successful return demonstration. Give example of sports heroes or movie stars with diabetes.

Teaching is one of the most positive experiences nurses can have. Teaching can be fun and rewarding, but it is hard work.

Nurses need to be prepared and skilled to teach. They must be able to adapt to the learning styles of the consumer by using a variety of styles and a flexible approach in meeting the educational goals. Selected learning preferences are shown in Box 14-6. Being knowledgeable in the subject and able to individualize the information to meet the

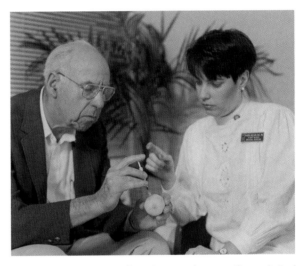

Successful consumer education requires excellent clinical teaching skills.

consumer's ability to learn are critical to quality teaching.

Patient-specific information must also be shared with family caregivers (Chang, 1999). Underscoring the importance of family teaching, Bailey and Mion (1997) developed the Caregiver Satisfaction with Information Questionnaire (Box 14-7).

LEADERSHIP

In Sigma Theta Tau's 1996 Arista II report on nursing leadership in the twenty-first century, participants asserted that enhancing the ability of nurse leaders to create and manage change is fundamen-

Exercise 14–5

Using one of the models presented, prepare a teaching plan based on your actual nursing experience.

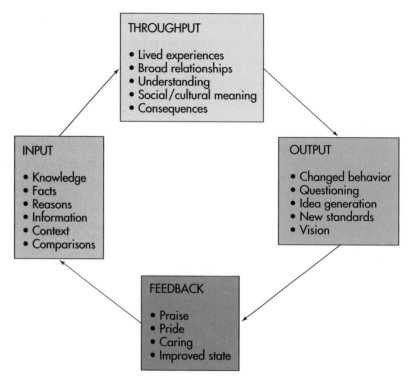

Figure 14-2   Teaching model adapted to general systems theory.

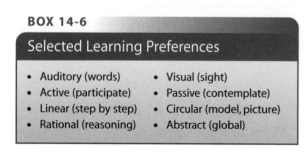

BOX 14-6

Selected Learning Preferences

- Auditory (words)
- Active (participate)
- Linear (step by step)
- Rational (reasoning)
- Visual (sight)
- Passive (contemplate)
- Circular (model, picture)
- Abstract (global)

tal to improving healthcare. Awareness and understanding of paradigm shifts in healthcare will equip nurse managers to participate in shaping healthcare organizations of the future. Trends include the following shifts:

1. From person as customer to population as customer (i.e., population-focused care)
2. From illness care to wellness care
3. From revenue management to cost management
4. From autonomy to interdependence of professionals (i.e., interdisciplinary approaches to care)
5. From continuity of provider to continuity of information

6. From patient as nonconsumer to patient as consumer of cost and quality information
7. From fee-for-service to capitated plans and managed care

According to the Institute of Medicine (2001), there is increasing attention to healthcare quality and error reduction. Nurse managers are in a pivotal position to influence the cost and the quality of care delivered by the staff. They set the tone for the vision and mission of the unit and the focus for the staff. They must believe in and model the consumer-based service philosophy. One who truly believes in the need to provide service that is satisfying to the consumer knows that each and every consumer is different. What will satisfy one person will not satisfy another. Being successful as leaders in nursing requires being open and flexible; leaders are expected not only to do things right but to do the right things. According to Fitzpatrick (2000), leadership requires (1) giving individualized attention to followers, (2) offering intellectual stimulation, (3) providing inspirational motivation, and (4) serving as a role model (idealized influence). Leadership also involves the ability to relinquish

BOX 14-7

Caregiver Satisfaction With Information Questionnaire

*1. In regard to ease of getting information, please rate the willingness of hospital staff to answer your questions.

*2. In regard to instructions, please rate how well the nurses and other staff explained about tests, treatments, and what to expect.

*3. In regard to informing family and friends, please rate how well family and friends were kept informed about the patient's condition and needs.

*4. In regard to information given by the nurses, please rate how well the nurses communicated with patients, families, and doctors.

†5. In regard to updates concerning the patient's condition, please rate how well the nurses informed you concerning the rest and comfort level of the patient.

†6. In regard to updates concerning the patient's condition, please rate how well the nurses informed you concerning the nutritional status of the patient.

†7. In regard to updates concerning the patient's condition, please rate how well the nurses informed you of the results of tests done for ongoing monitoring of the patient's illness (e.g., temperature, blood pressure, blood glucose monitoring).

†8. In regard to the patient's daily schedule, please rate how well the nurses informed you about the patient's actual and anticipated schedule each day.

*Items from the survey *Your Hospital Stay: The Patient's Viewpoint,* produced and distributed by NCG Research, Inc.
†Items developed by the authors.

control and a tolerance for ambiguity, as well as sudden and sometimes dramatic change.

Change is the modus operandi of the nursing environment in any healthcare setting. What works today may not work 6 months from now. Given the rapidly changing environment, the pressure to control costs, and advances in technology, science, and information, nurse managers need a whole new set of beliefs, behaviors, and skills. Selected examples of these are as follows:

1. Keep the consumer as the center of focus.
2. Recognize that each staff member has a unique contribution to make to the success of the unit. Allow staff to be creative and flexible in their work, ask for suggestions and new approaches to old problems, and seek participation in decision making. Managers set the tone; staff deliver the service.
3. Promote dignity, worth, caring, individual contributions, and cultural sensitivity in the staff. Successful managers recognize individual accomplishments and support failures. They accept that human beings are not perfect at all times and that it is okay to take a risk, look foolish, and fail. They implement hiring practices that foster selection of qualified racially and culturally diverse applicants.
4. Understand the economic value of service. Managers must believe that service will pay real

dollar dividends to justify the cost in terms of adequate quality and quantity of staff.
5. Evaluate patient outcomes and perceptions of care. It is imperative to ask patients about the services provided and how it felt to them, not after the fact but while they are receiving the service.

Patient outcomes or the notion of evidence-based standards and measurement of care are attracting greater attention and achieving much greater emphasis in the marketplace reform of healthcare. The focus of healthcare reform in the marketplace and of the movement toward managed care is the provision of quality care, but controlling costs is paramount. There is a growing collective voice among consumers that notes that healthcare institutions and professionals seem to be more focused on profits than on patient care (Grayson, 1997).

In the area of consumer relations, patient satisfaction with care is a particularly relevant measure. Patient satisfaction has been evaluated in the past with varying degrees of success. Current research efforts are aimed at developing valid and reliable patient outcome measures, including patient satisfaction. Nursing systems and nursing administration researchers are particularly interested in response to and satisfaction with nursing care. However, valid measurement of patient satisfaction is an evolving science; nurses do not always accurately gauge what factors are most important to patients, and satisfaction measures are often skewed in a positive direction.

Managers must be willing to give up direct control of every process. Staff must be given power and permission to be in control and to make decisions at the consumer-staff level of interaction. Some of our greatest successes come out of spontaneous actions. Giving up control involves being willing to take a risk and a belief in the other person's ability to perform.

Leadership behaviors contributing to individual and personal excellence include (1) allowing professionals more influence over their practice, (2) giving staff opportunities to learn new and varied skills, (3) giving recognition and reward for success and support and consolation for lack of success, and (4) fostering motivation and belief in the importance of each individual and the value of his or her contribution. The leader's role is to create within the worker a passion to do and contribute to the work effort successfully.

We do best those things that we know how to do skillfully and those things about which we feel passionately. Fitting the right person to the right job is important. Maximum contribution is required from each staff member in today's healthcare agencies. Because the leader is the one who sets the standard for the success or failure of the staff's contributions, it is important to assess each staff member carefully—what is his or her skill level and commitment level, and what can be done to assist in making a maximum contribution? Figure 14-3 is an example of a completed staff assessment tool. Nurse managers can compile similar information for members of their staff. The information can be used to form staff development plans.

When staff members know the leader is sincerely concerned about their welfare, they are better able to use their time, energy, and talents to serve the needs of the consumer. Staff members who are nurtured and cared for will be better able to nurture and care for the consumer.

◼ *Exercise 14–6*

Form small groups and assess each member of the group using the headings shown in the staff assessment tool (see Figure 14-3).

Staff Member	Skill Level	Commitment Level	Suggested Action
(1) S. Baker, RN	High technical competence Able to teach others Learns quickly Needs improved people skills	Appears bored Does only what is assigned No enthusiasm Critical of any change	Assign challenges to utilize technical strengths Provide situations in which teaching others occurs Plan: Team assign with D. Carroll
(2) D. Carroll, RN	6 mo post basic program Learns quickly Slow with technical skills Needs technical supervision Excellent people skills	Excited about work Asks for new experiences Accepting of new ideas Volunteers to help others	Improve technical skills Provide safe and successful learning experiences Plan: Team assign with S. Baker
(3) J. Ratke, RN	Moderate technical competence Works best alone Not interested in teaching co-worker Good people skills	Restless, distracted Looking for a change Accepts new ideas Self-commitment—not group-oriented	Set up an independent project of her choosing (e.g., unit research idea) Provide some special technical training to ↑ skills
(4) C. Thomas, RN	High level technical skills Enjoys helping others Excellent people skills Looks for challenges	Team player Interested in welfare of group Critical of poor performers Acts as cheerleader for change	Utilize willingness and group skills to plan and present a unit activity (e.g., inservice education production, unit open house)

Figure 14-3   Staff assessment tool.

The Solution

The vice president immediately met with the triage nurse and nurse manager. The nurse manager was surprised that her visit had not resolved the complaint. The vice president asked the triage nurse if she would have assessed a man with the same profile differently. Her immediate answer was "no." She stated that the staff was aware of the literary documents related to gender bias but that the protocol for assessing chest pain was well designed and very objective, without bias to gender. With the approval of the nurse manager and triage nurse, the vice president invited the husband into the meeting. The husband and the nurse talked through the scenario of events and conversation that occurred during triage, especially the husband's perception that the triage nurse dismissed his request for immediate attention. They agreed that the husband might have said, "Does she really have to register herself?" The triage nurse had not interpreted his statement as a request for immediate action. Each realized that a miscommunication had occurred. Furthermore, the nurse responded to the husband's concern about gender bias. She explained that there had been information in the medical literature, but that cardiologists, ethicists, and other healthcare experts had reviewed and approved the chest pain assessment protocol, ensuring no bias of gender. This situation was brought to resolution by an open line of communication. The result can often be "service recovery."

Several important points may be learned from this incident:

- Effective communication is a critical success factor. Clarification is always appropriate in situations of intensity and high emotion. Active listening is an essential component of effective communication.
- Imagine yourself in the patient's situation and environment when analyzing a communication exchange.
- Engage the involved persons in the evaluation and solution related to a miscommunication.
- Healthcare practices, policy, and procedure should be updated regularly to reflect new knowledge.
- Consumers are increasingly knowledgeable of healthcare; therefore expectations are more sophisticated, and maintaining public trust is of great concern.
- Leadership must exude missionary zeal in educating personnel to the expectations for behavior in terms of consumer satisfaction.

— Suzanne Freeman

 Would this be a suitable approach for you? Why?

CHAPTER CHECKLIST

Times have changed, as has the role of the nurse manager. The trend of healthcare moving into the community, home, clinic, and outpatient setting has placed a whole new perspective on how to provide quality, cost-effective nursing care. Patients must participate in their care and need service-oriented nurses to be teachers, advocates, and leaders on their behalf. Managing care delivery in these diverse settings requires the use of flexible and creative skills. The key is to keep the patient as the center of focus and provide cultural and racially sensitive nursing care.

- Consumer relationships in healthcare typically involve interactions between the consumer and the following:

- The physician
  - The physician-patient relationship is changing because of changes in the way medical care is delivered.
- The nurse
  - Nurses, as the healthcare providers who spend the most time with the consumer, set the tone for effective staff-patient interactions.
- The healthcare agency
  - The agency's approach to care is determined by its mission and philosophy.
- The healthcare payers
  - Insurance coverage and carriers usually dictate the services patients receive and where they receive them.

Continued

CHAPTER CHECKLIST—cont'd

- Because of their favorable status with consumers, nurses are in a unique position to promote positive consumer relationships.
- Four major responsibilities of nurses in promoting successful consumer relationships are as follows:
  - Service
  - Advocacy
  - Teaching
  - Leadership
- A service orientation is consumer driven and consumer focused, emphasizing the quality of the nurse-patient relationship and the delivery of services in a caring atmosphere.
  - Services differ from products:
    - Services are intangible, unpredictable, created and consumed simultaneously, and personal.
    - Products are tangible, predictable, produced and stored, and impersonal.
- The nurse can advocate by serving as a liaison between the consumer and the healthcare system.
  - Nurses can interpret the agency's rules and customs for the consumer and negotiate if conflicts arise.
  - Nurses also help secure culturally appropriate care and mediate cultural differences.
- Teaching is the sharing of information and education to help consumers become independent, self-responsible, and self-determining.
  - Nurses have an obligation to teach the consumer.
  - The three P's for successful consumer education are as follows:
    - Philosophy: Patient education is an investment with a significant positive return.
    - Priority: Education is important.
    - Performance: Clinical teaching excellence is a required skill for nurses.
  - Teaching can follow the five-step nursing process model.
- Leadership fosters decision making at the consumer-staff level of interaction. Effective leadership strategies for the nurse manager include the following:
  - Keeping the central focus on the consumer and remembering that the consumer may be a whole population

- Recognizing staff members' unique contributions and helping them maximize their personal excellence
- Promoting staff members' sense of dignity, worth, caring, cultural diversity, and sensitivity
- Understanding the economic value of service
- Valuing interdisciplinary approaches to care
- Evaluating patient outcomes and patients' perceptions of care

TIPS FOR BEING CUSTOMER FOCUSED

- Hire service-savvy people.
- Establish high standards of customer service.
- Help staff hear the voice of the customer.
- Remove barriers to serving customers.
- Reduce anxiety to increase satisfaction.
- Help staff cope with the stressful atmosphere of healthcare.
- Maintain the focus on service (Leebov, Scott, & Olson, 1998).

ADDITIONAL TIPS

- Ask yourself if this service or approach is one you would wish to receive.
- Remember that in the new pyramid of health services, it is the consumer who is the apex—the rest is there to support that person.
- Enter care relationships with the mindset of how to make care better from the receiver's perspective.
- Use the service, advocacy, teaching, leadership approach.

TERMS TO KNOW

consumer focus	high tech
cultural competence	high touch
gatekeeper	service
healthcare consumer	service lines
healthcare provider	

REFERENCES

Agency for Healthcare Research and Quality. (2001, January). Health plans need culturally and linguistically appropriate materials for non-English speaking patients. *ARHQ Research Activities, 245,* 11.

American Nurses Association (1999). *American Nurse.* Washington DC: Author

Bailey, D. A., & Mion, L. C. (1997). Improving caregivers' satisfaction with information received during hospitalization. *Journal of Nursing Administration, 27*(1), 21-27.

Bendall-Lyon, D., & Powers, T. L. (2001). The role of complaint management in the service recovery process. *Joint Commission Report on Quality Improvement, 27,* 278-286.

Brooks, A. M. (2001). Cultural diversity: Getting to a viewing point. *Journal of Professional Nursing, 17*(1), 4.

Broom, B. L. (2001). Assessing the value of the follow-through family project for students and families. *Journal of Nursing Education, 40*(2), 79-85.

Chang, B. L. (1999). Cognitive-behavioral intervention for homebound caregivers of persons with dementia. *Nursing Research, 48*(3), 173-182.

Doty, P., Kasper, J., & Litvak, S. (1996). Consumer-directed models of personal care: Lessons from Medicaid. *Milbank Quarterly, 74*(3), 377-409.

Fast, B., & Chapin, R. (1996). The strengths model in long-term care: Linking cost containment and consumer empowerment. *Journal of Case Management, 5*(2), 51-57.

Fitzpatrick, J. J. (2000). Reflections on achieving professional leadership. *Nursing Leadership Forum, 5*(1), 25-27.

Fitzpatrick, M. J., McElroy, M. J., & DeWoody, S. (2001). Building a strong nursing organization in a merged, service line structure. *Journal of Nursing Administration, 31*(1), 24-32.

Ford, R. C., & Fottler, M. D. (2000). Creating customer-focused healthcare organizations. *Health Care Management Review, 25*(4), 18-33.

Fottler, M. D., Ford, R. C., Roberts, V., & Ford, E. W. (2000). Creating a healing environment: The importance of the service setting in the new consumer-oriented healthcare system. *Journal of Healthcare Management, 45*(2), 91-107.

Geron, S. M., Smith, K., Tennstedt, S., Jette, A., Chassler, D., & Kasten, L. (2000). The home care satisfaction measure: A client-centered approach to assessing the satisfaction of frail older adults with home care services. *Journal of Gerontology B, 55*(5), 259-270.

Gerteis, M., Edgman-Levitan, S., Daley, J., & Debanco, T. L. (1993). *Through the patient's eyes: Understanding and promoting patient-centered care.* San Francisco: Jossey-Bass.

Grayson, M. (1997, February 20). Get the picture: Consumers sound off on health care. But you may not like what they tell you. *Hospitals & Health Networks, 71,* 30-32.

Henson, R. H. (1997). Analysis of the concept of mutuality. *Image, 29,* 77-81.

Institute of Medicine. (2001). *Informing the future: Critical issues in health.* Washington, DC: Author.

Kelly-Powell, M. L. (1997). Personalizing choices: Patients' experiences with making treatment decisions. *Research in Nursing & Health, 20,* 219-227.

Leebov, W., Scott, G., & Olson, L. (1998). *Achieving impressive customer service: Seven strategies for the healthcare manager.* Chicago: American Hospital Association Press.

Lewis, D., & Pesut, D. J. (2001). Emergence of consumer health care informatics. *Nursing Outlook, 49*(1), 7.

Malone, B. L. (1993). Caring for culturally diverse racial groups: An administrative matter. *Nursing Administration Quarterly, 17*(2), 21-29.

National Alliance for Hispanic Health. (2000). *Quality health services for Hispanics: The cultural competency component.* Washington, DC: Department of Health and Human Services.

O'Donnell, M., Parker, G., Proberts, M., Matthews, R., Fisher, D., Johnson, B., & Hadzi-Pravlovic. (1999). A study of client-focused case management and consumer advocacy: The community and consumer service project. *Australia New Zealand Journal of Psychiatry, 33*(5), 684-693.

Sigma Theta Tau International. (1996). Healthy people: Leaders in partnership. *Nursing Leadership in the 21st Century,* 7-11.

Stahl, D. A. (1997). Quality measures: Meeting consumer needs. *Nursing Management, 28*(8), 20-21.

Stubblefield, C. (1997). Persuasive communication: Marketing health promotion. *Nursing Outlook, 45,* 173-177.

U.S. Department of Health and Human Services, Bureau of Health Professions. (2001). *National sample survey of registered nurses.* Washington, DC: USDHHS.

VanderHenst, J. A. (1997). Client empowerment: A nursing challenge. *Clinical Nurse Specialist, 11*(3), 96-99.

Wilkes, M. S., Bell, R. A., & Kravitz, R. L. (2000). Direct-to-consumer prescription drug advertising: Trends, impact, and implications. *Health Affairs, 19*(2), 110-128.

Winslow, E. H. (2001). Patient education materials. *American Journal of Nursing, 101,* 33-38.

SUGGESTED READINGS

Baird, K. (2000). Customer service in health care: A grassroots approach to creating a culture of service excellence. San Francisco: Jossey-Bass.

Judkins, S. K., Barr, W. J., Clark, D., & Okimi, P. (2000). Consumer perception of the professional nursing role: Development and testing of a scale. Nurse Researcher, 7(3), 32-39.

McCall, T. B. (1996). A patient's guide to avoiding harmful medical care. Charleston, SC: Citadel Press.

Romano, C. A., Phyillaier, C. R., & Hinegardner, P. G. (2001). The nurses' guide to general health and medical websites. Nursing Leadership Forum, 5(4), 129-133.

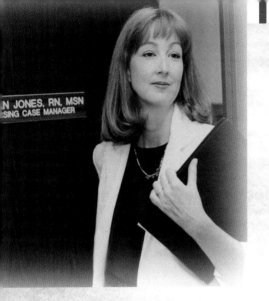

Chapter

15

Care Delivery Strategies

Karen A. Dadich

This chapter introduces nursing care delivery strategies that healthcare agencies currently use. The case method, functional nursing, team nursing, primary nursing, and nurse case management are presented. Patient-focused care, disease management, and differentiated practice are also discussed. This chapter defines and discusses each strategy, summarizes its benefits and disadvantages, and discusses the nurse manager's role and the staff nurse's perspective.

Objectives

- Specify and differentiate among five nursing care delivery strategies.
- Determine the role of the nurse manager and the staff nurse in each strategy.

- Describe the implementation of a disease management program.

- Summarize the differentiated nursing practice model.

Questions to Consider

- What method of nursing care delivery would you most enjoy working by and why?
- How does your level of nursing education affect the care you provide?
- How do you think a nurse manager influences the effectiveness of the nursing care delivery system?
- How do you think the staff nurse influences the implementation of each care delivery strategy?
- How do reimbursement strategies impact nursing care delivery strategies?

The Challenge

Laura Atkins, RN, BSN
Charge Nurse, Burn Intensive Care Unit, University Medical Center, Lubbock, Texas

As a new charge nurse on a 10-bed burn intensive care unit, I needed to assess the nursing staff in this critical care setting. Although we provide primary care to our patients, assessment of the staff's teamwork was essential. What was the level of their capabilities? It was immediately clear that the staff was clinically competent, but I was looking for more. Were there any leaders? How many teachers were among the group? After 8 months in the unit, I realized that several members of the staff were not using their full potential. Nurses with many years of experience were not being encouraged to share their knowledge. It seemed that some were tired, bored, and disenchanted with their position and their responsibilities. They bickered, gossiped, and did not try to foster a positive work environment. Collaboration with their peers and the many diverse members of the healthcare team required to provide care to our critically ill patients was minimal. I tried to determine what I could do to make a difference and potentially change the staff's perspective.

What do you think you would do if you were this nurse?

INTRODUCTION

A nursing **care delivery strategy** is the method used to provide care to patients. Because nursing care is viewed by some as a cost rather than a source of revenue, it is logical for institutions to evaluate their method of providing patient care for the purpose of saving money while still providing quality care. This chapter discusses five strategies of nursing care delivery: **case method, functional nursing, team nursing, primary nursing,** and the nurse **case management.** The influence of disease management programs and patient-focused care is introduced. Finally, the effect differentiated practice has on care delivery is described.

Each nursing care delivery model has advantages and disadvantages, and none is ideal. Some methods are conducive to large institutions, whereas other systems may work best in community settings. Managers in any organization must examine the organizational goals, the unit objectives, staff availability, and the budget when selecting a care delivery model.

CASE METHOD

The case method, or **total patient care** method, of nursing care delivery is the oldest method of providing care to a patient. The premise of the case method is that one nurse provides total care for one patient during the entire work period. This method was used in the era of Florence Nightingale when patients received total care in the home. Care also included meeting the needs of the whole family, including cooking and cleaning (Nelson, 2000). Total patient care is used in critical care settings where one nurse provides total care to a small group of critically ill patients. Nurse educators often select this method of care for students.

Advantages and Disadvantages

During an 8- or 12-hour shift, the patient receives consistent care from one nurse. The nurse, patient, and family exchange mutual trust and can work together toward specific goals. Usually, total patient care is comprehensive, continuous, and holistic. Changes in the patient's status are apparent to the nurse during the shift (Figure 15-1).

In today's costly healthcare economy, total patient care provided by a registered nurse (RN) is very expensive. The efficacy of this care delivery strategy is questionable. Is it realistic to use the highly skilled and extremely knowledgeable professional nurse to provide all the care required? In times of nursing shortages, there are not enough resources or nurses to use this model.

Total patient care is used in critical care settings where one nurse provides total care to a small group of critically ill patients. In the home setting, nursing care is supplemented by family members

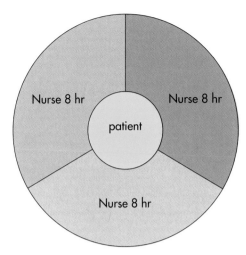

Figure 15-1   Case method of patient care for an 8-hour shift.

and home health aides in an effort to reduce the expense. Variations of the case method exist, and it is possible to identify similarities after reviewing other methods of patient care delivery described later in this chapter.

Nurse Manager's Role

When using the case method of delivery, the manager must consider the expense of the system. The manager must weigh the expense of an RN versus licensed practical (vocational) nurses (LPNs/LVNs) and **unlicensed assistive personnel.** Unlicensed assistive personnel are staff who are not licensed as healthcare providers. They are technicians, nurse aides, and certified nursing assistants. The patient may require 24-hour care; however, the manager must decide whether the patient needs to have RN care or RN-supervised care provided by LPNs/LVNs or unlicensed personnel. To provide cost-effective care to the patients, the staff must have adequate skills to provide total care.

The manager also needs to identify the level of education and communication skills of all staff. RNs must be educated in communicating and coordinating care, as well as supervising other staff members. LPNs/LVNs and unlicensed personnel also need continuing education to provide total care according to their level of practice.

Staff Nurse's Role

The staff nurse provides holistic care to a group of patients during a defined work time. The physical,

emotional, and technical aspects of care are the responsibility of the assigned nurse. Some nurses thrive on this care delivery model, whereas others wish to delegate simpler, less complex aspects of care to assistive personnel. This care delivery strategy requires the total patient care nurse to complete the complex functions of care, such as assessment and teaching the patient and family, as well as the less complex functional aspects of care.

FUNCTIONAL NURSING

The functional method of nursing care delivery became popular during World War II when there was a severe shortage of nurses in the United States. Many nurses entered the military to care for the soldiers. To provide care to patients at home, hospitals began to increase the number of LPNs/LVNs and unlicensed assistive personnel.

Functional nursing is a method of providing patient care by which each licensed and unlicensed staff member performs a specific task for a large group of patients. For example, the RN may administer all intravenous (IV) medications and do admissions, one LPN/LVN may provide treatments, another LPN/LVN may give all oral medication, one assistant may do all hygiene tasks, and another assistant may take all vital signs (Figure 15-2). This division of aspects of care is similar to the assembly line system used by industry. A **charge nurse** coordinates care and assignments and may ultimately be the only person familiar with all needs of any patient.

Advantages and Disadvantages

There are several advantages to this method of patient care delivery. First, each person becomes very

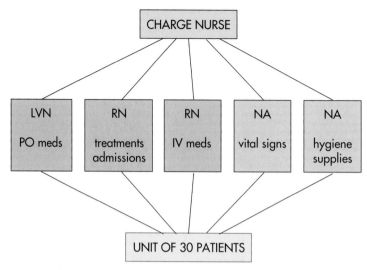

Figure 15-2 Functional method of nursing care delivery.

efficient at specific tasks and a great amount of work can be done in a short time. Another advantage is that unskilled workers can be trained to perform one or two specific tasks very well. The organization benefits financially from this strategy because patient care can be delivered to a large number of patients by mixing staff with a fixed number of RNs and a larger number of unlicensed assistive personnel. For example, a busy orthopedic unit may use the RN to do the patient assessments, the LVN/LPN to do the dressing changes, nurse aides to complete the bed baths, and physical therapy aides to do the ambulation.

Although financial savings may be the impetus for organizations to choose the functional system of delivering care, the disadvantages outweigh the savings (Figure 15-3). A major disadvantage is the fragmentation of care. The physical and technical aspects of care may be met, but the psychological and spiritual needs are often overlooked. Patients become confused with so many different care providers per shift. These different staff may be so busy with their assigned tasks that they do not have time to communicate with each other about the patient's progress. Because no one care provider sees patient care from beginning to the end, evaluation of the patient's response to care is difficult to assess. Critical changes in patient status may go unnoticed. Fragmented care and ineffective communication can lead to patient and family dissatisfaction and frustration. Exercise 15-2 provides an opportunity to imagine how a patient would react to the func-

tional method and also to imagine how the nurse may feel.

Exercise 15-2

Imagine you are a patient at a hospital that uses the functional method of patient care delivery. You just had surgery, and when you ask the nursing assistant for something for pain she says, "I'll tell the medication nurse." The medication nurse comes to your room and says that your medication is ordered IV and that the IV nurse will need to administer it. The IV nurse is busy starting an IV on another patient and will not be able to give your medication to you for 10 minutes. This whole communication process has taken 40 minutes, and you are still in pain. How do you feel about the functional method of patient care? How effective do you think communication between staff is when a patient has a problem?

Nurse Manager's Role

In the functional nursing method, the nurse manager must be sensitive to the quality of patient care delivered and the institution's budgetary constraints. Because staff members are responsible only for their specific task, the role of achieving **patient outcomes** becomes the nurse manager's responsibility. Staff members can view this system as autocratic and may become discontented with the lack of opportunity for input.

By using effective management and leadership skills, the nurse manager can improve the staff's perception of their lack of independence. The manager

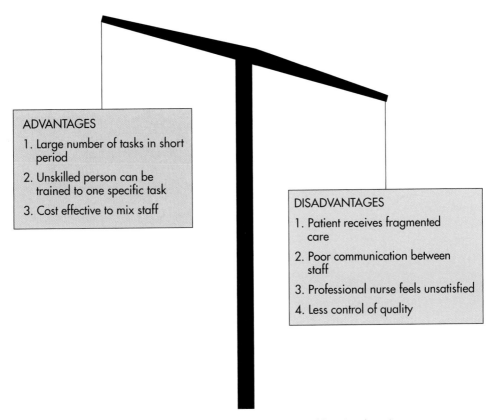

ADVANTAGES

1. Large number of tasks in short period
2. Unskilled person can be trained to one specific task
3. Cost effective to mix staff

DISADVANTAGES

1. Patient receives fragmented care
2. Poor communication between staff
3. Professional nurse feels unsatisfied
4. Less control of quality

Figure 15-3   Advantages and disadvantages of functional nursing.

can rotate assignments among staff within legal and organizational contexts to alleviate boredom with repetition. Staff meetings should be conducted frequently. This encourages staff to express concerns and empowers them with the ability to communicate about patient care and unit functions.

Staff Nurse's Role

The staff nurse becomes skilled at the tasks that are usually assigned. Staff follow clearly defined policies and procedures to complete the physical aspects of care in an efficient and economical manner. However, the functional method leaves the professional nurse feeling frustrated because of the task-oriented role. Nurses are educated to care for the patient holistically, and providing only a fragment of care to a patient results in unmet personal and professional expectations of nursing.

The functional method of care delivery works well in emergency and disaster situations. Each care provider knows the expectations of the assigned role and completes the tasks in a quick and efficient style. Subacute care agencies, extended care facilities, and ambulatory clinics use the functional method of care delivery. Severe budgetary cuts, reimbursement mechanisms, and nursing shortages have resulted in organizations changing the **staff mix** and increasing the proportion of unlicensed to licensed personnel. A modification of functional nursing is team nursing.

TEAM NURSING

After World War II the nursing shortage continued. Many nurses who were in the military came home to marry and have children instead of returning to the workforce. Because the functional method received criticism, a new system of team nursing was devised to improve patient satisfaction. "Care through others" became the hallmark of team nursing.

In team nursing a team leader is responsible for coordinating a group of licensed and unlicensed personnel to provide patient care to a small group of patients. The team leader, a highly skilled leader, manager, and practitioner, assigns each member specific

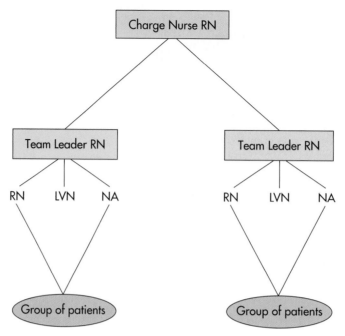

Figure 15-4   Team nursing.

responsibilities dependent on the role. Patients are assigned only to other RNs; care tasks can be assigned across a wide range of staff, depending on their roles and abilities. The members of the team report directly to the team leader, who then reports to the charge nurse or unit manager (Figure 15-4). There are several teams per unit, and patient assignments are made by each team leader. Communication is enhanced through the use of written patient assignments, the development of nursing care plans, and the use of regularly scheduled team conferences to discuss patient status and formulate revisions to the plan of care.

Advantages and Disadvantages

Some advantages of the team method are improved patient satisfaction, organizational decision making occurring at lower levels, and cost-effectiveness for the agency. Many institutions and community health agencies currently use the team nursing method.

Inpatient facilities may view team nursing as a cost-effective system because it works with an expected ratio of unlicensed to licensed personnel. Thus the organization has greater numbers of personnel for a designated amount of money.

The team method of patient care delivery is a good system, if implemented properly; however,

■ *Exercise 15–3*

Think of a time when you worked with a group of four to six people to achieve a specific goal or accomplish a task (perhaps in school you were grouped together to complete a project). How did your group achieve the goal? Was one person the organizer or leader who assigned each member a component, or did you each determine what skills you possessed that would most benefit the group? Did you experience any conflict while working on this project? How did the concepts of group dynamics and leadership skills affect how your group achieved its goal? What similarities do you see between the team nursing system of providing patient care and your group involvement to achieve a goal?

one major disadvantage arises if the team leader has poor leadership skills. The team leader must have excellent communication skills, delegation abilities, conflict resolution techniques, strong clinical skills, and effective decision-making abilities to provide a working "team" environment for the members. If a team environment does not exist, team members might not assume the individual accountability necessary to provide quality patient care (Watkins, 1993). Often, the team leader is not prepared for this role, and the team method becomes a miniature version of the functional method and the potential for fragmentation of care is high.

Nurse Manager's Role

The nurse manager, charge nurse, and team leaders must have management skills to effectively implement the team nursing method of patient care delivery. The unit manager must determine which RNs are skilled and who is interested in becoming a charge nurse or team leader. Because the baccalaureate-prepared RN's basic education emphasizes critical thinking and leadership concepts, they are likely candidates for such roles. The nurse manager should also provide adequate staff mix and orient team members to the team nursing system by providing continuing education about management techniques and group interaction. By addressing these factors, the manager is aiding the teams to function optimally. Managing other staff members' care is viewed as a way of maintaining clinical competence (Nelson, 2000). Do you agree?

The charge nurse functions as a liaison between the team leaders and other healthcare providers. Some charge nurses have a difficult time relinquishing authority; however, the charge nurse needs to encourage each team to solve its problems independently.

The team leader plans the care, delegates the work, and follows up with members to evaluate the quality of care. In the ideal circumstance the team leader updates the nursing care plans and facilitates patient care conferences. Time constraints during the shift may prevent scheduling daily patient care conferences.

The team leader must also face the challenge of changing team membership. Diverse work schedules may result in daily changes in the staff mix of a team and a daily assignment change for team members. The team leader assigns the professional, technical, and ancillary personnel to the type of patient care they are prepared to deliver.

Staff Nurse's Role

Team nursing uses the strengths of each caregiver. The staff nurses, as members of the team, develop strengths in care delivery. Some members become known for their expertise in the psychomotor aspects of care. If one nurse is skilled at starting IVs, she will start all IVs for her team of patients. If a nurse is especially skillful in motivating postoperative patients to use the incentive spirometer and ambulate, he or she should be assigned to the surgical patients. As a member of a group, each person strives to give the best care possible. Under the guidance and supervision of the team leader, the collective efforts of the team become greater than the functions of the individual caregiver.

Modular Method

A modification to team nursing is the modular method of patient care delivery. The modular method focuses on the geographic location of patient rooms and assignment of staff members (Magargal, 1987). The unit is divided into modules, or districts, and the same team of staff members are assigned consistently to the module. Each module has a modular, or team, leader RN who assigns the patients to module staff. Each module ideally consists of at least one RN, one LPN/LVN, and one nursing assistant. The charge nurse expects the module leaders to be accountable for patient care but assists in problem solving when necessary.

Bennett and Hylton (1990) found increased continuity of care when staff was consistently assigned to the same module, and the geographic closeness of the modular system saved nursing time. The modular system can also cost money because it requires a redesign of the work environment to allow medication carts, supplies, and charts to be located in each module. Traditional long corridors are not conducive to **modular nursing.**

The team nursing system originated to improve staff and patient satisfaction in the 1950s. However, RNs are educated to provide holistic care to patients, and they are not able to do this in the team method of patient care delivery. In the late 1960s, the nursing care delivery methods were reevaluated, and the primary nursing system evolved to provide increased autonomy for nurses.

 ## PRIMARY NURSING

A cultural revolution occurred in the United States during the 1960s. The revolution emphasized individual rights and independence from existing societal restrictions. This revolution also influenced the nursing profession because nurses were becoming dissatisfied with their lack of autonomy. Institutions were also aware of declining quality of patient care. The search for autonomy and quality care led to the primary nursing system of patient care delivery as a method to increase RN accountability for patient outcomes.

Primary nursing, an adaptation of the case method, was developed by Marie Manthey as a method of organizing patient care delivery in which one RN functions autonomously as the patient's **primary nurse** throughout the hospital stay. The primary nurse is responsible for 24-hour-a-day total patient care from admission through discharge. Conceptually, primary nursing care provides the patient and the family with coordinated, comprehensive, continuous care (Gray & Smedley, 1998).

Care is organized to use the elements of professional nursing practice (Pontin, 1999). The primary nurse collaborates, communicates, and coordinates all aspects of patient care (Pontin, 1999). Advocacy and assertiveness are leadership attributes desirable for this care delivery strategy.

The primary nurse, preferably baccalaureate prepared, is held accountable for meeting **outcome criteria** and communicating with all other healthcare providers about the patient (Figure 15-5). For example, a patient is admitted to a medical unit with pulmonary edema. His primary nurse admits him and then provides a written plan of care. When his primary nurse is not working, an **associate nurse** implements the plan. The associate nurse is an RN who has been delegated to provide care to the patient according to the primary nurse's specification. If the patient develops additional complications, the associate nurse notifies the primary nurse, who has 24-hour accountability and responsibility. The associate nurse inputs to the patient's plan of care and the primary nurse makes the appropriate alterations.

Advantages and Disadvantages

Primary nursing attracts a high-quality nursing staff who experience professional job satisfaction. Patients and families experience increased satisfaction with the quality of care. These experiences can advance the profession as a whole. Because of a decreased number of nonprofessional staff, healthcare agency costs are reduced.

RNs practicing primary nursing must possess a broad knowledge base and have highly developed nursing skills. In this system of care delivery, professionalism is promoted. Nurses experience a high level of job satisfaction because they are able to use their education to provide holistic and autonomous care for the patient. This high level of accountability for patient outcomes encourages RNs to further their knowledge and refine skills to provide optimal patient care. If the primary nurse is not motivated or feels unqualified to provide holistic care, job satisfaction may decrease.

In primary nursing, patients and families are satisfied with the care they receive because they establish a relationship with the primary nurse and identify the caregiver as "their nurse." Because the patient's primary nurse communicates the plan of care, the patient can move away from the sick role and begin to participate in his or her own recovery. By considering the sociocultural, psychological, and physical needs of the patient and family, the primary nurse can plan the most appropriate care with and for the patient and family.

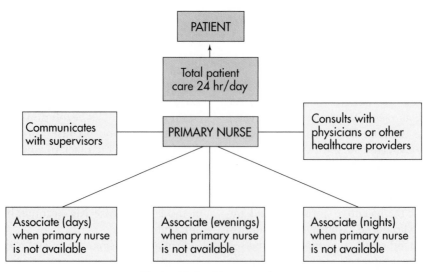

Figure 15-5 Primary nursing.

A professional advantage to the primary nursing method is a decrease in the number of unlicensed personnel. The ideal primary nursing system requires an all-RN staff. The RN can provide total care to the patient, from bed baths to patient education, even both at the same time! Unlicensed personnel are not qualified to provide this level of inclusive care (Figure 15-6).

A disadvantage of the primary nursing method is that the RN may not have the experience or educational background to provide total care. The agency needs to educate staff for an adequate transition from the previous role to the primary role. In addition, the RN may not be ready for or capable of handling the 24-hour responsibility for patient care. In times of nursing shortage, primary nursing may not be the strategy of choice (Jonsdottir, 1999). This strategy will not be effective with a large number of part-time RNs who are not available to assume the primary nurse role.

Exercise 15-4

Mr. Faulkner is admitted to the medical unit with exacerbated congestive heart failure. Mike Ross, RN, BSN, is Mr. Faulkner's primary nurse and will provide total care to Mr.

Faulkner. Mike notes this is Mr. Faulkner's third admission in 6 months for congestive heart failure–related symptoms. This is the first admission for which Mr. Faulkner has had a primary nurse. What do you think will be different about this admission with Mike providing primary nursing to Mr. Faulkner? Do you think there will be any difference in continuity of care? How involved do you think Mr. Faulkner will be with his own care in the primary nursing system?

With the arrival of managed care, patients' hospital stays are shorter than in the 1970s, when primary nursing became popular. Expedited stays make it challenging for primary nurses to adequately provide primary nursing. If the patient is admitted on Monday and discharged on Wednesday, the primary nurse has a difficult time meeting all patient needs before discharge if he or she is not working on Tuesday. The primary nurse must rely heavily on feedback from associates, which defeats the purpose of primary nursing.

Exercise 15-5

Imagine you are a primary nurse at an inpatient psychiatric facility. The patients you are assigned to are usually suicidal. How would you feel about the added responsibility for pa-

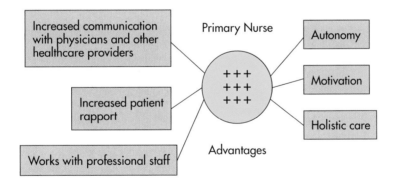

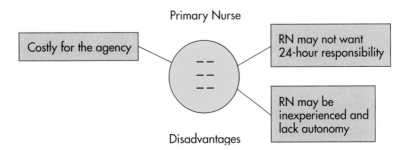

Figure 15-6   Advantages and disadvantages of the primary nursing strategy.

tients even when you were not at work? How would this responsibility affect your personal life? How would you make decisions?

Nurse Manager's Role

The primary nursing system can be modified to meet patient, nursing, and budgetary demands while maintaining the positive components that spawned its conception. The nurse manager needs to determine the desire of staff to become primary nurses and then educate them accordingly. The associate nurses and all other healthcare providers need clearly defined roles. They also need to be aware of the primary nurse's role and the importance of communicating concerns directly to that nurse.

The nurse manager who implements this care delivery strategy experiences some benefits. Primary nursing provides the nurse manager an opportunity to demonstrate leadership capabilities, clinical competencies, and teaching abilities to serve as a role model for professional practice. In addition, the role of budget controller and unit quality manager re-

main. The traditional roles of delegation and decision making must be relinquished to the autonomous primary nurse. The nurse manager functions as a role model, advocate, coach, and consultant. The Research Perspective focuses on the educational needs identified by nurse managers to maintain ongoing professional development.

Staff Nurse's Role

The primary nurse uses many facets of the professional role—caregiver, advocate, decision maker, teacher, collaborator, and manager. With 24-hour responsibility, the primary nurse has the autonomy and authority to deliver individualized, comprehensive, consistent care that is patient focused (Johnson & Tahan, 1997). The associate nurse provides care using the plan of care developed by the primary nurse. Changes to the plan of care can be made by the associate nurse in collaboration with the primary nurse. This strategy provides consistency between nurses and shifts. To function effectively in this setting, staff nurses will need experience and opportunities to be mentored in this role.

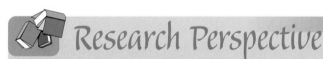 *Research Perspective*

Gould, D., Kelly, D., Goldstone, L., & Maidwell, A. (2001). The changing training needs of clinical nurse managers: Exploring issues for continuing professional development. *Journal of Advanced Nursing, 34*(1), 7-17.

This study surveys 197 clinical nurse managers in the United Kingdom to identify those learning needs required to maintain ongoing competency as a leader and manager of a nursing unit.

The authors' review of the literature revealed that there was no body of work to identify the specific ongoing professional development needs of clinical nurse managers. The nurse manager must possess a broad knowledge base, clinical competence, and the ability to lead and manage. The authors indicate that feelings of competence are related to job satisfaction and low staff turnover.

Sixty-five percent of the nurse managers responded and reported feelings of clinical competence but lacked confidence in a wide range of activities, including being a role model, being involved in clinical decision making, collaborating with medical staff, developing audits, being leaders, maintaining clinical standards, being cur-

rent with speed regarding disciplinary procedures, doing research, understanding risk management, and being involved in team building. The majority of the respondents were considered experienced; 52 had been in their present position for more than 3 years. The interviews also revealed levels of job satisfaction and its relationship to continuing professional development. The greater the number of topics identified as areas for improvement, the more likely the nurse managers were to report low levels of job satisfaction.

IMPLICATIONS FOR PRACTICE

The increasing complexity of leading and managing a nursing care setting requires unique knowledge and skill. The changing picture of healthcare requires ongoing professional development. Creating an environment that promotes lifelong learning will meet the ongoing professional needs of clinical nurse managers.

Because it is not usually financially possible for an agency to employ only RNs, true primary nursing rarely exists. Some institutions have modified the primary nursing concept and implemented a **partnership model** to incorporate their current staff mix.

PARTNERSHIP MODELS

In the partnership model (or coprimary nursing model) of providing patient care, an RN is paired with a technical assistant. The partner works with the RN consistently. When the partner is unlicensed, the RN allows the assistant to perform basic nursing functions. This frees the RN to provide "semiprimary care" to assigned patients. This strategy would be effective in a rehabilitative care setting.

A partnership between an RN and an LPN/LVN is different. The RN's role is to encourage growth in the LPN/LVN partner, and the two share the patient assignments. A study by Eriksen et al. (1992) indicated that the RN-LPN/LVN partnership model, implemented in an intensive care unit, decreased the reported level of stress experienced by the RNs and improved the quality of care provided to the patients. In some settings the partnership is legitimized with an official contract to formalize the relationship.

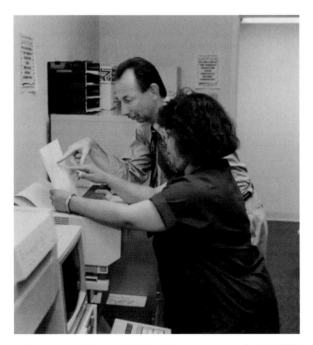

In the partnership model, the RN encourages the LPN/LVN partner's growth and the two share patient assignments.

Exercise 15-6

You are a primary nurse in a surgical intensive care unit of a small hospital. The unit you work on uses an RN-LPN/LVN partnership to decrease the number of RNs required per shift. You and your partner are assigned four surgical patients. Mr. Jones had a lobectomy 5 hours ago and is on a ventilator, Mrs. Martinez had a quadruple cardiac bypass 14 hours ago, Mr. Wong had a nephrectomy 2 days ago and is receiving continuous peritoneal dialysis, and Mr. Smith has a fractured pelvis and is comatose from a motor vehicle accident 24 hours ago. How would you distribute the staff to provide primary care to these four patients? Do you think it is possible to provide primary care in this situation? What responsibilities would you assume as the primary nurse, and what could you share with the LPN/LVN?

Primary nursing can be successful in clinic settings, home health settings, and research centers. There are professional advantages for the RN; however, most agencies are unable to afford a true primary nursing system. Another, relatively new system that is cost effective and allows the professional nurse to direct patient care is the patient-focused care model.

Another view of primary care is the care delivered in a **patient-focused care unit.** This strategy emphasizes quality, cost, and value (Reisdorfer, 1996). During a usual hospitalization, a patient may see dozens of personnel. In an effort to reduce the number of staff and tasks performed by staff, functions become centralized on a unit (Reisdorfer, 1996). Services on a unit can include pharmacy, radiology, dietary, physical therapy, occupational therapy, and social services.

The primary nurse in this model facilitates continuity of care; enhances collaboration with the patient, family, and interdisciplinary team; and controls practice through autonomous decisions (Johnson & Tahan, 1997). The multidisciplinary team formulates the plan of care after the primary nurse and the physician have assessed the patient.

Developed in the late 1980s, the patient-focused care unit strategy integrates principles from business and industry to decrease inefficiencies and create a plan that improves the quality of care, enhances patient and staff satisfaction, and reduces the cost of providing quality care. Like modular nursing discussed earlier, patient-focused care unit requires a change in the physical environment. Services required by patients are decentralized. Satellite laboratories, radiology facilities, pharmacies, and supply rooms are geographically proximate to the patient rooms (Seago, 1999). Original models of a patient-focused care unit included an RN paired with a cross-trained technician who provided bedside care, including respiratory therapy, phlebotomy, and electrocardiographs. Modifications in this nurse-managed model include team members who provide direct care activities such as recording vital signs, drawing blood, and bathing patients. Other support members of the team provide housekeeping and indirect caregiving activities (Seago, 1999).

In a patient-focused care unit, the role and scope of the nurse manager expand. No longer is the individual just a manager of nurses. Now the nurse manager assumes the accountability and responsibility to manage nurses and staff from other, traditionally centralized departments. Because care is focused on the needs of the patient and not the needs of the department, the role of the manager becomes more sophisticated. The nurse manager orchestrates all the care activities required by the patient and family during the hospitalization. Another nursing care delivery strategy that requires a complex set of expectations is the process of nursing case management.

NURSING CASE MANAGEMENT

Developed in 1985 as an outgrowth of primary care, nursing case management is a strategy to coordinate care, maintain quality, and contain costs while focusing on the outcomes of care (Cohen & Cesta, 2001). Nursing case management is a collaborative activity that focuses on comprehensive assessment and intervention and holistic care planning with appropriate referrals to meet the healthcare needs of the patient and the family (Figure 15-7).

"Within the walls," or internal, nursing case management coordinates care in the acute care setting. "Beyond the walls," or external, case management, originally developed in the 1970s by insurance companies in an attempt to control extremely expensive claims, is used by community agencies, outpatient settings, and health maintenance organizations.

The success of nursing case management models has been demonstrated in all healthcare settings, including acute, subacute, and ambulatory settings; long-term care facilities; and health insurance companies and the community. Table 15-1 identifies some of the service settings using this care delivery strategy.

The case management model of patient care delivery maintains quality care while streamlining costs and seeks the active involvement of the patient, the family, and diverse healthcare professionals. Healthcare organizations have tailored the case management system to meet their specific needs. The elements of the **case management method** are the **case manager** and the critical pathway.

Nurse Case Manager

The American Nurses Association recommends a baccalaureate in nursing with 3 years of clinical experience as the minimum preparation for a nurse case manager (NCM) (Bower, 1992). Many case management services prefer master's-prepared clinical nurse specialists who have advanced preparation with the specific populations being served. The case manager is client focused and outcome-oriented. He or she facilitates and promotes coordination of cost-

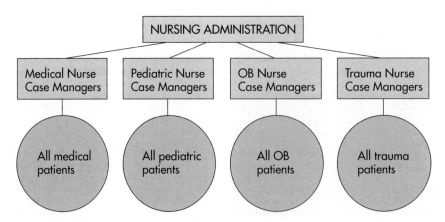

Figure 15-7 Nurse case management strategy in which all patients are assigned to a nurse case manager.

effective care, collaborates with members of the healthcare team, responds to needs of insurers, merges clinical and financial interests, and plays a role in the marketing strategies of the organization (Bower, 1992). In addition, the NCM serves as an advocate for the patient and the family.

Depending on the facility, there may be several case managers to coordinate care for all patients, or a case manager may be assigned to a specific high-risk population (see Figure 15-7). The case manager may be responsible to coordinate care for 20 patients. It is essential that the case manager have frequent interaction with the patient and the healthcare provider to achieve and evaluate **expected outcomes.**

In organizations that use this process, the NCM is assigned a patient on admission (or preadmission) based on the case manager's specialization. The NCM then coordinates patient care until discharge. The patient will have a specific **care MAP** (multidisciplinary action plan), or a **critical path,** based on a related diagnosis-related group (DRG) category. The case manager will implement the plan and be responsible for monitoring patient progress toward the desired outcome criteria. This progress is communicated to the physicians, nurses, and other healthcare providers. All healthcare providers work together to decrease the patient's length of stay while addressing patient problems.

Example:
Imagine you are the NCM responsible for pediatric patients. Margo, age 3, is admitted to the emergency room (ER) with severe shortness of breath and a history of asthma. You introduce yourself to Margo and her mother as the case manager responsible for

coordinating Margo's care throughout her hospital stay. You implement the care MAP used at your hospital and plan her care with the ER nurse and physician. After 2 hours Margo is transferred to the pediatric intensive care unit (ICU). The ICU nurses follow the care MAP, identifying patient problems and the normal tests and treatments expected on day 1 (Box 15-1). On day 3, Margo is transferred to the pediatric floor, where you will coordinate her care with her mother, the nurse, and the physician. The nurses follow the care MAP you initiated and discuss any variations with you. When Margo is ready for discharge on day 4, you talk with her mother and arrange a follow-up phone call. You have been the pivotal person for Margo and her mother throughout this admission. Your main goal is to expedite Margo's hospitalization and prevent a readmission. If Margo is readmitted, you will be her NCM.

CRITICAL PATHWAYS AND CARE MAPS

The tool case managers use to achieve patient outcomes is a critical path. Critical paths are grids that outline the critical or key events expected to happen each day of a patient's hospitalization (Cohen & Cesta, 2001). The critical path component is based on the DRG services provided by all disciplines for the patient's particular DRG classification. Box 15-1 lists the various components of a critical path.

Care MAPs are a combination of the nursing care plan and the critical path. The care plan component is similar to the care plans typically used, except a time is indicated for each intervention of the nursing diagnosis. (See the example in Box 15-1.)

Table 15-1 **NURSE CASE MANAGEMENT SERVICE AREAS**	
Category	**Service Setting**
Acute	Inpatient units: orthopedics, cardiovascular, critical care, high-risk perinatal, oncology
Subacute	Skilled nursing centers, rehabilitation units
Ambulatory	Physician's office, emergency rooms
Long-term care	Nursing homes, group homes, assisted-living facilities
Insurance companies	Health maintenance organizations (HMOs), preferred provider organizations (PPOs), workers' compensation, Medicaid, Medicare
Community	Nurse-managed centers, home health agencies, urgent care centers, schools, rural settings

Modified from information presented in Tahan (1999), Huber (2000), Cohen & Cesta (2001), and Stanton & Packa (2001).

BOX 15-1

Pediatric Asthma Care MAP (Example)

Critical Path

Care Category	Day 1	Day 2	Day 3	Day 4
Consults	None	None	None	None
Tests	CBC, theophylline level, BMP, PPD, chest x-ray, ABGs, urine dipstick, and specific gravity $\times$ 1	Theophylline level, ABGs if indicated	Theophylline level, check PPD	Theophylline level
Treatments	Pulse oximetry, postural drainage, peak expiratory flow if cooperative every shift, O_2 therapy if indicated, IVs if indicated	Peak flow every shift, chest PT every shift	Peak flow bid, chest PT every shift	Peak flow q24h; consider discharge if increased peak flow
Medications	(Amount according to weight) Aminophylline and/or Proventil NEB/PO and/or steroids	Steroids may be discontinued within 48 hr or taper over 7-10 days; assess for change to PO medications	Assess change to PO medications	Consider discharge home within 24 hr of initiation of PO medications
Activity	As tolerated	As tolerated	As tolerated	As tolerated
Nutrition	As tolerated	As tolerated	As tolerated	As tolerated
Discharge Plan	Inquire whether family used home care before admission; begin initial discharge plan	Initiate social work consult as indicated	Monitor progress on discharge plan, consult with physician, social worker, home health care; physician to give 24-hr notice to patient and write official discharge order	Before discharge confirm home plan with parents, social worker, and home health care

Patient Variance (includes variances in response to treatment or special needs on admission; for example, the patient may also have an infection)

Patient Problems/Potential Problems

	Day 1	Day2	Day 3	Day 4
Alteration in breathing patterns	a. Auscultate breath sounds for rales, wheezing, stridor, rhonchi	a. Auscultate breath sounds	a. Auscultate breath sounds, check color, retractions, nasal flaring q8h and prn	a. Auscultate breath sounds, check color, retractions, nasal flaring q8h and prn
	b. Assess skin and mucous membrane color and nasal flaring q4h	b. Assess color changes	b. Monitor and record vital signs q8h	b. Monitor and record vital signs q8h

BOX 15-1

Pediatric Asthma Care MAP (Example)—cont'd

Patient Problems/Potential Problems—cont'd

	Day 1	Day2	Day 3	Day 4
Alteration in breathing patterns—cont'd	c. Note agitation, anxiety	c. Assess for retractions, nasal flaring q6h	c. Assess for retractions, O_2 saturation; determine discharge readiness	c. Assess for retractions, O_2 saturation; determine discharge readiness
	d. Note changes in vital signs or O_2 saturation	d. Note changes in vital signs and O_2 to discharge oximeter	d. Chest PT every shift unless contraindicated	d. Chest PT every shift unless contraindicated
	e. Monitor response to treatment (notify physician of headache, agitation, tachycardia, respiratory distress)	e. Chest PT every shift	e. Observe response to nebulizer treatment and check with physician	e. Observe response to nebulizer treatment and check with physician
	f. Chest PT every shift, position for chest expansion	f. Monitor response to treatment (report to physician changes, headache, increased respirations, distress, agitation, tachycardia)	f. Assess response to activity	f. Assess response to activity
	g. Encourage PO fluids, assess hydration status	g. Assess peak flow every shift	g. Assess clinical state, increased peak flow, tolerance of PO medications, theophylline level therapeutic	g. Assess clinical state, increased peak flow, tolerance of PO medications, theophylline level therapeutic
		h. Assess patient's response to activity		
		i. Encourage PO fluids		
Knowledge deficit	a. Orient to environment	a. Assess family and patient teaching needs for disease process and begin discharge teaching	a. Continue discharge teaching regarding medications, treatment, and importance of follow-up	a. Discharge planning

Modified from Cohen, E. L., & Cesta, T. G. (1993). *Nursing case management: From concept to evaluation.* St. Louis: Mosby.
ABGs, Arterial blood gases; *BMP,* basic metabolic profile; *CBC,* complete blood count; *ER,* emergency room; *IV,* intravenous; *PPD,* purified protein derivative; *PT,* physiotherapy.

Continued

BOX 15-1

Pediatric Asthma Care MAP (Example)—cont'd

Patient Problems/Potential Problems—cont'd

	Day 1	Day2	Day 3	Day 4
Knowledge deficit —cont'd	b. Assess parent and child level of understanding	b. Assess need for visiting nurse, community referrals	b. Discharge plan with parents to minimize respiratory irritants at home and in the environment	b. Medication review
	c. Familiarize with hospital protocol (e.g., IV pump, medications, treatment)			c. Signs and symptoms of respiratory distress review
				d. Identify precipitating factors for asthma attack
				e. Exercise regimen
				f. Follow-up care
				g. When to call physician/ come to ER
Anxiety	a. Provide calm environment	a. Encourage family to state feelings, fears, and anxieties	a. Continue to encourage verbalization of concerns	a. Reevaluate level of anxiety and provide support
	b. Explore stressors and coping mechanisms	b. Evaluate anxiety level and provide supportive measures prn	b. Reevaluate level of anxiety	b. Reassure parents/child regarding knowledge of asthma
	c. Assess family dynamics			
	d. Encourage parent to stay with child			

Modified from Cohen, E. L., & Cesta, T. G. (1993). *Nursing case management: From concept to evaluation.* St. Louis: Mosby.
ABGs, Arterial blood gases; *BMP,* basic metabolic profile; *CBC,* complete blood count; *ER,* emergency room; *IV,* intravenous; *PPD,* purified protein derivative; *PT,* physiotherapy.

The primary reason to implement a care MAP is to provide a written system for identifying patient and family needs. All healthcare providers follow the care MAP to improve the quality of care, decrease the length of stay, change practice patterns to increase efficiency, facilitate outcomes, and reduce costs.

Development of critical paths and care MAPs can occur in various ways. Organizations can purchase paths for high-volume case types and individualize them according to the practice patterns within the organization, or the staff of a healthcare agency can develop its own care path/MAP. Accomplishing this process involves a number of steps.

Initially, the diagnosis for MAP development is determined. This decision is usually based on the volume of patients admitted with a particular diagnosis. For example, patients with myocardial infarction, chronic obstructive pulmonary disease, or joint replacement might be a first choice. The standards of care for the particular healthcare problem are reviewed. Retrospective chart review or concurrent chart review of patients currently receiving services for selected case types can identify patterns that can be incorporated into the path (Cardinal, Kraushar, & Wagie, 1994). This audit of charts can also identify costs associated with the treatment. Pathway/MAP development teams are organized to develop the tool. Membership on the team will include members from diverse departments involved in the care of the patient. For example, a team might include a physician, nurse manager, staff nurse, social worker, dietitian, occupational therapist, and pharmacist.

Following the audit, key patient care expectations and critical events are identified for incorporation into the path (Klenner, 2000). Small groups within the development team work to refine the elements of the path/MAP. Documentation strategies and discharge planning and instructions are affected by path/MAP development and may require revision. Newly developed tools can be tested on previously admitted patients. In essence, the patient's hospital stay is "redocumented" to identify usability of the tool (Klenner, 2000). Implementation of the tool can be enhanced through the networking of the development team members with their respective colleagues. Team cooperation and collaboration for path/MAP development improves utilization because all team members authored the tool and have a vested interest in the process (Berry, Cranston, & Fox, 2000).

If a patient's progress deviates from the normal path/MAP, a variance is indicated. A **variance** is anything that occurs to alter the patient's progress through the normal critical path. Analysis of variance is essential for effective utilization of a path/MAP. Circumstances that can cause a variance include operational, provider, patient, or clinical elements (Cohen & Cesta, 2001). Operational causes include broken equipment or interdepartmental delays. Changes in the practice pattern of the healthcare provider can affect the pathway and cause a variance. Complications in the patient's condition, such as a hemorrhage into the joint af-

ter total knee replacement, may increase total hospital days. A complication can inhibit the ability of the patient to meet the clinical indicator as described in the path/MAP. A patient or family's refusal of a specific component of care can create a variance.

Variances can be positive or negative. A negative variance is an undesired outcome, whereas a positive variance is an outcome that is achieved before it is expected (Cohen & Cesta, 2001). A patient undergoing a second hip replacement who attended preoperative classes and engaged in activities to "ready himself" for the surgery may actually leave the hospital sooner than predicted on the care MAP. The NCM on the orthopedic unit and the insurance company's case manager would view this as a positive variance.

Advantages and Disadvantages

Nursing case management is a process for providing comprehensive care for those with complex health problems. Case management provides a well-coordinated care experience that can improve the care outcome, decrease the length of stay, and use multiple disciplines and services efficiently. Families and patients receive care across a continuum of settings, often from diverse institutions. NCMs can break down invisible institutional barriers for the client (Guttman, 1999). Nurses receive a sense of satisfaction knowing that the patient and family received coordinated, quality care in a cost-effective manner across the spectrum of the illness or injury.

Nursing leaders across the country and in diverse health settings identified major obstacles in the implementation of case management services. Financial barriers, lack of administrative support, human resource inequities, turf battles, and the lack of information support systems have been identified as obstacles in the implementation of case management services (Rantz & Bopp, 1996). Case management is not a revenue-generating activity, but rather a "revenue-protecting" activity. It minimizes costs for those case types with the potential of high resource consumption (Rantz & Bopp, 1996). Consequently, case management can be seen as an expense.

The development of collaborative models of healthcare management incorporating nurses, social workers, and utilization case managers have demonstrated significant cost savings. Some institutions have developed departments of healthcare case management. In this setting the NCM works with the "medically complex," the social worker with the "socially complex," and utilization management for utilization review. This team of case managers, each with identified core functions, also has specialty functions based on the specific scope of responsibility (Cohen & Cesta, 2001). Collaboration among these case managers has positively affected health delivery costs.

Education and preparation of case managers is a major human resource issue. Inadequately educated staff may be assigned as case managers. The ideal case manager is a clinical nurse specialist. Performance appraisal of the case manager presents another human resource challenge. The case manager does not manage other employees; rather the case manager manages patients and their care. How is this individual's performance evaluated? As with any other nursing position, performance appraisal criteria must be developed before the implementation of the process.

Who should be the case manager is a hotly contested question. Physicians see themselves as the managers of care. Social workers lay claim to this role. Nursing staff may see case management as utilization review. Nursing case management is a professionally autonomous role that requires expert clinical knowledge and decision-making skills. Publications by the American Nurses Association have served to clarify the role, scope, and function of the NCM (Bower, 1992).

Disease management programs take the role of the NCM to another level of responsibility (Goldstein, 1998). Disease management is population based, focused on improving the quality of life, reducing hospital readmissions, and enhancing longevity through ongoing management of chronic conditions (Brown, 2000; Goldstein, 1998). Those with chronic conditions who are high consumers of healthcare dollars are the recipients of disease-managed care. Chronic illnesses such as arthritis, asthma, cardiovascular disease, congestive heart disease, and diabetes are the prime focus of disease management programs (Given, 2001). All chronic and hereditary conditions are predicted to be disease managed in an attempt to reduce extensive costs associated with these conditions (Goldstein, 1998).

Disease management consists of assessment, comprehensive patient and family education, medical management based on treatment algorithms, and focused visits with the healthcare team in an ambulatory setting to assist with adherence to the treatment protocol (Cohen & Cesta, 2001). NCMs often decide whether a patient meets the specific criteria for a disease-managed program. Patients with complex healthcare needs and multiple diagnoses will continue to need extensive nursing case management and will not be eligible for a specific disease management program (Goldstein, 1998).

Nurse Manager's Role

The nurse manager has increased demands when leading the case management system. Quality improvement is constantly assessed to ensure the care MAP is DRG appropriate and that case managers are adequately managing their caseloads. Reimbursement for the care delivered is tied to effective planning and care delivery within the case management process. Patient satisfaction is also pertinent to evaluate for quality. If the patients are not satisfied with the system, the census may decline.

Communication among all systems must be coordinated. Because the NCM works with all departments, the nurse manager may need to facilitate interdepartmental communication. Educating the staff of other departments about the NCM's role and responsibilities will increase the effectiveness of the case management process.

Staff Nurse's Role

The staff nurse provides patient care according to the case manager's specifications and must know the extent of the case manager's role. The case management system of patient care delivery is designed to move a patient from the illness state to optimal wellness as quickly as possible.

It is a concern that the art of nursing may vanish with an increased emphasis on moving patients quickly through the **care delivery system** to save money. The prospective payment system common in the managed care environment dictates that nursing must develop new systems of care delivery to maintain quality care. One way to facilitate quality care is to consider the different abilities and education of the nurses caring for the patient. According to the American Association of Colleges of Nursing (AACN), it is no longer reasonable or useful to prepare a nurse to be all things to all people (Billingsley, 1995).

DIFFERENTIATED NURSING PRACTICE

Differentiated nursing practice acknowledges the education, skill mix, and competency of each RN. Clearly defined competencies for the various levels of nurses are the foundation for differentiated practice (Foss & Koerner, 1997). Nurses prepared at the associate/diploma, baccalaureate, master's, and doctorate level are integrated in the differentiated practice model. Each defined role is different and complementary. Nurses choose the role based on their competency, skill, desire, and education (Foss & Koerner, 1997).

Refinements in differentiated practice have been in place in various clinical settings. Sioux Valley Hospital in Sioux Falls, South Dakota, has used a differentiated practice model in combination with a case management mode. Associate, primary, and advanced practice nurses were the cornerstone of the model. The associate nurse in the Sioux Valley Model was responsible for the assigned patient during a shift (Foss & Koerner, 1997). Critical paths guided the care delivered. The primary nurse coordinated care from admission to discharge for those with complex psychosocial, educational, or discharge planning needs (Foss & Koerner, 1997). Clinical nurse specialists and nurse practitioners, the advanced practice nurses, were responsible for care throughout the illness episode. The advanced practice nurse interacted and collaborated with multiple disciplines to coordinate ongoing care across all healthcare settings (Foss & Koerner, 1997).

Incentives for implementing differentiated practice have been identified and include (1) the ability to identify the differences in preparation of nurses by level of education; (2) the ability to use different levels of nurses to meet the total needs of the patient; (3) improved clinical outcomes that are cost effective; (4) enhanced prestige of nursing through the identification of different levels of nursing to the public, the payers, and healthcare administration; (5) effective utilization of nursing resources to meet the diverse needs of managed care; and (6) career satisfaction with equitable compensation (Bellack & Loquist, 1999).

As the complexity of healthcare increases and the pressures of managed care exert their influence, areas such as communication and critical thinking will become more paramount. Differentiated practice in nursing can respond to these changing healthcare systems, payment strategies, and rising acuities and complex healthcare needs seen in patients and their families.

Nurse Manager's Role

Implementation of the differentiated practice model requires a shift in managerial style. Use of participatory managerial behaviors becomes essential. The nurse manager has the responsibility as a role model and mentor to encourage the professional growth of the staff. Collaborating with the staff to expand decision making, problem solving, and goal setting becomes essential. The manager becomes a teacher, coach, and facilitator. Leadership behaviors of the manager in a differentiated practice setting become vital to the success of the organization. Successful managers demonstrate mutual trust, respect for ideas, and consideration of feelings. This leadership and management style expands the freedom of the nursing care delivered.

Staff Nurse's Role

Nursing staff practicing in the differentiated model find opportunities for more meaningful work. Increased autonomy, authority, and accountability provide opportunities to gain control over nursing practice. With greater control and responsibility comes a sense of empowerment.

Nursing competency and education can also determine advancement. Many organizations use clinical ladders for advancement. If a specific level is attainable with certain skills and education, a nurse can advance in position and salary according to the organization's structure. The differentiated model of care delivery describes a system of organizing nursing practice according to the education, clinical experience, competency, and decision making required by the patient and family needs.

COMPARISONS OF DELIVERY STRATEGIES

Each patient care delivery strategy has identified strengths and weaknesses. There is no perfect method of delivering nursing care to groups of patients and their families. No strategy is used in its "pure form." Patient care delivery must be individualized to the care setting. With modification, each strategy can be used by hospitals, clinics, and home health and community agencies.

The Solution

As a charge nurse, I am required to know about all the patients and have the ability to make assignments according to the knowledge, strengths, and capabilities of the staff. As a result of my individualized assessment of each person's ability, I learned that several of the staff, including the LVN/LPNs, were really terrific nurses. However, they were performing at a level to minimally meet expectations of the position held. Some staff felt isolated from their colleagues who worked the other 12 hours of the day. Others voiced a sense of isolation from other critical care nurses. Working with each person allowed me to discover that these nurses wanted to expand their body of knowledge. Some even indicated a desire to return to school. How did this happen?

I tried to empower the nurses by getting them to teach me things I didn't know. I taught them aspects of care they were not accustomed to performing. Today, these nurses are more involved with the diverse elements of the unit's operation. The staff appear more satisfied with their positions. As the nurses began to feel empowered, it became easier to bring up and discuss issues with the assistant nurse manager and the nurse manager. Problems and concerns are now being addressed. The staff on our shift have become part of the solution. We have begun to discuss strategies to assist the day shift to do the same.

— Laura Atkins

 Would this approach be suitable for you? Why?

CHAPTER CHECKLIST

The roles of the nurse manager and staff nurse vary with each nursing care delivery strategy. Regardless of the strategy, the nurse manager must have strong leadership and management skills for the strategy to be effective. Numerous issues must be considered when a care delivery strategy is implemented. Without a competent manager, none of the discussed strategies would be effective.

- A care delivery strategy is the method nurses use to provide care to patients.
- There are five strategies of patient care delivery, each with its advantages and disadvantages:
  - The case method focuses on total patient care for a specific time period.
    - The nurse manager must consider the expense of this system and identify all staff members' level of education and communication skills.
  - The functional method emphasizes task-oriented care for a large group of patients.
    - The nurse manager is responsible for achieving patient outcomes, whereas staff members are responsible only for their specific tasks.
    - The functional method is most often used in subacute care facilities.
  - In the team method, a small team provides care to a small group of patients.
    - The nurse manager in this strategy needs strong management, critical thinking, and leadership skills.
    - The modular method is a modification of team nursing that focuses on the geographic location of patient rooms and assignments of staff members.
  - In the primary nursing method, a primary nurse provides total patient care and directs patient care from admission to discharge.
    - The nurse manager functions as role model, advocate, coach, consultant, budget controller, and unit quality manager.
    - The partnership model, or coprimary nursing model, pairs an RN with a technical assistant.
    - The patient-focused care unit employs a primary nurse and multiskilled team members.
  - The nursing case management system is outcome based and is facilitated by a case manager, who directs unit-based care using a critical path/care MAP.
    - The nurse manager in this care delivery system faces increased demands and pressure to move the patient through the system as quickly as possible.
    - Managed care is a way of organizing patient care delivery with cost savings as the main goal.

- The nurse manager and charge nurse are responsible for directing patient care regardless of the delivery system. Key leadership and management concepts for directing patient care include the following:
  - Accountability
  - Delegation
  - Critical thinking
  - Communication
  - Promotion of autonomy
  - Collaboration
- The concept of differentiated practice emphasizes two levels of nursing practice: technical and professional.
  - Each level has specific roles and responsibilities that depend on the nurse's educational preparation, experience, and clinical expertise.
  - All the nursing roles complement each other.

TIPS FOR CARE DELIVERY STRATEGIES

- Look at the organization and the population being served when selecting a care delivery strategy.
- The mission and philosophy of an organization will affect the selection process.
- Evaluate staff mix trends to determine whether there is a potential impact on your care delivery approach.
- There are advantages and disadvantages to any strategy; there is no ideal approach.

- Know that every strategy has specific expectations for both managers and staff.

TERMS TO KNOW

associate nurse
care delivery strategy
care MAP
case management method
case manager
case method
charge nurse
critical path
differentiated nursing practice
expected outcomes
functional nursing
modular nursing
outcome criteria
partnership model
patient-focused care unit
patient outcomes
primary nurse
primary nursing
staff mix
team nursing
total patient care
unlicensed assistive personnel
variance

REFERENCES

Bellack, J. P., & Loquist, R. S. (1999). Employer responses to differentiated nursing education. *Journal of Nursing Administration, 29*(9), 4-8, 32.

Bennett, M., & Hylton, J. (1990). Modular nursing: Partners in professional practice. *Nursing Management, 21*(3), 20-24.

Berry, V., Cranston, B., & Fox, T. (2000). Caremapping: "What's in it for nurses?" *Nursing Case Management, 5*(2), 63-72.

Billingsley, M. (1995). The differentiated nurse. *Nursing Connections, 8*(2), 12-13.

Bower, K. A. (1992). *Case management by nurses.* Washington, DC: American Nurses Publishing.

Brown, M. J. (2000). Stroke management: Beginnings. *Outcomes Management for Nursing Practice, 4*(1), 34-38.

Cardinal, J., Kraushar, V. K., & Wagie, T. (1994). Implementation of episodic case management in a managed care organization. In R. S. Howe (Ed.), *Case management for health care professionals.* Chicago: Precept Press.

Cohen, E. L., & Cesta, T. G. (1993). *Nursing case management: From concept to evaluation.* St. Louis: Mosby.

Cohen, E. L., & Cesta, T. G. (2001). *Nursing case management: From essentials to advanced practice applications* (3rd ed.). St. Louis: Mosby.

Eriksen, L., Quandt, B., Teinert, D., Look, D., Loosle, R., Mackey, G., & Strout, B. (1992). A registered nurse-licensed vocational nurse partnership model for critical care nursing. *Journal of Nursing Administration, 22*(12), 28-37.

Foss, N., & Koerner, J. (1997). The advanced practice nurse's role in differentiated practice: Martha's story. *AACN Clinical Issues, 8,* 262-270.

Given, B. A. (2001). Nurse practitioners: Issues within a managed care environment. In J. M. Dochterman & H. K. Grace (Eds.), *Current issues in nursing* (6th ed.). St. Louis: Mosby.

Goldstein, R. (1998). The disease management approach to cost containment. *Nursing Case Management, 3*(3), 99-103.

Gould, D., Kelly, D., Goldstone, L., & Maidwell, A. (2001). The changing training needs of clinical nurse managers: Exploring issues for continuing professional development. *Journal of Advanced Nursing, 34*(1), 7-17.

Gray, R., & Smedley, N. (1998). Assessing primary nursing in mental health. *Nursing Standard, 12*(21), 35-36.

Guttman, R. (1999). Case management of the frail elderly in the community. *Clinical Nurse Specialist, 13,* 174-178.

Huber, D. (2000). The diversity of case management models. *Lippincott's Case Management, 5,* 248-255.

Johnson, T., & Tahan, H. (1997). Care management: Outcomes-based practice for the primary nurse. *Journal of Nursing Care Quality, 11*(5), 55-68.

Jonsdottir, H. (1999). Outcomes of implementing primary nursing in the care of people with chronic lung diseases: The nurses' experience. *Journal of Nursing Management, 7,* 235-242.

Klenner, S. (2000). Mapping out a clinical pathway. *RN, 63*(6), 33-36.

Magargal, P. (1987). Modular nursing: Nurses rediscover nursing. *Nursing Management, 18*(11), 98-104.

Nelson, J. W. ((2000). Models of nursing care: A century of vacillation. *Journal of Nursing Administration, 30*(4), 156, 184.

Pontin, D. (1999). Primary nursing: a mode of care or a philosophy of nursing? *Journal of Advanced Nursing, 29,* 584-591.

Rantz, M. J., & Bopp, K. D. (1996). Issues of design and implementation from acute care, long term care and community based settings. In E. L. Cohen (Ed.), *Nurse case management in the 21st century.* St. Louis: Mosby.

Reisdorfer, J. T. (1996). Building a patient-focused care unit. *Nursing Management, 27*(10), 38, 40, 42, 44.

Seago, J. A. (1999). Evaluation of a hospital work redesign: Patient-focused care. *Journal of Nursing Administration, 29*(11), 31-38.

Stanton, M. P., & Packa, D. (2001). Nursing case management: A rural practice model. *Lippincott's Case Management, 6*(3), 96-103.

Tahan, H. A. (1999). Clarifying case management: What is in a label? *Nursing Case Management, 4,* 268-278.

Watkins, S. (1993). Team spirit. *Nursing Times, 89*(1), 59-60.

SUGGESTED READINGS

Cole, L., & Houston, S. (1999). Structured care methodologies: Evolution and use in patient care delivery. *Outcomes Management for Nursing Practice, 3*(2), 53-59.

Cook, T. H. (1998). The effectiveness of inpatient case management. *Journal of Nursing Administration, 28*(4), 36-46.

Coughlin, C. (2000). Management case studies: Is now the time to design new care delivery models? *Journal of Nursing Administration, 30*(9), 403-404.

Davidhizar, R., Dowd, S., & Brownson, K. (1998). An equitable nursing assignment structure, *Nursing Management, 29*(4), 33-36.

Marks, L., Dennis, R., Borozny, M., & Ferrone, K. (1999). The new team triad. *Nursing Management, 30*(2), 44-46.

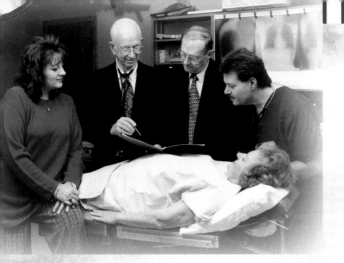

Staffing and Scheduling

Catherine M. Kirk

This chapter explains key concepts related to staffing and scheduling. It defines and discusses the interrelationship between the personnel budget and the staffing plan and reviews measures for evaluating unit productivity. It also discusses the impact of various staffing and scheduling strategies on overall nursing satisfaction and continuity of patient care. These key points are critical to nurse managers' ability to deliver safe and effective care and services in their areas of responsibility while maintaining a high degree of employee satisfaction and controlling the unit's labor expenses. Nurse managers' ability to use this information is critical to their ability to lead productive services.

Objectives

- Identify key external and internal organizational variables that affect staffing plans.
- Analyze activity reports to determine the effectiveness of a unit's productivity.
- Examine personal scheduling needs in relation to the patient's need for continuity of care and the nurse manager's need to create a schedule that is balanced and fair for all team members.
- Relate floating, mandatory overtime, and the use of supplemental agency staff to staff satisfaction and patient care outcomes.

Questions to Consider

- What activity measures can be used to assess unit workload levels?
- How do managers know that staffing on their units is adequate for the units' workload?
- What factors need to be considered by a manager to ensure that a schedule is both balanced and equitable?

The Challenge

Catherine Kirk, RN, MSN
Executive Director of Heart and Lung Services, All Saints Healthcare System, Racine, Wisconsin

The intensive care unit (ICU) at Saint Mary's Medical Center in Racine, Wisconsin, is a very busy 15-bed unit. The ICU staff work 12-hour shifts and every third weekend but are often requested to add hours above their full-time equivalent (FTE; regular schedule) to accommodate a census that has been trending upward for many months. The staff are very involved in the scheduling process, using a staffing committee and a modified approach to self-scheduling to create the unit's monthly schedule. Night-shift staffing has been inadequate for more than 12 months, resulting in all ICU staff floating to the night shift on a regular basis to meet staffing needs. Staff who float to the night shift are often on overtime or bonus pay, a fact that has created significant undesirable variances in the ICU staffing budget. Floating to the night shift has been a source of staff dissatisfaction and has contributed to some recent unit turnover.

Experienced ICU candidates inquiring about night-shift positions are a rare occurrence at Saint Mary's. Thus, when a registered nurse with 12 years of ICU experience moved to the community and applied for a full-time night-shift position, both the manager and the ICU staffing committee were elated. There was just one catch. The potential employee revealed in her application that she had two scheduling requirements that must be met if she was to take a position in this unit. First, she could work only 8-hour shifts because of child care needs. Second, she would require every Saturday off for religious reasons but would be willing to work every Sunday in exchange for this consideration. The manager had to decide what actions to take.

 What do you think you would do if you were this nurse?

INTRODUCTION

Healthcare costs are escalating at a furious pace. Healthcare organizations have recognized that controlling labor costs is one of the most effective strategies for overall cost reduction. Because nursing salaries constitute one of the major drivers of labor costs in a healthcare organization, nurse leaders are increasingly challenged to tightly manage staffing and scheduling within nursing cost centers. Nurse managers must make skilled staffing and scheduling decisions to ensure that safe and cost-effective care is provided by the appropriate level of caregiver. No matter what the practice setting—acute care, home care, or long-term care—there is an increased focus on manager accountability for establishing and monitoring effective and efficient staffing systems.

STAFFING

Nurse managers' roles are complex and demanding. Of the many responsibilities and challenges the roles entail, staffing remains one of the most pivotal to daily unit operations, to patient and family satisfaction with care and services, and to employee satisfaction. Staffing issues often cause nurse managers great concern.

Staffing is a function of planning for hiring and deploying qualified human resources to meet the needs of patients for care and services. Nurse managers have several opportunities to influence the use of staffing resources in the unit. First, nurse managers are accountable for projecting the staffing needs of a unit each year during the preparation of a unit's personnel budget. Second, nurse managers are accountable for using the approved personnel budget to prepare a balanced staffing plan and schedule for a unit. Finally, nurse managers are responsible for monitoring, evaluating, and modifying the staffing plan over the course of the year based on a unit's volume and acuity trends.

THE STAFFING PROCESS

Because the staffing process guides the development of a unit's staffing plan for the year, it is typically conducted in conjunction with the development of the personnel budget. Nurse managers must consider a number of variables that affect both the staffing process and the personnel budget.

External Variables That Affect Staffing Plans

Nurse managers must consider a number of external variables when preparing the personnel budget and projecting the unit's staffing needs. The external variables that are considered are highlighted in the following sections.

State Licensing Standards

An important source for guidance in projecting staffing requirements is the licensing regulations of the state department of health. **Staffing regulations** or recommendations usually relate to the minimum number of professional nurses required on a unit at a given time or to the amount of minimum staffing in an extended care facility or prison. Most states establish broad guidelines for minimum nurse staffing levels. However, a number of states, responding to the concerns of healthcare professionals and the public, have mandated or are attempting to mandate what the minimum nurse staffing level must be through the legislative process (nursingworld.org).

JCAHO and Other Regulatory Agency Standards

There are a number of national organizations with the mission to continuously improve the safety and quality of healthcare provided to the public. The Joint Commission on Accreditation of Healthcare Organizations (JCAHO) is an example of this type of organization. JCAHO works to support performance improvement in healthcare organizations through establishing standards and survey accreditation. To comply with the 2001 JCAHO patient care standards related to staffing, for example, an institution must "provide an adequate number of staff members with the experience and training needed." JCAHO is not prescriptive as to what constitutes "adequate" staffing. However, in response to increasing public concerns about patient care safety and quality, JCAHO has initiated an effort to begin correlating an organization's clinical outcome data with its staffing ratios to determine the effectiveness of the overall staffing plan.

During the JCAHO accreditation process, the surveyor reviews the staffing plans developed by the nurse manager for any obvious staffing deficiencies—for example, a shift without a registered nurse (RN) assigned to the unit. The surveyor also interviews staff nurses outside of the presence of nurse managers to inquire about staff perceptions of units' staffing adequacy (JCAHO, 2001). Nurse managers are well advised to prepare a balanced staffing plan that supports a unit's unique patient care needs and the scrutiny of the JCAHO survey process.

Additional regulatory agencies that provide accreditation services similar to those provided by JCAHO include the Center for Accreditation of Rehabilitation Facilities (CARF), the Accreditation Association for Ambulatory Health Care (AAAHC), the National Committee for Quality Assurance in Behavioral Health, and the Community Health Accreditation Program.

American Nurses Association Standards

The debate over what constitutes minimum staffing is polarizing nurses and the organizations that employ them. The American Nurses Association (ANA) speaks on behalf of professional nurses working in the United States. The ANA has established a number of standards for professional nursing practice, including principles for safe staffing (Box 16-1), that apply to all clinical care settings. Nurse managers must consider the relationship between these standards of care and their staffing plans as they develop the unit budgets because managers are as accountable for the safe provision of quality patient care as they are for fiscal management of the unit.

Although the ANA is not prescriptive relative to optimal staffing levels, they have supported research over the last decade to determine the effect of minimizing professional nursing positions in a staffing plan. Nursing researchers and others established a correlation between RN staffing levels and the quality of patient care outcomes, such as length of hospital stay, postoperative infection, and the development of hospital-acquired complications (e.g. pneumonia, urinary tract infections, pressure ulcers) (American Nurses Association, 2000b). Noting that these quality indicators show improvement with more RN involvement in patient care, professional nursing organizations such as the ANA are encouraging nurses to demand higher RN-to-patient ratios in clinical practice settings.

Meanwhile, healthcare organizations continue efforts to reduce rising labor costs by undertaking major reengineering of traditional nursing staffing models to decrease the RN-to-patient ratios. As a

BOX 16-1

ANA Principles for Nurse Staffing

Principles

The nine principles identified by the expert panel for nurse staffing and adopted by the ANA Board of Directors on November 24, 1998, are listed below. A discussion of each of the three categories is available through ANA.

I. Patient Care Unit Related

a. Appropriate staffing levels for a patient care unit reflect analysis of individual and aggregate patient needs.

b. There is a critical need to either retire or seriously question the usefulness of the concept of nursing hours per patient day (HPPD).

c. Unit functions necessary to support delivery of quality patient care must also be considered in determining staffing levels.

II. Staff Related

a. The specific needs of various patient populations should determine the appropriate clinical competencies required of the nurse practicing in that area.

b. Registered nurses must have nursing management support and representation at both the operational level and the executive level.

c. Clinical support from experienced RNs should be readily available to those RNs with less proficiency.

III. Institution/Organization Related

a. Organizational policy should reflect an organizational climate that values registered nurses and other employees as strategic assets and exhibit a true commitment to filling budgeted positions in a timely manner.

b. All institutions should have documented competencies for nursing staff, including agency or supplemental and traveling RNs, for those activities that they have been authorized to perform.

c. Organizational policies should recognize the myriad needs of both patients and nursing staff.

From American Nurses Association. (1999). *Principles for nurse staffing.* Washington, DC: Author.

result of these competing concerns, staff nurses and their professional nursing organizations may find themselves in disagreement with the healthcare organization regarding what constitutes a minimum safe staffing level, and nurse managers may feel torn between these opposing views when preparing and proposing a unit's personnel budget.

Consumer Expectations

Exceeding the expectations of consumers for care and services has become a major strategy for maintaining and improving the financial viability of the healthcare organization (Health Care Advisory Board, 1999). Recognizing that the patient expects to receive high-quality nursing care, delivered promptly and efficiently by nurses who appear to be satisfied with their workload, creates another variable that nurse managers must consider as they prepare their budgets. Proposing an extremely tight personnel budget that has no ability to flex up when patient acuity or volumes increase may satisfy the organization's finance department. However, there are negative consequences of preparing an overly tight budget. Declining patient satisfaction scores, dealing with increased patient and staff complaints, or managing the potential legal and financial consequences of a serious patient error that can be attributed to an understaffed unit can all result from chronically understaffing a unit. Nurse managers are advised to consider these less tangible variables when preparing the personnel budget.

■ *Exercise 16-1*

Review an organization's policies and procedures for assigning staff. Review a specific unit's staffing plan and current work schedule. Is the unit's actual schedule reflective of the organization's staffing policies? Is the unit's actual schedule consistent with the staffing plan? Interview two or three staff nurses on the unit as though you were a state or other regulatory surveyor and ask them if they believe the unit usually has adequate staffing. What would these nurses' answers reveal to the surveyor?

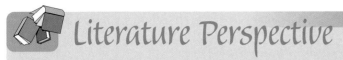

Literature Perspective

Bordoloi, S. K., & Weatherby, E. J. (1999). Managerial implications of calculating optimum nurse staffing in medical units. *Health Care Management Review, 21*(4), 35-44.

A tool was developed for managers to apply qualitative judgments to the staffing policies. This tool allowed the developing hospital to adjust staffing mix as educational/training levels and skills changed. This tool is useful where censuses fluctuate in a predictable manner.

IMPLICATIONS FOR PRACTICE
The use of a model to "number crunch" based on qualitative judgments and changing staff expertise would be useful guidance in determining needed staffing for given shifts and units.

Internal Organization Variables That Affect Staffing Plans

Nurse managers must also consider a number of internal organizational variables when preparing the personnel budget and projecting the unit's staffing needs. The internal organizational variables that are considered are highlighted in the following sections. Organizational financing assumptions (see Chapter 13) are a key element.

Organizational Staffing Policies

Nurse managers will be guided in their development of unit personnel budgets by the organization's staffing policies. For example, the organization establishes the rate at which an employee earns overtime and what other benefit time will be paid for by the organization. Organizational staffing policies must comply with federal and state labor laws. Thus nurse managers will be in compliance with these laws if they adhere to their organizational staffing policies. An opportunity to apply qualitative judgment to policies was the basis of the article described in the Literature Perspective.

Structure and Philosophy of the Nursing Services Department

A nursing philosophy statement outlines the values and beliefs about the practice of nursing and the provision of patient care within the organization. The philosophy statement is used to guide the practice of nursing in the various nursing units on a daily basis. Nurse managers must propose a staffing plan and a personnel budget that allows for consistency between the written philosophy statement and the observable practice of nursing on their

units. It is very demoralizing for nurses to feel they cannot comply with their nursing philosophy statement because of problems associated with consistently inadequate staffing.

The philosophy statement also guides the establishment of the overall structure of the nursing service department and the staffing models that are used within the organization. The **staffing model** adopted by the organization plays a major role in determining the mix of professional and assistive staff needed to provide patient care. Examples of the advantages and disadvantages of some staffing models used in healthcare today are summarized in Box 16-2 and are described in greater depth in Chapter 15.

Determining the staffing skill mix that best meets the needs of the unit requires nurse managers to consider the intensity of nursing care generally required by unit patients. To determine the intensity of care, managers consider factors such as the severity of patient illnesses, the complexity of nursing care and procedures, the degree of patient dependency on the nursing staff, and the amount of time generally required to provide patient care. Reducing the complement of professional staff in the skill mix has become a major cost-saving strategy in many organizations (McGillis-Hall, 1998).

Organizational Support Systems

Another critical, but often overlooked, variable that affects the development of the nursing personnel budget is the presence, or absence, of organizational systems that support the nurse in providing care. If the organization has recognized the need to keep the professional nurse at the bedside, support systems to allow that to happen will be evident. Examples of

BOX 16-2

Advantages and Disadvantages of Various Staffing Models

Total Patient Care: The registered nurse (RN) assumes total responsibility for meeting the patient's care needs during the assigned shift.

- Advantages:
  - Increased nursing autonomy
  - Increased nursing accountability for the shift
  - Holistic care enhanced for the shift
- Disadvantages:
  - Patient experiences care variation across shifts
  - Costly care with RNs doing non-RN work
  - Decreased accountability for the total patient experience

Functional Nursing: The RN organizes assignments around the provision of patient care tasks.

- Advantages:
  - Increased task proficiency
  - Maximal efficiency of different levels of caregivers on the unit
  - Highly efficient use of resources
- Disadvantages:
  - Patient experiences fragmentation of care
  - Staff lack a holistic perspective on care needs
  - Patient and staff dissatisfaction

Team Nursing (modular nursing): The RN is responsible for assigning and supervising a team of caregivers who share a patient assignment.

- Advantages:
  - Increased productivity of the RN
  - Increased interaction between RN and patient focused on professional nursing activities
  - Cost effective

- Disadvantages:
  - RNs may lack skills in delegation and supervision
  - RNs may spend more time in supervision than in interacting with patients
  - Good team planning requires time
  - Patients perceive fragmentation of care
  - Lines of responsibility and accountability may blur

Primary Nursing: The RN assumes responsibility for planning care for the patient for a 24-hour period or longer.

- Advantages:
  - Increased nurse job satisfaction
  - Increased nursing accountability and responsibility
  - Increased nursing autonomy
- Disadvantages:
  - Newer/less experienced nurses unable to plan adequately for care
  - Requires a level of organizational sophistication to implement and maintain

support systems that enhance the nurse's ability to remain on the unit and provide direct care to patients include transporter services, clerical support services, and hospitality services (Ashley, 2000).

However, professional nurses often work in organizations that require them to function in the role of a multipurpose worker. Because nurses are generally scheduled in hospitals 24 hours a day, 7 days a week, they may be required to provide services for other professionals who provide more limited hours of care to patients. Professional nurses may assume the functions of respiratory therapists, physical therapists, clinical dietitians, and pharmacists on weekends, evenings, and nights. It is wise for nurse

managers to identify what costs are being incurred in the unit as a result of the absence of adequate organizational support systems and to develop strategies to put those systems into place or justify the budget accordingly.

Changes in Services That Will Be Offered

Nurse managers must also consider organizational plans to expand existing clinical services or to develop new services or programs when preparing the personnel budget. For example, a manager of an inpatient surgical unit must consider the potential effect of offering a new surgical procedure to the community. What projections have been made for this market? What is the expected length of stay for patients undergoing this new procedure? What are the national standards for care for this type of patient? A nurse manager will use this information to project added staff to manage these changes in service.

Conversely, nurse managers must also be aware of any organizational plans to delete an existing service that their new unit supports. For example, if a nurse manager in a home care setting knows that reimbursement for a certain procedure in the home has declined to the point that this service must be discontinued, allowances for fewer required staffing resources in the coming year must be made.

Projected Units of Service

The amount of work performed by a nursing unit, or **cost center,** is referred to as its **workload.** Workload is measured in terms of the **units of service** defined by the cost center (see Chapter 13). Nurse managers must understand the nature of the work in their area of responsibility to define the units of service that will be used as their workload statistic and to **forecast,** or project, the volume of work that will be performed by their cost center during the upcoming year (or validate the projection made by someone else) to propose an adequate personnel budget.

FORECASTING UNIT WORKLOAD

Nurse managers consider a number of factors besides projected units of service when beginning the process of forecasting the unit's workload for the upcoming year, including the following:

1. Historical staffing requirements
2. Effectiveness of the current staffing plan
3. Trends in acuity on the unit
4. Anticipated skill mix or other personnel changes
5. New physicians, programs, services, or technology anticipated to affect staffing

Nurse managers use this information and the information available in the unit's activity report to predict daily staffing needs for the upcoming budget period.

The Unit Activity Report

Nurse managers rely on the unit's **activity report** for obtaining key statistics that can be used to project units of service for the upcoming year and for monitoring the unit's current productivity performance.

BOX 16-3

Typical Report Indicators

- Volume statistic: number of units of service for the reporting period
- Capacity statistic: number of beds or blocks of time available for providing services
- Percentage of occupancy: number of occupied beds for the reporting period
- ADC (average daily census): average number of patients cared for per day for the reporting period
- ALOS (average length of stay): average number of days that a patient remained in an occupied bed

---

BOX 16-4

Formulas for Calculating Volume Statistics

- **ADC:** patient days for a given time period divided by the number of days in the time period
  566 patient days in June =
  $$566 \text{ patient days}/30 \text{ days} = \text{ADC of } 18.9$$
- **Percentage of Occupancy:** daily patient census divided by the number of beds in the unit
  18 patients in a 20-bed unit =
  $$18 \text{ patients}/20 \text{ beds} = 90\% \text{ occupancy}$$
- **ALOS:** the number of patient days for a specified period divided by the number of discharges for the same period
  There are 566 patient days and 98 discharges in June
  566 patient days divided by 98 discharges = 5.77 ALOS

Institutionwide reports are generated that provide nurse managers with a variety of measures of unit workload. Although the format of these reports may vary, the kinds of information typically available to nurse managers in an activity report are included in Box 16-3.

In the inpatient setting, the **average daily census (ADC)** is one measure considered by nurse managers to project the potential workload of the unit. The ADC is a simple measure of the average number of patients being cared for in the available beds on the unit trended over a specific period. The formula for calculating the ADC is found in Box 16-4.

If a unit's ADC is trending upward, the nurse manager will propose additional personnel to manage this increase in patient volume. If the ADC is trending downward, the nurse manager will propose the need for fewer resources to manage this downward census trend. In the acute care setting, a unit's ADC can be extremely volatile based on the patterns of admissions, transfers, and discharges on the unit; in a long-term care setting, however, the unit's ADC may be very stable over prolonged periods. Nurse managers may note census trends based on a particular shift, the day of the week, or the season of the year. The addition of new physicians, the creation of new programs or services, and many other variables may also affect a unit's average daily census. The number of admissions and discharges per shift also increases staffing demands. Nurse managers must maintain a strong grasp on this measure of workload to prepare an adequate staffing plan for their unit.

Another way of assessing a unit's activity level is to calculate the **percentage of occupancy.** The unit's occupancy rate can be calculated for a specific shift, on a daily basis, or as a monthly or annual statistic. The formula for calculating the percentage of occupancy is found in Box 16-4. Nurse managers use the percentage of occupancy to develop the unit's staffing plan. Optimal occupancy rates may vary by practice setting. In long-term care the organization would desire 100% occupancy rates. However, in acute care, 85% occupancy rates would ensure the best potential for patient throughput to the unit.

Another measure of unit activity that may be considered by nurse managers is the **average length of stay** (ALOS), or the number of days each patient stays in the occupied bed. As reimbursement dollars have decreased, so have lengths of stay. The cost of treating the patient has not decreased as dramatically because the patient's acuity is greater; essentially, we need to provide more care in less time for fewer dollars with the same, if not better, outcomes. For this reason, as a unit's ALOS trends downward, the need for staffing resources may not change substantially, or it may actually climb. The formula for calculating the average length of stay is also found in Box 16-4.

FORECASTING UNIT STAFFING REQUIREMENTS

Calculation of Full-Time Equivalents

Nurse managers use the unit's forecasted workload to calculate the number of **full-time equivalents** (FTEs) that will be needed to construct the unit's overall staffing plan. It is important to remember that there

is a distinction between an employee in a position and an FTE. Chapter 13 describes FTEs and how they are calculated. To achieve a balanced staffing plan, nurse managers must determine the correct combination of full-time and part-time positions that will be needed.

Nurse managers must also consider the effect of productive and non-productive hours when projecting the FTE needs of the unit. **Productive time** (see Chapter 13) is the paid hours that are actually worked on the unit. Productive hours can be further defined as direct or indirect. Direct care hours are used to pay for the care of patients. Indirect hours are used to pay for other required unit activities, such as staff meetings or continuing education attendance.

Nonproductive time (see Chapter 13) includes those hours of benefit time that are paid to an employee for vacation, holiday, personal, or sick time or for an employee attending orientation or continuing education activities. In most practice settings, nurses must be replaced when they are off duty and accessing their paid benefit time off. Managers must be aware of the average benefit hours required for their unit, or they will understate their FTE needs. This requires nurse managers to carefully consider how to allocate their budgeted FTEs into full-time and part-time positions to meet the staffing requirements for the unit when a portion of the staff are taking paid time off. In addition, looking at the number of employees being paid for any specific day may not reflect the number actually providing care.

■ *Exercise 16–2*

Select a community health organization and determine the hours of operation for this organization. Assess what the master scheduling plan is. Determine how many RNs need to be employed to ensure that each shift area of operation has one RN present. Assuming that a 40-hour work week will equal one FTE, convert the required number of registered nurse positions to FTEs.

Distribution of FTEs

Nurse managers must consider a number of variables when they begin the process of distributing FTEs into the **master staffing plan** for the unit. The master staffing plan, which is based on the unit's approved personnel budget, will serve as a guide for creating the unit's schedules for the upcoming year. Variables that must be considered by managers when creating master staffing plans include the following:

1. The hours of operation of the unit
2. The basic shift length for the unit

3. Known activity patterns for the unit at various times of day
4. Maximum work stretch for each employee
5. Shift rotation requirements
6. Weekend requirements

Each of these variables interrelates with the others, so few "absolutes" are possible. For example, initially one might think that a 24/7 unit might require more staff than a 7 AM to 6 PM area. If the first, however, is providing basic care all day and few activities at night (e.g., a long-term care facility), fewer staff might be needed than in the second if that were, for example, a day surgery unit.

The master staffing plan must consider the distribution of **fixed FTEs** in the plan. Fixed FTEs are held by those employees who will be scheduled to work, no matter what the volume of activity in the unit is. These employees generally hold an exempt or salaried position, meaning their compensation does not depend on the unit's workload. Examples of employees who typically hold a fixed FTE include the nurse manager, the clinical specialist, and the unit educator.

The manager then distributes the **variable FTEs** into a master staffing plan. Variable FTEs are held by those employees who are scheduled to work based on the workload of the unit. These employees are considered nonexempt or hourly wage employees, meaning their compensation depends on the actual number of hours worked in a given pay period. Examples of employees who typically hold a variable FTE position include staff nurses, clerical staff, and other ancillary support staff assigned to the unit.

SCHEDULING

The Nursing Executive Center of the Advisory Board Company is a nationally recognized think-tank that studies complex or emerging issues confronting nursing administrators. Nursing retention and recruitment have been at the forefront of their research for the past several years. In a comprehensive study of the employment attributes most likely to result in nursing turnover in a hospital setting, the Nursing Executive Center found that having limited scheduling options was second only to inadequate compensation as a factor leading to nursing turnover.

Scheduling is a function of implementing the staffing plan by assigning unit personnel to work specific hours and specific days of the week. The nurse manager is greatly challenged to take the FTEs that are allotted through the personnel budget, distribute them appropriately across the day of the week and time of day, and create a master schedule for the unit that also meets each employee's personal schedule. Although completely satisfying each individual staff member is not always possible, a schedule can usually be created that is both fair and balanced from the employee's perspective while still meeting the care needs of the unit. Creating a flexible schedule with a variety of scheduling options that leads to work schedule stability for each employee is one mechanism for retaining staff within the control of nurse managers (Shader, Broome, Broome, West, & Nash, 2001).

Variables That Affect Staffing Schedules

Nurse managers must consider many variables to create a fair and balanced schedule. Examples of variables nurse managers can anticipate and must consider as they prepare the unit's schedule are found in Box 16-5.

> ■ Exercise 16–3
> Assume you are going on a job interview. Considering your personal preferred work schedule, what scheduling practices would be most satisfying to you and might lead you to accept employment with the organization? What scheduling practices might cause you to look elsewhere for a job? Develop a list of questions to ask your potential employer regarding scheduling practices in their organization.

Other unanticipated variables can complicate the best-prepared schedule. When faced with call-ins for illness, funeral leaves, jury duty, or an emergent

BOX 16-5

Anticipated Scheduling Variables

- Hours of operation
- Shift rotations
- Weekend rotations
- Approved benefit time for the schedule period—vacations, holidays, etc.
- Approved leaves of absence/short-term disability
- Approved seminar, orientation, or continuing education time
- Scheduled meetings for the schedule period
- Current filled positions and current staffing vacancies
- Number of part-time employees

need for a leave of absence (LOA), nurse managers must attempt to fill a shift vacancy on short notice. Requesting staff to add hours over their planned commitment, floating staff in from another unit or securing someone from a staffing pool, contracting with agency nursing staff, or mandating overtime are examples of strategies that nurse managers may be compelled to use to ensure safe staffing of their units. However, many potential negative consequences are associated with using these strategies. For example, some states have passed legislation regarding mandatory overtime. The strategies for adding supplemental staff to the unit are examined more carefully in the following sections.

Increasing Staff FTEs

Upon being hired, employees create an implied contract with the organization for the FTEs they will work. Generally, full-time and part-time staff agree to work the FTEs that best meet their personal needs for income, benefits, time worked, and time off. When nurse managers are faced with an unanticipated staffing vacancy, the easiest remedy for fixing this problem may be to ask a staff member to work a double shift or to call an off-duty staff member and ask that person to come in on a scheduled day off. However, when nurse managers use this strategy, they are violating the contract the organization has with the employee, although staff will be compensated for the inconvenience of adding hours above their FTE, and may even earn added bonus pay or overtime pay for the effort. Staff may ultimately become dissatisfied with this approach to managing staffing on the unit—especially if this is a recurring problem.

> ### Exercise 16-4
> Assume you are the senior staff leader working in the charge role of the shift. One of the staff assigned to work with you becomes ill and must go home suddenly, leaving the designated patient assignment undone. As a unit leader, what factors would you consider as you determine how to reassign this work to other nurses? As a co-worker on the shift, what effective follower behaviors might you demonstrate to support the leader in this situation? Can you identify any behaviors that would complicate the staffing situation further?

Floating Staff

Another strategy that may be used to deal with unanticipated staff vacancies involves floating nurses from one clinical unit to another to fill the staffing vacancy. This can be an effective strategy if the nurses are being deployed from a centralized flexible staffing pool and they have the competencies to work on the unit to which they are assigned. Nurses working as float nurses are generally very experienced nurses who maintain a broad range of clinical competencies. They usually receive added compensation for their willingness to be flexible and to float to a variety of units on short notice. Nurse managers are fortunate if they have a strong flexible staffing pool to draw upon when faced with unanticipated staffing vacancies.

However, when an organization does not have a vital flexible staffing pool, nurses may be expected to float across clinical units just to fill the shift vacancy. There are several areas of concern related to this strategy for meeting unanticipated staffing needs. First, the floating nurse may not have the required competencies for working on a unit. Just as a psychiatrist would never be asked to cover for a cardiac surgeon, a behavioral health nurse should not be required to work in the intensive care unit. Specialized nursing competencies do not necessarily transfer across clinical practice settings. Floating a nurse should always raise the question about the practitioner's competence to provide safe care to patients in the unfamiliar unit.

Second, floating a nurse to an unfamiliar setting raises that nurse's anxiety level, which may contribute to errors made during the shift. Sometimes floating requires multiple reassignments to fit nursing skills with patient needs. There is a risk management component to floating that nurse managers may overlook in their eagerness to fill the shift vacancy (Trossman, 1999). Finally, required floating may be in violation of state board of nursing or other regulatory standards for ensuring that patients will be assigned safely to a competent practitioner. Many states have developed guidelines for floating safely that are available for licensed professionals to follow when confronted with a request to float.

Use of Agency Staff

Many nurses choose to work for staffing agencies. They may be hired by the nursing unit as independent contractors for a shift, a week, or a longer period. There are advantages to working for an agency, such as higher hourly rates of pay, diversity in work assignments, exposure to a variety of work teams, and the ability to travel. Use of agency nursing staff is one of the primary methods used by nurse managers to fill temporary staff vacancies.

Despite advantages to using agency staff, nurse managers must consider the potential negative aspects of depending on supplemental staff to meet the unit's staffing plan. First, patients may be unable to distinguish agency staff from unit staff. The professional behavior and clinical performance of the agency staff member will then be seen as a reflection of the care provided on the unit. For this reason, nurse managers must expect agency staff to function as competent professionals in their unit.

Second, it is difficult to monitor the performance of agency staff because they may work for only one shift in the unit before moving on to another unit or another facility. Managers may have difficulty documenting errors with agency staff members because of the sporadic nature of their assignment to a given unit.

Finally, if managers identify concerns about the competency of an agency employee, they may elect not to have that individual return to the unit in the future. However, if they do not communicate their performance concerns to that person's employer, the agency staff may not receive the necessary performance counseling. In that case, the agency employee may move from institution to institution perpetuating poor clinical performance practices until a serious patient outcome results. The use of agency personnel requires a high degree of supervision by nurse managers.

Mandatory Overtime

Requiring staff to stay on duty after their shift ends to fill staffing vacancies is called *mandatory overtime*. The issue of mandatory overtime is being discussed by professional nursing organizations and state boards of nursing across the country, and it has become a major negotiating point for nurses in unionized settings. Legislation prohibiting mandatory overtime has been adopted in some states and is pending in others. Mandatory overtime is a staffing strategy that is opposed by the ANA and many other professional nursing organizations because it is seen as a risk to both patients and nurses. Tired and overworked nurses are more likely to have compromised decision-making abilities and technical skills as a result of fatigue. Thus they are more likely to make mistakes leading to patient harm and compromised patient outcomes (American Nurses Association, 2000a). For many nurses, fear of litigation and loss of nursing licensure because of errors made in an exhausted state is a strong motivating factor in refusing to work mandatory overtime hours on their unit.

Once again, nurse managers may feel conflicted over this issue. Managers may feel compelled to require staff to work overtime out of a belief that a tired nurse is better than no nurse at all. When faced with an unsafe staffing situation, managers may believe no other options exist for providing care to the patients. Organizations generally have policies regarding their right to mandate overtime. The policies may specify that refusing to work the required overtime constitutes patient abandonment and is punishable with corrective discipline. However, some states have made clear that refusing mandatory overtime does not constitute patient abandonment.

Exercise 16-5

Review a healthcare organization's policies on overtime. Is mandatory overtime covered in the policy? Are the consequences for failing to work mandatory overtime when requested to do so by a supervisor outlined in the policy? What does the state board of nursing allow regarding mandatory overtime? How would you respond to a nurse manager who required you to stay on the job after your shift was over? Develop a list of questions you might ask on a job interview relating to use of overtime in the organization.

Constructing the Schedule

Mechanisms are typically in place within an organization for staff to use in requesting days off and to know when the final schedule will be posted. In addition, most organizations have written policies and procedures that must be followed by nurse managers to ensure compliance with state and federal labor laws relative to scheduling. These policies also aid managers in making scheduling decisions that will be perceived as fair and equitable by all employees.

Schedules are usually constructed for a predetermined block of time based on organizational policy—for example, weekly, biweekly, or monthly. The unit schedule may be prepared in a decentralized fashion by nurse managers or by unit staff through a self-scheduling method. However, centralized staffing coordinators may oversee all of the schedules prepared for the patient care units. Each method of schedule preparation has pros and cons. The Research Perspective offers some conclusions about the method to select.

Decentralized Scheduling—Nurse Manager

One decentralized method for preparing the schedule involves nurse managers developing the schedule in isolation from all other units. In this model nurse

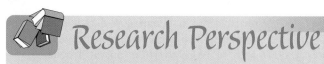

Research Perspective

Silvestro, R., & Silvestro, C. (2000). An evaluation of nurse rostering practices in the National Health Service. *Journal of Advanced Nursing, 32*, 525-535.

Nurse rostering (scheduling) was examined in the National Health Service (UK). This study developed out of the trend toward self-scheduling, which has been viewed as empowering for staff. Fifty NHS wards were surveyed; 9 wards had in-depth case studies. Benefits and limitations were found. The author found that the operational context was an important determinant of how to approach scheduling issues. Specifically, ward size (number of beds), demand variability, demand predictability, and complexity of skill mix must be considered. Unit-based or centralized staffing is recommended for large, complex units (70 staff or more); team scheduling (unit-based or subunit teams) seems appropriate for medium-sized wards; and self-scheduling fits well for small wards (up to 35 staff).

IMPLICATIONS FOR PRACTICE

Staffing is a complex issue that should be re-search-based, especially when new approaches are introduced.

---

managers approve all schedule changes and actually spend time on a regular basis drafting the staff schedule considering only the staffing needs of the unit. In other decentralized models, managers do the preliminary work on schedules and then submit them to a centralized staffing office for review and for the addition of any needed supplemental staff. The advantage of this decentralized model is that the accountability for submitting a schedule in alignment with the established staffing plan rests with managers. These individuals are ultimately the ones accountable for maintaining unit productivity in line with the personnel budget, so the incentive to manage the schedule tightly is strong. The negative aspect of this decentralized method relates to the inability of any individual nurse manager to know the "big picture" related to staffing across multiple patient care units. Requests for time off are approved in isolation from all other units, and there is a very real potential with this model that each manager will make a decision at the unit level that will be felt in aggregate as a "staffing shortage" across multiple units.

Staff Self-Scheduling

A self-scheduling process has the potential to promote staff autonomy and to increase staff accountability for productivity on the unit. In addition, team communication, problem-solving skills, and negotiating skills can be enhanced through the self-scheduling process. Successful self-scheduling is achieved when each individual's personal schedule

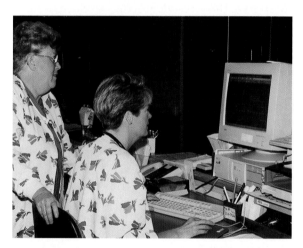

Computerized programming has dramtically reduced the amount of time spent preparing staffing schedules.

is balanced with the unit's staffing needs. Several factors can influence the successful implementation of self-scheduling (Ruflin, Matlock, Holy, Sorbello, Nadzan, & Selden, 1999):

- Committee structure
- Staff education
- Staff negotiation skills
- Managerial support

Self-scheduling has become more complicated in the wake of care delivery changes and the decentralization of many activities to the individual patient care units. The professional nursing staff cannot work in isolation of other care members when creating a schedule. Assessing the readiness of support staff to participate in this type of initiative is critical as resource utilization and cost containment continue to be major focal points of concern.

Centralized Scheduling

One benefit to centralized scheduling is that the staffing coordinator is usually aware of the abilities, qualifications, and availability of supplemental personnel who may be needed to complete the schedule. In many organizations the centralized staffing coordinator is also aware of each unit's personnel budget and any constraints it may impose on the schedule. On the other hand, a disadvantage to centralized staffing is the limited knowledge the coordinator has relative to changing patient acuity needs or other patient-related activities on the unit. Developing a mechanism for the centralized staffing coordinator to share unit-specific knowledge with the respective nurse manager can resolve this disadvantage satisfactorily.

Many organizations have invested in computer software designed to create optimal schedules based on the approved staffing plans for individual units. The centralized staffing coordinator maintains the integrity of the computerized databank for each unit; enters schedule variances daily; generates planning sheets, drafts, and final schedules; and runs any specialized productivity reports requested by nurse managers. Nurse managers review the initial schedule created by the computer, make necessary modifications, and approve the final schedule.

The process for creating schedules selected by the organization depends on a large number of variables, including the size of the organization and the complexity of the staffing that must be produced.

EVALUATING UNIT PRODUCTIVITY

Nurse managers are increasingly pressed to justify their staffing decisions. Managers have budgeted nursing salary dollars in the personnel budget based on the estimated units of service that will be provided in the unit. For each dollar spent, there is an expected return. If managers are able to provide more care to more patients while spending the same or fewer salary dollars, they have increased their unit produc-

tivity. Conversely, if the same or more salary dollars are spent to provide less care to fewer patients, managers have decreased their unit productivity.

Calculating nursing productivity is challenging for nurse managers because it is difficult to quantify the efficiency and effectiveness of individual nurses providing care to patients. Individual nurses can vary greatly in their critical-thinking abilities, their skill levels, and their ability to make timely and accurate decisions that affect patient outcomes. Because patient care is an extremely dynamic process, patient acuity trending with a classification system is one method that can be used by nurse managers to project daily staffing needs and justify unit productivity.

Patient Classification Systems

One of the most commonly cited reasons for exceeding a unit's staffing plan is the increased acuity of the patients on that unit. However, the dynamic nature of patient care often makes it difficult to quantify and qualify the care needs of patients at any given time.

Patient classification systems have been developed in an effort to give nurse managers the tools and language for describing the acuity of patients on their unit. Sicker patients receive higher classification scores, indicating that more nursing resources are required to provide patient care. Nurse managers use the classification data to make adjustments to the unit's staffing plan for a given time or for quantifying acuity trends over longer periods as they forecast their staffing needs during the budget process.

Patient Classification Types

Two basic types of patient classification systems exist: prototype and factor. A **prototype evaluation system** is considered both subjective and descriptive. It classifies patients into broad categories and uses these categories to predict the patient care needs. The relative intensity measures (RIMs) system is a prototype system. This system classifies patient care needs based on their diagnosis related group (DRG). This system was first tried unsuccessfully in the early 1980s. Since then, Yale New Haven Hospital in New Haven, Connecticut, has developed a RIMs system that is used to measure both workload and productivity. The data are then fed to a decision support system that integrates the clinical and financial information.

A **factor evaluation system** is considered more objective. It takes tasks, thought processes, and patient care activities and gives each one a time or rating. These associations are then summed to determine the hours of direct care required, or they are weighted for each individual patient. The Nursing Intervention Classification (NIC) system is a factor system that takes into consideration different interventions specific to each individual patient (McCloskey & Bulechek, 2000). Each intervention is given a name and a definition and is further broken down to incorporate a list of all associated interventional activities. The list of interventions is comprehensive and applicable to inpatient, outpatient, home care, and long-term care patients.

It is not unusual for organizations to use a combination of systems. Some patient types with a single healthcare focus, such as maternal deliveries or outpatient surgical procedure patients, would be appropriately classified with a prototype system. Patients with more complex care needs and a less predictable disease course, such as those with pneumonia or stroke, are more appropriately evaluated with a factor system.

Advantages of Patient Classification Systems

On a broad scale, patient classification data can provide nurse managers with additional information that can be used when preparing the personnel budget. Acuity trending can help managers determine whether the unit's staffing model or skill mix should change. The system may also help managers determine the cost of care being provided to patients and may help justify changes in patient charges for services. On a daily basis, patient classification data can be used to fine-tune daily staffing requirements.

Disadvantages of Patient Classification Systems

There are a number of potential problems with patient classification systems. The issue most often raised by the organization's administrators relates to the questionable reliability and validity of the data collected through a self-reporting mechanism. Nurses are often charged with the responsibility of classifying their patients. When this activity is done retrospectively, after the shift's work has been completed, the evaluator may be fatigued and may perceive that staff have worked harder than usual during the shift. This fatigue may be used to justify classifying the patient into a higher acuity category.

Recent research compared actual time and motion studies, in which a single observer continuously timed the occurrences and duration of nursing activities, with self-reporting by nursing staff of the time and duration of each task performed. Biases of self-reporting were found to be no greater than observer-induced bias in time-and-motion measurement (Burke, McKee, Wilson, Donahue, Batenhorst, & Pathak, 2000). However, bias continues to be identified as a concern by administrators; therefore ongoing quality monitoring programs must be developed to randomly audit the patient classification system to seek out bias.

Another concern with patient classification data relates to the inability of the organization to

---

BOX 16-6

Analysis of Labor Costs per Unit of Service

1. Manager of a cardiac telemetry unit proposes the following in the personnel budget. These are the unit's productivity targets.
   - Total patient days: 5840
   - ADC = 16

   Staffing plan for ADC of 16:
   - Day shift: 3 RNs and 3 UAPs (50% RN skill mix)
   - Evening shift: 3 RNs and 3 UAPs (50% RN skill mix)
   - Night shift: 3 RNs and 1 UAP (75% skill mix)

   Direct care labor costs are also projected by the manager based on the average RN and UAP salaries for this unit.
   - Target = $139.32 per patient, or $2229.12 per day

2. Manager actually staffs as follows:
   - ADC = 16
   - Actual staffing for ADC of 16
   - Day shift: 4 RNs and 2 UAPs (66% RN skill mix)
   - Evening shift: 4 RNs and 2 UAPs (66% RN skill mix)
   - Night shift: 3 RNs (100% RN skill mix)
   - Direct labor costs for this day = $145.44 per patient, or $2327.04 per day.

3. Manager has incurred a variance:
   - Exceed target by $6.12 per patient, or $97.92 for the day.

ADC, Average daily census; *RN*, registered nurse; *UAP*, unlicensed assistive personnel.

staff to meet the prescribed staffing levels outlined by the patient classification system. Administrators worry that they risk potential liability if they do not follow the staffing recommendations of the patient classification system. If the classification data indicates that six caregivers are needed for the upcoming shift, but the organization can provide only five caregivers, what are the potential consequences for the organization if an untoward event occurs? Concern over the accuracy of biased data and the inability to meet predicted staffing levels outlined by the patient classification systems have caused many healthcare organizations to abandon patient classification as a mechanism for determining appropriate staffing levels.

Labor Cost Per Unit of Service

Organizations that distrust patient classification systems are moving toward the use of another measure of nursing productivity. **Labor cost per unit of service** is a simple measure that compares budgeted salary costs per budgeted volume of service (productivity target) with actual salary costs per actual volume of service (productivity performance). This measure requires managers to staff according to their staffing plan because the plan reflects the approved personnel budget. If managers compare their actual productivity performance to their productivity target and the two numbers match, managers know they have staffed productively (but a match could also be a result of less care provided). Box 16-6 provides an analysis of labor costs per unit of service.

If managers compare the two numbers and the actual productivity performance number is higher than the target, they have spent more money for care than they budgeted. Managers must explain change in productivity to the finance department in a **variance report.** A number of variables may cause the labor costs to be higher than anticipated, such as increased overtime, paying bonus pay for regular staff, using costly agency resources, or a higher-than-anticipated amount of indirect educational or orientation time.

If managers compare the two numbers and the actual productivity performance number is lower than the target, they have spent less money for care than they budgeted. Managers must also explain this high degree of productivity. One variable that may cause the labor costs to be lower than anticipated is an increased nonprofessional skill mix. However, managers can also create lower labor costs by consistently understaffing their unit. Managers who routinely use this strategy to improve the financial performance of the unit do so at the risk of increased staff and patient dissatisfaction, staff turnover, and decreased unit and patient quality outcomes.

Impact of Leadership on Productivity

Nurse managers must possess staffing and scheduling skills to accurately prepare a staffing plan that balances organizational directives with unit needs for care and services. They must spend time each month evaluating their unit's productivity performance. Yet recent research has shown that nurse managers can best improve unit productivity by spending more of their work time coaching and mentoring staff and providing them with clear information and direction related to meeting unit productivity goals. In fact, nurse managers who spend the majority of work time managing operational issues, such as staffing and scheduling, may actually be contributing to a decrease in unit productivity by reducing those work hours remaining in the day for unit leadership activities (Fox, Fox, & Wells, 1999).

The Solution

The manager called a team meeting with the entire ICU staff to discuss the potential employee's request. During this discussion, several of the current staff nurses identified that 12-hour shifts were also becoming problematic for them. They were also in favor of looking at an 8-hour scheduling option for personal reasons, but expressed concern that a mixture of 8- and 12-hour shifts could lead to disrupted continuity of care for ICU patients. Staff were uncertain how the potential employee's accommodation for weekend hours would affect the overall balance of weekend staffing but were open to considering this request because the desire to attract an experienced nurse and reduce staff floating to the night shift was so strong.

Staff helped the manager construct a list of pros and cons related to modifying the existing ICU schedule. Benefits included less floating to the night shift for current

Continued

The Solution—cont'd

ICU staff, increasing the complement of experienced nurses on the night shift, accommodating current staff desires for more schedule flexibility, and reducing overtime and bonus pay. Negatives included potential continuity of care issues for patients, potential staffing imbalance on Saturday and Sunday nights, and establishment of a precedent for allowing individual scheduling needs to disrupt other team member schedules.

The manager took the input from the staff and constructed a draft schedule that did include a mixture of shift options and accommodated the weekend schedule needs for the applicant. While reevaluating the current schedule, the manager was able to identify a number of other opportunities for enhancing schedule flexibility for all staff. Continuity of care was addressed by scheduling staff in work units that equalled 24 hours of care. Nurses desiring 8-hour shifts were scheduled in work units of three staff assigned to day, evening, and night shifts on the same days. Those nurses desiring 12-hour shifts were scheduled in work units of two staff for day and night shifts on the same days. Each work unit, whether it was constructed of 8- or 12-hour staff, was able to care for its patient assignment for a full 24-hour period. Staff reviewed the draft schedule and approved it with a few minor modifications, and the applicant was contacted and offered the position.

Shortly after implementing the new schedule, staff were surveyed regarding their satisfaction with the schedule changes. The response was overwhelmingly positive. Floating to the night shift was significantly reduced, as was overtime and bonus pay for added hours. The new employee was viewed by the rest of the ICU staff as a very strong addition to their team. The solution had a beneficial impact for all staff and demonstrated the importance of manager solicitation of staff involvement in solving problems that will directly impact them.

— Catherine Kirk

 Would this be a suitable approach for you? Why?

CHAPTER CHECKLIST

This chapter addresses the managerial functions of staffing and scheduling and asserts that skill in both functions are needed by the manager to maintain unit productivity and patient staff satisfaction.

- The nurse manager must consider the following external variables when developing the personnel budget and staffing plan:
  - State licensing regulations
  - JCAHO and other regulatory agency standards
  - ANA and other standards
  - Consumer expectations
- The nurse manager must also consider the following internal variables when preparing the budget and the unit staffing plan:
  - Organizational financial assumptions
  - Organizational staffing policies
  - Structure and philosophy of the nursing services department
  - Organizational support services

- Changes in services and programs
- Projected units of service
- When forecasting the personnel needs for the unit, the nurse manager must consider the following:
  - The staffing model of the unit
  - The skill mix of the nursing staff
  - The number of positions and FTEs needed to meet the anticipated units of service
  - The amount of nonproductive paid-benefit time allotted to each staff member
- When constructing the unit schedule, the nurse manager must consider the following:
  - Unit hours of operation
  - Shift or weekend rotations required in the unit
  - Approved paid time off for vacations, holidays, or other benefit hours
  - Staffing vacancies
- When evaluating unit productivity, the nurse manager should consider the following:
  - Acuity trends identified through patient classification systems
  - Labor cost per unit of service
  - Periodic unit activity reports

TIPS FOR STAFFING AND SCHEDULING

- Know state and federal laws regarding staffing and voluntary accreditation (professional society and institutional) standards for staffing.
- Understand current demands for staff and anticipate externally imposed changes, such as services offered, availability of registered nurses, and licensed practical/vocational nurses.
- Value the various responses to short staffing from the manager, staff, and patient perspectives.
- Understand the complexity of staffing issues and how they relate to staff satisfaction, community perception, budget, and accreditation standards.

TERMS TO KNOW

activity report
average daily census (ADC)
average length of stay
cost center
factor evaluation system
fixed FTEs
forecast
full-time equivalents (FTE)
labor cost per unit of service
master staffing plan
nonproductive time
percentage of occupancy
productive time
prototype evaluation system
scheduling
staffing
staffing model
staffing regulations
units of service
variable FTEs
variance report
workload

REFERENCES

American Nurses Association. (1999). *Principles for Nurse Staffing.* Washington, DC: Author.

American Nurses Association. (2000a, June 28). *ANA house of delegates sends strong message on mandatory overtime and nurse staffing.* Press release, Washington, DC: American Nurses Association.

American Nurses Association. (2000b, May 2). *New ANA study provides more proof of link between RN staffing and quality patient care.* Press release, Washington, DC: American Nurses Association.

Ashley, J. S. (2000). People behind the health care delivery system: The key to quality improvement and expense reduction. *Nursing Administration Quarterly, 24*(4), 1-10.

Bordoloi, S. K., & Weatherby, E. J. (1999). Managerial implications of calculating optimum nurse staffing in medical units. *Health Care Management Review, 21*(4), 35-44.

Burke, T., McKee, J., Wilson, H., Donohue, R., Batenhorst, A., & Pathak, D. (2000). A comparison of time-and-motion and self-reporting methods of work measurement. *Journal of Nursing Administration, 30*(3), 118-125.

Fox, R.T., Fox, D. H., & Wells, P (1999). Performance of first-line management functions on productivity of hospital unit personnel. *Journal of Nursing Administration, 29*(9), 12-18.

Health Care Advisory Board. (1999). *Hardwiring for service excellence.* Washington, DC: Author

Joint Commission on Accreditation of Healthcare Organizations, Section 2, Human Resources. (2000). *CAMH: Comprehensive Accreditation Manual for Hospitals: The official handbook.* Oakbrook Terrace, IL: JCAHO

Joint Commission on Accreditation of Healthcare Organizations. (2001, January 11). *Joint commission to develop a new approach to assessing the effectiveness of staffing in health care organizations.* Press release. Chicago.

McCloskey, J., & Bulechek, G. (2000). *Nursing Interventions Classification (NIC)* (3rd ed.). St. Louis: Mosby.

McGillis-Hall, L. (1998). Policy implications when changing staff mix. *Nursing Economics, 16*(6), 291-312.

Ruflin, P., Matlock, R., Holy, C., Sorbello, S., Nadzan, L., & Selden, T. (1999). Closed unit staffing speaks volumes. *Nursing Management, 30*(6), 37-40.

Russell, S. (2001, March 13). Battle afoot to decide staffing levels for nurses. *San Francisco Chronicle.*

Shader, K., Broome, M., Broome, C., West, M. E., & Nash, M. (2001). Factors influencing satisfaction and anticipated turnover for nurses in an academic medical center. *Journal of Nursing Administration, 31*(4), 210-216.

Silvestro, R., & Silvestro, C. (2000). An evaluation of nurse rostering practices in the National Health Service. *Journal of Advanced Nursing, 32,* 525-535.

Trossman, S. (1999). Staffing smart: A difficult proposition. *American Nurse, 31*(1), 1-2.

SUGGESTED READINGS

Aiken, L. H., & Patrician, P. A. (2000). Measuring organizational traits of hospitals: The revised nursing work index. *Nursing Research, 49*(3), 146-153.

Anthony, M. K., Standing, T., & Hertz, J. E. (2000). Factors influencing outcomes after delegation to unlicensed assistive personnel. *Journal of Nursing Administration, 30*(10), 474-481.

Blegan, M., Goode, C., & Reed, L. (1998). Nurse staffing and patient outcomes. *Nursing Research, 47*(1), 43-49.

Dugan, J., Lauer, E., Bouquot, Z., Dutro, B., Smith, M., & Widmeyer, G. (1996). Stressful nurses: The effect on patient outcomes. *Journal of Nursing Care Quality, 10*(3), 46-58.

Harrington, C. Swan, J. H., Mullen, J., & Carrillo, H. (1999). *Predicting nursing staffing in nursing homes in the U.S.* Wichita, KS: Department of Health Services Organization and Policy, College of Health Professions, Wichita State University.

Larrabee, J. (1995). The changing role of the consumer in health care quality. *Journal of Nursing Care Quality, 9*(2), 8-15.

MacPhee, M. (2000). Hospital networking: Comparing the work of nurses with flexible and traditional schedules. *Journal of Nursing Administration, 30*(4), 190-198.

Mailey, S., Charles, J., Piper, S., Hunt-McCool, J., Wilborne-Davis, P., & Baigis, J. (2000). Analysis of the nursing workforce compared with national trends. *Journal of Nursing Administration, 30*(10), 482-489.

Reed, L., & Blegan, M. A. (1998). Adverse patient occurrences as a measure of nursing care quality. *Journal of Nursing Administration, 28*(5), 62-69.

Schaffner, J., Alleman, S., Ludwig-Beymer, P., Muzynski, J., King, D., & Pacura, L. (1999). Developing a patient care model for an integrated delivery system. *Journal of Nursing Administration, 29*(9), 43-50.

Silberzweig, J., & Giguere, B. (1996). Redesign for patient satisfaction. *Journal of Nursing Care Quality, 11*(2), 25-33.

Terry, D. (1999). Effective employee relations in reengineered organizations. *Journal of Nursing Administration: Healthcare Law, Ethics, And Regulation, 1*(3), 33-40.

Upenieks, V. (2000). The relationship of nursing practice models and job satisfaction outcomes. *Journal of Nursing Administration, 30*(6), 330-335.

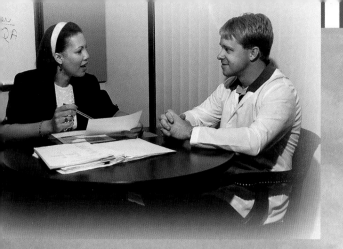

Chapter 17

Selecting, Developing, and Evaluating Staff

Cynthia Whittig Roach

*T*his chapter illustrates the importance of selecting the right employees for an organization and ensuring that individual employees understand clearly what is expected of them. Emphasis is placed on the selection interview and the importance of the orientation process for new staff. Role theory is a useful organizing framework for the manager and the employee to follow throughout all aspects of role performance. Effective communication of roles and role expectations among all members can facilitate improved performance, increased worker satisfaction, and most important, improved quality of care delivered. The role of the manager as a coach who empowers employees to grow as followers and develop their leadership skills in a learning environment is explored.

Objectives

- Apply current philosophies of performance appraisal to a variety of situations.
- Relate concepts of role theory to performance.
- Differentiate five appraisal strategies.
- Examine specific guidelines for performance feedback.
- Distinguish key points for the appraisal interview.
- Identify components of the coaching process to develop followers.

Questions to Consider

- *How does a manager select and hire the right person for a position?*
- *How does a manager develop new staff?*
- *How does a manager coach staff and create a learning environment?*
- *How does a manager empower staff members?*
- *What is your role at work? at home? at school?*
- *How do you deal with conflict in these roles?*
- *What are some of your assumptions about performance appraisals?*
- *What type of appraisal methods are you familiar with?*
- *How would you improve performance appraisals?*
- *What do you believe empowers you to improve your performance?*

The Challenge

Linda Gates, RN, BSN
Clinical Nurse Manager, Memorial Hospital, Colorado Springs, Colorado

The nursing units were tasked with improving evaluations for all nurses. The staff wanted more specific guidelines that validated competencies unique to their units. They also wanted professional recognition of their work on various committees with the hospital and activities within local, state, and national organizations. The managers were challenged to develop an improved and more comprehensive evaluation method that would incorporate the overall goals of the organization, evaluate the competencies critical to each specific nursing unit, and serve to develop the professionalism of the staff.

What do you think you would do if you were this nurse?

INTRODUCTION

Healthcare delivery systems are businesses that are economically driven. Whether the setting is inpatient or outpatient, the emphasis is on providing the highest quality care at an affordable price. The nurse manager is a key individual whose leadership can directly influence many environmental functions. These factors begin with the selection of the right person for the right position and having the manager function in the role of coach. As a coach, the nurse manager can assist and encourage employees to perform at their highest levels with an empowered and self-directed manner. The nurse manager also functions to clarify the organization's mission and expectations. The role of follower cannot be underrated; a strong patient care unit has both effective leadership and team members who understand their role in meeting the goals for quality patient care. Professional healthcare providers must clearly understand what is expected of their performance, as well as the ramifications if they do not meet those expectations. This can be achieved only when all members of the organization have clearly defined roles and overall objectives. Ambiguous roles are more detrimental to role performance and employee work satisfaction than conflict within the role.

Role ambiguity in the workplace creates an environment for misunderstanding and hinders effective communication. In this situation individuals do not have a clear understanding of what is expected of their performance or how they will be evaluated. In contrast, **role conflict** is easier to recognize. Employees know what is expected of them, but they are either unwilling or unable to meet the requirements.

Human beings create the work environment. Clear expectations and positive attitudes by all individuals, both leaders and followers, are essential to deliver quality patient care. Employees who are empowered by a supportive leader and manager have unlimited potential to provide the best care possible for their patients.

SELECTING STAFF

The selection of staff would seem to be a relatively simple process. The manager wants the most qualified individual for the position. Choosing the right individual is the challenge! This individual must "fit" within the organization and within the specific work group. The applicant and the manager must agree on what defines quality care and the manner in which it should be delivered. The manager must also decide whether members of the existing staff are to be included in the screening and interview process for new employees. The following guidelines are suggestions for the manager and staff, as well as for the prospective employee.

The manager's focus before and during the interview is to be prepared and have well-thought-out questions. The environment should be comfortable and provide privacy without interruptions. The interview questions can be related to the applicant's prior experience or be directed to evaluate values and critical-thinking skills. This may be accomplished by asking the applicant to describe his or her reactions to challenging situations previously experienced. Some technical skills may be important for the work environment and therefore also must be discussed or validated, such as specific certifications. The applicant may be given a case study to read and discuss with the interviewer. The case study could describe a situation for the unit in which the applicant is being interviewed; it could also contain content that would require the applicant to prioritize the care of one patient or a group of patients. Ideally, this case study would evaluate critical thinking. Questions from the applicant should be answered honestly. Staff members may also be included in the interview and can provide information to the applicant as appropriate. At the conclusion of the interview, it is important for the nurse manager to thank the applicant for the interview and inform him or her when the decision will be made. The manager should also inform the applicant if the decision will be made in writing or by telephone.

The applicant also has responsibilities in preparation for the employment interview. It is important to be on time and appropriately dressed. Conservative dress is always acceptable. A uniform is not necessary and usually not even preferable. First impressions may be lasting impressions. Prior review of the organization's goals and mission statement, as well as a review of the **position description** for which the interview is being conducted, is also appropriate. The applicant should be prepared to answer each question honestly and thoughtfully. It is equally important to the prospective employee to make the right decisions as it is to the employer. The manager and the applicant must have a clear understanding of the values and organizational goals for nursing care for there to be a good fit within the role. The applicant should keep to the subject at hand and avoid irrelevant conversations. The individual must prepare in advance for any questions that might be discussed. In addition to describing previous situations and how they were handled, the applicant may be asked to describe personal strengths and weaknesses. At the end of the interview, the applicant should thank the manager for his or her time and verify when the selection will be made and how it will be communicated. It is also appropriate

to send the manager a brief note of appreciation for the interview. Preparation for interviews is discussed further in Chapter 26.

DEVELOPING STAFF

Once the interview and offer are completed and an applicant has accepted the position, orientation should be planned. Orientation to the organization usually is a structured program that is generally applicable to all new employees. It may include outlining the mission, benefits, safety programs, and other specific topics. Orientation to the work area usually depends on the specialty area involved, the skills that need to be verified, and the environment itself. Every individual brings to a new position various experiences and skills. It is imperative that the orientation period be used efficiently for both the employee and the organization. Orientation is a very expensive endeavor for the organization, and everyone should use the time wisely.

Orientation can accomplish a variety of things. It is a time for the new employee to learn the work environment and the staff. Many institutions provide a preceptor who is considered an expert clinician and resource. In fact, the Kolb (1985) Learning Style Inventory (LSI) may be administered to the new employee and the information then shared with the preceptor and the new employee. If the preceptor understands the new employee's learning style, he or she can provide a better focus for implementation of the orientation goals. After the learning style has been identified, the new employee then works with a preceptor who understands how to specifically address the individualized learning needs of the new employee in a manner that enhances learning.

Continued development of the staff is a unique role of the nurse manager. It is a challenge to merge a group of individuals with varying levels of expertise and experience. If the focus is centered on professional socialization and development, a common thread will "weave" itself throughout all employees. That common thread may be a particular philosophy of care delivery, further development of critical-thinking skills for a specific specialty, or political activities in which members are involved. Some units encourage a monthly journal club or a brief presentation by employees to summarize information learned from a conference. One nursing unit could send a staff member to the monthly open meeting of the state board of nursing. This staff member then could give a summary of the report of the meeting to the staff—an exciting way to keep informed of the role of professional nursing.

Empowerment strategies are useful for individual professional development, as well as overall staff development. Empowerment is a process that acknowledges the values and judgment of individuals and trusts that their decisions will be the correct ones. In this chapter's Challenge and Solution, employee self-development and professional empowerment were the results of intervention.

For an individual to feel empowered, the environment must be open and the individuals must feel safe to explore and develop their own potential. Kinsman (1998) states that there must be a desire for self-development that includes intellectual, emotional, and spiritual changes. The organizational environment must allow the individual the freedom of making decisions but retain the accountability for the consequences of those decisions. Management must release control to followers so that they might perform work more effectively, individually and as a team. Employee attitudes, feelings of empowerment, and performance within roles can be influenced by specific environmental challenges and situations. These challenges can affect commitment to the organization and individual work satisfaction. Positive feedback or **coaching,** achievement recognition, and support for new ideas may en-

hance the employee's feeling of empowerment and his or her ability to perform effectively. The Research Perspective describes some recent research that focuses on using the best that people have to offer in their work situation.

One strategy for staff empowerment includes providing timely feedback for performance contributions, not simply during the annual **performance appraisal.** Supporting the implementation of innovative ideas and providing opportunities for mentoring relationships are also valuable approaches for the manager and staff. Many organizations use shared governance as a guide for accountability. A premise of shared governance is that power, control, and decision making can empower staff and enhance individual and group accountability.

Implementation of empowerment strategies that incorporate staff work-decision involvement can enhance performance and provide an atmosphere that promotes work satisfaction (Laschinger, Sabiston, & Kutszcher, 1997). Employees must have clear role expectations and perceive that their contributions are valued. Empowerment and control for certain aspects of the environment have been linked to increased personal health, job satisfaction, and individual performance. They are then more likely to be committed to the organization and to provide a higher level of patient care. These principles are applicable to both managers and staff members.

 Research Perspective

Buckingham, M., & Clifton, D. O. (2001). *Now, discover your strengths.* New York: The Free Press.

Driven by the issue of knowing that each employee is different, the authors set about to identify how organizations can capitalize on these differences. Asking 198,000 employees working in 36 different companies, "At work do you have the opportunity to do what you do best every day?", created some distinctive differences. Respondents with the response "strongly agree" were more likely to work in areas with lower employee turnover, higher productivity, and more customer satisfaction. The basic premise is that each of us can be more successful in life and in our careers if we can typically use our strengths to approach various situations. Using 34 dominant "themes,"

the StrengthsFinder Profile provides feedback to individuals about their specific strengths. These 34 themes include such aspects as achiever, activator, communicator, developer, futuristic, learner, maximizer, and strategist. This Gallup study has now incorporated more than 2 million people.

IMPLICATIONS FOR PRACTICE

Leaders, managers, and followers can be more productive when focusing on their individual strengths and those of their co-workers. Using strengths to develop staff potentially has positive outcomes for the individual, the work unit, and the patients we serve.

ROLE CONCEPTS AND THE POSITION DESCRIPTION

The acquisition of a role requires an individual to assume the personal, as well as the formal, expectations of a specified role or position. Many individuals function within multiple roles. As discussed in the Theory box, **role theory** provides an appreciable framework for the development and evaluation of staff. Today's professional nurse is often a parent, spouse, and community volunteer and maintains full-time employment outside the home. Many skills are necessary for each role. In addition, the role-taker (i.e., the individual actually performing the role) has specified performance objectives within the social context in which the role is acted out. The social context includes the physical and social environment. Acquisition of the role is time dependent; individuals apply their life experiences to each role and interpret the role within their own value system. As roles become more complex, the individual may take longer to assimilate the components of each particular role. Nursing graduates enter the profession with various levels of educational and life experiences. The nurse manager plays an integral role in assisting these individuals in the development and acquisition of the complex

role of the professional nurse. The important thing to remember is that role development evolves over time and with consideration to individual needs. Coaching is a technique that the manager can use to facilitate individual development; this technique is discussed later in this chapter within the context of performance appraisal.

What does all of this have to do with a position description? Everything! The position description provides written guidelines describing the roles and responsibilities of a specific position within the organizational context. The position description reflects functions and obligations of a specific work position. It is a contract for the individual that describes responsibilities of the work assignment, as well as to whom the individual reports. The position description should reflect current practice guidelines for individuals and may have competency-based requirements. As paradigms of nursing delivery systems shift to the home and community, professional nurses must have a clear understanding of the performance that is expected. The nurse is also responsible for clearly understanding the position descriptions of the paraprofessionals to whom care is delegated. Clear and concise position descriptions for all employees are extremely important because they provide the basis for roles within the organiza-

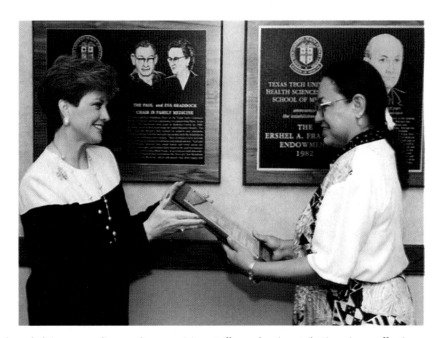

Acknowledging, rewarding, and reorganizing staff members' contributions is an effective way to empower the workforce.

Theory Box

ROLE THEORY

THEORY/CONTRIBUTOR	KEY IDEAS	APPLICATION TO PRACTICE
Role Theory and Role Dynamics in Organizations Kahn et al. (1964) developed this theory.	Roles within organizations affect an individual's interactions with others. Acquisition of these roles is time dependent and varies based on individual experiences and value systems. For effective communication to take place, role expectations for performance must be understood by all individuals involved.	The role of the professional nurse is complex. Role acquisition, role clarity, and role performance are enhanced by the use of clear position descriptions and evaluation standards.

BOX 17-1

Excerpts From a Position Description

- Responsible for the provision of direct patient care to all age groups
- Must have current certification in advanced cardiac life support (ACLS) and pediatric advanced life support (PALS)
- Required to accurately assess and prioritize patient care needs and delegate care appropriately to paraprofessionals, including LPNs/LVNs (licensed practical nurses/licensed vocational nurses) and EMTs (emergency medical technicians)
- Responsible for therapeutic communication to patients, families, and staff

---

tion. Excerpts from a position description for a staff nurse in the emergency room appear in Box 17-1.

Exercise 17–1

Obtain a position description for a registered nurse from a community nursing service and a hospital. Compare them. Analyze the general categories (e.g., communication, responsibilities) and the specific behaviors. What competencies do you already have? How will you develop other competencies?

PERFORMANCE APPRAISALS

Providing feedback to employees regarding their performance is one of the strongest rewards an organization can provide. Performance appraisals are individual evaluations of work performance. Evaluations are usually done annually but also may be required after a scheduled orientation period for new employees. Ideally, evaluations are conducted on an ongoing basis, not at the conclusion of a predetermined period. As the Literature Perspective illustrates, addressing evaluation as a system is important.

The process of providing feedback, for either above-average or below-average performance, is best received at a time closest to the incident(s) being evaluated. The actual appraisal is sometimes viewed as a negative experience. Many nurse managers perceive the appraisal as a time-consuming process of endless paperwork. Instead, the emphasis should be placed on role clarification (if necessary), evaluation of competency-based performance outcomes, and the contributions the employee has made to the organization. Performance appraisals provide the basis for many administrative decisions, including promotions, salary increases, and disciplinary actions. Appraisals should be designed so that they can be supported in court should the need arise. Court decisions can be made based on the evidence, or lack of evidence, presented in the evaluation instrument. Consider, for example, the individual who has been fired for reasons of poor work performance. The employee must be provided written notice that performance is unsatisfactory and that notice must specify what the employee must accomplish for satisfactory performance. This simple condition can make the difference for either the employee or the employer to justify the fairness for termination. Performance appraisals can be either formal or informal. Performance appraisals may

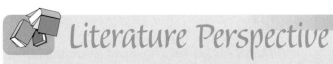

Literature Perspective

Barnes, B., Leis, S., Brammer, J. M., Gustin, T. J., & Lupo, T. C. (1999). A developmental evaluation process for nurses: Enhancing professional excellence. *Journal for Nursing Administration, 29*(4), 25-32.

Challenged with dissatisfaction of the evaluation process, a project for redesign was implemented over a 2-year period in one Midwestern hospital. Focus groups of middle managers, shift managers, and clinical staff nurses met to identify problems with the current performance appraisal system and to define behaviors to "exceed standards." Essential components were divided into five categories: professional practice development, citizenship, research/performance improvement, customer relations, and clinical practice/continuum of care. Benefits of this process enabled the staff to collaborate, plan future projects, develop a self-assessment tool, and improve work satisfaction. This process of redesign encouraged a significant change throughout the institution.

also include personal and peer evaluations as well as managerial components.

An informal appraisal might be as simple as immediately praising the individual for performance recognized. A compliment from a family member or patient might be conveyed. Some units have a specific bulletin board for thank-you notes from patients and their families. Sometimes a simple "Thank you for all your hard work today!" can be extended from the manager to the staff. In addition, staff members have a responsibility to show the manager their appreciation and give positive and negative feedback.

The formal performance appraisal involves written documentation according to specific organization guidelines. Whether the evaluation is informal or formal, it does not preclude interim evaluations. The primary reason for an interim evaluation is so that praise or corrections be made as close to an episode as possible.

Brief anecdotal notes entered into the employee's file on a regular basis are important. These anecdotal notes, when accumulated over time, provide a more accurate cumulative appraisal. The anecdotal note describes an occurrence, either favorable or unfavorable, in a brief and concise manner. The purpose is to assist the manager with information throughout an entire rating period. An example of a brief anecdotal note follows.

These notes, combined with variance reporting, are another means of documenting employee performance and provide a more conclusive appraisal that reflects the entire rating period. Variance reporting identifies specific occurrences, based on benchmarks or specific standards. As an example, "The employee will have CPR certification by January 1." If the employee does not meet this deadline, a variance is recorded along with the specific circumstances or discipline planned. This topic is explored further in Chapter 22.

Example of an Anecdotal Note: Nurse "Smith"

2/14/03: Patient (Samuel Karruthers) and family stated how much they appreciated Ms. Smith's nursing care during this hospitalization. Her coordination of rehabilitation services in a competent and caring manner decreased their anxiety and assisted them in learning what they needed to know for care in the home. Ms. Smith had the family demonstrate dressing changes and transfer techniques under her supervision to establish their confidence and competence in being able to care for the patient in their home. She made the patient feel "special," not like just another number. Compliment relayed to employee. Note in employee's anecdotal record.

Additional methods may also be incorporated into the performance appraisal in the form of competency assessment tools. These may include observation of daily work, case studies, exemplars, self-assessment, mock events, presentations, return demonstrations, and quality improvement monitors (Wright, 1998). Integration of competency assessment data into the evaluation process further enhances the individual employee's sense of empowerment, as well as accountability for the evaluation process. Staff should be encouraged to maintain their own portfolios of accomplishments (Bradley, 2001).

The overall evaluative process can be enhanced if the manager employs the technique of coaching.

Coaching is a process that involves the development of individuals within an organization. This coaching process is a personal approach in which the manager and the employee interact on a frequent and regular basis with the ultimate outcome that the employee performs at an optimum level. Coaching can be individual or may involve a team approach; when implemented in a planned and organized manner, it can promote team building and optimal performance of the employees. Coaching is a learned behavior for the nurse manager and takes time and effort to be developed. The rewards for both the employee and the nurse manager are significant; communication is enhanced and the performance appraisal process is an active one between the employee and the manager. Coaching is a management technique that can facilitate continual development and promote team building. (Antonioni, 2000; Kennedy, 2000; Lachman, 2000; Sethi, 1999).

Exercise 17-2

Select a partner. Observe some behavior and prepare an anecdotal note. Ask your partner for feedback about the content.

The formal performance appraisal usually involves some type of predetermined evaluation tool or instrument. The tool may be a simple one or may involve the integration of a variety of measuring methods. The instrument(s) should reflect the philosophy of the organization and be as objective and specific regarding the employee's performance as possible. Numerous instruments and a variety of simple to complex scoring methods for each exist. The new employee must have a clear understanding of timing and the content of the appraisal tool at the onset of employment. The example in Box 17-2 illustrates a type of peer appraisal method in which a staff nurse could evaluate another staff nurse within the area-specific context of assessment documentation.

Exercise 17-3

Think back to your last performance appraisal, either in the clinical situation as a professional nurse or in the role of nursing student. Did you feel you were fairly and adequately evaluated? Were the comments reflective of your current practice and made by someone who had directly observed the care that you provided? What was the environment like for the interview? Were you comfortable with the evaluator? Was feedback given, both positive and negative? How did you feel at the conclusion of the interview? Taking the time to think about the answers to these questions might pro-

---

BOX 17-2

Peer Performance Appraisal, Staff Nurse

Area of Responsibility:

Assessment/Diagnosis: Provides continuous holistic assessment to include physical, psychosocial, spiritual, and educational needs. Directs outcome criteria so that discharge plans are timely and optimum quality care is delivered.

a. Database (history/physical assessment) completed within 12 hours of admission (Score 4)

b. Documentation reflective of continuous assessment per unit guidelines (e.g., neurovascular assessment of extremity following cardiac catheterization) (Score 3)

c. Initiates plan of care according to critical path guidelines within 12 hours of admission (Score 4)

d. Provides for safe environment (Score 4)

---

vide you insight and direction before your next performance appraisal interview.

The scoring procedures for evaluations can be as simple as satisfactory/unsatisfactory. A more complex scoring system that includes a numerical rating scheme (using a range of 1 to 4, with 1 meaning "rarely meets standards," to 4 meaning "always exceeds standards") also appears in Box 17-2. The results from the peer-review process are then summarized and incorporated into the manager's formal performance appraisal.

PERFORMANCE APPRAISAL TOOLS

The type of appraisal tool used is not as important as how it is used. A formal written tool may have specific guidelines or a more open-ended format. General topics may be addressed in an anecdotal or "incident" type of format. The tool or evaluation form should facilitate accurate appraisal of the individual's performance and provide an opportunity to identify personal goals of the individual and goals of the organization.

There are primarily two categories of performance appraisal tools: structured and flexible. Table 17-1 summarizes examples of structured and flexible tools.

Table 17-1	STRUCTURED AND FLEXIBLE PERFORMANCE APPRAISAL TOOLS	
Structured (Traditional Method)	**Flexible (Collaborative Method)**
Forced distribution scale	Behaviorally anchored rating scales (BARS)
Graphic rating scale	Management by objectives (MBO)
	Peer review

STRUCTURED (TRADITIONAL) METHODS

The forced distribution scale is a norm-referenced tool that prevents the evaluator from rating all individuals in the same manner. The evaluator is provided a schematic diagram (Figure 17-1) and asked to rate the individual according to all individuals the manager evaluates. As depicted in the figure, the evaluator has indicated that the individual rated is in the top 10% of employees but is not the best employee. This scale also provides the employee with a brief visual picture of how this evaluator has ranked performance in reference to others. It further illustrates that this particular evaluator has an even distribution of scores for the evaluation summary of all employees. This type of scale can undermine group cohesion and communication effectiveness by its very nature of rank-ordering individual performance. This employee should feel positive about the evaluation. In reality, however, the employee is likely to feel just the opposite. The employee can see how many other employees, above him or her on the scale, are perceived as being better. The forced distribution scale can also undermine morale and group cohesion, as well as stifle creativity or the uniqueness of the individual employee.

Graphic rating scales are another example of a structured approach to evaluation. They comprise a numbering system that indicates low and high values for evaluating performance. The rating scale is popular because it is easy to construct and easy to use. Problems with this type of scale are that it lacks specificity and may promote a **halo** or **recency effect**. The halo effect describes an evaluation based

on the presumption that if the employee does well in several known areas, he or she is doing well in all areas. The recency effect describes a phenomenon in which performance closer to the rating session is better remembered than that from previous months. For example, the employee performs in a satisfactory or less than satisfactory manner up until the month before the evaluation is due and then becomes "superemployee." If the majority of the information used for an evaluation is collected during the last month of the rating period, it may not accurately reflect the total performance. The evaluation then reflects the "best" behavior rather than behavior that occurred during the majority of time in the rating period. Supervisors tend to rate people the same from one rating period to the next. Thus there is the potential for overinflation of the evaluation if the recent performance is all that is included. Anecdotal notes compiled consistently over the entire rating period are a much more equitable method for providing an accurate summary of the employee's performance. Some managers use small notes with adhesive backs to place inside an employee's file to document behaviors quickly as situations warrant. A sheet of paper for notes placed in the front of each file would also serve the same purpose. The manager might also keep secured electronic data files for the same purpose. Security of the files, electronic or paper, is important to maintain confidentiality.

Rating scales are relatively easy to construct and easy to complete (Table 17-2). On the downside, they usually consist of generalizations, not specific behaviors, and the rating is relatively subjective in nature. Some managers never give a "5," with the rationale that no employee always exceeds expectations.

Flexible (Collaborative) Method

The evaluation focus can also be conducted with a collaborative approach. How can the manager assist the individual to develop professionally? One method that has been used for many years is management by objectives (MBO). This method is also termed *the establishment of learning goals*, which are mutually established by the employee and the manager. Progress regarding the accomplishment of these goals is documented throughout the rating period. The MBO method is similar to learning goals but is more rigid in structure. An MBO approach requires that the employee establish clear and measurable objectives at the beginning of each

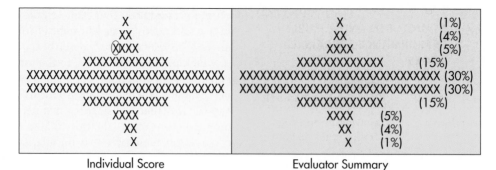

Figure 17-1   Forced distribution scale. *X*, Employee; ⊗, individual whom the employer is rating (evaluation history).

Individual Score	Evaluator Summary

Table 17-2 EXAMPLE OF A RATING SCALE

Criteria	Almost Never				Always Exceeds
1. Completes nursing care in a professional and competent manner	1	2	3	4	5
2. Is reliable; comes to work on time	1	2	3	4	5
3. Provides patient teaching as appropriate	1	2	3	4	5

---

rating period. These objectives are then addressed individually and in writing by both the employee and the manager during the performance appraisal evaluation. Learning goals are easier to define for both individuals because they are usually stated in broader terms. Both approaches support evaluation of employee performance. Then, in effect, the employee has created a "performance contract," as well as having defined definite goals for future professional performance. Box 17-3 illustrates goals and accomplishments.

Behaviorally anchored rating scales (BARS) can also be implemented as a collaborative or flexible approach. The focus is on behavior and should include employees in the development. BARS combine ratings with critical incidents (specific examples that have occurred) or criterion references (examples usually based on standards of practice or competency-based standards). The criteria used for this scale are specific to the specialty of nursing delivered and preestablished outcomes. This scale is also considered more advantageous in terms of litigation. BARS describes the employee's performance both quantitatively and qualitatively. Staff who are involved in the development of these instruments

---

BOX 17-3

Learning Goals and Accomplishments

Learning Goals:
1. Prepare for and take advanced cardiac life support (ACLS) certification examination
2. Participate in shared governance committee as unit representative

Accomplishments (12 months later—summary):
1. Successfully passed certification examination
2. Participated in monthly meetings; chaired task force for development and implementation of new delivery system; presented inservice class to staff on several units

---

are more likely to understand the importance of evaluation for each criterion selected and to have an understanding of their performance expectations. This is another example of clarification of roles and role expectations within the organization. The primary drawback of this scale is that it is expensive to develop and time consuming to implement; it must be designed for each specific position description or

BOX 17-4

Example of a Behaviorally Anchored Rating Scale

Emergency room (ER) staff nurse responsibilities for patient admitted with chest pain: (ER records evaluated per protocol; minimum 10/rating period). Met/Unmet

1. Vital signs recorded within 5 min of admission
   _____

2. Cardiac monitor, IV, lab tests, and ECG done within 15 min _____

3. If sublingual nitroglycerin given, vital signs recorded every 5 min for 30 min _____
   a. Chest pain changes evaluated per protocol
      _____
   b. Post–chest pain 12-lead ECG documented
      _____

standard of practice. However, it provides the manager with concrete information regarding an employee's performance, with minimal subjective interference. Box 17-4 provides an example of how established nursing standards of practice, or protocols for practice, can be incorporated into the appraisal process using peer review. The data might also be used in an outcome review process as a component of a continuous quality improvement program. The final result would be summarized by the manager and incorporated into the employee's performance appraisal.

Peer review is also a flexible or contemporary strategy. If the guidelines are developed collaboratively, peer review may also be considered a developmental method of evaluation. That is, employees are involved in the development and implementation process. This method has increased in popularity in the United States and internationally (Vuorinen, Tarkka, & Meretoja, 2000). Nurses tend to function in their normal patterns in the presence of peers, and this can be a very solid rating method. However, it is important to obtain objective ratings based on performance, not subjective ratings based on personal friendships. This method should not be used if the manager is attempting to institute team-building strategies or if the unit is unstable and employees do not like each other. The employees must trust and respect each other to willingly participate in the peer appraisal process.

Summary of Appraisal Instruments

Which instrument/method of appraisal is best? The missions and goals of the organization determine the tool(s) used. A combination of several tools is most likely superior to any one method. The primary success of any performance appraisal lies in the skills and communication abilities of the manager. Role ambiguity and uncertainty of standards of practice and methods for evaluation are significant contributors to decreased work satisfaction. The best-designed instrument will fail if the manager is ineffective and unable to communicate with the employee.

Exercise 17-4

Obtain a performance appraisal tool from the local healthcare organization from which you obtained a position description. Based on the descriptions provided, how would you characterize it? Is it structured or flexible? Is it quantitatively based, qualitatively based, or both? How does the tool reflect the position description?

Appraisal Interview Environment

The appraisal instrument is not the only factor in the evaluation process. The environment in which the appraisal is conducted is as important as the actual interview (Cohen, 2000). The interview should be conducted professionally and in a positive manner. It is an ideal time for communication between the employee and the manager. There should be no interruptions, if possible. This time is important for clarification of employee and organizational goals. Evaluation of employee performance should be objective and nonemotional. The evaluation instruments should be clearly completed, and time should be allowed for discussion. Future goals may be established. The manager and the employee should sign the appraisal form(s) and each be provided a copy. The effectiveness of the entire appraisal method relies on the manner in which the manager uses the tools and the feedback that the employee receives. Effective communication between the manager and employees can prevent potential performance problems on a unit. Specific behaviors by the manager enhance the actual appraisal process (Box 17-5).

Exercise 17-5

Find a partner. Using an audio tape recorder or a videotape recorder (preferred), conduct a performance appraisal. Seek feedback using the key behaviors in Box 17-5.

BOX 17-5

Key Behaviors for the Performance Appraisal Session

- Provide a quiet, controlled environment, without interruptions.
- Maintain a relaxed but professional atmosphere.
- Put the employee at ease; the overall objective is for the best job to be done.
- Review specific examples for both positive and negative behavior (keep an anecdotal file for each employee).
- Allow the employee to express opinions, verbally and in writing.

- Write future plans and goals, training needs, etc. (a "performance contract" for the future).
- Set follow-up date as necessary to monitor improvements, if cited.
- Show the employee confidence in his or her performance.
- Be sincere and constructive both in praise and in criticism.

The Solution

The managers decided to apply the performance appraisal principles and develop guidelines for comprehensive portfolio development. The clinical portfolio represents a strategy to manage and achieve quality outcomes. The planning and implementation of the portfolio included (1) analysis of existing evaluation components; (2) current institutional requirements (e.g. fire, safety, immunizations, certifications); (3) collaboration of the nurse manager committee and professional development committee; (4) integration of previous department-specific competency components; (5) evidence of continuing education; (6) peer-review evaluations; (7) personal notes from patients, families, and staff; and (8) a personal reflective self-evaluation.

The managers and staff believe that this comprehensive approach provides a more complete picture of the employee's performance for the entire rating period. Portfolio development is the responsibility of each employee and thus mandates employee accountability and responsibility for the inclusion of the information as listed above.

— Linda Gates

 Would this be a suitable approach for you? Why?

CHAPTER CHECKLIST

The manager plays a key role in the selection and development of staff. As a role model, the manager is also key in the establishment of the type of work environment that exists. Managers must be supportive and develop their staff to their highest potential. They must have accurate position descriptions and tools for evaluation of employee performance. These are integral to role development and professional socialization. Managers must also use various communication methods to empower their employees. Coaching and implementation of empowerment strategies positively contribute to overall staff performance as well.

- The interviewer should do the following:
  - Prescreen the applicants.
  - Prepare questions in advance.
  - Control the environment.
  - Provide role clarification.
  - Be a good listener.
  - Give honest answers to questions.
  - Provide closure.
  - Inform the applicant when he or she will be notified.
- The applicant should do the following:
  - Be on time and dressed appropriately.
  - Review the organization's mission and goals.
  - Prepare questions in advance.

- Answer questions honestly and completely.
- Note appreciation for the interview.
■ Development of the staff includes the following:
  - Organized and efficient orientation
  - Plans for education, team building, and professional socialization
  - Active coaching
  - Implementation of empowerment strategies
■ Development of accurate position descriptions and tools for evaluation of employees is integral to role development and professional socialization. Nurse managers should use various communication methods, including coaching techniques.
■ Role theory describes how individuals perceive their position in an organization.
  - Distinction and clarity among the various positions are imperative if partnerships in quality patient care are to exist.
  - The position description serves several purposes:
    - Provides written guidelines that describe roles and responsibilities
    - Reflects the position's overall function and obligations
    - Serves as a contract between manager and employee
    - Reflects current practice guidelines for the position
■ Performance appraisals are a method of providing feedback to the employee in relation to individual performance.
  - Types of structured (traditional) performance appraisals include the following:
    - Graphic rating scales
    - Forced distribution method

- Types of flexible (collaborative) performance appraisals include the following:
  - Behaviorally anchored rating scales (BARS)
  - Learning goals/management by objective (MBO)
  - Peer review

TIPS FOR CONDUCTING AN INTERVIEW

■ Prescreen the application and schedule a time for the interview.
■ Prepare questions in advance. Be concise but thorough.
■ Control the environment for noise and interruptions.
■ Explain and clarify the role for which the applicant is interviewing.
■ Be a good listener.
■ Answer questions honestly.
■ Inform the applicant when he or she will be informed of the decision.

TERMS TO KNOW

coaching	position description
empowerment	role ambiguity
halo or recency effect	role conflict
performance appraisal	role theory

REFERENCES

Antonioni, D. (2000). Leading, managing, and coaching. *Industrial Management, 42*(5), 27-33.

Barnes, B., Leis, S., Brammer, J. M., Gustin, T. J., & Lupo, T. C. (1999). A developmental evaluation process for nurses: Enhancing professional excellence. *Journal for Nursing Administration, 29*(4), 25-32.

Bradley, C. A. (2001). Your role in your annual performance evaluation. *American Journal of Nursing, 101*(7), 71-73.

Buckingham, M., & Clifton, D. O. (2001). *Now, discover your strengths.* New York: The Free Press.

Cohen, S. (2000). Prepare for your best employee evaluation yet. *Nursing Management, 31*(10), 8.

Kahn, R. L., Wolfe, D. M., Quinn, R. P., Snoek, J. D., & Rosenthal, R. A. (1964). *Occupational stress: Studies in role conflict and ambiguity.* New York: Wiley.

Kennedy, M. (2000). How do you motivate your staff? *OR Manager, 16*(8), 19.

Kinsman, F. (1998). Leadership from alongside. In J. Adams (Ed.), *Transforming leadership.* Alexandria, VA: Miles River Press.

Kolb, D. A. (1985). *Learning-style inventory.* Boston: McBer.

Lachman, V. (2000). Enrich your performance coaching techniques. *Nursing Management, 31*(1), 14-19.

Laschinger, H. K. S., Sabiston, J. A., & Kutszcher, L. (1997). Empowerment and staff nurse decision involvement in nursing work environments: Testing Kanter's theory of structural power in organizations. *Research in Nursing and Health, 20,* 341-352.

Sethi, D. (1999). Leading from the middle. *Human Resource Planning, 22*(3), 9-10.

Vuorinen, R., Tarkka, M., Meretoja, R. (2000). Peer evaluation in nurses' professional development: A pilot study to investigate the issues. *Journal of Clinical Nursing, 9,* 273-281.

Wright, D. (1998). *The ultimate guide to competency assessment in healthcare* (2nd ed.). Eau Claire, WI: PESI Health Care.

SUGGESTED READINGS

Benner, P. (1984). *From novice to expert: Power and excellence in nursing practice.* Menlo Park, CA: Addison-Wesley.

Biddle, B. J. (1979). *Role theory: Expectations, identities, and behaviors.* New York: Academic Press.

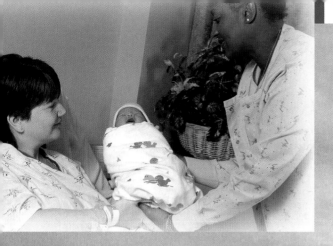

Chapter

18

Cultural Diversity in Healthcare

Dorothy A. Otto

Ana M. Valadez

T his chapter focuses on the importance of cultural considerations for patients and staff. Although it does not address comprehensive details about any specific culture, it does provide guidelines for actively incorporating cultural aspects into the roles of leading and managing. It presents concepts and principles of transculturalism, describes techniques for managing a culturally diverse workforce, emphasizes the importance of respecting different lifestyles, and discusses the effects of diversity on staff performance. Scenarios and exercises to promote an appreciation of cultural richness are also included.

Objectives

- Use concepts and principles of culture, cultural diversity, and cultural sensitivity in leading and managing situations.
- Analyze differences between cross-cultural, transcultural, multicultural, and intracultural concepts.
- Describe common characteristics of any culture.
- Illustrate the richness of cultures as they relate to staff and patients through storytelling.
- Evaluate individual and societal factors involved with cultural diversity.
- Compare and contrast values and beliefs about illness that

affect management of nursing care interventions involving patients from specific cultures.

- Use tools to address staff and patient cultural diversity.

Questions to Consider

- Why is it necessary to understand values, beliefs, and rituals held by culturally diverse staff and patients?
- What implications would "cultural sensitivity" have for you as a nurse leader or manager?
- In what ways do health-related or personal problems vary with the culture of patients and staff?
- What specific tools could you use to incorporate cultural diversity into your practice setting?

The Challenge

Marilyn E. Tompkins, RN, MSN, FNP-C
Assistant Professor of Clinical Nursing, University of Texas Health Science Center—Houston, School of Nursing; Nurse Practitioner—Student Health Center, University of Houston, Downtown Campus, Houston, Texas

Many international students who come to the Student Health Center for treatment of a viral respiratory infection do not know the acuity level of their illness. They often come from cultures in which the mother would determine the level of illness; thus they visit the center within the first 24 hours of having a "common cold." After the assessment, the nurse practitioner is the key source of information for teaching the signs and symptoms of illness, which may be self-limiting. Those symptoms that require medical intervention receive appropriate therapy.

 What do you think you would do if you were this nurse?

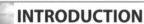

INTRODUCTION

Nurse leaders and managers are concerned with **cultural diversity** from two perspectives: the care of a diverse patient population and positive work experiences in a culturally diverse workforce. The American Nurses Association (ANA, 1993, 1997, 2000) has a long and radiant history supporting human rights. As early as 1972 the profession supported numerous efforts to eliminate discriminatory practices against specific patients and nurses. In 1993 the ANA took further action that provided a giant step for ensuring human rights for everyone. In 1997 the Ohio Nurses Association put forth a resolution that was adopted by the House of Delegates (HOD). The resolution addressed elimination of racism in the nursing workplace. In 2000 the HOD introduced an action report addressing international nursing partnerships. The action report spoke to the ANA bylaws that reflect activities related to international healthcare issues. The HOD agreed to explore possibilities for an exchange program with at least one national nurses association and engage in collaborative exchanges with colleagues from the international community to accomplish several outcomes, one of them being inclusiveness and vision. This action is reflective of how the United States' healthcare system is viewed worldwide.

American healthcare has consistently focused on individuals and their health problems, yet we have failed some people as a group in recognizing their cultural differences, beliefs, symbolism, and interpretation of illness. Commonly, the patients whom healthcare practitioners care for are newcomers to healthcare in the United States. This is true also for new staff. They are neither acculturated nor assimilated into the cultural values of the dominant **culture.** The knowledge base necessary for providers to recognize and manage cultural differences of patients and staff must be addressed. For example, consider what communication barriers might occur when an Egyptian physician, a Russian nursing student, and an American faculty member take care of a Mexican National patient receiving chemotherapy.

In its report to the Secretary of Health & Human Resources and Congress, the National Advisory Council on Nurse Education and Practice (NACNEP, 2000) addressed the need for a culturally diverse workforce to meet the healthcare needs of our nation. The Council defined that a national action-oriented agenda is needed to address the underrepresentation of racial-ethnic minorities in the workforce. To this end the NACNEP solicited, through the Division of Nursing, an Expert Workgroup on Diversity to advise them on the development of the National Agenda. The workgroup based their recommendations on four overarching goals. The four goals addressed (1) enhancing efforts to increase the recruitment, retention, and subsequent graduation of minority nurses; (2) promoting leadership development for minority nurses; (3) developing a practice environment that promotes diversity; and (4) promoting the preparation of all nurses so that culturally competent care can be provided.

Lipson, Dibble, and Minarik (1996) indicated that culture is influenced by intersections of forces larger than the individual and by shared values of what constitutes ethical professional practice. These authors provided a set of general guidelines to alert nurses in the hospital or community settings to the similarities and differences within and among the groups represented in the guidebook.

The ANA *Code of Ethics for Nurses with Interpretative Statements,* Provision 8 states, "The nurse collaborates with other health professionals and the public in promoting community, national, and international efforts to meet health needs" (2001, p. 23). This provision helps the nurse recognize that healthcare must be provided to culturally diverse populations in the United States and in all continents of the world. Even though a nurse may have the inclination to impose his or her own cultural values on others, avoiding this imposition affirms the respect and sensitivity for the values and healthcare practices associated with different cultures. Participating in a medical mission trip to provide primary care and treatment with "American drugs" to Indian family members in the mountainous villages of Honduras where natural sources are used to treat injuries, illnesses, and diseases is an imposition of healthcare views.

Nurses need to research healthcare disparities of disadvantaged patient groups. Clinical research models should incorporate collegial partnerships that provide links between global views and local "site" actions.

Meaning of Diversity in the Organization

The 2000 National Sample Survey of Registered Nurses (Bureau of Health Professions Division of Nursing, 2001) revealed that of the approximately 2.7 million registered nurses (RNs) in the United States, 86.6% reported their racial/ethnic origin as white; the remaining classified themselves in a racial/ethnic minority group. The reported groups included Hispanic, Asia/Pacific Islander, black, and American Indian/Alaskan Native. For comparison of the RN data with Census 2000, the resident population estimates in the United States by gender, race, and Hispanic origin information is available on these websites: http://www.censtus.gov/population/estimates/nation or http://www.census.gov/Press-Release/www/2001/cb01cn61.html.

Leading and managing cultural diversity in an organization means managing personal thinking and helping others to think in new ways. Managing

issues that involve culture—whether institutional, ethnic, gender, religious, or any other kind—requires patience, persistence, and much understanding. An organization's culture is significantly affected by the stories that circulate within it. Stories have symbolic power. Each person's behaviors have an effect on others.

Exercise 18-1

Think of a recent event in your workplace, such as a project, task force, celebration, or something similar. What meaning did people give the event? Was it viewed as being a symbol of some quality of the workplace, such as its effectiveness, its values and beliefs, or its innovations?

Staff who know what is valuable to the patients and to themselves can act accordingly and feel good about it. Having a clear mission, goals, rewards, and acknowledgment of efforts leads to a greater productivity and work effort from a culturally diverse staff that aspires to unity and uniqueness.

When assessing staff diversity, the nurse leader or manager can ask these three questions:

- What is the composition of the unit's workforce?
- What is the cultural representation of the workforce?
- What kind of team-building activities are needed to create a cohesive workforce for effective healthcare delivery?

Box 18-1 lists some of the techniques that may be effective when managing a culturally diverse workforce.

CONCEPTS AND PRINCIPLES

What is *culture*? Does it exhibit certain characteristics? What is *cultural diversity,* and what do we think of when we refer to *cultural sensitivity*? Are *culture* and *ethnicity* the same? Various authors have different views. Spector (2000) specified that cultural background is a fundamental component of one's ethnic background. **Ethnicity** includes, but is not limited to, characteristics such as "migratory status, . . . race, . . . language and dialect, . . . an internal sense of distinctiveness, and . . . an external perception of distinctiveness" (p. 81).

Inherent characteristics of culture are often identified with the following four factors: (1) It develops over time and is responsive to its members

BOX 18-1

Techniques for Managing a Culturally Diverse Workforce

- Have patience. Treat all questions as equally important even though they may be common everyday knowledge to you.
- Be cognizant that foreign or minority staff may not consider themselves deprived or of lesser socioeconomic status than the majority.
- Do not treat gender bias or those with different lifestyles as needing intervening techniques to change behaviors. Assume they are happy with their choice.
- Do not assume emotional outbursts represent anger. This may be a natural communication style for different groups.
- Treat compliments from your staff with respect. Avoid feeling that they are trying to request a special favor from you. In some cultures, compliments are used quite often to demonstrate respect.
- Do not assume that physical features denote a specific race or ethnic identify. Some Hispanics demonstrate Asian features, whereas some Puerto Ricans or Jamaicans may be mistaken for African blacks.
- Take the time to know your colleagues. Make time for conversational chats that will facilitate learning about each other.
- Always remember that the less you know about your staff, the more difficult your job will be as an effective manager.
- Be aware that people in your workforce may at one time or another have actually felt a part of an oppressed group. Give them a feeling of value and dignity.

and their familial and social environments, (2) its members learn it and share it, (3) it is essential for survival and acceptance, and (4) it changes with difficulty. For the nurse leader or manager, the characteristics of ethnicity and culture are important to keep in mind because the underlying thread in all of them is that staff's and patients' culture and ethnicity have been with them all of their lives. They view their cultural background as normal; the challenge is for others to view it also as normal and to assimilate it into the existing workforce.

Purnell and Paulanka's (1998) Model for Cultural Competence was constructed using a circle with the outer zone representing global society,

the second zone representing community, the third zone representing family, and the inner zone representing the person. The interior of the circle is divided into 12 pie-shaped wedges delineating cultural domains and their concepts, for example, workplace issues, family organization, and healthcare practices. The innermost center circle is black, representing unknown phenomena. Cultural consciousness is expressed in behaviors from "unconsciously incompetent—consciously incompetent—consciously competent to unconsciously competent." The usefulness of this model is derived from its concise structure, applicability to any setting, and wide range of experiences that can foster inductive and deductive thinking when assessing cultural domains.

Camphina-Bacote (1999) expanded her culturally competent model of care to five constructs: (1) awareness, (2) knowledge, (3) skill, (4) encounters, and (5) desire. She defined **cultural competence** as "the process in which the healthcare provider continuously strives to achieve the ability to effectively work within the cultural context of a client (individual, family or community)" (1999, p. 203). Individuals must examine their own biases and prejudices toward other cultures during the awareness process. Cultural knowledge requires acquisition of a sound educational foundation about various worldviews of different cultures: "One's world view can be considered a paradigm or way of viewing the world and phenomena in it" (p. 204). The skill of conducting a cultural assessment is learned while assessing one's values, beliefs, and practices to provide culturally competent services. The process of cultural encounters encourages direct engagement in cross-cultural interactions with individuals from other cultures. This process allows the person to validate, negate, or modify his or her existing cultural knowledge. It provides culturally specific knowledge bases from which the individual can develop culturally relevant interventions. Cultural desire requires the intrinsic qualities of motivation and genuine caring of the healthcare provider to "want to" engage in becoming culturally competent. Some of Camphina-Bacote's constructs are reflected in the Research Perspective.

Dochterman and Kennedy-Grace (2001) wrote of culture as being a system of learned patterns of behavior unique to members of a group. Culture encompasses more than ethnicity and might include multiple cultures.

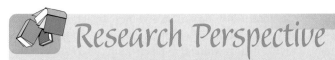
Research Perspective

Napholz, L. (1999, February). A comparison of self-reported cultural competency skills among two groups of nursing students: Implications for nursing education. *Journal of Nursing Education, 38*(2), 81-83.

Using a convenience sample of 66 junior-level nursing students, researchers designed this study to determine whether an additional cultural sensitivity intervention facilitated greater self-perceived cultural competency skills. The students were divided into two groups, and both groups received the traditional teaching approach related to cultural diversity. In addition, the treatment group received three 2-hour on-site consultations from a cultural nursing expert. Although uneven sample size of the groups precluded conclusive statements, the findings nonetheless offer some instructive guidance. The content on cultural aspects of care has been revised. Students must now view a videotape on clinical nursing aspects of culture. In addition, the inclusion of other culturally related content must be reflected on the students' anecdotal records and during their clinical conference discussions.

IMPLICATIONS FOR PRACTICE
- Faculty need to provide students with cultural learning experiences that explore attitudes for culturally competent care, a skill needed by the practicing nurse.
- Students who are more aware of their cultural beliefs and how they affect care tend to develop more culturally relevant care plans, an everyday tool used by the practicing nurse.
- Students, the practitioners of the future, need to be fully cognizant of how culture affects healthcare delivery.

Cultural diversity is the term currently used to describe a vast range of cultural differences among individuals or groups. *Cultural sensitivity* describes the affective behaviors in individuals—the capacity to feel, convey, or react to ideas, habits, customs, or traditions unique to a group of people.

Cultural differences are particularly important to Hispanics, whether they originate from Spain, Mexico, or Central or South America. Castillo (1996) wrote of first-generation groups having stronger ties to traditions and customs from their country of origin than second and third generations. Values change as new generations of a culture group adopt the new country's views over time.

A strong family value system exists in the black culture. Blacks are more likely to be an integral part of the family structure, receive support from family, and be viewed positively by younger blacks. In addition, blacks have a high affiliation and belief in religion, and the church is used as a support system for daily life and during a crisis. Data have shown that some black persons have lifelong disadvantages of lower economic status, less education, substandard housing, and poorer health status. Consider this question: How will a growing population of black female elders, who will need assistance with daily living and management of health problems, influence the family support network, change the treatment of the aged, and be the family caregiver (Sayles-Cross, 1996)?

Nurse leaders and managers who ascribe to a positive view of culture and its characteristics acknowledge cultural diversity among patients and staff. This includes providing culturally sensitive care to patients while simultaneously balancing a culturally diverse staff. For example, cultural diversity might mean being sensitive to or being able to embrace the emotions of a large **multicultural** group comprised of staff and patients. Unless we understand the differences, we cannot come together and make decisions in the best interest of the patient.

Exercise 18-2

Think about differences in people's values and how they affect healthcare. What do people who are 20 years old value as compared with those who are 50? What are the values of two people of the same age who have very different socioeconomic status? Visit the public library and look through magazines that are geared toward men and those geared toward women. What about those devoted to outdoor life and those geared to "fine" living? What values do you see reflected there? How does all of this affect healthcare?

Transculturalism sometimes has been considered in a narrow sense as a comparison of health beliefs and practices of people from different countries or geographic regions. However, culture can be construed more broadly to include differences in health beliefs and practices by gender, race, ethnicity, economic status, gender preference, age, and disability or physical challenge. Thus, when concepts of transcultural care are discussed, we should consider differences in health beliefs and practices not just between and among countries, but between genders and among races, ethnic groups, different economic strata, and so on. This requires us to consider multiple factors about all individuals.

The range of attitudes toward culturally diverse groups can be viewed along a continuum of intensity (Lenburg et al., 1995, p. 4): hate . . . contempt . . . tolerance . . . respect . . . celebration/affirmation.

Two questions that are addressed by Lenburg et al. (1995) regarding becoming culturally competent should be considered by practicing nurses (p. 10):

- What has more influence on health and illness behavior—a group's cultural characteristics or the political and economic context in which it exists?
- Is it the cultural characteristics of patients that affect their behavior in the healthcare system or the knowledge and behavior of providers?

Variables that may influence the nurse's response may include how the illness is perceived by the culture and the cultural competency of the healthcare provider. Leininger (1990) identified several major theoretical premises relating to transcultural nursing theory that nurse managers and staff can follow (Theory box):

Culturally based care values, beliefs, and practices are essential to human growth. Living and survival, health values, beliefs, and practices are derived from the culture and vary between and within cultures. Health and care concepts are identifiable by cultural groups and are linked together by cultural values and action patterns. Features of social structure are powerful forces influencing health and care in any culture, and folk and professional care and health values and action patterns are identifiable in a given culture.

According to Parker and Nichols (2001), nurses who choose to work with the Native American population must understand the complexities of tribal governance of the Native Americans and Alaska Natives in the United States to provide effective healthcare to their populations. *Trust, responsibility, tribal sovereignty, tribal politics,* and *self-governance* are commonly used terms in Indian communities, including in their healthcare programs; these concepts affect the nurses' roles when working in tribal settings. Cantone (2001) acknowledged that traditions vary from tribe to tribe and even among members of the same tribe who live in different regions. Basic Native American beliefs about health that extend beyond tribal boundaries include the importance of prayer, the treatment received from the traditional medicine man or woman, and the reverence of elders for their life experiences and wisdom.

To understand, value, and use diversity, nurse managers need to approach every staff person as an individual. Although staff of different cultural groups may be diverse in appearance, values, beliefs, communication patterns, and mannerisms, they have many things in common. Staff members

Theory Box

CULTURAL CARE THEORY

THEORY/CONTRIBUTOR	KEY IDEA	APPLICATION TO PRACTICE
Leininger (1991) is credited with developing a theory of culture care.	The theoretical framework embraces the idea that cultural constructs are embedded in each other and their application is broad and holistic. Care is viewed as culturally defined in every culture, with predictors defining health or illness.	When patients are given "human caring," the person's cultural characteristics will be addressed and incorporated into the overall plan of care.

want to be accepted by others and to succeed on their jobs (Blank & Slipp, 1994). Nurse managers should openly support the competencies and contributions of staff members from all cultural groups. Nurse managers hold the key to allowing the full potential of each person on the staff.

Sullivan and Decker (2001) described the importance of communication and how cultural attitudes, beliefs, and behavior affect communication. Body movements, gestures, verbal tone, and physical closeness when communicating are all part of a person's culture. For the nurse manager, understanding these cultural behaviors is imperative in accomplishing effective communication within the diverse workforce population. Tappen (2001) addressed differences across cultures that the nurse leader/manager needs to monitor. These differences include relationships to people in authority, spatial differences, eye contact, expressions of feelings, meaning of different language versions, thinking modes, evidence-based decision making, and preferred leadership/management style. Nurses need to ensure that ineffective communication by staff with patients and others does not lead to misunderstandings and eventual alienation.

Exercise 18−3

Consider a patient who is admitted to the postpartum unit after delivery of her third baby. You see that the mother has no right forearm or hand. The patient is aware of your observation, and she comments, "We have our first daughter." What are your reactions to the mother's physical disability? What would you say in response to the patient's comment?

The use of a bilingual health professional interpreter can be an effective strategy when caring for non-English speaking patients. As an example, the "LanguageLine" Services offers healthcare providers over-the-phone interpretation services and document translation (www.LanguageLine.com).

Exercise 18−4

During one of your group meetings, have everyone share with each other at least one or two slang words that may have a different meaning for different groups of people. Following this meeting have one of your group post a list of the words and meanings discussed in the meeting (similar to the list shown in Box 18-2). Allow everyone to continue to add slang words that patients or staff use that may create confusion or misunderstanding. Reviewing the list regularly allows staff to understand phrases and, in

some instances, to gain a cultural perspective connected to the phrase.

INDIVIDUAL AND SOCIETAL FACTORS

Nurse managers must work with staff to foster respect of different lifestyles. To do this, nurse managers need to accept three key principles: multiculturalism, which refers to maintaining several different cultures; cross-culturalism, which means mediating between/among cultures; and transculturalism, which denotes bridging significant differences in cultural practices.

Exercise 18−5

Consider doing a group exercise to enhance cultural sensitivity. Ask each group member to write down four to six cultural beliefs that he or she values. When everyone has finished writing, have the group members exchange their lists and discuss why these beliefs are valued. When everyone has had a chance to share their lists, have a volunteer compile an all-encompassing list that reflects the values of your workforce. (The key to this exercise is that many of the values are similar or perhaps even identical.)

Cultural differences among groups should not be taken in the context that all members of a certain group or subgroup are indistinguishable. Tappen

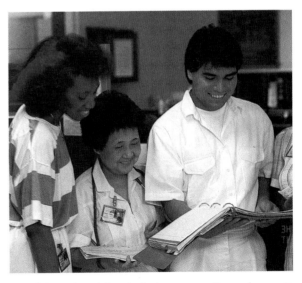

Respecting cultural diversity fosters cooperation and supports sound decision making.

BOX 18-2

Slang Terms and Their Meanings

Term	Meaning
"Spent weekend on the Chesterfield," Canada	On the sofa
"That's a fool," Caucasian	Ridiculous, mindless
"niz-hon I," Native American	Acceptable, goodness
"Shalom," Jewish	Peace, hello, or goodbye
"I feel you," African-American	I sympathize with you
"Chill out; chillin," African-American	Relax; down time
"Running off," Appalachian	Diarrhea
"High blood," Appalachian	Hypertension
"Birds don't marry fishes," Japanese mother	Don't marry outside your race
"It's a disaster," various cultures	Chaos
"Peace out," African-American	Goodbye, see you later
"Lip lard," southern United States	Lipstick
"Down with my homies," African-American	Out with friends
"Yo," African-American	What's up?
"Bakwas," India	Nonsense talk
"Ciao," Italy	Good-bye
"Puti," Philippines	White American
"De poca madre," Mexico	Cool, neat mother
"Ay que quapo," Mexico	Wow, how cute

Respecting cultural diversity fosters cooperation and supports sound decision making.

(2001) described this "indistinguishable" phenomenon and recommended that cultural differences be viewed as group tendencies. For example, in the arena of gender differences, women are perceived to have a more participative management style; however, this does not mean that all male managers use an authoritative management model. Likewise, women managers may use multiple sources of information to make decisions, and this does not mean that all male managers make decisions on limited data. Thus the norm for gender recognition should be that females and males be hired, promoted, rewarded, and respected for how successfully they do the job, not because of who they are, where they come from, or whom they know.

In today's workplace, female-male collaboration should provide efficacious models for the future. Gender does not determine response in any given situation. However, men reportedly seem to be better at figuring out what needs to be done, whereas women are best in collaborating and getting others to collaborate in accomplishing a task. Men tend to take neutral, logical, and objective stands on problems, whereas women become involved in how the problems affect people. It is important to recognize that women and men bring separate perspectives to resolving problems, which can help them function more effectively as a team on the nursing unit. Men and women must learn to work together and value the contributions of the other and the differences they bring to any situation.

Accessibility to healthcare in the United States is linked to specific social strata. This challenges nurse leaders, managers, and followers who strive for worth, recognition, and individuality for patients and staff regardless of their ascribed economic and social standing. Beginning nurse leaders, managers, and followers may sense that the knowledge they bring to their job lacks "real-life" experiences that provide the springboard to address staff and patient needs. In reality, although lack of experience may be slightly hampering, it is by no means an obstacle to addressing individualized attention to staff and patients. The key is that if the nurse manager and staff respect people and their needs, economic and social standing becomes a moot point. Nurse managers must be cognizant of divergent views about healthcare as a right for all people rather than a privilege for a few. Healthcare services are moving from a largely unicultural to a multicultural approach. Andrews (1998) reported the increasingly growing diverse healthcare workforce. She advocated the development of a **transcultural nursing administration.** Shared values and beliefs, although part of the corporate culture, often are measured by perceptions or feelings. If nursing administrators are committed to transcultural management, they should actively promote recruitment of diverse staff and be alert to signs of prejudice in their organization. Likewise, mission statements and policies should be reviewed to reflect the workforce diversity.

Ethnocentrism, believing one's own values are the best, most desired, or preferred, is the basis of "cultural imposition," according to Leininger (1990). Ethnocentrism is viewed as a major concern in nursing. Leininger defined *cultural imposition* as "the tendency of nurses to impose their values, beliefs, and practices on another culture" (p. 55). Such practice occurs from nurses' lack of awareness about different cultures and nurses' ethnocentric tendencies.

Failure to address cultural diversity leads to negative effects on performance and staff interactions. Nurse managers can find many ways to address this issue. For example, in relation to performance, a nurse manager can make sure messages about patient care are received. This might be accomplished by sitting down with the staff nurse and analyzing the situation to make sure that understanding has occurred. In addition, the nurse manager might use a communication notebook that allows the nurse to slowly "digest" information by writing down communication areas that may be unclear. For effective staff interaction, the nurse manager also can make a special effort to pair mentors and mentees who have different ethnic backgrounds.

The complexities of culture strongly influence perceptions, opinions, and generalizations. Mancini (1997) wrote about the need for nurse managers and supervisors to be ever vigilant of attitudes and behaviors that encourage racial or ethnic stereotypes and inhibit communication and trust. She believes a culturally skilled manager who understands and values differences can ultimately build trust and enhance communication, as well as production and motivation in the team. Culturally skilled nurse managers can provide "cultural safety" to patients

by examining their cultural beliefs and attitudes and how they affect others (Meleis, Isenberg, Koerner, Lacey, & Stern, 1995). Ultimately, experience working with diverse staff and patients may be the best educational environment for learning culture, other than living as a "resident" within a culture group for the purpose of acculturation. Managers can help eliminate stereotyping by presenting alternative views or referring to the lists of commonalities among the staff.

Nurse managers must address communication and motivational issues when working with employees of different backgrounds. Lowenstein and Glanville (1996) challenge nurse managers to use their pivotal positions to confront cultural conflict and render effective conflict resolution. Although nurse managers must set the tone, the staff (followers) share in the responsibility for creating a climate that lends itself to open discussions about cultural differences.

RICHNESS OF CULTURES

In many health facilities the staff members, as well as the patients, have a variety of culturally diverse backgrounds. Nurses must understand and appreciate the richness of cultures. They should work toward consensus building that offers employees a practice area that promotes quality care for patients.

Although the literature has addressed multicultural needs of patients, it is sparse in identifying effective methods for nurse managers to use when dealing with multicultural staff. Differences in education and culture can impede patient care, and uncomfortable situations may emerge from such differences. For example, staff members may be reluctant to admit language problems that hamper their written communication. They may also be reluctant to admit their lack of understanding when interpreting directions. Psychosocial skills may be troublesome as well because non-Westernized countries encourage emotional restraint. Staff may have difficulty addressing issues that relate to private family matters. Non-Asian nurses may have difficulty accepting the intensified family involvement of Asian cultures. The lack of assertiveness and the subservient physician-nurse relationships of some cultures are other issues that provide challenges for nurse managers. Unit-oriented workshops arranged by the nurse manager to address effective assertive techniques and family involvement as it relates to cultural differences are two ways of assisting staff with cultural work situations.

Exercise 18-6

As part of your team-building activities, plan a luncheon with a group that includes each team member's favorite "homemade" recipe. Ask each person to briefly write or discuss why the recipe is meaningful, such as, "we always had it at Christmas," "my grandmother said it cured all ailments," or "my dad thought it was gourmet cooking." Share recipes if requested.

Husting (1995) believes that management has a responsibility to address cultural issues because healthcare workforces are changing rapidly. All workers bring to the workplace their own values, beliefs, and behaviors. Diversity of these values and beliefs can be in conflict and create a work environment that is not conducive to worker effectiveness and quality patient care. Husting proposed a model that can help management address a culturally diverse workforce and assist in moving them to a culturally congruent workplace environment. The model's characteristics include discussing ethnocentricity and moving on to recognizing and respecting diverse views of culture. The outcome of the model is equal worker partnerships, that is, capitalizing on the best aspects of all cultures for an effective harmonious work setting.

The Canadian Nurses Association *Code of Ethics for Registered Nurses* (1997) identifies "fairness" as one of its values and states, "Nurses provide care in response to need regardless of such factors as race, ethnicity, culture, spiritual beliefs, social or marital status, gender, sexual orientation, age, health status, lifestyle or physical attributes of the client" (p. 17). This comprehensive statement has salient implications of applicability in any country.

Providing quality of life and human care is difficult to accomplish if the nurse does not have knowledge of the recipient's culture as it relates to care (Leininger, 1994). Leininger's view of cultural care is from a transcultural perspective, that is, examining values, beliefs, and symbols of particular cultures. Accordingly, "quality of life" must be addressed from an emic (inside) cultural viewpoint and compared with an etic (outsider) professional's perspective. By comparing and contrasting these two viewpoints, more meaningful nursing practice interventions will evolve. This comparative analysis will require nurses to include in their cultural stud-

ies worldwide, global views that take into account the social and environmental context of different cultures.

Exercise 18-7

Assess several clinical settings. Do these settings have programs related to cultural diversity? Why? What are the programs like? If there are no programs, why do you think they have not been implemented?

DEALING EFFECTIVELY WITH CULTURAL DIVERSITY

Andrews (1998) reported the increasingly growing diverse healthcare workforce. She advocated development of a transcultural nursing administration. Shared values and beliefs, although part of the corporate culture, often are measured by perceptions or feelings. If nursing administrators are committed to transcultural management, they should actively promote recruitment of diverse staff and be alert to signs of prejudice in their organization. Likewise, mission statements and policies should be reviewed to reflect the workforce diversity.

Nurse managers hold the key to making the best use of cultural diversity. Managers have positions of power to begin programs that enrich the diversity among staff. For example, capitalizing on the knowledge that all staff bring to the patient is possible for better quality care outcomes. One method that can be used is to allow staff to verbalize their feelings about particular cultures in relationship to personal beliefs.

Generalizations can lead to stereotypes, such as believing that all Hispanics are Roman Catholics, all Jewish people are orthodox in their dietary practices, all whites are WASPs (white, Anglo-Saxon Protestants), or all Asians eat rice. Nurse managers must develop synergism and high morale for a culturally diverse staff. An excellent way to do this is for the nurse manager to use group projects. For example, two or three staff members could be present at a patient care conference. The nurse manager can facilitate the presentation by providing coffee and a relaxed environment. Buttons that convey messages such as, "I'm on a winning team" or "Caring is my job," are high morale boosters for staff.

Exercise 18-8

Holiday celebrations have cultural significance. What is the cultural meaning of the specific holiday? How do staff or

Table 18-1 EXAMPLES OF HOLIDAY CELEBRATIONS OF CULTURAL SIGNIFICANCE

Term	Country	Date
Araw Ng Mga Patay	All Saints Day, Philippines	November 1
Chinese New Year	China, Chinatowns	January or February (varies with Chinese Calendar)
Cinco de Mayo	Independence Day, Mexico	May 5
Ramadan	Muslim/Islamic festival, India	Ninth month of Muslim year
Dipavali/Diwali	Hindu festival of lights, India	October-November
Hanukkah/Chanukah	Jewish festival of lights, US	December
Christmas	Compare countries and dates, U.S.	December 25
Kwanzaa	African-American, U.S.	Between Christmas and New Year's Day
Boxing Day	Worker's Recognition, Canada, Australia, Great Britain	December 26
Martin Luther King, Jr.	Civil rights, U.S.	January 20

others celebrate these days? Table 18-1 provides some examples.

The establishment of mentoring programs should be done so that all staff can expand their knowledge about cultural diversity. Vance and Olson (1998) addressed mentoring international colleagues and students. Although their emphasis was on the educational aspect of mentoring, the underlying principles for mentoring in the service settings are the same: (1) Mentors are living role models, (2) if the mentor has firsthand experience with the mentee's country and culture, the relationship will be strengthened, and (3) both mentor and mentee should have an understanding of each other's culture and language. Programs that address the staff's cultural diversity should not try to make people of different cultures pattern their behavior after the prevailing culture. Nurse managers must carefully select those mentors who ascribe to transcultural, rather than ethnocentric, values and beliefs. A much richer staff exists when nurse managers build on the valuable culture of all staff and when diversity is rewarded. The pacesetter for the cultural norm of the unit is the nurse manager. For example, to demonstrate commitment to cultural diversity, a nurse manager might make a special effort to ensure that African-American, Asian-American, and Hispanic holidays or other cultural representations on the unit are recognized by the staff. Staff who are active participants in these pro-

grams can then be given positive reinforcement by the nurse manager. These activities promote a better understanding and appreciation of individuals' cultural heritage.

Continuing-education programs should assist nurses in learning about the care of different ethnic groups. Meleis et al. (1995) identified 10 recommendations for enhancing the development of knowledge related to culturally competent care for diverse and marginalized populations (Box 18-3). For example, with other appropriate organizations (e.g., Philippine Nurses Association of Metropolitan Houston) and institutions (e.g., M.D. Anderson Cancer Center), sponsor or encourage the development of a yearly workshop or conference on cross-cultural nursing for faculty and nursing service staff who have had limited preparation in the area of cultural care or cultural beliefs in healing.

Exercise 18-9

Identify a situation in which care to a culturally diverse patient had positive or negative outcomes of care. If a negative outcome resulted, what could you have done to make it a positive one?

Sensitive or controversial issues are often addressed by behaviors that represent avoidance or coercion. The similarities or differences about the issue or person are not acknowledged, either subconsciously or consciously. Avoidance precludes any opportunities for open discussion and potential

BOX 18-3

Recommendations for Action Related to Culturally Competent Care

1. Make a commitment to provide equitable, culturally competent care.
2. Sustain disciplinary culturally competent knowledge.
3. Identify mechanisms that allow integration of all existing knowledge pertaining to nursing care of different disadvantaged populations.
4. Develop a base of transdisciplinary knowledge that mirrors heterogeneous healthcare practices within cultural groups.
5. Develop knowledgeable healthcare for disadvantaged groups using appropriate theories and frameworks.
6. Explore organizational structures that create environments that foster cooperative working relationships and knowledge related to disadvantaged populations.
7. Use proven effective models when delivering care to disadvantaged populations.
8. Develop policies that support content addressing diversity in nursing curricula with the cooperation of curriculum committees and state regulatory bodies.
9. Develop methodologies to address adequate faculty and student preparation in culturally competent nursing practices on the local, regional, national, and international levels.
10. Work with ethnic minority nursing organizations to recruit and retain a diverse nurse population.

BOX 18-4

Problem-Solving Communication: Honoring Cultural Attitudes Toward Death and Dying

Scenario 1: Staff and a Patient's Family

What nurses often call interference with the care of a patient commonly reflects family attitudes toward death and dying. Often, Hispanic families rush to the hospital as soon as they hear of a relative's illness. Because most Hispanics believe that death is the passing of an individual to a life that offers tranquility and everlasting happiness, being at the bedside offering prayers and encouragement is the norm rather than the unusual exception. The nurse manager in this situation, herself a non–American-educated nurse manager, had worked extensively at helping her staff to understand different cultures. A consensus compromise was worked out between the staff and one such Hispanic family. The family, consisting of three generations, was given the authority to decide what family members could stay at the loved one's bedside and for how long. By doing this, the family felt they had control of the environment and quickly developed a priority list of family members who could stay no more than 5 minutes at the patient's bedside. As the family member left the bedside, his or her task was to report the condition of their loved one to other family members "camping" in the visitors' lounge. Although their loved one did not survive a massive intracranial hemorrhage, all of the family felt a part of the "passage of life" by their loved one.

Scenario 2: A Nurse Manager and Another Staff Member

Eastern world cultures that profess Catholicism as their faith celebrate the death of a loved one 40 days after the death. The nurse manager needs to recognize that time off for the nurse involved in this celebration is imperative. Such an occurrence had to be addressed by a nurse manager of Asian descent. The nurse manager quickly realized that the nurse, whose mother died in India, did not ask for any time off to make the necessary burial arrangements, but rather waited 40 days to celebrate his mother's death. The celebration included formal invitations to a church service, as well as a dinner after the service. One day during early morning rounds the nurse explained how death is celebrated by Eastern world Catholics. The Bible's description of the Ascension of the Lord into heaven 40 days after his death served as the conceptual framework for the loved one's death. The grieving family believed their loved one's spirit would stay on earth for 40 days. During these 40 days the family held prayer sessions meant to assist the "spirit" to prepare for its ascension into heaven. When the 40 days have passed, the celebration previously described marks the ascension of their loved one's spirit into heaven.

Because this particular unit truly espoused a multicultural concept, the nurses had no difficulty in allowing the Indian nurse 2 weeks of unplanned vacation so that his mother's "passage of life" celebration could be accomplished in a respectful, dignified manner.

for change. Avoidance can be a powerful and controlling strategy, but situations do not vanish because they are avoided. Aspects of the situations may eventually resurface. If the situation becomes intolerable, frustration and anger most likely will occur. Various responses are possible, and insistence that the issue is no longer visible in the setting does not imply its resolution.

Coercion is acted out through the use of power or status to persuade people to act in specific ways. Although coercion is not a negative behavior, it can lead to negative consequences through the inequity of power. Coercive tactics limit choices and may result in powerlessness, although the importance of the outcome varies greatly. For example, the use of coercion in a situation may result in anger, which is a normal response to feelings of powerlessness that result from being or feeling controlled. Passivity and aggression often perpetuate the situation, and individuals may not recognize the effect of their actions.

Choices, decisions, and behaviors reflect learned beliefs, values, ideals, and preferences. The goal of communication is maintenance or restoration of personal integrity and recognition of worth and respect of individuals or groups.

The two scenarios described in Box 18-4 illustrate how problem-solving communication can promote mutual understanding and respect. The first scenario involves a compromise between staff members and a patient's family, and the second involves a nurse manager and a staff member from a different culture.

Exercise 18–10

Identify a situation involving a staff member in which a request was made that required a culturally sensitive decision. What did you observe about religious or ethnic practices in regard to this decision?

Passages of life that culminate in happy events also can challenge the nurse manager—for example, the quinceñera observed by Hispanic families. This event is the celebration for 15-year-old girls to be introduced into society. The nurse whose daughter is celebrating this event must have time to make plans for this festive celebration. Because of the significance of the celebration and the pride that the parents take in their daughter, inviting "key" staff to the quinceñera is common. Nurse managers who understand and value cultural rituals can help individuals meet their needs and help staff, in general, learn and accept various cultural practices and perspectives.

The Solution

The nurse practitioner provides teaching and reinforcement with instruction sheets that list serious signs and symptoms for the student's recognition and decision about seeking further medical treatment. At the orientation for new students and international students, the services available at the student health center are explained and small groups are formed to discuss the services offered and the opportunities for visits to the "self-care station" to obtain a day's supply of free over-the-counter medications, teaching sheets for various minor illnesses, or to make an appointment with the nurse practitioner. Interpreters are available for the international students with English a second language.

— Marilyn E. Tompkins

 Would this be a suitable approach for you? Why?

CHAPTER CHECKLIST

All potential or current nurse leaders or managers must acknowledge and address cultural diversity among staff and patients. Culture lives in each of us. It determines how we think, what we value, how we behave, and how we communicate with each other. In everyday work activities, the nurse manager must be able to do the following:

■ Assess staff diversity and use techniques to manage a culturally diverse workforce.

Continued

CHAPTER CHECKLIST—cont'd

- Lead staff with a clear understanding of principles that embrace culture, cultural diversity, and cultural sensitivity.
- Be able to communicate effectively with staff and patients from diverse cultural backgrounds:
  - Recognize slang terms that have different meanings in different cultures.
  - Understand that nonverbal behaviors also carry different connotations depending on one's culture.
- Select basic characteristics of any culture.
- Appraise factors, both individual and societal, inherent in cultural diversity:
  - Three key principles relate to respect for different lifestyles:
    - Multiculturalism refers to maintaining several different cultures simultaneously.
    - Cross-culturalism refers to mediating between two cultures (one's own and another).
    - Transculturalism denotes bridging significant differences in cultural practices.
  - Sexual orientation and gender recognition are important factors to consider in dealing fairly with all patients and staff members.
- Use tools that clarify staff and patient cultural diversity effectively:
  - Mentoring programs can help staff expand their knowledge of cultural diversity.
  - Continuing education programs can help nurses learn about caring for different ethnic groups in ways that honor their beliefs.
- Appreciate the cultural richness found among staff and patients.

TIPS FOR DEALING WITH CULTURAL DIVERSITY

Being a nurse manager in a country that views its strength in its population's cultural diversity requires special skills. The nurse manager needs to do the following:
- Ascribe to effective techniques for managing a culturally diverse workforce.
- Appreciate and encourage programs that address cultural diversity of staff.
- Assist staff in problem solving special cultural needs of patients.
- Embrace three key principles relating to culture: multiculturalism, cross-culturalism, and transculturalism.
- Commit to lifelong learning about culture for self and staff.

TERMS TO KNOW

cultural competence
cultural diversity
culture
ethnicity
ethnocentrism
multicultural
transculturalism
transcultural nursing administration

REFERENCES

American Nurses Association. (1993). *Summary of proceedings of 1993 House of Delegates*. Washington, DC: Author.

American Nurses Association. (1997). *Summary of proceedings of 1997 House of Delegates*. Washington, DC: Author.

American Nurses Association. (2000, June 23-28). *Summary of proceedings of 2000 House of Delegates*. Indianapolis: Author.

American Nurses Association. (2001). *Code of ethics for nurses with interpretative statements*. Washington, DC: American Nurses Publishing.

Andrews, M. M. (November 1998). Transcultural perspectives in nursing administration. *Journal of Nursing Administration, 28*(11), 30-38.

Blank, R., & Slipp, S. (1994). *Voices of diversity: Real people talk about problems and solutions in a workplace where everyone is not alike*. New York: AMACON (American Management Association).

Bureau of Health Professions, Division of Nursing. (2001, February). *The Registered Nurse Population, National Sample Survey of Registered Nurses—2000. Preliminary Findings*. Rockville, MD: U.S. Department of Health and Human Resources, Health Resources and Services Administration.

Camphina-Bacote, J. (1999, May). A model and instrument for addressing cultural competence in health care. *Journal of Nursing Education, 38*(5), 203-207.

Canadian Nurses Association. (1997, March). *Code of ethics for registered nurses*. Ottawa, Ontario: Author. Available at http://www.can-nurses.ca/pages/ethics/ethics.htm

Cantone, J. A. (2001, Winter). Earth, wind, fire and water. *Minority Nurse*, pp. 24-29. (CASS Recruitment Media Publication.)

Castillo, H. M. (1996). Cultural diversity: Implications for nursing. In S. Torres (Ed.), *Hispanic voices: Hispanic health educators speak out.* New York: NLN Press.

Census 2000. Retrieved from http://www.census.gov/population/estimates/nation and http://census.gov/PressRelease/www/2001/cb01cn61.html

Dochterman, J. M., & Kennedy-Grace, H. K. (2001). *Current issues in nursing*, 6th ed. St. Louis: Mosby.

Husting, P. M. (1995, August). Managing a culturally diverse workforce. *Nursing Management, 26*(8), 26, 28-29.

Leininger, M. M. (1990). Culture: The conspicuous missing link to understanding ethical and moral dimensions of human care. In M. Leininger (Ed.), *Ethical and moral dimensions of care.* Detroit: Wayne State University.

Leininger, M. M. (1991). *Culture care diversity and universality: A theory of nursing.* New York: National League for Nursing. Pub No. 15-2402.

Leininger, M. M. (1994, Spring). Quality of life from a transcultural nursing perspective. *Nursing Science Quarterly, 7*(1), 22-28.

Lenburg, C. B., Lipson, J. G., Demi, A. S., Blaney, D. R., Stern, P. N., Schultz, P. R., & Gage, L. (1995). *Promoting cultural competence in and through nursing education: A critical review and comprehensive plan for action.* Washington, DC: American Academy of Nursing.

Lipson, J. G., Dibble, S. L., & Minarik, P. A. (1996). *Culture and nursing care: A pocket guide.* San Francisco: UCSF Nursing Press.

Lowenstein, A. J., & Glanville, C. (1996). Cultural diversity and conflict in the health care workplace. *Nursing Economics, 13*(4), 203-209, 247.

Mancini, M. E. (1997). Managing cultural diversity. In K. W. Vestal. *Nursing management: Concepts and issues*, 2nd ed. Philadelphia: Lippincott.

Meleis, A. I., Isenberg, M., Koerner, J. E., Lacey, B., & Stern, P. (1995). *Diversity, marginalization, and culturally competent health care issues in knowledge development.* Washington, DC: American Academy of Nursing.

Napholz, L. (1999, February). A comparison of self-reported cultural competency skills among two groups of nursing students: Implications for nursing education. *Journal of Nursing Education, 38*(2), 81-83.

National Advisory Council on Nurse Education and Practice. (2000). *A national agenda for nursing workforce, racial/ethnic diversity.* Washington, DC: U.S. Department of Health and Human Services, Health Resources & Service Administration, Bureau of Health Professions.

Parker, J. G., & Nichols, L. A. (2001, Summer). Second opinion: Tribes know best. *Minority Nurse.* (CASS Recruitment Media Publication.)

Purnell, L. D., & Paulanka, B. J. (1998). *Transcultural health care: A culturally competent approach.* Philadelphia: FA Davis.

Sayles-Cross, S. (1996). Aging, care giving effects and black family caregivers. In R. W. Johnson (Ed.), *African American voices: African American health educators speak out.* New York: NLN Press.

Spector, R. E. (2000). *Cultural diversity in health and illness*, 5th ed. Upper Saddle River, NJ: Prentice Hall Health.

Sullivan, E. J., & Decker, P. J. (2001). *Effective leadership and management in nursing*, 5th ed. Upper Saddle River, NJ: Prentice Hall.

Tappen, R. (2001). *Nursing leadership and management: Concepts and practice*, 4th ed. Philadelphia: FA Davis.

Vance, C., & Olson, R. K. (Eds.). (1998). *The mentor connection in nursing.* New York: Springer.

SUGGESTED READINGS

Bonder, B., Martin, L., Miracle, A. (2002). *Culture in clinical care.* Thorofare, NJ: Slack.

Camphina-Bacote, J. (1994, March). Cultural competence in psychiatric mental health nursing: A conceptual model. *Nursing Clinics of North America, 29*(1), 1-8.

Corlese, I. B., Nicholas, P. K., & Nokes, K. M. (2001, First Quarter). Issues in cross-cultural quality-life research. *Journal of Nursing Scholarship, 33*(1), 15-20.

Giger, J. N., & Davidhizar, R. E. (1999). *Transcultural nursing: Assessment & intervention*, 3rd ed. St. Louis: Mosby.

Greenberg, J., & Baron, R. A. (2000). *Behavior in organizations: Understanding and managing the human side of work*, 7th ed. Upper Saddle River, NJ: Prentice Hall.

Guido, G. W. (2001). Employment laws: Corporate liability issues. In *Legal and ethical issues in nursing*, 3rd ed. Upper Saddle River, NJ: Prentice Hall.

Hilfinger Messias, D. K. (2001, First Quarter). Globalization, nursing, and health care for all. *Journal of Nursing Scholarship, 33*(1), 9-11.

Leininger, M. M. (1991). *Culture care diversity & universality: A theory of nursing.* New York: National League for Nursing.

Zemke, R., Raines, C., & Filipczak, B. (2000). *Generations at work: Managing the clash of veterans, boomers, Xers and nexters in your workplace.* New York: AMACOM.

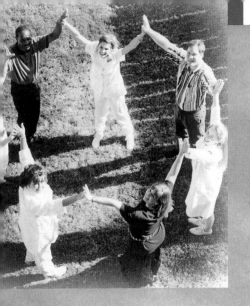

Chapter 19

Building Teams Through Communication and Partnerships

Karren Kowalski

*T*his chapter explains major concepts and presents tools with which to create and maintain a smoothly functioning **team.** *Life requires that we work together in a smooth and efficient manner, communicate effectively, and develop relationships that produce partnerships. Many important team efforts occur in the work setting. Such teams often include members with various backgrounds and educational preparation (e.g., physicians, nurses, administrators, allied health professionals, and support staff such as housekeeping and dietary staff members). Each team member has something valuable to contribute and deserves to be treated honorably and with respect. When teams are not working, all team members must change how they communicate and interact within the team.*

Objectives

- Distinguish between a group and a team.
- Identify four key concepts of teams.
- Demonstrate an effective communication interaction.
- Identify at least five communication pitfalls.
- Apply the guidelines for acknowledgment to a situation in your clinical setting.
- Compare a setting that uses the "rules of the game" with your current clinical setting.
- Develop an example of a team that functions synergistically, including the results such a team would produce.

Questions to Consider

- *What differentiates a team from a group? How is it created?*
- *What are the most common communication breakdowns?*
- *What are key aspects of a well-functioning team?*
- *What are the key issues or questions team members want to know?*
- *How are communication and self-worth connected?*
- *What role do agreements or guidelines play in a team?*
- *What are the behaviors and attitudes that destroy teams?*
- *Do teams go through stages of development?*

The Challenge

From Diane Gallagher, RN, MS
Director, Women's and Children's Services, Rush-Presbyterian-St. Luke's Medical Center, Chicago, Illinois

An extensive "team" of people works together to care for the neonate in a neonatal intensive care unit (NICU). They include physicians, registered nurses, respiratory therapists, physical therapists, social workers, neonatal nurse practitioners, and ancillary staff. Occasionally, specialists are consulted for specific cardiac, neurological, or gastrointestinal problems. These are intermittent "team" members who play a crucial role in the baby's care.

Recently, a new group of specialists joined our team. They were identified as a top-notch group who would, by virtue of their expertise and reputation, increase the census and revenues for the hospital. Our team was excited to have this opportunity to grow in an area where we had infrequent experience. However, things did not go smoothly. There were clinical disagreements, communication breakdowns, and interpersonal conflicts. The experience evolved into mutual distrust and control issues.

As disagreements, insults, and complaints escalated on both sides, the situation came to a defining moment when the director of the specialty group said, "I'm never bringing any of our patients here. I'm sending them to the PICU." The response from the NICU team was, "Fine with us; we don't need you, your patients, or the hassle." It seemed reasonable to not work together because in fact, functionally, we were already not working together. This response was in direct conflict with our belief that we could provide a valuable service and make a difference for both the patients and their families. This posed a dilemma for the staff, but everyone felt the situation was hopeless.

No one believed we could function as a team, and therefore further efforts to work together were futile. We had tried and failed. Let's just cut our losses and move on. How does one create a team when no one believes it is possible and some believe it's not even necessary?

 What do you think you would do if you were this nurse?

INTRODUCTION

As we experience changes such as cost cutting and downsizing in healthcare, teamwork becomes critical. The adage "If we do not all hang together we will all hang separately" was never more true than now as we move through an era in which healthcare is rapidly changing. To create finely tuned teams, communication skills must improve. Each team member must focus on improving his or her own skills, as well as supporting other team members, to grow in **effective communication.**

In our society, where so much emphasis is placed on the individual and individual achievement, teamwork is the quintessential contradiction. In other words, with all the focus on individuals, we still need individuals to work together in **groups** to accomplish goals. Everybody knows and understands this, particularly individuals who spend their Sundays watching football or basketball. These team sports are premier models of cooperation and competition. They are the model for teamwork for

business today, and they represent a group following their respective leader or "coach" (Parcells, 2000).

GROUPS AND TEAMS

The definition of *group* is a number of individuals assembled together or having some unifying relationship. Groups could be all the parents in an elementary school, all the members of a specific church, or all the students in a school of nursing because the members of these various groups are related in some way to one another by definition of their involvement in a certain endeavor. A *team*, on the other hand, is a number of persons associated together in specific work or activity. Not every group is a team, and not every team is effective.

A group of people does not constitute a team. From Parker's (1990) perspective, a team is a group of people with a high degree of interdependence geared toward the achievement of a goal or a task.

Often, we can recognize intuitively when the so-called team is not functioning effectively. We say things such as, "We need to be more like a team" or "I'd like to see more team players around here." Consequently, in the process of defining *team,* effective versus ineffective teams should be considered. Teams are groups that have defined objectives, ongoing positive relationships, and a supportive environment and that are focused on accomplishing a specific task. Teams are essential in providing cost-effective, high-quality healthcare. As resources are expended more prudently, patient care teams must develop clearly defined goals, use creative problem solving, and demonstrate mutual respect and support. Facilities with ineffective teams will find themselves out of business.

■ Exercise 19–1

Think of the last team or group of which you were a part. Think about what went on in that team or group. Specifically think about what worked for you and what didn't work. Use the "Team Assessment Questionnaire" in Table 19-1 to evaluate these aspects more specifically. When you have finished answering the questions, use the scoring mechanism at the bottom to discover how well your team or group functioned in terms of roles, activities, relationships, and general environment.

When a team functions effectively, a significant difference is evident in the entire work atmosphere, the way in which discussions progress, the level of understanding of the team-specific goals and tasks, the willingness of members to listen, the manner in which disagreements are handled, the use of consensus, and the way in which feedback is given and received. The original work done by McGregor (1960) sheds light on some of these significant differences, which are summarized in Table 19-2.

Ineffective teams are often dominated by a few members, leaving others bored, resentful, or uninvolved. Leadership tends to be autocratic and rigid, and the team's communication style may be overly stiff and formal. Members tend to be uncomfortable with conflict or disagreement, avoiding and suppressing it rather than using it as a catalyst for change. When criticism is offered, it may be destructive, personal, and hurtful rather than constructive and problem-centered. Team members may begin to "stuff" their feelings of resentment or disagreement inside, sensing that they are "dangerous." This creates the potential for later eruptions

and discord. Similarly, the team avoids examining its own inner workings, or members may wait until after meetings to voice their thoughts and feelings about what went wrong and why.

In contrast, the effective team is characterized by its clarity of purpose, informality and congeniality, **commitment,** and high level of participation. The members' ability to listen respectfully to each other and communicate openly helps them handle disagreements in a civilized manner and work through them rather than suppress them. Through ample discussion of issues, they reach decisions by consensus. Roles and work assignments are clear, but members share the leadership role, recognizing that each person brings his or her own unique strengths to the group effort. This diversity of styles helps the team adapt to changes and challenges, as does the team's ability and willingness to assess its own strengths and weaknesses and respond to them appropriately.

The challenges encountered in today's healthcare systems are prodigious. Ongoing rounds of downsizing budget cuts, declining patient days, reduced payments, and staff layoffs abound. Effective teams participate in effective problem solving, increased creativity, and improved healthcare.

COMMUNICATING EFFECTIVELY

When new graduates go through a facility orientation, communication skills are often reviewed. Many nurses view this as a waste of time that could be used to further technical skills; yet, at evaluation time, communication skills are often seen as an area for improvement (Buckman, Korsch, Baile, & Jason, 2000). The only thing human beings do more often than communicate is breathe. It is the most important component of daily activities. It is essential to clinical practice, to building teams, and to leadership. A person cannot *not* communicate. Because communication consists of both verbal and nonverbal signals, humans are continuously communicating not just thoughts, ideas, and opinions but also feelings and emotions (Morreale, Spitzberge, & Barge, 2001). Once the message is sent, it cannot be retracted; it can be amended, but the first impression of the communication usually is lasting. Yet as important as this initial impression is, it is often an unconscious response or reaction.

How we communicate is also a reflection of self-worth: Once a human being has arrived on this

Table 19-1 TEAM ASSESSMENT QUESTIONNAIRE

Circle the appropriate number using the following scale.
(1, Not at all; 2, limited extent; 3, some extent; 4, considerable extent.)

1. People are clear about goals for the group.	1 2 3 4
2. Unnecessary procedures, policies, and formality are minimized.	1 2 3 4
3. Team members feel free to develop and experiment with new ideas and approaches.	1 2 3 4
4. The allocation of rewards is perceived to be based on excellent performance.	1 2 3 4
5. Recognition and praise outweigh threats and criticism.	1 2 3 4
6. Calculated risk taking is encouraged.	1 2 3 4
7. People are clear about their responsibilities and expectations for performance.	1 2 3 4
8. People are clear about how their roles and responsibilities interrelate with those of others.	1 2 3 4
9. People perceive others in the work group to be high performers.	1 2 3 4
10. People are clear about what personal characteristics/competencies are necessary for superior performance in their jobs.	1 2 3 4
11. The team produces high-quality decisions, products, and/or services.	1 2 3 4
12. The team is able to conduct effective meetings.	1 2 3 4
13. The team achieves its goals.	1 2 3 4
14. The team and its individual members are able to interact effectively with others outside the team.	1 2 3 4
15. The team makes decisions and produces output in a timely fashion.	1 2 3 4
16. The team members truly support each other in carrying out their respective responsibilities.	1 2 3 4
17. Team members are open in their communications with each other.	1 2 3 4
18. Team members follow through on commitments.	1 2 3 4
19. Team members trust each other.	1 2 3 4
20. All team members are equal contributors to the team process.	1 2 3 4
21. The group often evaluates how effectively it is functioning.	1 2 3 4
22. Individual members feel committed to the team.	1 2 3 4

If you'd like to score your team assessment questionnaire, enter the score you selected for each question. Next, take the scores for each area; then calculate the average score.

Roles Item/Score	Activities Item/Score	Relationships Item/Score	Environment Item/Score
7 ___	2 ___	5 ___	1 ___
8 ___	3 ___	14 ___	2 ___
9 ___	11 ___	16 ___	3 ___
10 ___	12 ___	17 ___	4 ___
18 ___	13 ___	19 ___	5 ___
20 ___	15 ___	22 ___	6 ___
21 ___			
Total Score ___	Total Score ___	Total Score ___	Total Score ___
Average Score = ___ (Total Score ÷ by 7)	Average Score = ___ (Total Score ÷ by 6)	Average Score = ___ (Total Score ÷ by 6)	Average Score = ___ (Total Score ÷ by 6)

If the average for a column (e.g., Activities) was 3.5, it means the group is fairly productive in its activity, falling halfway between "some extent" and "considerable extent." If the average for the relationships column was 1.5, it indicates the respondent believes that team members have not been effective in developing relationships with one another that are clearly defined, effective, or respectful of one another.

From Dubnicki, C. (1991, May-June). Building high-performance management teams. *Healthcare Forum Journal, 34*, 19-24.

Table 19-2 ATTRIBUTES OF EFFECTIVE AND INEFFECTIVE TEAMS

Attribute	Effective Team	Ineffective Team
Working environment	• Informal, comfortable, relaxed	• Indifferent, bored; tense, stiff
Discussion	• Focused • Shared by almost everyone	• Frequently unfocused • Dominated by a few
Objectives	• Well understood and accepted	• Unclear, or many personal agendas
Listening	• Respectful—encourages participation	• Judgmental—much interruption and "grandstanding"
Ability to handle conflict	• Comfortable with disagreement • Open discussion of conflicts	• Uncomfortable with disagreement • Disagreement usually suppressed, or one group aggressively dominates
Decision making	• Usually reached by consensus • Formal voting kept to a minimum • General agreement is necessary for action; dissenters are free to voice opinions	• Often occurs prematurely • Formal voting occurs frequently • Simple majority is sufficient for action; minority is expected to go along
Criticism	• Frequent, frank, relatively comfortable, constructive • Directed toward removing obstacle	• Embarrassing and tension-producing; destructive • Directed personally at others
Leadership	• Shared; shifts from time to time	• Autocratic; remains clearly with committee chairperson
Assignments	• Clearly stated • Accepted by all despite disagreements	• Unclear • Resented by dissenting members
Feelings	• Freely expressed, open for discussion	• Hidden, considered "explosive" and inappropriate for discussion
Self-regulation	• Frequent and ongoing, focused on solutions	• Infrequent, or occurs outside meetings

Modified from McGregor, D. (1960). *The human side of enterprise.* New York: McGraw-Hill.

earth, communication is the largest single factor determining what kinds of relationships she or he makes with others and what happens to each in the world (Satir, 1988, p. 51). Self-worth is a major influence in all communication. Stress results whenever self-worth is threatened.

Communication is learned from watching others. A host of poor examples can be seen in movies and television. Poor communication leads to relationship breakdowns, misunderstandings, high levels of emotion, judgment, and an excess of drama. Nursing programs teach therapeutic communications with patients and their families. However, little focus is placed on effective communication in the workplace, although communication is essential to building and maintaining smoothly functioning teams.

A basic model of communication patterns between the sender and the receiver is found in Figure 19-1. Effective communication develops a rhythm in which messages are sent and received in a productive, respectful, and supportive manner (Wilson, 1999). Communication begins to break down as the rhythm is disrupted. The sender-receiver pattern disintegrates into a nonrhythmic event, as described in Figure 19-1. When nonrhythmic patterns develop, the participants may feel disrespected, upset, and even fearful.

Stress

Satir (1988) has identified the connection between stress and self-worth that can evolve as a result of a breakdown in communication. She defines stress as a threat to positive self-worth. Human beings tend to feel stress or anxiety whenever there is an unconscious linking of feelings, behaviors, or comments from others to a lowering of self-esteem or an

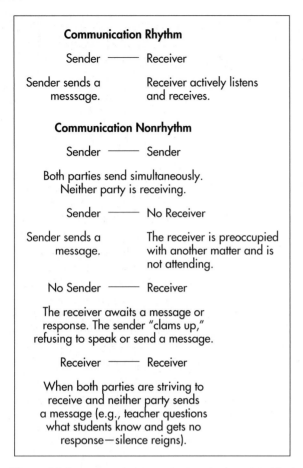

Communication Rhythm

Sender ———— Receiver

Sender sends a   Receiver actively listens
messsage.   and receives.

Communication Nonrhythm

Sender ———— Sender

Both parties send simultaneously.
Neither party is receiving.

Sender ———— No Receiver

Sender sends a   The receiver is preoccupied
message.   with another matter and is
                        not attending.

No Sender ———— Receiver

The receiver awaits a message or
response. The sender "clams up,"
refusing to speak or send a message.

Receiver ———— Receiver

When both parties are striving to
receive and neither party sends
a message (e.g., teacher questions
what students know and gets no
response—silence reigns).

Figure 19-1   Potential communication rhythms. (Modified from Satir, V. [1988]. *The new peoplemaking.* Mountain View, CA. Science & Behavior Books; and Olen, D. [1993]. *Communicating speaking & listening to end misunderstanding and promote friendship.* Germantown, WI: JODA Communications.)

attack on self-worth. A conscious effort should be made to relieve stress through activities such as ensuring specific/scheduled quiet time, requesting peer support, keeping a journal, treating yourself to something special, or going for a walk (Weiss, 2001).

Stress Response Model

When this threat is identified, the receiver often reacts using one of the five communication patterns: attribution of blame, placation, constrained cool headedness, immaterial irrelevance, or congruence (Bradley & Edinberg, 1990; Satir, 1988). Each pattern interaction and the source of the interaction are described with examples of each pattern in Table 19-3. The pattern that produces effective communication, the one to strive for, is congruence. Congruent communication occurs when both the verbal and nonverbal actions fit the inner feelings of

the sender and are appropriate to the context of the message. This communication pattern creates the kind of connection between the sender and the receiver that fosters respect, support, and the creation of relationship.

Communication Barriers

In today's busy world, many interruptions and interferences to clear, focused, effective communication create breakdowns. According to Ceccio and Ceccio (1982), to be aware of these potential problems allows both sender and receiver to be prepared to minimize such barriers.

- *Distractions:* Distractions most commonly come through sensory perceptions, such as poor lighting or background noise, including music, talking, ringing phones, and interruptions by others. Papers, reports, and heavy workloads can also be distracting.
- *Inadequate knowledge:* The sender and receiver may be at different levels of knowledge, particularly in this time of highly specialized and technical knowledge bases. For multiple reasons, one person may not seek clarity from the other.
- *Poor planning:* The process of organizing, planning, and clearly thinking through what needs to be communicated is very helpful. If the interaction is more spontaneous, it can more easily fall into a nonrhythmic pattern.
- *Differences in perception:* Both the sender and the receiver have their individual mental filters—the way in which they see the world. Because of this individuality, no two filters are the same. Thus the same message is interpreted differently. Add to this sociocultural, ethnic, and educational differences, to name a few, and it is easy to see how these differences can occur.
- *Emotions and personality:* Someone who is experiencing distress may not be able to receive another message or may have difficulty keeping his or her emotions out of an unrelated message. Most humans, at some point, bring distress or problems from home to the workplace. If these remain unconscious, they can influence the work setting in a negative or nonproductive way.

Communication Pitfalls

Effective communication suggests that the interaction is a rhythmic pattern that is respectful and clear, promotes trust, and encourages the expression of feelings and viewpoints. On the other hand,

Table 19-3 COMMUNICATION PATTERNS

Pattern	Interaction	Source	Example
Attribution of blame	Sender blames receiver	Fault-finder dictator acts superior as camouflage for fear and low self-esteem	Mostly "you" messages; for example, "You really blew it!"
Placation	Sender placates receiver	Sender's low self-worth: puts herself/himself down	"I was wrong. I'm sorry. It's all my fault."
Constrained cool headedness	Sender is correct and very reasonable without feeling or emotion	Feelings of vulnerability covered by cool analytical thinking	"Studies have shown that in 75% of cases the patient is correct. I decided to use research data in coming to a solution."
Irrelevant	Sender is avoiding the issue, ignoring own feelings and feelings of the receiver	Fear, loneliness, and purposelessness	"Wait a minute. Let me tell you about…"(changes the subject)
Congruence	Sender's words and actions are congruent; inner feelings match the message	Any tension is decreased and self-worth is at a high level	"For now, I feel concerned about the anger and hostility exhibited by Dr. X. I'm wondering what approach would de-escalate him?"

Modified from Satir, V. (1988). *The new peoplemaking.* Mountain View, CA: Science & Behavior Books; and Bradley, J., & Edinberg, M. (1990). *Communication in the nursing context* (3rd ed.). Norwalk, CT: Appleton & Lange.

pitfalls in communication comprise actions, behaviors, and words that create distrust, are dishonoring, and decrease the feelings of self-worth in the receiver. Box 19-1 lists the major pitfalls of communication. These pitfalls lead to communication breakdowns that affect not only the team but also the quality of care to patients (Jason, 2000).

Communication Guidelines

There are effective guidelines that can be used when communicating. These are used mostly to facilitate a positive outcome and to create an environment in which the communicator can achieve the desired outcome. Unconscious use of any of the pitfalls will most likely result in thwarting the desired outcome. Box 19-2 lists effective guidelines for communication.

 Exercise 19–2

In pairs or small groups, compare and contrast the effective guidelines for communication with the communication pitfalls. Give examples of each from your own recent personal experience. Hypothesize how you could have changed the pitfalls into a positive interaction.

KEY CONCEPTS OF TEAMS

In rare instances, a team may produce teamwork spontaneously, like kids in a school yard at recess. However, most management teams learn about teamwork because they need and want to work together. This kind of working together requires that they observe how they are together in a group and that they unlearn ingrained self-limiting assumptions about the glory of individual effort and authority that are contrary to cooperation and teamwork. Keys to the concept of team include the following:

- Conflict resolution
- Singleness of mission
- Willingness to cooperate
- Commitment

Conflict Resolution

The word *team* is usually reserved for a very special type of working together. This working together requires communication in which the members understand how to conduct interpersonal relationships

BOX 19-1

Communication Pitfalls

1. **Advice giving**

   It is so tempting to give advice when a co-worker comes with an issue or problem. *Don't!* Most often what the person wants is to work through the issue by talking out loud. Just listen.

2. **Making others wrong**

   When telling others "our" story of distress, the adversary is always "wrong." The telling of the story to a third party only reinforces how right "I" am and how wrong, bad, or terrible the other person is. If you have an issue or problem, take the problem to the person with whom you are upset. "Take the mail to the correct address." Don't gossip!

3. **Defensiveness**

   Defensiveness occurs when you do not listen, are hostile or aggressive, or respond as if attacked when there was no attack. Look for a physiological signal in your body so that you can identify your own distress. Stop. Breathe. Acknowledge that the message did not come out the way you intended and begin again.

   Also, defensiveness can occur when met with hostile, aggressive behavior from another. Rather than choose an emotional response or react to the attack, know that the other person's behavior has nothing to do with you personally but is the response chosen by that person in a moment of stress. Any one of a dozen other responses could have been chosen. Understand the person is motivated by fear or hurt.

4. **Judging the other person**

   Evaluating another person as "good" or "bad," or someone you like or don't like, or judging their actions or behavior as "stupid" or "crazy" or "inappropriate" is a reflection of how you judge yourself. Who is the hardest person on you? Of course, you are. Know that you can have feelings about situations or behaviors without judging the other person in a negative way. Rather, you can feel compassion for their stress and fear, which often drives behavior. This is true particularly when a supervisor or physician is reprimanding you.

5. **Patronizing**

   Speaking to another as if they are less than human or in need of custodial care fails to honor them as a human being. You do not have to be condescending or seek to humiliate in an overly sweet voice. These are merely other versions of judging or making the person wrong. Another approach is to question what is at issue for them in the moment.

6. **Giving False Reassurance**

   One of the great temptations of nurses is to "fix" things and make them better, to rescue the situation or the person involved. To accomplish this goal, sometimes we reassure inappropriately. Know that you do not have to fix every situation. You can support people to work through the situation themselves.

7. **Asking Why Questions**

   When working in the team, refrain from asking why questions. These tend to create a defensive response in the other person. Instead, ask "What makes you think…"

8. **Blaming Others**

   Saying things such as "You make me so angry" is blaming the other person for your feelings, which you choose at any given time. In nearly every situation, the responsibility for communication breakdown is a joint responsibility. You can always choose your response, even if that response is to say, "I can't discuss this with you now. I would like to talk about this later when I am more calm."

with their peers in thoughtful, supportive, and meaningful ways. It requires that team members be able to resolve conflicts among themselves and to do so in ways that enhance rather than inhibit their working together. In addition, team members must be able to trust that they will receive what they need while being able to count on one another to complete tasks related to team functioning and outcomes. To communicate effectively, people must be willing to confront issues and to openly express their ideas and feelings—

to use interactive skills to accomplish tasks. In nursing, constructive confrontation has not been a well-used skill. Consequently, if communication patterns are to improve, the onus is on each of us as individuals to change communication patterns. In essence, for things to change, each of us must change.

Singleness of Mission

Each and every team must have a purpose—that is, a plan, aim, or intention. However, the most suc-

BOX 19-2

Guidelines for Communication

Approach each interaction as though the other person has no knowledge of effective communication. Assume responsibility for creating the sender-receiver rhythm.

Share your thoughts and feelings. Be self-revealing.

Casual conversation or "small talk" can be important to relationships, particularly when it is light and humorous. It balances the deep meaningful talk.

Acknowledging, praising, and encouraging the other person is supportive and brings life and energy to the relationship.

Present messages in a way that the other person can receive them.

When you have a problem or issue with another, take responsibility for the problem and speak about it as your problem also.

Use language of equality even when position titles are not of the same level.

Modified from Olen, D. (1993). *Communicating speaking & listening to end misunderstanding and promote friendship.* Germantown, WI: JODA Communications.

cessful teams have a mission—some special work or service to which the team is 100% committed. The sense of mission and purpose must be clearly understood and agreed to by all (Fisher & Thomas, 1996). The more powerful and visionary the mission is, the more energizing it will be to the team. The more energy and excitement are engendered, the more motivated all members will be to do the necessary work.

Willingness to Cooperate

Just because a group of people has a regular reporting relationship within an organizational chart does not mean the members are a team. Boxes and arrows are not in any way related to the technical and interpersonal coordination or the emotional investment required of a true team. Most of us have been involved in organizations in which people could accomplish assigned tasks but were not successful in their interpersonal relationships. In essence, these employees received a salary for not getting along with a certain person or persons. Some of these employees have not worked cooperatively for years! Organizations can no longer afford to pay people to not work together. Personal friendship or socialization is not required, but cooperation is a necessity.

Commitment

Commitment is a state of being emotionally impelled and is demonstrated when there is a sense of passion and dedication to a project or event—a mission. Often, this passion looks a little crazy. In other words, people go the extra mile because of their commitment. They do whatever it takes to accomplish the goals or see the project through to completion. An example of commitment is discussed by Charles Garfield when he talks about being a part of the team that created the lunar landing module for the first man to walk on the moon. People did all kinds of things that looked crazy, including working extended hours and shifts, calling in to see how the project was progressing, and sleeping over at their work station so as not to be separated from the project—all because everybody knew they were a part of something that was much bigger than themselves. They were a part of sending a man to the moon, something that human beings had been dreaming about for thousands of years. It was a historical moment, and people were intensely committed to making it happen.

Many people go through their entire lives hating every single day of work. Needless to say, most of them are not committed. Because we spend an extensive amount of time in the work setting, it is critically important to both physical and mental well-being that people enjoy what they do. If this is not the case for you, then try to find a different job or profession—one you might love. Life is too short to do something that you hate doing every day. While you are moving into whatever you decide you love doing, commit to yourself to do your best at whatever you are now doing. Be 100% present wherever you are. Do the best work you are capable of doing. This honors you as a human being, and it honors your co-workers and patients.

Exercise 19-3

Box 19-3 contains eight questions. Spend at least 20 minutes in a quiet place thinking about and writing answers to these eight questions. Pay particular notice to question 7.

There are many examples of commitment, such as that of Jan Skaggs, the Vietnam veteran who was the driving force behind the building of the Vietnam War Memorial. He was a clerk in the Washington, DC, bureaucracy who attended a veterans' meeting and decided there needed to be a memorial to those who lost their lives in Vietnam, a memorial that had all 58,000 names inscribed on it. He had only a

BOX 19-3

Exploring Commitment

The key to finding your compelling mission/passion that will lead you to success and peak performance is to ask yourself the right questions. Your answers to these questions will help you understand what you need to know about yourself. Read each question, then think carefully for a few minutes and answer each question honestly. Do not censor or edit out anything, even if it seems impossible or unrealistic—allow yourself to be surprised. Let your imagination soar.

1. Am I deriving any satisfaction out of the work I am now doing?
2. If they didn't reward (praise or pay) me to do what I now do, would I still do it?
3. What is it that I really love to do?
4. What do I want to pursue with my time and energy that is worthwhile?
5. What motivates me to reach out and do my very best, to excel?
6. What is it that only I can say to the world? What needs to be done that can best be done only by me?
7. If I won $10 million in the lottery tomorrow, how would I live? What would I do each day and for the rest of my life?
8. If I were to write my own obituary right now, what would be my most significant accomplishment? Is that enough?

Repeating this exercise often will give you additional insights and information about what you really want and love to do. If taken seriously, the exercise should help you to have an understanding of why you selected this profession and whether or not you have the stamina to do whatever it takes to make a contribution and to make a difference in the practice of nursing.

high school diploma and did not even own a suit, but 5 years and $7 million later, the wall was dedicated (Lopes, 1987). This is a demonstration that one does not have to have a college degree to be committed. Sometimes a college degree can inhibit people from accomplishing their goals because they become diverted from a purpose, from a mission, or from life goals by things such as good grades. Rather than understanding grades as a tool of measurement, they see it as an end in itself.

Almost anyone can be taught the technical aspects of what needs to be done in most patient care settings. Teaching people to love what they do or to care about patients and their families—even the most difficult and unique patients and families—is far more difficult.

TOOLS AND ISSUES THAT SUPPORT TEAMS

When individuals come together in a group, they spend a fair amount of their time in group process or social dynamics, which allows the group to advance toward becoming a team and completing a goal. Each person within the group struggles with three key questions that must continually be reevaluated and renegotiated. These three questions, according to Weisburg's classic work (1988), are as follows:

1. Am I in or out?
2. Do I have any power or control?
3. Can I use, develop, and be appreciated for my skills and resources?

This chapter's Literature Perspective focuses on the classic work of Weisburg (1988).

"In" Groups and "Out" Groups

Most of us want to be valued and recognized by others as a part of the group, one who "knows" or understands. Most people want to be at the core of decision making, power, and influence. In other words, they want to be part of the "in" group, and researchers have demonstrated that those who feel "in" cooperate more, work harder and more effectively, and bring enthusiasm to the group. The more we feel we are not a part of the key group, the more "out" we feel and the more we withdraw, work alone, daydream, and engage in self-defeating behaviors. Often, intergroup conflict results when individuals who feel they are "out" and want to be "in" create a schism or a division that prohibits the team from accomplishing its goals.

Power and Control

Everybody wants at least some power, and everybody wants to feel they are in control. When faced with changes that we are unable to influence, we feel impotent and experience a loss of self-esteem. Consequently, all of us want to feel we are in control of our immediate environment and that we have enough power and influence to get our needs met. When a situation or an event arises that we are unable to handle, we attempt to compensate for it

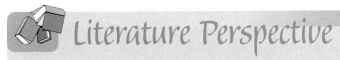

Literature Perspective

From Weisburg, M. R. (1988). Team work: Building productive relationships. In W. B. Reddy & K. Jamison (Eds.), *Team building blueprints for productivity and satisfaction* (pp. 62-71). Alexandria, VA: NTL Institute for Applied Behavioral Sciences; and San Diego: University Associates.

Building productive relationships in the workplace is critical to team success. Increasing productivity requires observing team members at work and unlearning deeply ingrained, self-limiting assumptions about individual effort and authority that work against cooperation. In some respects, this is an ongoing process of renewal that cannot occur without some disarray and confusion.

IMPLICATIONS FOR PRACTICE

Every team member must deal with three key issues: (1) Am I in or out? (2) Do I have any power and control? (2) Can I use, develop, and be appreciated for my skills and resources? These issues must be addressed periodically if trust, motivation, and commitment are to be maintained in the team. Differences of opinion must be expressed constructively with honor and respect for each other.

in some way; most of these ways are not productive to smoothly functioning teams.

Exercise 19-4

Think about a time when you or a small group of classmates wanted to change a class, an assignment, or the grading curve of a test and the faculty or the school administration adamantly refused. How did you feel? What was the response? Did you engage in gossip to make the faculty or the administration appear wrong? You may have been "right," but the sense of a loss of control or power is very uncomfortable, sometimes resulting in stress and fear. Very mature behavior is required to maintain a positive, problem-solving approach.

Positive Communication Model

Whenever human beings are in distress or are having an emotional reaction to a situation or the actions of another, a conditioned response is to move into one or all of the following: *blame, judgment,* or *demand*. These are depicted in the awareness model found in Figure 19-2. With effort and practice, it is possible to create a communication interaction that produces a significantly improved outcome.

- When an individual is reacting at the feeling level, he or she tends to move unconsciously to blame. By taking accountability for these feelings, one can move out of blame and own one's feelings by stating, "I feel . . ."
- Likewise, when an individual is trapped in distress or reaction at the thinking level, he or she most often turns to judgment. By thinking compassionately, one can dismantle the judgment and

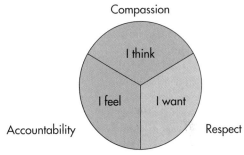
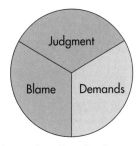

Figure 19-2 Awareness model: differentiating between conscious and unconscious responses. (Modified from St. Charles Medical Center. [1993]. *People centered teams.* Bend, OR: SCMC.)

state what one thinks in a compassionate way: "I think. . ."
- Finally, when in distress, we make demands that are often unreasonable. By calming oneself, one can find respect for the other human being and make a request: "I want. . ."

Most broken relationships are stuck in blame, judgment, and demand. Being accountable, compassionate, and respectful helps clarify what goes on inside each of us.

Everyone needs to feel as though their skills, tools, and contributions are needed and valued and that they are respected for what they have to offer to the workplace, team, or group. Everyone has weaknesses, and there is no need to emphasize these or to spend time in ongoing correction. Rather, focus should be placed on people's strengths, specifically, acknowledging and emphasizing what people do well.

Part of focusing on people's strengths is being willing to acknowledge peers, faculty, and the other significant people in one's life (Roman, 2001). In contrast, many role models focus on correction. Consequently, many of us spend a large portion of our time correcting others rather than appreciating people for all the wonderful things they are. We seem to believe a finite number of available **acknowledgments** exists, and we must not give out too many of them because they must be held in reserve for very important events. In addition, we do not always give acknowledgments in a way they can be received and valued. Box 19-4 can serve as a guide for giving acknowledgment.

To deal with the three personal issues discussed in this section, team members must learn how to state openly what is on their minds and be responsive and respectful as other members of the team do the same. In other words, team members must give and receive feedback constructively. These are essential elements that must be in place for people to be able to give and receive feedback in constructive ways.

BOX 19-4

Guidelines for Acknowledgment

1. Acknowledgments must be specific. The specific behavior or action that is appreciated must be identified in the acknowledgment; for example, "Thank you for taking notes for me when I had to go to the dentist. You identified three key points that appeared on the test."
2. Acknowledgments must be "eye to eye," or personal. Look the person in the eye when you thank them. Do not run down the hall and say "Thanks" over your shoulder. Written appreciation also qualifies as "eye to eye."
3. Acknowledgments must be sincere, that is, from the heart. Each of us recognizes insincerity. If you do not truly appreciate a behavior or action, do not say anything. Insincerity often makes people angry or upset, thus defeating the goal.
4. Acknowledgments are more powerful when they are given in public. Most people receive pleasure from public acknowledgment and remember these occasions for a long time. For people who are shy and may prefer no public acknowledgment, this is an opportunity to work on a personal growth issue with them. Public acknowledgment is an opportunity to communicate what is valued.
5. Acknowledgments need to be timely. The less time that elapses between the event and the acknowledgment, the more powerful and effective it is and the more the acknowledgment is appreciated by the recipient.

Working cooperatively, an effective team produces extraordinary results that no one team member could have achieved alone.

■ *Exercise 19–5*

Within the next 3 days, find three opportunities to acknowledge a peer or acquaintance using the five guidelines for acknowledgment shown in Box 19-4. In addition, use the guidelines to accept at least one self-acknowledgment.

Group Agreements

One of the most helpful tools available is to have the team members come to an agreement about the ground rules concerning their relationships with one another (Mears, 1997). This can take place in various ways. There are even multiple kinds of guidelines or rules that can be used to set the context for how people relate. One example of a set of guidelines can be found in Box 19-5. These are called "The Rules of the Game." They have gone through multiple transitions and redesign, but the basic tenets are essentially the same. People must agree on the goals and mission with which they are involved. They have to reach some understanding of how they will exist together. Tenets or rules such as "We will speak supportively" go a long way to avoid gossiping, backbiting, bickering, and misinterpreting others. As you review these group agreements, keep in mind that a part of this process is the willingness of members of the team to be accountable for upholding the agreements and to give feedback when the

BOX 19-5

"Rules of the Game" for Women's and Children's Hospital, Rush-Presbyterian–St. Luke's Medical Center

These "Rules of the Game" were adapted from a San Francisco real estate broker who was the founder and president of Hawthorn-Stone. Dr. Karren Kowalski proposes that we use them not only among ourselves but with each new person who joins the organization, asking if we/they are willing and able to do the very best we/they can to support the rules.

1. BE WILLING TO SUPPORT RUSH'S PURPOSE, GAMES, RULES, AND GOALS

    By first asking if people will support the rules, we have their agreement that they can be held accountable for times when they violate the "rules of the game."

2. SPEAK SUPPORTIVELY

    This means no swearing; if it does not serve, do not say it; if it does not support, do not say it; do not make other people wrong; you may choose not to say negative things. Language either empowers or limits people in terms of achieving their potential. How we speak about a colleague, the institution, our job, the workplace, and so forth, does make a difference.

3. CORRECT SUPPORTIVELY

    Dr. Kowalski says, "Make corrections without invalidation or correct without crucifixion."

4. ACKNOWLEDGE THAT WHATEVER IS BEING COMMUNICATED IS TRUE FOR THE SPEAKER AT THAT MOMENT

    Most of the time people make comments because they truly believe them. Therefore it is important not to judge what is being said and misinterpret it, but to listen so that we can understand what is being said. Emphasis is on active listening.

5. COMPLETE YOUR AGREEMENT

    Only make agreements that you intend to and are willing to keep. This is especially important for those who (1) procrastinate and (2) say "yes" to everything. If you must break an agreement, communicate this information as soon as possible.

6. IF A PROBLEM ARISES, FIRST USE THE SYSTEM FOR CORRECTIONS, THEN COMMUNICATE THE PROBLEM WITH OPTIONAL SOLUTIONS TO THE PERSON WHO CAN DO SOMETHING ABOUT THE PROBLEM

    This is another way to eliminate gossip, judgment, and self-righteousness.

7. BE EFFECTIVE AND EFFICIENT

8. OPTIMIZE EVERY EVENT—CREATE MORE WITH LESS

    Items 7 and 8 go together. Look for value in every event. Focus on what can be learned or done; use "lateral thinking" to create effective options.

9. HAVE THE WILLINGNESS TO WIN AND TO ALLOW OTHERS TO WIN

    "Win/lose" is a "zero sum game." Effective problem solving allows everyone to win—to get their needs met.

10. FOCUS ON WHAT WORKS

    The corollary is, get beyond what's not working. Be willing to try something new. When it's broke, fix it!

11. WHEN IN DOUBT, CHECK OUT FEELINGS

    When there seem to be blocks to communication or progress, it is often related to how people are feeling. Check this out, ask the person/people in question. Get the feelings out in the open where they can be checked out, tested, responded to.

12. AGREE TO DISAGREE UNTIL REACHING CONSENSUS

    Commit to working together toward mutually agreeable solutions. This keeps things in a forward motion without judgment. It keeps things hopeful.

13. TELL THE TRUTH FROM THE POINT OF VIEW OF PERSONAL RESPONSIBILITY

    Always begin with the pretense that you are willing to assume 50% of the responsibility. This eliminates "you, you, you" messages and allows you to work with others toward a solution, not toward blame.

Modified from Thurber, M. (1973). *Rules of the game.* San Francisco: Hawthorne-Stone Real Estate.

agreements have been violated. Without rules, people have implicit permission to behave in any manner they choose toward one another, including angry, hurtful acting-out behavior.

Trust

Trust is the basis by which leaders/managers facilitate the activities and the progress of the team. Hogan defines *leadership* as "the ability to persuade a group to set aside individual preoccupations in order to pursue a common goal, and leadership should be evaluated in terms of how a group performs vis-à-vis the other groups with which it competes" (1997, p. 1). Hogan concludes that the essential task of leadership is to build high-performance teams. Thus the key sign that leaders/managers are performing poorly is the degree to which their team members do not trust them.

Trust is also a major issue among group members, and one of the first questions to come up in the group concerns whom one can trust or not trust. In the early days of organizational development, McGregor (1967) defined *trust* in the following way:

> Trust means: "I know that you will not—deliberately or accidentally, consciously or unconsciously—take unfair advantage of me." It means, "I can put my situation at the moment, my status and self esteem in this group, relationship, my job, my career, even my life, in your hands with complete confidence" (p. 163).

One can see from this description how critical trust is within a team (Druskat & Wolff, 2001). The leader models trust through behaviors such as setting the ground rules by which the team will function and holding team members accountable for adhering to the rules. Trust is probably the most delicate aspect within relationships and is influenced far more by actions than by words. In other words, what people do is more powerful than what they say. Trust is a fragile thread that can be severed by one act. Once destroyed, trust is more difficult to reestablish than its initial creation.

CREATING SYNERGY

Teams function with varying levels of effectiveness. The interesting part of this is that effectiveness can be created systematically. Truly effective teams are ones in which people work together to produce ex-

traordinary results that could not have been achieved by any one individual (Mears, 1997). This phenomenon is often described as **synergy**. In the physical sciences, synergy is found in metal alloys. Bronze, the first alloy, was a combination of copper and tin and was found to be much harder and stronger than either copper or tin separately and the tensile strength of bronze can be predicted by merely adding the tensile strength of tin and of copper.

We see the same properties of synergy in human endeavors, for example, in the 1980 U.S. hockey team. Many people remember this hockey game, in which the Americans defeated the Russians. The team consisted of a group of college kids, none of whom could establish a successful career in the National Hockey League. However, for 2 weeks they were the best hockey team in the world—and they were the best because they knew how to work together to produce extraordinary results. Likewise, Jackson (1995) describes the creation of a synergistic kind of team in his book about coaching the Chicago Bulls basketball team.

To consistently create synergy, one must follow some basic rules:

- Establish a clear purpose.
- Listen actively.
- Be compassionate.
- Tell the truth.
- Be flexible.
- Commit to resolution.

Establish a Clear Purpose

Creative synergy requires a clear purpose. Each member of the team must understand the reason they are together, determine what he or she wishes to accomplish (as delineated by defined goals and objectives), and express his or her belief in both the value and feasibility of the goals and tasks. Teams function best when the members can not only tell others about their purpose but also define and operationalize succinctly the meaning and value of this purpose.

Listen Actively

Listening actively means that one is completely focused and tuned in to the individual who is speaking. It means listening without judgment. It means listening to the essence of the conversation so that you can actually repeat to the speaker most of the speaker's intended meaning. It means being 100% present in the communication (For guidelines to active listening, see Box 19-6). It does not mean developing a defensive response or argument in your head while the other person is still speaking. To listen actively, a person must be absolutely focused on the speaker, absorbing words, posture, tone of voice, and all the clues accompanying the message, so that the intent of the communication can be re-

ceived. Specific purposes used in **active listening**, including examples, are found in Table 19-4.

Be Compassionate

To be compassionate means to have a sympathetic consciousness of another's distress and a desire to alleviate the distress. Consequently, it is inappropriate

---

BOX 19-6

Guidelines for Active Listening

1. Slow down your internal processes and seek data. Do not interrupt the speaker.
2. The more information you acquire through listening, the less interpretation you do (making up the missing pieces or motivations). The less information you have, the more interpretation you do.
3. Realize that the first words from the other person are not necessarily representative of inner thoughts and feelings. Be patient.
4. When listening, suspend your own beliefs and views and judgments, at least temporarily. Attempt to under-

stand the perspective of the other person, particularly if it is different from yours.
5. Realize that any judgments or "labels" strongly influence the manner in which you listen to the other person.
6. Appreciate the difference between understanding other people's perspective and agreeing with them. First strive to understand. Then you may agree or disagree.
7. Effective listening is based on an inner desire to learn about another's unique experience of the world.

Modified from Olen, D. (1993). *Communicating speaking & listening to end misunderstanding and promote friendship.* Germantown, WI: JODA Communications.

Table 19-4 ACTIVE LISTENING

Use of Active Listening	Examples
To convey interest in what the other person is saying	I see! I get it. I hear what you're saying.
To encourage the individual to expand further on his or her thinking	Yes, go on. Tell us more.
To help the individual clarify the problem in his or her own thinking	Then the problem as you see it is . . .
To get the individual to hear what he or she has said in the way it sounded to others	This is your decision, then, and the reasons are . . . If I understand you correctly, you are saying that we should . . .
To pull out the key ideas from a long statement or discussion	Your major point is . . . You feel that we should . . .
To respond to a person's feelings more than to his or her words	You feel strongly that . . . You do not believe that . . .
To summarize specific points of agreement and disagreement as a basis for further discussion	We seem to be agreed on the following points . . . But we seem to need further clarification on these points . . .
To express a consensus of group feeling	As a result of this discussion, we as a group seem to feel that . . .

to focus time and energy on making the other person wrong, especially when your perspective differs from his or hers. It means listening from a caring perspective—one that is focused on understanding the viewpoint of the other person rather than insisting on the "rightness" of one's own point of view.

Tell the Truth

To tell the truth means to speak clearly to personal points and perspectives while acknowledging that they are, merely, a personal perspective. If an observation is made about the tone or behavior of a speaker that affects the ability of others to hear the message, feedback can be provided in a way that does not make the speaker wrong. This is accomplished in an objective rather than subjective manner using neither a cynical nor a critical tone of voice. To be effective, one must own—be responsible for—personal opinions and attitudes.

Be Flexible

Flexibility and openness to another person's viewpoint are critical for a team to work well together. No single person has all the right answers. Therefore acknowledging that each person has something to contribute and must be heard is important. Flexibility reflects a willingness to hear another team member's point of view rather than being committed to the "rightness" of a personal point of view.

Commit to Resolution

To commit to resolution means that one can agree to disagree with someone even when that perspective is different. Rather than assuming the person is wrong, this is a commitment to hear his or her perspective, listen to the real message, identify differences, and creatively seek solutions to resolve the areas of differences so that there can be a common understanding and shared commitment to the issue. Both parties need to then agree that they feel heard and agree to the resolution. This differs greatly from compromise and majority vote seen in the democratic process. When compromise exists, there is acquiescence or relinquishing of a significant portion of what was desired. This generally leaves both parties feeling negative about themselves or the agreement. Consequently, most compromises must be reworked at some future date. Working on conflict and its resolution (Table 19-5) is time consuming yet essential to effectively functioning teams (Eisenhardt, Kahwajy, & Bourgeois, 1997).

Synergy cannot occur when one team member becomes a self-proclaimed expert who has the "right" answer. Nor can synergy occur when people refuse to speak. Each team member has good ideas, and these need to be shared. They are not shared, however, when someone feels uncomfortable in the team. It is difficult to speak up and appear wrong or inadequate. The challenge each person faces is to push through discomfort and become a full partici-

Table 19-5 ASPECTS OF CONFLICT	
Destructive	**Constructive**
Diverts energy from more important activities and issues	Opens up issues of importance, resulting in their clarification
Destroys the morale of people or reinforces poor self-concepts	Results in the solution of problems
Polarizes groups so they increase internal cohesiveness and reduce intergroup cooperation	Increases the involvement of individuals in issues of importance to them
Deepens differences in values	Causes authentic communication to occur
Produces irresponsible and regrettable behavior such as name-calling and fighting	Serves as a release for pent-up emotion, anxiety, and stress
	Helps build cohesiveness among people sharing the conflict, celebrating in its settlement, and learning more about each other
	Helps individuals grow personally and apply what they learn to future situations

Modified from Hart, L. B. (1980). *Learning from conflict.* Reading, MA: Addison-Wesley.

pant in problem identification and resolution for the overall benefit of the team.

Our society tends to be dualistic in nature. **Dualism** means that most situations are viewed as right or wrong, black or white. Answers to questions are often reduced to yes or no. As a result, we sometimes forget there is a broad spectrum of possibilities. Exercising creativity and exploring numerous possibilities are important. This allows the team to operate at its optimal level.

We have all known people who were self-proclaimed experts, to whom it was critically important that they be right and acknowledged as right, who become judgmental of others whose perspective and opinions differ from theirs. Consequently, being able to tell the truth to one's synergistic team and to encourage them to stretch and look at different ways of functioning is vital. This requires strong skills in good negotiation and conflict resolution, something for which few of us have been trained. If self-proclaimed experts think we are judging them, they will not hear the questions, the observations, or the "truth" because the message seems to be making them wrong rather than originating from compassion. The most valuable contribution an individual can make to an organization is a passionate commitment to the creation of synergistic teams.

THE VALUE OF TEAM BUILDING

The value of team building is to enhance functioning in any one or all of the following processes (Herman & Reichelt, 1998):

- The establishment of goals and objectives
- The allocation of the work to be performed
- The manner in which a group works: its processes, norms, decision-making processes, and communication patterns
- The relationships among the people doing the work

When things are not going well in an organization and there are problems that need to be resolved, the first intervention people think of is "team building." Naturally, for teams (a collection of people relying on each other) to be effective, they must function smoothly. The difficulty is that when organizations are feeling stress and facing difficulties, they generally do not have teams whose members function well together. Team building can ad-

dress any one of the aforementioned activities, depending on the available time and other resources. A team-building consultant can teach a team how to set goals and priorities; help a team analyze the distribution of the workload using various team members' strengths; examine a team's process, norms, decision-making processes, and communication patterns; and promote resolution of interpersonal conflicts or problems within the team.

Regardless of which areas are problematic, appropriate assessment of the team is essential. The problems may be in priority or goal setting, allocation of the work, team decision making, or interpersonal relationships among the members. The success of the team depends on its members and its leadership.

Team building has grown out of an area of social psychology that focused on group dynamics. In the late 1950s and early 1960s, group dynamics centered on an entity called *training groups*, or "T" groups. As is often the case with new technology, some people did not have positive experiences with T groups, and as a result, such groups acquired a questionable reputation. The notoriety focused on the confrontational style and lack of sensitivity in sharing observations and information. People within the groups felt they were considered to be wrong about various behaviors, attitudes, and activities. As a result, distrust often predominated.

Druskat and Wolff (2001) build a strong case for dealing constructively with building an underlying foundation for teams. They believe three major components of smoothly functioning teams must be created:

- Mutual trust among the members
- A strong sense of team identity (that the team is unique and worthwhile)
- A sense of team efficacy (that the team performs well and its members are synergistic in their manner of working together)

At the heart of these components are the emotions we often work so hard to keep out of the workplace. However, as human beings we function in the same way in both work and personal lives. Mutual trust can be developed only when each team member tells the truth about feelings, thoughts, and wants *and* listens and supports other members of the team to do likewise.

Understandable anxiety exists concerning the safety of being vulnerable and exposed if personal

Interview Questions for Team Building

1. What do you see as the problems currently facing your team?
2. What are the current strengths of your institution or work group? What are you currently doing well?
3. Does your boss do anything that prevents you from being as effective as you would like to be?
4. Does anybody else in this group do anything that prevents you from being as effective as you would like to be?
5. What would you like to accomplish at your upcoming team-building session? What changes would you be willing to make that would facilitate a smoother-functioning team and accomplishment of the team goals?

issues are revealed. That is why it is helpful for the team-building facilitator to make a thorough assessment of major issues and the willingness on the part of members to work on issues. One approach is to interview members of the team individually to discover what the critical issues are. The kinds of questions that might be asked are found in Box 19-7.

The kind of tool presented in Box 19-7 enables the leader of the team to understand what the issues are before going into the team-building exercise so that he or she is not surprised and does not become defensive. It also gives the facilitator some sense of what the major issues are within the group so that he or she has a better understanding of how to work with the group.

MANAGING EMOTIONS

Probably one of the greatest fears in team-building exercises is that people will become emotional, that they will lose control of themselves or the environment, or that they will appear weakened or vulnerable. Men have a particularly difficult time with this fear, but many women also want to appear strong and are hesitant to be open and vulnerable. Although many people acknowledge that we are all thinking and feeling persons, management/leadership is usually more willing to deal with the "thinking" side than the "feeling" side of individuals within the team.

Because people spend such a large percentage of their time in the work setting, it would be unrealis-

tic to believe that they always and continually appear in an unemotional and controlled state. Human beings simply do not function that way. What is observed is people's aspirations, their achievements, their hopes, and their social consciousness; they are observed falling in love; falling in hate and anger; winning and losing; and being excited, sad, fearful, anxious, and jealous. Consequently, these "feelings" are important components of organizational life and do much to undermine work effectiveness. Most of us know of situations in which, because of an emotional disagreement, two individuals have avoided each other for years. Because of the power of emotions and the inevitability of their presence, their effect on interpersonal relationships, and their influence on productivity and the quality of work, emotions should be a high priority when examining the functioning of the team. Fortunately, research is now appearing that addresses the importance to teams of emphasizing the "emotional intelligence" of individuals and teams (Druskat & Wolff, 2001). Those teams that address these issues are much more successful and create a positive work environment.

According to Bocialetti (1988), people are sensitive to what happens when emotions are revealed. When people yell or get angry or upset, and when goals, objectives, and tasks are disputed, employees see the following:

- A member intimidating and frightening others within the group
- Embarrassment
- A member overstating or exaggerating another's view to appear right
- Provocation of defensive and hostile responses
- Overconcern with one's self—self-absorption
- Gossip
- Loss of control
- A member distracting others from "real work"
- Disruption or termination of relationships within a group

These are behaviors that destroy any hope of creating a smoothly functioning team, one that supports its members to grow and learn and provide quality patient care. On the other hand, the cost of suppressing emotions or "feelings" includes the following:

- Physical and psychological stress
- Withdrawal from participation
- Loss of energy and depression
- Reduction of learning

- Hiding of important data because of fear
- Festering problems and emotions
- Prevention of others from being acknowledged
- Decreased motivation
- Weakening of the ability to receive constructive feedback
- The loss of one's influence

These kinds of outcomes lead to the conclusion that suppressing emotions at work is neither healthy nor constructive for team members.

When emotions are handled appropriately within the team, there are several positive outcomes for work setting. One creates a sense of internal comfort with the workings of the team and the organization. When stress is lowered and kept at lower levels on average, problems are much more easily resolved. This phenomenon is similar to releasing steam slowly with a steam valve rather than having the gasket blow. Interpersonal relationships on the team are more stable and people have a sense of closer ties and collegiality when emotions are addressed. Fewer negative relationships or interactions develop, which results in more effective and pleasant working relationships all around.

Work group effectiveness improves when the team is functioning smoothly and emotions and "feelings" are being addressed on a routine basis rather than waiting for a volcanic eruption. Problems of withdrawal, boredom, and frustration are much less likely to overwhelm the team and lead to its breakdown (Turpin, 2000). The skills and tools previously discussed (e.g., speaking supportively) are the basic tools one needs to handle the emotional aspects of the team. Choosing to cope with emotional upset must be a conscious choice, one that requires practice to improve the skill.

THE ROLE OF LEADERSHIP

Teams usually have a leader. In addition, teams function within large organizations that have leaders. Without the approval and the support of the leader, team building, which can be a costly endeavor in terms of consultation fees as well as work time and resources of the team, is difficult to undertake and of questionable effectiveness. Although very strong teams may be able to educate themselves regarding some of the issues, such as establishing goals and priorities or clarifying their own

team process, addressing any kind of relationship issue among team members without a more objective outside party facilitating the process is exceedingly difficult.

Because leadership is such a pivotal part of smoothly functioning teams, it is illuminating to examine leaders more carefully. Truly progressive leaders understand that leadership and followership are not necessarily a set of skills; rather, these are qualities of character, a manifestation of a person's own being (Tracey & Hinkin, 1998). On speaking specifically to leadership, we are not talking about "putting on a role." In actuality, leaders realize more fully their capacity for influence, risk taking, and decision making. Leadership, and to some degree followership, is as much about character and development as it is about education. According to Peter Vaill (1989), leadership is concerned with bringing out the very best in people. For a leader who truly believes this, team building is a natural outgrowth. This type of leader understands that the very best in a person is tied intimately to the individual's deepest sense of himself or herself—to one's spirit. The efforts of leaders must touch the spiritual aspect in themselves and others. Warren Bennis (1989) once said that leaders simply care about more people. Consequently, this caring manifests itself in doing whatever it takes to improve team functioning. This may imply involving oneself in team building with the team. The risk in such an endeavor is that the team leader is open to being vulnerable, to being judged by others, and to being wrong. However, if the leader has modeled the "rules of the game" and has held people to these rules, as well as holding himself or herself to them, the team-building exercise will not degenerate into judging and placing blame.

If true leadership is about character development as much as anything, then character development is also beneficial for followers—that is, members of the team. The areas of character development often addressed include communication, particularly those aspects of speaking supportively that avoid placing blame and justifying and enhance understanding the other person's message. Box 19-8 highlights an example of character development, which the chapter author relates from her own Vietnam experience.

Leaders understand the multiple aspects of the issue of control. They take control of their lives rather than being at the mercy of others—rather than being victims. They have clarity regarding their own control issues. They focus time and energy primarily and almost exclusively on those issues, events, and behaviors over which they have control. Their activities are thus primarily focused on areas relating directly to them—not on world

events or other happenings over which they have neither influence nor control.

Confidence, which loosely translates as faith or belief that one will act in a correct and effective way, is a key aspect of character. Thus it follows

BOX 19-8

The "Can Do" Brigade: An Army Nurse's Study in Character Development

As life events are reviewed, important or pivotal learning can be identified. One life event that significantly affected me was the year I spent as an Army Nurse Corps officer in South Vietnam. This was the first time I remember an awareness and understanding of confidence in the face of incredible obstacles. I had spent the first 10 months of my nursing career in labor and delivery at Indiana University before volunteering for a guaranteed assignment to Vietnam. I went to Fort Sam Houston for 6 weeks of basic training, where they taught me really important things like how to salute, how to march, and how many men are in a battalion. No one ever asked me if I could start an IV or draw a tube of blood. This was important because Indiana University had the largest medical school class in the United States at that time and nurses did nothing that interfered with medical education. Therefore I had never started an IV or drawn blood. When I arrived in Saigon, they put me in a sedan with another nurse and sent me up to the Third Surgical Hospital, one not unlike the one in MASH. We even had a Major Burns—that was not his name but it was his function. Surgical hospitals receive only battle casualties; their purpose is to stabilize and to transport.

The Third Surgical Hospital was located in the middle of the 173rd Airborne Brigade, whose job it was to defend the Bein Hoi Air Base, where all the sorties in the south were flown during the war. We were stopped at the gate by an MP who stepped up and saluted very snappily. He knew that a staff car must contain either a very-high-ranking officer or, if it was his lucky day, females.

While I was in Vietnam, 500 American women and 500,000 American men were there. He looked in the window, saluted snappily, and said "Afternoon, ma'am!" He wanted to know where we were going; he talked to us for a few minutes and assured us if there was anything he could do for us we should just give him a call. He saluted us and said, "CAN DO." I didn't understand because I didn't know that there are units with very high esprit de corps who attach snappy little sayings at the end of things like salutes, phone conversations, memos, and so forth.

The 173rd was the "CAN DO" brigade. When we got to the hospital and met the chief nurse, she took us down to the mess hall and introduced us to all the doctors and nurses. We were sitting and having coffee when the field phone rang in the kitchen and the mess sergeant yelled out, "Incoming wounded." Everybody got up and started to leave for the preop area. I just sat there until the chief nurse said, "Come on." I said, "You don't understand, I deliver babies." She was not impressed! She took me by the arm and led me to preop.

When we got there, we discovered there weren't just a few incoming wounded, there were more than 30 and some were very seriously injured. She immediately told the sergeant to call headquarters battalion of the 173rd Airborne and tell them that the Third Surg needed blood. She turned to me and said, "Lieutenant, you are responsible for drawing 50 units of fresh whole blood." I was shocked! I had never drawn a tube of blood, but I found in the back section of preop a Specialist 4th class who was already setting up "saw horses" and stretchers, putting up IV poles, and hanging plastic blood sets. I started to help and soon I heard trucks out back. I opened the door and looked outside. There were two huge Army trucks and out of the back of these were jumping kids, 17, 18, 19, and 20 years old. They were covered with red mud from the bottom of their boots to the tops of their helmets. I looked at them and I looked at the clean cement floor, and in an instant my mother came to me. I put my hand on my hip and said, "Where have you boys been?" One PFC stepped forward and saluted me very snappily and said, "Ma'am, we just came in this afternoon from 30 days in the field, we have been out in the rice paddies chasing the Viet Cong, we have not had a hot meal, and we've not had a shower but Sergeant Major said the Third Surg needs blood!" He saluted smartly and said, "CAN DO!" They were very clear. After 30 days of chasing and being chased by the Viet Cong, giving a unit of blood was easy. "CAN DO!" They were confident. They were kids who had looked into the face of death. At that moment, I knew if they CAN DO, I Can Do! Life requires confidence; with confidence, you can make your dreams come true!

that confidence in oneself can be closely tied to self-esteem, which is satisfaction with oneself. The greatest deterrent to self-esteem and self-confidence is fear. Fear is described by some as "false evidence appearing real" (see box at right). Susan Jeffers (1987) believes the core fear—the one that rules our lives—is one of "I can't handle it." So the core of our fears is "I can't handle it," and it is exactly the opposite of being confident or holding oneself in high esteem. Working on self-confidence requires an attitude of belief, of confidence, of I "CAN DO" whatever is required (see Box 19-8) (Fisher & Thomas, 1996).

> **False**
> **Evidence**
> **Appearing**
> **Real**

Simply caring about more people translates into a willingness to focus time and energy on members of the team. From one perspective, caring is risking being with someone and sharing both suffering and joy. Healing often emerges from caring. Behaviors that demonstrate caring include giving of oneself in terms of warmth and love and particularly giving one's time. The second aspect of caring is truly listening to team members and hearing and understanding them. The third aspect includes being 100% present for them. The fourth is to honor the other person—to see their wholeness, their possibilities, their hopes, and their dreams.

Leading the team is clearly not the easiest thing to do, but neither is being an active, fully participating member of the team. Both require taking risks, including being in a relationship. Being in a team-building experience and hearing those things that have not worked for people in their interactions with peers and the leader can be scary but worthwhile. It requires a focus on personal and professional growth. It requires building character.

Exercise 19–6

The "Gordian Knot": A Team-Building Game

Gordian knot is a term sometimes used to describe a problem that cannot be solved. However, teamwork can sometimes solve seemingly impossible problems, as this game will illustrate.

In a group of 8 to 10 people, form a tight circle with your shoulders touching and your hands placed in the center. Take the hand of two other people across the circle from you. The goal is to unwind the knot until the entire circle is holding hands side by side. You may not let go of hands to unwind the knot unless your instructor gives you special permission to do so!

Debriefing

After your group has unwound its knot, together choose one or two categories of questions from Part I of the "Team-Building Discussion" outline that follows. Discuss these questions, writing down your answers as you go so that you can report to the class later. Be sure to support your answers with examples from your group's experience with the game. Then, complete all questions in Part II.

PART I

LEADERSHIP AND BUILDING TEAMWORK

What did it feel like not to have a designated leader? _____

Who became the leader? _____

How? _____

Did the leadership process work? _____

How did you feel about it? _____

Who came up with new ideas? _____

Did the team support this process? _____

How were conflicts resolved and problems solved? _____

How did you build a sense of teamwork? _____

TEAM MEMBERSHIP

Did you feel a part of the team? _____

Why or why not? _____

Did your team have a good mix of skills and abilities? _____

Did you adapt to the needs of others or to the needs of the team? _____

Continued

■ *Exercise 19–6—cont'd*

Did you adapt to the needs of others or to the needs of the team? _____

Did you meet your objectives without wasting time and energy? _____

What role did you play as a team member? _____

TRUST AND OPENNESS

What was the team's level of trust and open communication? _____

Great Deal = 10   Much = 7   Some = 5   Little = 3   None = 0

What contributed to this level of trust? _____

Did you deal with issues candidly and honestly? _____

What was your level of trust? _____

What would have increased the team's level of trust and openness? _____

CONTRIBUTION TO THE TEAM-DEVELOPING RELATIONSHIPS

Did you all know and agree to the mission of the team? _____

How were decisions made? _____

Who participated in making them? _____

When did you need to make decisions? _____

Were they primarily about what to do (tasks) or how to do it (process)? _____

Did you use each other as resources? _____

Did you work well together? _____

How did your relationships develop and strengthen? _____

How do you feel about each other now? _____

CULTIVATING A FEELING OF SATISFACTION ABOUT YOUR TEAM

Do you feel proud of your team? _____

How do/did you feel rewarded by being a member of this team? _____

Did you have fun? _____

Did the challenge cease to be fun? _____

How did the team handle this? _____

Are you satisfied with your results? _____

DEVELOPING THE TEAM THROUGH RISK TAKING

Did you, individually or as a team, try out any new or uncomfortable communications or behavior? Give examples.

_____

Did that feel safe? _____

Did you support each other in your risk taking? _____

PART II

EVALUATE AND SHARE WITH THE REST OF THE TEAM HOW YOU FEEL YOU DID AS A PARTICIPANT

Consider the following:

Was I active or passive? _____

Did I communicate clearly? _____

Did I take risks? _____

Did I support others? _____

Did I ask for help or support from others? _____

Was my behavior typical for me? _____

How would I do it differently? _____

Give each other honest and helpful feedback on the congruency of self-perception versus the perception of other team members.

Debriefing exercise courtesy Walter Kowalski, BreakThroughs, Inc., Englewood, CO.

The Solution

The first question that needed to be asked was, "Were we committed to providing the most optimal care for the neonate?" In other words, why would teamwork be important in this situation? What's the vision or mission? After achieving agreement among the NICU team, we strategized on how to create a "team" with the specialists. Making your intent clear is very important. A meeting with the director of the specialty team, the NICU medical director, and nursing leadership was arranged. We discovered that we shared a common goal: to provide the best care possible for the baby. Keeping that goal as the focus, we then identified areas of mutual respect. From there, both sides were willing to listen to each other's concerns. Care guidelines could be identified, as well as areas of responsibility. Ideas on how to improve the communication process were also discussed. A plan based on patient needs, complete with agreements, was implemented.

Were we a team yet? The answer is no. There was still a little skepticism and reserve. Everyone seemed to have a "wait-and-see" attitude. The first big chance was identified when the specialty group insisted a patient of theirs be admitted to the NICU because they believed it was the best place for the baby to be. Another measurable outcome was having the agreements honored. This reinforced to everyone that their concerns had been heard and respected. Mutual trust was building, and a collegial relationship began. A year later, it is hard to imagine that this situation ever occurred. There is enthusiasm for this specialty's physicians and their patients. It is certainly a change in attitude.

There are many components to team building, but the most important component is to be clear about your mission and intention when working with potential team members. The intention to provide the best care possible assisted each one of us to be more open, creative, and trusting. These are all necessary components of team building. Remember, teams are made up of individuals. Ask yourself if you are willing to accept responsibility for your response and actions. Be the change that you want to see.

— Diane Gallagher

 Would this be a suitable approach for you? Why?

CHAPTER CHECKLIST

Nurse managers must help build teams. Although the manager does not have to lead the team, the manager must ensure that the group can function effectively as a team. The team members must be able to communicate with each other effectively, share a single mission, be willing to cooperate with each other, and be committed to achieving their objectives. Successful teamwork requires leadership, trust, and willingness to take risks.

- A team is a highly interdependent group of people that has the following characteristics:
  - Has defined goals and objectives
  - Communicates effectively with one another
  - Has an ongoing relationship
  - Is focused on accomplishing a task
- Attributes of effective teams include the following:
  - Clarity of purpose
  - Informality
  - Effective communication
  - Participation
  - Listening
  - Civilized disagreement
  - Consensus decisions
  - Clear roles and work assignments
  - Shared leadership
  - Diversity of styles
  - Self-assessment and self-regulation
- Each team member deals continually with three questions:
  - Am I in the "in" group or the "out" group?
  - Do I have any power or control?
  - Can I use, develop, and be appreciated for my skills and resources?
- Focusing on team members' strengths and acknowledging what they do well are two of the keys to team building.
  - To be effective, acknowledgments must be the following:
    - Specific
    - Personal

Continued

CHAPTER CHECKLIST—cont'd

- – Sincere
- – Timely
- – Public
- One of the most helpful tools for teams is a set of ground rules that govern how members will interact with each other.
- Trust is essential for successful teamwork.
- Synergy allows a team to produce results that could not have been achieved by any one individual. Creating it requires the following:
  - Active listening
  - Compassion
  - Honesty
  - Flexibility
  - Commitment to resolution of conflicts
- Managing emotions is a key strategy in team building.
- Leadership is a pivotal part of a smoothly functioning team.
  - Leadership relies on personal character development as much as on education.
  - Confidence is a key aspect of the leader's character.

- – A "can do" attitude is one of the most important confidence-building strategies a leader can adopt.
- Taking a risk and experimenting with a new behavior is the most effective way to change behavior.

TIPS FOR TEAM BUILDING

- Commit to the purpose of the team.
- Develop team relationships of mutual respect.
- Communicate effectively and actively listen.
- Create and adhere to team agreements concerning function and process.
- Build trust.

TERMS TO KNOW

acknowledgment	group
active listening	sender-receiver
commitment	synergy
dualism	team
effective communication	

REFERENCES

Bennis, W. (1989). *On becoming a leader.* Reading, MA: Addison-Wesley.

Bocialetti, G. (1988). Teams and management of emotion. In W. B. Reddy & K. Jamison (Eds.), *Team building blueprints for productivity and satisfaction* (pp. 62-71). Alexandria, VA: NTL Institute for Applied Behavioral Sciences; and San Diego: University Associates.

Bradley, J., & Edinberg, M. (1990). *Communication in the nursing context* (3rd ed.). Norwalk, CT: Appleton & Lange.

Buckman, R., Korsch, B., Baile, W., & Jason, H. (2000). Review and commentary: A practical guide to communication skills in clinical practice. *Education for Health,* 13(2), 221-227.

Ceccio, J., & Ceccio, C. (1982). *Effective communication in nursing: Theory and practice.* New York: John Wiley & Sons.

Druskat, V., & Wolff, S. (2001). Building the emotional intelligence of groups. *Harvard Business Review,* 79(3), 81-91.

Dubnicki, C. (1991, May-June). Building high-performance management teams. *Healthcare Forum Journal,* 34, 19-24.

Eisenhardt, K., Kahwajy, J., & Bourgeois, L. (1997, July-August). How management teams can have a good fight. *Harvard Business Review,* 75, 77-85.

Fisher, B., & Thomas, B. (1996). *Real dream teams: Seven practices used by world class team leaders to achieve extraordinary results.* Delray Beach, FL: St. Lucia Press.

Hart, L. B. (1980). *Learning from conflict.* Reading, MA: Addison-Wesley.

Herman, J., & Reichelt, P. (1998). Are first line nurse managers prepared for team building? *Nursing Management,* 29(10), 68-72.

Hogan, R. (1997). What we know about leadership. *Academic Leader,* 13(12), 1.

Jackson, P. (1995). *Sacred hoops: Spiritual lessons of a hardwood warrior.* New York: Hyperion.

Jason, H. (2000). Communication skills are vital in all we do as educators and clinicians. *Education for Health,* 13(2), 157-161.

Jeffers, S. (1987). *Feel the FEAR and DO IT anyway.* Columbia, NY: Fawcett.

Lopes, S. (1987). *The wall.* New York: Collins.

McGregor, D. (1960). *The human side of enterprise.* New York: McGraw-Hill.

McGregor, D. (1967). *The professional manager.* New York: McGraw-Hill.

Mears, P. (1997). *Healthcare teams: Building continuous quality improvement.* Boca Raton, FL: St. Lucia Press.

Morreale, S., Spitzberg, B., & Barge, K. (2001). *Human communication: Motivation, knowledge, & skills.* Belmont, CA: Wadsworth.

Olen, D. (1993). *Communicating speaking & listening to end misunderstanding and promote friendship.* Germantown, WI: JODA Communications.

Parcells, B. (2000). The tough work of turning around a team. *Harvard Business Review,* 78(6), 179-184.

Parker, G. M. (1990). *Team players and teamwork.* San Francisco: Jossey-Bass.

Roman, M. (2001). Teams, teammates, and team building. *MedSurg Nursing*, 10(4), 161-165.

Satir, V. (1988). *The new peoplemaking*. Mountain View, CA: Science & Behavior Books.

Thurber, M. (1973). *Rules of the game*. San Francisco: Hawthorne-Stone Real Estate.

Tracey, J., & Hinkin, T. (1998). Transformational leadership or effective managerial practices? *Group & Organizational Management*, 23(3), 220-237.

Turpin, C. (2000). Creating winning teams. *Nephrology Nursing Journal*, 27(2), 171.

Vaill, P. (1989). *Managing as a performing art*. San Francisco: Jossey-Bass.

Weisburg, M. (1988). Team work: Building productive relationships. In W. B. Reddy & K. Jamison (Eds.), *Team building blueprints for productivity and satisfaction*. Alexandria, VA: NTL Institute for Applied Behavioral Sciences; and San Diego: University Associates.

Weiss, W. (2001). Attitude: A major managerial challenge. *Supervision*, 62(6), 3-7.

Wilson, J. (1999). Improving communication skills. *Management Accounting*, 77(3), 88.

SUGGESTED READINGS

Dubnicki, C. (1991, May-June). Tuning up your team. *Healthcare Forum Journal*, 34, 25-28.

Dyer, W. (1987). *Team building issues and alternatives*. Reading, MA: Addison-Wesley.

Francis, D., & Young, D. (1979). *Improving work groups: A practical manual for team building*. San Diego: University Associates.

Jeffers, S. (1992). *Dare to connect: Reaching out in romance, friendship and the workplace*. Columbia, NY: Fawcett.

Nanus, B. (1992). *Visionary leadership*. San Francisco: Jossey-Bass.

Schmieding, N. J. (1993). Nurse empowerment through context structure and process. *Journal of Professional Nursing*, 9, 239-245.

Sibbet, D., & O'Hara-Devereaux, M. (1991). The language of teamwork. *Healthcare Forum Journal*, 34, 27-30.

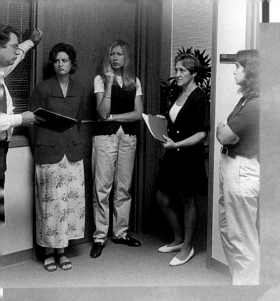

Chapter

20

Conflict: The Cutting Edge of Change

Mary Ann T. Donohue

This chapter focuses on maximizing the nurse leader's and manager's ability to deal with conflict by providing effective strategies for conflict resolution. To resolve conflicts, nurses must be able to determine the nature of the particular conflicts, choose the most appropriate approach for each situation, and implement an appropriate course of action. Therefore an understanding of organizational culture, personality theory, and stress will help the nurse leader and manager accept the nature of individual differences and capitalize on the group members' collective strengths. Because some conflicts are, by nature, unresolvable, an understanding of polarities and polarity management will also help the nurse leader and manager capitalize on the positives in a difficult situation.

Objectives

- Use a model of the conflict process to determine the nature and sources of hypothetical and actual conflict.
- Assess your preferred approaches to conflict and commit to be more effective in resolving future conflict.
- Determine which of the five optional approaches to conflict is the most appropriate in hypothetical and real situations.

- Diagram the structure and dynamics of important polarities

(unresolvable conflicts) and identify ways to manage them.

Questions to Consider

- *What situations, issues, and people trigger conflict for you? Why? How do you trigger conflict for others?*
- *How do you usually determine why people are having conflict? How do you usually react to and resolve conflict?*
- *What typical consequences occur from conflicts in which you are involved?*
- *How have you tended to handle unresolvable or recurring conflicts in the past? How could you handle them in the future?*

The Challenge

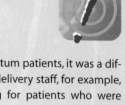

Denyse J. Addison, MSN, RN
Nurse Manager, Hackensack University Medical Center, Hackensack, New Jersey

In our institution, the obstetrical population encompasses labor and delivery, postpartum, and antepartum care. Traditionally, the high-risk antepartum patients, any pregnant women with medical complications, were cared for on the mother-baby unit. As the volume of antepartum patients increased, especially those experiencing preterm labor, the department had an opportunity to expand its services. An eight-bed semiprivate antepartum unit was proposed, to be managed by the nurse manager of the labor and delivery unit.

Plans were made to immediately begin hiring new staff into this area. However, there was an urgent need to initiate the service, so staff from both the labor and delivery and mother-baby units were assigned. Although both staffs had previously been trained and maintained competencies in the care of antepartum patients, it was a difficult transition. The labor and delivery staff, for example, were more comfortable caring for patients who were high-risk antepartum and were either delivered or were sent to another unit for continued treatment. Rarely would the maximum length of stay for both units exceed 3 or 4 days, whereas the antepartum patient may stay weeks, even months.

The conflict was that neither staff wanted to leave their "home base" unit and float to the newly created antepartum unit, creating tension on each side.

 What do you think you would do if you were this nurse?

INTRODUCTION

Much has been written and said about how to solve problems and how to resolve **conflicts** rationally, logically, and effectively. The error in this reasoning is the assumption that such rational processes lead to solutions and resolutions in all situations. Peterson (2000, p. 1) illustrates this "trap" when she outlines seven "simple" steps toward resolving conflict:

1. Identify the problem.
2. Communicate with the appropriate people about the problem.
3. Develop a set of possible solutions.
4. Decide on one of the options.
5. Carry out the action required.
6. Monitor to guarantee the action is taken.
7. Evaluate the effectiveness of your decision-making process.

Conflict arises from a perception of incompatibility. In other words, conflict primarily stems from differences in beliefs, values, attitudes, goals, priorities, methods, information, commitments, ideas, interpretations of reality, personalities, backgrounds, needs, interests, and/or motives (Scott, 1990).

Conflicts are more than just debates or negotiations. They represent an escalation of everyday competition and discussion into an arena of hostile or emotion-provoking encounters that strain personal or interpersonal tranquility, or both (Scott, 1990, p. 1). Perhaps the most difficult aspect to accept is that some conflict is permanent and may be, in fact, normal (Porter-O'Grady, 1999). Some of the first authors on **organizational conflict** (Blake & Mouton, 1964) claimed that complete resolution of conflict may be undesirable because conflict may in fact stimulate growth, creativity, and change for the better.

Stress in the workplace may also account for an increase in conflict among workers (Calabrese, 2000). In the modern healthcare environment, workers are exposed to very high levels of stress resulting from increased demands on an ever-limited staffing supply, a decrease in available resources, and a more acutely ill patient population. A growing body of literature has already tied a reduced nursing workforce to negative outcomes for both staff and their patients (Aiken, Sloane, Lake, Sochalski, & Weber, 1999; Bolsin, 2000; Kovner & Gergen, 1998; Tarnow-Mordi, Hau, Warden, & Shearer, 2000). Traditionally, members of the healthcare team have not been accustomed to admitting to having a vulnerability to the effects of stress and fatigue. Furthermore, nursing administrators have not been accustomed to making changes that might respect staff members' concerns about stress in the workplace. Other stressful occupations, such as the aviation field, have conscientiously created a culture whereby fatigue, stress, and error are readily identified as areas for continuous improvement (Sexton, Thomas, & Helmreich, 2000). Such strategies, borrowed from business and industry, have not yet permeated the healthcare arena. Unfortunately, one report (Farrell, 1999) indicates that nurses were more fearful and concerned about staff-staff aggression as a distress factor when compared with other workplace issues. Nurses and women are more known for their use of compromise and avoidance, as opposed to a more open acknowledgment of the factors contributing to the issues causing the conflict (Valentine, 1995) and may thus be unwitting saboteurs of the resolution process.

TYPES OF CONFLICT

Conflict occurs in all areas of our lives and in three broad categories. Conflict can be intrapersonal, interpersonal, or organizational in nature.

Intrapersonal conflict occurs within a person. Questions often arise that create a conflict over priorities, ethical standards, and different ways to act. When a nurse manager decides what to do about the future (e.g., "Do I really want to study for a higher degree or should we start our family now?"), there are conflicts between personal and professional priorities. Some issues present a conflict over comfortably maintaining the status quo (e.g., "My relationship with the experienced nurses on the unit is pretty smooth right now, and I don't want to rock the boat") or taking risks to make suggestions and confront people when needed (e.g., "Would telling them their way of doing things can be improved and suggesting new ones like I learned in school jeopardize my rapport with them?").

Interpersonal conflict occurs when we realize that everybody does not see the world exactly the same way. There are conflicts between and among patients, nurses, care teams, family members, physicians, and other staff members. A manager may be called on to assist two nurses in resolving a scheduling conflict or determining whether sharing particular information would be a violation of confi-

dentiality. Patients resist suggestions for changing their diet, exercise, and health habits. Members of healthcare teams often have disputes over the best way to treat particular cases. Interpersonal conflict is common and can create the energy to build important relationships and teams.

Organizational conflict occurs when confronting policies and procedures in patient care and personnel management and accepted norms of behavior and communication. Some organizational conflict is related to hierarchical structure and role differentiation among employees, such as labor and management negotiations and financial administrators' and department chairs' arguments over decisions about cutting costs. Nurse managers can become enmeshed in institutionwide conflict concerning cost reductions and quality of care, advances in technology and research versus expansion of access to care, and increasing profitable services while reducing unprofitable ones.

A major source of organizational conflict stems from new systems that promote more participation and autonomy of staff nurses. Increasingly, nurses are charged with both determining and carrying out direct patient care and fulfilling institutional goals to bring about quality patient care. The Magnet studies demonstrate that staff nurses who share in the governance process experience job satisfaction, an important measure of personal fulfillment and organizational success. Yet an empowered nursing staff simultaneously revise their roles and relationships with nurse managers (Keenan, Hurst, & Olnhausen, 1993). As staff nurses assume more autonomy and accountability for identifying areas for quality improvement in patient care, they may desire more of a voice in organizationwide politics. At the same time, managers' span of control steadily increases, so previously clear roles become even more blurred and subsequently need to be redefined. All such change involves organizational conflict mixed with intrapersonal and interpersonal conflict, as well as the management of change and stability.

Another source of conflict has to do with the **allocation of scarce resources**. In the past, it was assumed that moral and ethical standards would always override financial concerns. However, increased expenditures have not always demonstrated the best results. The reform measures introduced in the last decade, aimed at containing healthcare costs, introduced new sources of conflict for nurses (Maddox, 1998). Nurses may find themselves unprepared to provide direct care concurrently with articulating their complex needs to wary providers who may be unwilling to extend hospital stays, or even allow expensive, inpatient admissions in the first place. According to Tim Porter-O'Grady (1999, p. 7), nurse leaders must become accustomed to linking nursing practice and quality outcomes in the following way:

How can we quantify it?

What can we do about it?

What evidence will show that we've achieved the desired outcome?

THE CONFLICT PROCESS

Conflict proceeds through four stages: frustration, conceptualization, action, and outcomes (Hurst & Kinney, 1989; Kinney & Hurst, 1989). The ability to resolve conflicts productively depends on understanding this process (Figure 20-1) and on developing creative ways to deal with conflict. Notice how the arrows in Figure 20-1 flow both ways between stages. This illustrates that moving into a subsequent stage may lead to a return to and change in a previous stage. For instance, two nurses view the conflict (conceptualize it) as a fight to control, whereas a third thinks it is about professional standards. A nurse leader/manager gets them all to talk. They have expressed much frustration and mistrust. All agree that the real conflict comes from a difference in goals, which leads to less negative emotion and a much clearer understanding of all the issues.

Frustration

When people or groups perceive that their goals may be blocked, they feel frustrated. This frustration may escalate into stronger emotions, such as anger and deep resignation. This frustration comes from what people believe to be true, even though there may not be a real conflict at all! For example, a nurse may perceive that a patient is uncooperative when in reality the patient is afraid or has a different set of priorities from those of the nurse. At the

same time, the patient may view the nurse as controlling and insensitive. When such frustrations occur, it is a cue to stop and clarify the nature of major differences.

Conceptualization

Everyone involved develops an idea or picture of what the conflict is about. This may be an instantaneous "snapshot," or it may develop over time. This concept of the conflict may be very clear in people's minds, or it may be very fuzzy. Everyone involved has an individual interpretation of what the conflict is and why it is occurring. Most often, these interpretations are different and involve the person's own perspective, which is based on personal values, beliefs, and culture.

Regardless of its clarity or accuracy, however, conceptualization forms the basis for everyone's reactions to the frustration. The way the individuals perceive and define the conflict has a great deal of influence on the creative resolution and productive outcomes to follow. For example, within the same conflict situation, some individuals may see the conflict as insubordination and become angry, whereas others view it as trivial bickering and withdraw. Such differences in conceptualizing the issue could block its resolution. Thus it is important for each person to clarify "the conflict as I see it" and "how it makes me feel" before all the people involved can define the conflict (i.e., develop an accurate conceptualization together) and proceed to resolve their differences.

People are not likely to reach outcomes that truly resolve the conflict and satisfy them unless they have a clear understanding of the differences among them. During the conceptualization process, we can ask two very powerful questions:

1. What is the nature of our differences?
2. What are the reasons for those differences?

People may differ on four aspects of a conflict: facts; goals; methods to achieve goals; and the values or standards used to select goals, priorities, and methods.

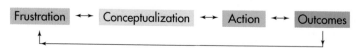

Figure 20-1   Stages of the conflict process.

Providing accurate information is usually easier than working out differences in values, priorities, methodology, and standards. Disagreements over facts may uncover conflicts over goals, means, and values, which may lead to the conflict expanding or even escalating out of control. Values, opinions, and beliefs are more personal, thus generating disagreements that can be threatening and adversarial. The more accurately any conflict is defined, the more likely it will be resolved.

Action

Intentions, strategies, plans, and behavior "flow" out of the conceptualization. A pattern of interaction among the individuals involved is set in motion (e.g., "Let's work together" or "We're not getting any place this way"). As actions are taken to resolve the conflict, the way that some or all parties conceptualize the conflict may change. The important point is that people are always taking some action regarding the conflict, even if that action is **avoiding** it or deciding to do nothing.

There are five distinct action-oriented approaches to resolving conflict (see p. 354). The longer ineffective actions continue, the more likely people will experience frustration, resistance, or even hostility. The more the actions appropriately match the nature of the conflict, the more likely it will be resolved with desirable results.

Outcomes

Tangible and intangible consequences, or "outcomes," result from the actions taken. The conflict may be resolved with a new plan that incorporates the goals of two or more people to ensure that no one loses. Productivity and efficiency may increase, decrease, or stay the same. Emotions may be high, and anger and resistance may remain, resulting in further conflicts. Relationships may be strengthened, weakened, or ended. Such outcomes have very important consequences in the work setting. Assessing the degree of conflict resolution (Box 20-1) is useful for improving individual and group skills in resolutions.

▪ *Exercise 20–1*
Recall a situation in which conflict was apparent. Note arguments each person/side makes and how each responds to the other's comments. What was the outcome? Was the conflict resolved? Was anything left unresolved?

Two general outcomes are considered when assessing the degree to which a conflict has been resolved: the degree to which important goals were achieved and the nature of the subsequent relationships among those involved (Boxes 20-2 and 20-3). Four questions can be asked about the nature of the subsequent relationships (Johnson & Johnson, 1997): (1) Are the relationships stronger and are people better able to interact? (2) Do the members like and trust each other more? (3) Are all the members satisfied with the results of the conflict? (4) Have group members become more able to resolve future conflicts with one another?

▪ *Exercise 20–2*
It is time to assess your tendencies to approach conflict. As you read and answer the 30-item conflict survey in Box 20-3, think of how you face and respond to conflict in professional situations. After completing the survey, tally, total, and reflect on your scores for each of the five approaches. Consider the following questions:
- Which approach(es) do you prefer? Which do you use least?
- Why do you think you tend to act that way?
- Considering the types of conflicts you tend to have, what are the strengths and weaknesses of your pattern?

As you read the rest of this section, use this pattern of scores and your reflections to examine the appropriate uses of each approach, assess your use of each approach more extensively, and commit to new behaviors to increase your future effectiveness.

BOX 20-1

Assessing the Degree of Conflict Resolution

I. Quality of decisions
   A. How creative are resulting plans?
   B. How practical and realistic are they?
   C. How well were intended goals achieved?
   D. What surprising results were achieved?
II. Quality of relationships
   A. How much understanding has been created?
   B. How willing are people to work together?
   C. How much mutual respect, empathy, concern, and cooperation has been generated?

Modified from Hurst, J., & Kinney, M. (1989). *Empowering self and others.* Toledo, OH: University of Toledo.

BOX 20-2

Snapshot of Two Conflicts

Unproductive

Suppose I perceive a conflict between you and me because you disagree with my ideas about how to motivate others to accomplish quality improvement projects. Looking at the four stages in the process of conflict, we might find the following in an unproductive conflict:

1. **I am frustrated** working together on the quality improvement committee because you usually put down my ideas for change. **You** are frustrated because you perceive that I do not support your goals for improved patient care.

2. **I see (conceptualize)** the conflict as your ignorance of new concepts and research findings. Besides, you want things pretty much your way. **You** see it as my eagerness to "shake up" people, promote myself as a leader, and increase my power.

3. **My** view leads to my being forceful **(action)** with you and sharing new research studies and articles that I have found to prove my point, which confirms your judgment of me. **You** resist me with your considerations about why the new techniques will not work and by refusing to read the articles.

4. The **outcome** is that **we** have created a **defensive climate** and a lack of desire to work together. We have clouded the real issue and generated hostility among all of the group. The committee submits a compromise plan to which no one is committed and it then disbands. **The project essentially has failed.**

Productive

The same conflict could present itself and evolve through the same process with different outcomes.

1. **I feel frustrated** that we have to work on the same committee together because I believe that you tend to resist and disagree with my ideas for change. **You** seem to think that what the organization is doing now works just fine.

2. As **we talk,** we realize **(conceptualize)** that we want the same thing: incentives to support quality improvement projects.

3. Our commitment to getting these incentives spurs us to identify critical areas for study. At the same time, **we decide (action)** that we need to look at new plans and research to suggest improvements and additions for our quality improvement endeavors. I say, "If you look at current and new plans, I will work on securing supporting research." We agree and others on the committee agree to do other necessary tasks.

4. The committee then prioritizes areas for study and develops a time frame **(outcomes).** It creates an incentive program **combining the strengths** of our plan with some new ideas to promote internal motivation and productivity and recommends it to the personnel committee. The committee continues and the **project is successful.**

MODES OF CONFLICT RESOLUTION

Five general, distinct approaches can be used in conflict resolution: avoiding, accommodating, **competing, compromising,** and collaborating (Johnson & Johnson, 1997; Thomas & Kilmann, 1973). These approaches can be viewed along two different continua: from uncooperative to highly cooperative and from unassertive to highly assertive (Thomas, 1975). (See the Conflict Self-Assessment in Box 20-3.)

On the cooperative continuum, actions can range from complete competition to total cooperation. Two nurses might compete for a manager position on the one extreme while teaming cooperatively to institute the expansion of their unit. On the as-

sertiveness continuum, actions range from ignoring one's own goals (highly unassertive) to doing what it takes to get what one intends (highly assertive). A nurse might forgo asking for time off (unassertive) at a time when the clinical manager predicts the unit will be understaffed and overly busy (assertive).

It is unlikely that anyone would select any one approach to the exclusion of the others. In fact, as we examine later in the discussion of polarity management, people tend to move horizontally or vertically between these continua in some combined action that is appropriately assertive and cooperative, depending on the nature of the conflict situation.

Avoiding

Avoiding, or withdrawing, is very unassertive and uncooperative because avoiders neither pursue their

BOX 20-3

Conflict Self-Assessment

Directions: Read each of the following statements. Assess yourself in terms of how often you tend to act similarly during conflict at work. Place the number of the most appropriate response in the blank in front of each statement. Put 1 if the behavior is never typical of how you act during a conflict, 2 if it is seldom typical, 3 if it is occasionally typical, 4 if it is frequently typical, or 5 if it is very typical of how you act during conflict.

_____ 1. Create new possibilities to address all important concerns.

_____ 2. Persuade others to see it and/or do it my way.

_____ 3. Work out some sort of give-and-take agreement.

_____ 4. Let other people have their way.

_____ 5. Wait and let the conflict take care of itself.

_____ 6. Find ways that everyone can win.

_____ 7. Use whatever power I have to get what I want.

_____ 8. Find an agreeable compromise among people involved.

_____ 9. Give in so others get what they think is important.

_____10. Withdraw from the situation.

_____11. Assertively cooperate until everyone's needs are met.

_____12. Compete until I either win or lose.

_____13. Engage in "give a little and get a little" bargaining.

_____14. Let others' needs be met more than my own needs.

_____15. Avoid taking any action for as long as I can.

_____16. Partner with others to find the most inclusive solution.

_____17. Put my foot down assertively for a quick solution.

_____18. Negotiate for what all sides value and can live without.

_____19. Agree to what others want to create harmony.

_____20. Keep as far away from others involved as possible.

_____21. Stick with it to get everyone's highest priorities.

_____22. Argue and debate over the best way.

_____23. Create some middle position everyone agrees to.

_____24. Put my priorities below those of other people.

_____25. Hope the issue does not come up.

_____26. Collaborate with others to achieve our goals together.

_____27. Compete with others for scarce resources.

_____28. Emphasize compromise and trade-offs.

_____29. Cool things down by letting others do it their way.

_____30. Change the subject to avoid the fighting.

Conflict Self-Assessment Scoring

Look at the numbers you placed in the blanks on the conflict assessment. Write the number you placed in each blank on the appropriate line below. Add up your total for each column, and enter that total on the appropriate line. The greater your total is for each approach, the more often you tend to use that approach when conflict occurs at work. The lower the score, the less often you tend to use that approach when conflict occurs at work.

Collaborating	Competing	Compromising	Accommodating	Avoiding
1._____	2._____	3._____	4._____	5._____
6._____	7._____	8._____	9._____	10._____
11._____	12._____	13._____	14._____	15._____
16._____	17._____	18._____	19._____	20._____
21._____	22._____	23._____	24._____	25._____
26._____	27._____	28._____	29._____	30._____
TOTAL _____	TOTAL _____	TOTAL _____	TOTAL _____	TOTAL _____

Throughout the rest of this section, there are descriptions of each approach and related self-assessment and commitment-to-action activities. Use these totals to stimulate your thinking about how you do and could handle conflict at work. Most important, consider if your pattern of frequency tends to be consistent, or inconsistent, with the types of conflicts you face. That is, does your way of dealing with conflict tend to match the situations in which that approach is most useful?

From Hurst, J. B. (1993). Human Resource Development Center, University of Toledo, OH.

own needs, goals, and concerns immediately nor assist others to pursue theirs. The positive side of withdrawing may take the form of diplomatically side-stepping or postponing an issue until a better time or simply walking away from a "no-win" situation (Box 20-4). The self-assessment in Box 20-5 will help you recognize your own avoidance behaviors and use them more effectively.

Accommodating/Smoothing

When accommodating, people neglect their own needs, goals, and concerns (unassertive) while trying to satisfy those of others (cooperative). This approach has an element about it of being self-sacrificing and simply obeying orders or serving other people. For example, sometimes we do not care where we eat, but others in our group do. So we say, "Fine, let's eat there! I like all kinds of food. I'm really hungry, so let's go." Box 20-6 lists some appropriate uses of **accommodation.**

Accommodators often feel disappointment and resentment because they "get nothing in return." This is a built-in by-product of the overuse of this approach. The self-assessment in Box 20-7 asks you to examine your present use of accommodation and challenges you to think of new ways to use it more effectively.

Competing/Coercing

During competition, people pursue their own needs and goals at the expense of others. Sometimes people use whatever power, creativeness, or strategies are available to "win." Competing may also take the form of standing up for your rights, defending important principles, and contending for limited funds (Box 20-8).

People who compete well often may not be able to hear the truth, have others disagree, or be challenged, even when they are wrong. They often react by feeling threatened or acting defensive or aggressive. Competition within work groups can generate ill will, a win-lose stance, and commitment to inaction. Use Box 20-9 to help you learn to use competing more effectively.

Negotiating/Compromising

Negotiating involves both assertiveness and cooperation on the part of everyone and requires skill. The Theory box illustrates the key ideas behind negotiation. A give-and-take relationship results in conflict resolution, with each person meeting his or her most important priorities as much as possible. Compromising is often an exchange of concessions or creation of a middle position. This is the preferred means of conflict resolution during union ne-

BOX 20-4

Appropriate Uses for the Avoiding Approach

1. When facing trivial and/or temporary issues, or when other far more important issues are pressing (e.g., tangential issues are only symptoms of deeper conflicts)
2. When there is no chance to obtain what one wants or needs, or when others could resolve the conflict more efficiently and effectively
3. When the potential negative results of initiating and acting on a conflict are much greater than the benefits of its resolution
4. When people need to "cool down," distance themselves, or gather more information, perhaps gaining a hindsight or meaningful view

BOX 20-5

Avoidance: Self-Assessment and Commitment to Action

If you tend to use avoidance often, ask yourself the following questions:

1. Do people have difficulty getting my input into and understanding my view of conflicts?
2. Do I block cooperative efforts to resolve issues?
3. Am I distancing myself from significant others?
4. Are important issues being left unidentified and unresolved?

If you seldom use avoidance, ask yourself the following questions:

1. Do I find myself overwhelmed by a large number of conflicts and a need to say "no"?
2. Do I assert myself even when things do not matter that much? Do others view me as an aggressor?
3. Do I lack a clear view of what my priorities are?
4. Do I stir up conflicts and fights for some reason?

Commitment to Action
What two new behaviors would increase your effective use of avoidance?
1.
2.

gotiations, in which each side is appeased to some degree. In this mode nobody gets everything they think they need.

Negotiation and compromise are valued approaches. They are chosen when less accommodating or avoiding is appropriate (Box 20-10). Compromising is a blend of both assertive and cooperative behaviors, although it calls for less finely honed skills for each behavior than does **collaboration.** Negotiation is more like trading (e.g., "You can have this if I can have that"). Compromise is one of the most frequently selected behaviors used by nurse managers because it supports a balance of power between themselves and others in the work setting. The self-assessment in Box 20-11 will help you become more aware of your own use of negotiation and compromise and improve it.

Collaborating

Collaborating, the opposite of both avoiding and competing, is the creative stance. It is both assertive and cooperative because people work creatively and openly to find the solution that most fully satisfies all important concerns and goals to be achieved. Collaboration involves analyzing situations and defining the conflict at a higher level where shared "superordinate" goals are identified and commit-

ment to work together is generated (Box 20-12). For example, when nurses and physicians work together, they can collaborate by replacing "Who's in charge?" with "What does the patient require?" and "Where does each of us fit into the plan?" This requires discussion about the plan (superordinate

---

BOX 20-6

Appropriate Uses of Accommodation

1. When other people's ideas and solutions appear to be better or when you have made a mistake
2. When the issue is far more important to the other(s) than it is to you (This is a natural, logical step to cooperation and collaboration.)
3. When you see that accommodating now "builds up some important credits" for later issues
4. When you are outmatched and/or losing anyway; when continued competition would only damage the relationships and productivity of the group and jeopardize accomplishing major purpose(s) and maintaining credibility
5. When preserving harmonious relationships and avoiding defensiveness and hostility are very important
6. When letting others learn from their mistakes and/or increased responsibility is possible without severe damage (and you are able to avoid saying, "I told you so!")

BOX 20-7

Accommodation: Self-Assessment and Commitment to Action

If you use accommodation often, ask yourself the following questions:
1. Do I feel that my needs, goals, concerns, and ideas are not being attended to by others?
2. Am I depriving myself of influence, recognition, and respect?
3. When I am in charge, is "discipline" lax?
4. Do I think people are using me?

Infrequent use of accommodation may result in your being viewed as unreasonable or insensitive.

If you seldom use accommodation, ask yourself the following questions:
1. Am I building goodwill with others during conflict?
2. Do I admit when I've made a mistake?
3. Do I recognize legitimate exceptions?
4. Do I know when to give in, or do I assert myself at all costs?

Commitment to Action
What two new behaviors would increase your effective use of accommodation?
1.
2.

BOX 20-8

Appropriate Uses of Competing

1. When quick, decisive action is necessary
2. When important, unpopular action needs to be taken, or when trade-offs may result in long-range, continued conflict
3. When an individual or group is right about issues that are vital to group welfare
4. When an individual or group has had others take advantage of the individual's or group's noncompetitive behavior and now feel obliged to compete

BOX 20-9

Competing: Self-Assessment and Commitment to Action

If you use competing often, ask yourself the following questions:

1. Am I surrounded by people who agree with me all the time and who avoid confronting me?
2. Are others afraid to share themselves and their needs for growth with me?
3. Am I out to win at all costs? If so, what are the costs and benefits of competing?

If you seldom compete, ask yourself the following questions:

1. How often do I avoid taking a strong stand and then feel a sense of powerlessness?
2. Do I avoid taking a stand so that I can escape risk?
3. Am I fearful and unassertive to the point that important decisions are delayed and people suffer?

Commitment to Action

What two new behaviors would increase your effective use of competition?

1.
2.

BOX 20-10

Appropriate Uses of Compromise

1. When two powerful sides are committed strongly to perceived mutually exclusive goals
2. When temporary solutions to complex issues need to be implemented
3. When conflicting goals are "moderately important" and not worth a major confrontation (coercion/competing)
4. When time pressures people to expedite a workable solution
5. When collaborating and competing fail

BOX 20-11

Negotiation/Compromise Self-Assessment and Commitment to Action

If you tend to use negotiation often, ask yourself the following questions:

1. Do I ignore large, important issues while trying to work out creative, practical compromises?
2. Is there a "gamesmanship" in my/our negotiations?
3. Am I sincerely committed to compromise or negotiated solutions?

If you seldom use negotiation, ask yourself the following questions:

1. Do I find it difficult to make concessions?
2. Am I often engaged in strong disagreements or do I withdraw when I see no way to get out?
3. Do I feel embarrassed, sensitive, self-conscious, or pressured to negotiate, compromise, and bargain?

Commitment to Action

What two new behaviors would increase your compromising effectiveness?

1.
2.

goals), how this will be accomplished, and who will make what contributions to achieving the plan.

The same scenario fits for patients and families as well. What is their superordinate goal? Who will do what so that they can reach this goal? The stakes are high (quality patient care) when all stakeholders (e.g., patient, nurse, family, physician) agree to work together.

Trivial issues do not require collaboration and consensus seeking. Some people favor collaboration to reduce their risk-taking and to spread responsibility. Use the self-assessment in Box 20-13 that follows to determine your own use of collaboration.

At the onset of conflict, involved individuals can carefully analyze situations to identify the nature and reasons for conflict and choose an appropriate approach for promoting collaboration. In other words, we can collaborate on the decision to withdraw, compete, or negotiate. For example, suppose you and I are disagreeing about the timing of procedures for patients under your care. At the point that we both agree that it is your responsibility and decision to make, we collaborate and agree.

I say, "I see your point, so let's do it that way." Or we might talk and subsequently agree that you are too emotionally involved with a patient's problem and that it may be time for you to withdraw from providing the care and enlist the skills of another nurse. This discussion can result in collaborative efforts for you to withdraw. Another, less desirable choice could be to compete and let the winner's po-

Theory Box

NEGOTIATING THEORIES

THEORY/CONTRIBUTOR	KEY IDEA	APPLICATION TO PRACTICE
Getting to Yes: Negotiating agreement, principled negotiation, or negotiation on merits theories were developed by Fisher and Vry (1991).	Principled negotiation can produce mutually acceptable agreements in every type of conflict. The method involves four steps: (1) Separate the people from the problem; (2) focus on interests, not positions; (3) invent options for mutual gain; and (4) insist on using objective criteria.	Negotiation requires extra efforts to communicate: Speak and listen for mutual understanding. Getting to yes comes from building a working relationship and creatively developing options from which those involved will benefit.

From Fisher, R. S., & Vry, W. (1991). *Getting to yes: Negotiating agreement without giving in.* New York: Penguin Books.

BOX 20-12

Appropriate Uses for Collaboration

1. When seeking creative, integrative solutions where both sides' goals and needs are important, thus developing group commitment and a consensual decision
2. When learning and growing through cooperative problem solving, resulting in greater understanding and empathy
3. When identifying, sharing, and merging vastly different viewpoints
4. When being honest about and working through difficult emotional issues that interfere with morale, productivity, and growth; compromise supports a balance of power between self and others in the workplace

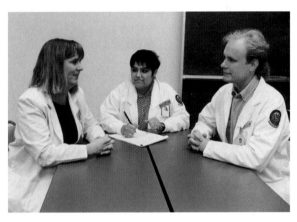

Compromise supports a balance of power between self and others in the workplace.

sition stand (e.g., "Do as I say" or "I'm in charge of this patient"). The decision to compete or collaborate depends on both parties involved.

The nature of the differences, underlying reasons, importance of the issue, strength of feelings, commitment, and goals involved all have to be considered when selecting an approach to resolving conflict. Preferred and previously effective approaches can be considered, but they need to match the situation. Sometimes, a third party may be introduced into a conflict so that **mediation** can occur. Mediation is a learned skill for which advanced training and/or certification is available. The mediator is usually an impartial helper who assists each party in the conflict to better hear and understand

the other. This is thought to empower those involved in the problem because resolution occurs only when they gain the insight, the perspective, and eventually, the ability to solve it (Somma, 1999). The Research Perspective provides an example of positive outcomes.

MANAGING UNRESOLVABLE CONFLICTS

Not all of the conflicts confronting people are resolvable. In fact, most of our own present problems and conflicts, especially the continuing or reappearing ones, are probably unresolvable. Such conflicts

BOX 20-13

Collaboration Self-Assessment and Commitment to Action

If you tend to collaborate often, ask yourself the following questions:

1. Do I spend valuable group time and energy on issues that do not warrant or deserve it?
2. Do I postpone needed action to get consensus and avoid making key decisions?
3. When I initiate collaboration, do others really respond that way? (Are there hidden agendas, unspoken hostility, and/or manipulation in the group?)

If you seldom collaborate, ask yourself the following questions:

1. Do I ignore opportunities to cooperate, take risks, and creatively confront conflict?
2. Do I tend to be pessimistic, distrusting, withdrawing, and/or competitive?
3. Am I involving others in important decisions, eliciting commitment, and empowering them?

Commitment to Action

What two new behaviors would increase your collaboration effectiveness?

1.
2.

cannot be resolved by the right amounts of money, time, resources, staff, support networks, state-of-the-art technology, diet, exercise, vacation time, teamwork, courage, training, rational thinking, and/or leadership (Box 20-14). They are inherently unresolvable (Hurst, 1996; Johnson, 1992).

Many conflicts (and problems) are inherently unresolvable because they consist of two interdependent, dynamic polar opposites that require a shifting emphasis from pole to pole over time, rather than the selection of the one "best" option. Resolvable conflicts (and solvable problems) tend to be either/or choices that lead to some end. Unresolvable conflicts, or **polarities**, involve a both/and decision of when to emphasize one pole and when to emphasize its opposite. For instance, a manager's need to give clear direction to a team automatically places less emphasis on the team deciding on the direction themselves. However, for the team to be successful, sooner or later that manager will experience the need for the team to work on its own, setting its own direction. Johnson (1992) has identified several common polarities with which

people deal continually. These include self and others, individual and team, individual and organizational responsibility, control and participatory management, specific and general communication, tasks and relationships, centralization and decentralization, and stability and change. Others you are probably confronting include "me and my department," personal life and professional life, stimulation (stress) and tranquility, conditional acceptance (love) and unconditional acceptance (love), cost and quality, efficiency and effectiveness, management and leadership, and planning and acting.

Polarity Structure

Polarities have six important elements (Figure 20-2), including two neutral, interdependent poles; two sets of resulting positive consequences ("upsides"), one for each pole; and two sets of associated negative consequences ("downsides"). To determine the nature of the unresolvable conflicts, one has to ask five basic questions, as shown in Box 20-15.

By answering the basic questions in Box 20-15, an individual or team can diagram the specifics of any polarity situation. Typically, people see only half of the situation—the upside of their preferred pole and the downside of its opposite—and are therefore blind to the other two quadrants—their preferred pole's downside and its opposite's upside (Johnson, 1992). This blindness, coupled with the need to be right, leads to much conflict with those who favor the opposite pole and see only the other two quadrants. The awareness that there are such things as polarities and diagramming important ones tend to increase collaboration and "win-win" thinking because people learn that fighting over one pole leads to experiencing its downside consequences (Hurst & Vander Veen, 1995; Johnson, 1992).

Polarity Dynamics

Visually, a polarity diagram consists of the two polar opposites on a horizontal axis divided into four quadrants of results by a vertical line. Although simple in form, polarity diagrams clearly picture the consequences to be experienced and the nature of its historical and predictable flow.

Notice in Figure 20-2 that polarities naturally and predictably "flow" (arrows represent a plot of changes in results) from the downside of pole L toward the upside of pole R, then into the downside of pole R, then toward the upside of pole L, and finally back to the downside of L where it all began. For example, a nurse manager was confronted by an angry team because they felt they were being

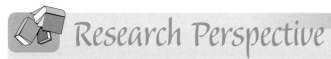
Research Perspective

Saulo, M., & Wagener, R. J. (2000). Mediation training enhances conflict management by healthcare personnel. *The American Journal of Managed Care, 6*(4), 473-483.

The purpose of this study was to evaluate the effectiveness of mediation training on a diverse group of healthcare professionals and ancillary staff who were participants in an intensive educational program. All were employees at either a community-based not-for-profit hospital, a health maintenance organization (HMO), a managed care insurance company, or a skilled nursing rehabilitation company. The program consisted of 25 hours in training that included 11 hours of didactic content, 10 hours of mock mediation exercises and simulations, and 4 hours of homework. Group members were also introduced to concepts related to cultural competency and ethical issues such as end-of-life decision making.

Mediation was defined as "the process by which a neutral or impartial person(s) assists parties in isolating the issues or concerns that comprise or surround their dispute" (p. 476). The mediator facilitates the communication process so that the parties are able to develop options, evaluate options against mutually agreed-on criteria, and reach a consensus that addresses their expressed needs and interests. The mediator facilitates a three-stage process, in which participants have an opportunity to express concerns, fears, expectations, and goals. Ground rules (stage 1) help establish a balance of power between the participants, and emphasis is placed on mutual interests rather than on adversarial positions. In stage 2 the parties improve their understanding of the other's perspective, leading to an agreement in stage 3.

The outcomes of the training were measured in three ways:

1. *Comfort level before and after training:* A Likert-scale instrument was developed to measure perceived differences in comfort level with conflict before and after training and the transfer of mediation skills to other settings. Participants were able to rank their comfort level with conflict, pretraining, and posttraining, on a Likert scale that ranged from 1 (low) to 10 (high).

2. *Transfer of mediation skills to the workplace:* After their training, the participants were asked to review a list of mediation skills that were covered in the sessions and to rank them on a Likert-scale, ranging from 1 (seldom) to 5 (frequently), based on the extent to which they used a particular skill in the workplace and with their own families. Two months after training, the participants were contacted and asked to rate on a Likert scale ranging from 1 (not useful) to 5 (useful), again based on the extent to which the mediation skills were useful in the workplace, with co-workers and with patients, and in their families at home.

3. *Observation and interviews:* In one setting with 16 participants, the investigators were permitted to observe staff at their workplace and identify the mediation skills used by the employees. These individuals were also interviewed and asked to enumerate the ways in which mediation training had made a difference in their work lives.

A statistically significant increase in the comfort level of the participants with conflict was reported after mediation training. The skills used most often were active listening, summarizing, reframing, neutrality, and balancing power, as well as the common good. The training participants had used their newly acquired mediation skills very effectively to acknowledge and empathize with frustrated consumers. In all cases the participants were able to look beyond the actual presenting issue and to more clearly identify issues that had consequences not only for the individual plan members but also for the organization.

IMPLICATIONS FOR PRACTICE

Tensions and stress in modern healthcare settings will undoubtedly continue, and even escalate. Because mediation training is effective and readily accessible, mediation training should be available in all clinical settings to be used to resolve conflict, decrease stress, and help avoid costly litigation.

BOX 20-14

How to Tell if a Conflict May Be Unresolvable

PROBABLY IS UNRESOLVABLE	ASK THESE QUESTIONS ABOUT THE SITUATION	PROBABLY IS RESOLVABLE
Answer is yes	Is this difficulty ongoing?	Answer is no
Answer is yes	Are there two interdependent poles?	Answer is no
Answer is yes	Does choosing one need to incorporate the other to succeed?	Answer is no
Answer is yes	Is this really a both/and decision?	Answer is no

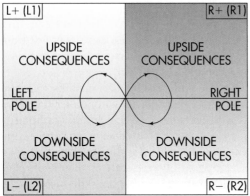

Figure 20-2 Generic structure and predictable flow of polarities.

BOX 20-15

Basic Polarity Questions

1. What neutral terms describe the two polar opposites involved?
2. What are the positive consequences of actions emphasizing the first pole?
3. What are the negative consequences of action overemphasizing that pole to the exclusion of its opposite?
4. What are the positive consequences of actions taken toward the second pole?
5. What are the negative consequences of action overemphasizing the second pole while excluding the first?

treated like children and told what to do all the time (control management's downside, L2). Working together, they initiated team meetings and decision-making procedures (actions emphasizing participatory management) that resulted in more ideas, ownership of the area, and self-direction from the team and its individual members (participatory upside, R1). However, after a few months of overemphasizing participation, the team began to lose its focus and cohesiveness (participatory downside, R2) and came to the manager for direction. The manager listened and provided clarification (action emphasizing control management), and the team regained its focus and efficiency (upside of control management, L1). Polarities have this infinite-type swing to them, as represented by the shape of the flow of the arrows in Figure 20-2.

Wide, rapid, or very prolonged swings usually lead to disruptions in the smooth conduct of activity. When any polar opposites like change and stability are approached as separate independent problems or conflicts—as they generally are—the outcomes tend to reflect the greater amount of time and intensity of consequences in the downside "quadrants" (Figure 20-3). Sometimes people hang onto one pole so long—usually for fear of the other pole's downside—that they either are forced to change their emphasis or do so very rapidly and extremely. This leads to a "flip" from the downside of the original pole to the downside of the new pole, almost without experiencing the upside on the way (Johnson, 1992). This hanging onto one pole to reap the benefits of its upside and avoid its opposite's downside is what Johnson (1992) calls "the one pole myth," or being "stuck" (p. 156).

The polarity diagram in Figure 20-4 was generated by a team of college students working on assertiveness ("crusading" away from the passive downside toward the assertive upside). They drew this on a chart pad by asking these questions: (L2) With what negative results of passiveness are we dissatisfied? (R1) To what positive outcomes of assertiveness are we committed? (R2) What negative consequences would occur from overemphasizing

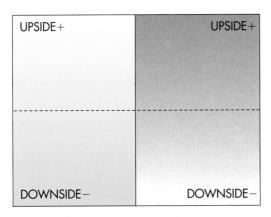

Figure 20-3   Polarity diagram.

assertiveness (excluding any passive acceptance)? (L1) What are the positive consequences of being passively accepting?

Exercise 20-3

After rereading the section on polarity dynamics, answer the questions listed in Box 20-15 and fill out the blank polarity diagram shown in Figure 20-3 in relation to a conflict you would describe as "ongoing" in a clinical setting. Be specific about the upside and downside consequences of each pole. Then draw a time line through the quadrants, starting in the lower left quadrant and moving through the upper right, down into the lower right, up toward the upper left, and finally back into the lower left. Shape the line to conform with how the organization has moved through this polarity over time. Talk to some people who have been around for a while to get their historical perspective on this issue. Then consider the following questions:

- Who tends to crusade for what pole? What are their positions and years of experience?
- How are resources, time, and personnel wasted on mismanaging this polarity?
- What blocks the effective management of this polarity?
- What already aids in its management?
- What new things and actions would add to its management in the future?

By seeing the total picture, the involved parties can take steps to make changes flexibly, without overemphasizing any one pole for too long. Most important, they can draw the results line (arrows) that best represented how this polarity usually flowed. They can see how stuck they had been, especially with almost every assertive act "feeling" negative and being resisted by others and almost every positive passive act lumped in with the negatives of "giving in." Input from as many people as possible is important when drawing such diagrams.

Polarity Management

"The objective of polarity management is to get the best of both opposites while avoiding the limits of each" (Johnson, 1992, p. xii). In other words, once people determine their conflict is a polarity, they can act to maximize both poles' upsides and minimize both poles' downsides. This is called *polarity management,* which requires a shifting focus from pole to pole when cues of approaching downside consequences are noted. The key to effective polarity management is to sense oncoming downside consequences, or to be sensitive to feedback that there are negative consequences occurring, and take action toward the opposite pole. One nurse manager noticed that two teams had been functioning so long that individual members were complaining about being overlooked and that their creativity was stifled by the group. The manager scheduled a luncheon party, presented individual awards to each member, and initiated a creative suggestion box for staff to contribute individual and team ideas for improving quality and efficiency.

Polarity management involves two opposing groups that usually are in conflict. "Crusaders" are dissatisfied with the downsides of the present pole and advocate action toward its opposite. "Tradition bearers" prefer the present pole, citing its upsides, and point to the downsides of the crusaders' preferred pole as reasons to keep the emphasis where it is. Typically, the communication between crusaders and tradition bearers is argumentative, competitive, and defensive. Both sides know they are right and the other side is wrong. Polarity management alters this communication to a mood of cooperation, collaboration, and support because both sides realize that any decision to emphasize one pole results in everyone experiencing the downside of that pole and, if stuck at that pole long enough, experiencing the downsides of both poles at once (Johnson, 1992).

A manager and an organization can do several things to begin managing polarities more collaboratively and effectively. Many of them are listed in Box 20-16.

As a rule, the more skilled people are at problem solving and conflict resolution, the more likely they will mismanage polarities. This happens when people treat both/and decisions like either/or ones, thus looking for the right choice. Yet no one right choice exists, at least in the long run. Partnering with others and shifting action to what is needed next in a timely manner are important to manage polarities effectively.

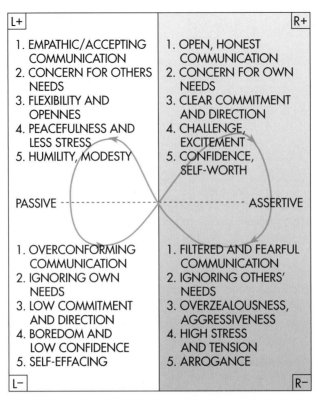

Figure 20-4 The passive acceptance and assertive polarity.

BOX 20-16

Actions for Managing a Polarity

The following list of actions exemplifies steps in the management of any polarity:

- Note that the situation involves at least one continuous both/and polarity.
- Diagram, in writing, the polarity's poles, upsides, and downsides.
- Draw a timeline (arrows representing its past, present, and predictable future flow) with dates to identify the history of this particular polarity.
- Listen carefully to people with preferences for the opposite pole. Solicit their input regularly.
- Identify key individuals and groups who are "crusading" for the new pole and "traditionally supporting" staying at the present pole. Involve them in analyzing and managing this polarity.
- State major goals and objectives in terms of maximizing the upside consequences.

- Determine what present policies, procedures, committee structures, and typical actions (1) block the effective management of this polarity (shifting from pole to pole) and (2) exemplify and/or support managing this polarity effectively. Then create new ones that would facilitate managing this polarity in the future.
- Note which people are most accurately sensitive to any changes in results toward either downside and encourage and listen to their ongoing feedback.
- Identify and create flexible ways to shift resources to either pole and to monitor results.
- Continually diagram polarities and monitor their flow.
- Value crusaders' and tradition bearers' viewpoints, their ongoing collaboration, and healthy competition between them.

The Solution

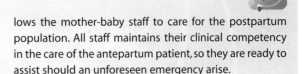

The nurse managers of labor and delivery and the mother-baby unit collaborated to solve the problem. They formed an alliance to allow the staff to work together and feel comfortable. They matched schedules and provided coverage for the unit. The staff was allowed to freely "vent" their concerns and were asked to come up with any innovative ideas that might help the new unit grow. The ultimate goal was eventually realized: The labor and delivery nurses provided the care for the antepartum patients and were able to hire additional staff to increase their numbers. This plan is very successful because it allows the mother-baby staff to care for the postpartum population. All staff maintains their clinical competency in the care of the antepartum patient, so they are ready to assist should an unforeseen emergency arise.

— Denyse J. Add

 Would this be a suitable approach for you? Why?

CHAPTER CHECKLIST

Conflicts may be resolvable or unresolvable, and they are common in healthcare and when dealing with people. To resolve conflict, parties need to identify their differences, priorities, and common goals; determine which approach to conflict is most appropriate; and act in that way to resolve it. When conflicts involve polarities, parties need to analyze their structure and dynamics, identify ways to shift emphasis among opposite poles, and partner with others concerned.

- The three types of conflict are as follows:
  - Intrapersonal
  - Interpersonal
  - Organizational
- The conflict process flows among four stages:
  - Frustration
    - Blocked goals lead to frustration.
    - Frustration is a cue to stop and clarify differences.
  - Conceptualization
    - The way a person perceives a conflict determines how he or she reacts to the frustration.
    - Differences in conceptualizing an issue can block resolution.
  - Action
    - Intentions, strategies, plans, and behavior flow out of conceptualization.
  - Outcome (may be both tangible and intangible)
- When assessing how well a conflict has been resolved, one must consider the following:
  - The degree to which important goals were achieved by assessing the outcomes

- The nature of subsequent relationships among those involved in the conflict
- The five modes of conflict resolution are as follows:
  - Avoiding
  - Accommodating
  - Competing
  - Compromising
  - Collaborating
- Each mode of conflict resolution can be viewed along two different continua:
  - From uncooperative to highly cooperative
  - From unassertive to highly assertive
- A conflict probably is unresolvable in the following circumstances:
  - The difficulty is ongoing.
  - There are two interdependent, polar-opposite positions.
  - One pole needs to incorporate the other to succeed.
  - It is a both/and rather than either/or decision.
- Polarities are unresolvable conflicts.
  - Polarities have six important elements:
    - Two neutral, interdependent poles
    - Two sets of resulting positive consequences (upsides)
    - Two sets of associated negative consequences (downsides)
  - Polarity management requires a shifting focus from one pole to the other when cues of the approaching downside consequences become evident.

Continued

TIPS FOR ADDRESSING CONFLICT

- Communicate to yourself and others that conflict is a necessary and beneficial process typically marked by frustration, different conceptualizations, a variety of approaches to resolving it, and ongoing outcomes.
- In sorting out the different conceptualizations of a conflict situation, determine any similarities and differences in facts, goals, methods, and values.
- To assess the degree of conflict resolution, ask questions about the quality of decisions (e.g., creativity, practicality, achievement of goals, breakthrough results) and quality of the relationships (e.g., understanding, willingness to work together, mutual respect and cooperation).
- Remind yourself of your preferences for perceiving and resolving conflict (e.g., which of the five approaches do you avoid and which do you overuse?) and assess each situation to match the best approach for that type of conflict regardless of which is your favorite approach.
- Assist others around you in assessing conflict situations and determining how they can best approach them.

- Persistent and recurring problems and conflicts often are polarities that inherently are unresolvable. Approach them by mapping their upsides and downsides and creating ways to balance actions toward each pole when appropriate.

TERMS TO KNOW

accommodation
allocation of scarce resources
avoiding
collaboration
competing
compromising
conflict
interpersonal conflict
intrapersonal conflict
mediation
negotiating
organizational conflict
polarities

REFERENCES

Aiken, L. H., Sloane, D. M., Lake, E. T., Sochalski, J., & Weber, A. L. (1999). Organization and outcomes of inpatient AIDS care. *Medical Care, 37*(8), 760-772.

Blake, R. R., & Mouton, J. S. (1964). *The managerial grid.* Houston: Gulf.

Bolsin, S. N. (2000). Routes to quality assurance: Risk adjusted outcomes and personal professional monitoring. *Journal for Quality in Healthcare, 12*(5), 367-369.

Calabrese, K. R. (2000). Interpersonal conflict and sarcasm in the workplace. *Genetic, Social & General Psychology Monographs, 126*(4), 459-495.

Farrell, G. A. (1999). Aggression in clinical settings: Nurses' views—A follow-up study. *Journal of Advanced Nursing, 29*(3), 532-541.

Fisher, R. S., & Vry, W. (1991). *Getting to yes: Negotiating agreement without giving in.* New York: Penguin Books.

Hurst, J. B. (1993). Human Resource Development Center, University of Toledo, OH.

Hurst, J. (1996). Assisting clients to maximize polarities and stop trying to solve unsolvable problems. *Guidance & Counseling, 11*(4), 23-26.

Hurst, J., & Kinney, M. (1989). *Empowering self and others.* Toledo, OH: University of Toledo.

Hurst, J. S., & VanderVeen, N. (1995). Polarity analysis and management: An alternative approach to unsolvable conflicts. *CACD Journal, 15,* 11-16.

Johnson, B. (1992). *Polarity management: Identifying and managing unsolvable problems.* Amherst, MA: HRD Press.

Johnson, D. W., & Johnson, F. P. (1997). *Joining together: Group theory and group skills* (6th ed.). Englewood Cliffs, NJ: Prentice Hall.

Keenan, M. J., Hurst, J. B., Olnhausen, K. (1993). Polarity management for quality care: Self-direction and manager direction. *Nursing Administrator Quarterly, 18*(1), 23-29.

Kinney, M., & Hurst, J. (1989). *Group process in education.* Lexington, MA: Ginn Custom Publishers.

Kovner, C., & Gergen, M. (1998). Nurse staffing levels and adverse events following surgery in US hospitals. *Image: Journal of Nursing Scholarship, 30*(4), 315-321.

Maddox, P. J. (1998). Administrative ethics and the allocation of scarce resources. *Online Journal of Issues in Nursing,* 1-10.

Peterson, G. (2000). *Seven steps toward resolving conflict.* Retrieved from www.parentsplace.com/health/adulthealth/gen/0,3375,12307,00 html (IVillage.com).

Porter-O'Grady, T. (1999). The leader as mediator. *Aspen's Advisor for Nurse Executives, 14*(7), 1-5.

Saulo, M., & Wagener, R. J. (2000). Mediation training enhances conflict management by healthcare personnel. *The American Journal of Managed Care, 6*(4), 473-483.

Scott, G. G. (1990). *Resolving conflict with others and within yourself.* Oakland, CA: New Harbinger.

Sexton, J. B., Thomas, E. J., Helmreich, R. L. (2000). Error, stress and teamwork in medicine and aviation: Cross sectional surveys. *British Medical Journal, 320,* 745-749.

Somma, C. T. (1999). Mediation: A positive alternative in conflict resolution for clinical laboratories. *MLO, 31*(1), 42-45, 54.

Tarnow-Mordi, W. O., Hau, C., Warden, A., & Shearer, A. J. (2000). Hospital mortality in relation to staff workload: A 4 year study in an adult ICU. *Lancet, 356,* 185-189.

Thomas, K. (1975). Conflict and conflict management. In M. Dunnette (Ed.), *The handbook of industrial psychology.* Chicago: Rand McNally.

Thomas, K. W., & Kilmann, R. H. (1973). Thomas-Kilmann conflict mode instrument. In J. W. Pfieffer, R. Heslin, & J. E. Jones (Eds.), *Instrumentation in human relations training* (pp. 266-268). San Diego: University Associates.

Valentine, P. E. B. (1995). Management of conflict: Do nurses/women handle it differently? *Journal of Advanced Nursing, 22,* 142-149.

SUGGESTED READINGS

Alvarez, C. (2000). When a staff member is causing conflict. *Clinical Nurse Specialist, 14*(6), 260.

Arnetz, B. (1999). Staff perception of the impact of health care transformation on quality of care. *International Journal for Quality in Health Care, 11*(4), 345-351.

Ashworth, P. (2000). Nurse-doctor relationships: conflict, competition or collaboration. *Intensive and Critical Care Nursing, 16*(3), 127-128.

Bakker, A. B., Killmer, C. H., Siegrist, J., & Schaufeli, W. B. (2000). Effort-reward imbalance and burnout among nurses. *Journal of Advanced Nursing, 31*(4), 884-891.

Bragg, T. (2000). Ten ways to deal with turf wars. *Occupational Health & Safety, 69*(2), 26-28, 30.

Burkhalter, D. K., Farmer-Dougan, V. A., & Nordstrom, C. R. (1997). Targeted goal setting: Helping nurses manage a turbulent work environment. *Journal of Nursing Management, 5,* 89-96.

Byrnes, J. D. (2000). The aggression continuum: A paradigm shift. *Occupational Health & Safety, 69*(2), 70-71.

Casantino, C. A., & Merchant, C. S. (1995). *Designing conflict management systems.* San Francisco: Jossey-Bass.

Cooper, J. (1999). Managing workplace stress in outpatient nursing. *Professional Nurse, 14*(8), 540-543.

Couch, M. Z. (1999). Is there an elephant in the copy room? Bold remedies for resolving hidden issues at work. Lubbock, TX: Perelandra.

Curtin, L. (1993). Empowerment: On eagle's wings. *Nursing Management, 24*(6), 7-9.

Eason, F. R. (1999). Conflict management: Assessing educational needs. *Journal for Nurses in Staff Development, 15*(3), 92-96.

Felder, L. (1999). *Does someone at work treat you badly?* New York: Berkley.

Fitzpatrick, J. M. (1999). Shift work and its impact upon nurse performance: Current knowledge and research issues. *Journal of Advanced Nursing, 29*(1), 18-27.

Flanagan, L. (1999). Conflict 101. *Family Practice Management, 6*(2), 64.

Flarey, D. L. (1993). The social climate of work environments. *Journal of Nursing Administration, 23*(6), 9-15.

Forte, P. S. (1997). The high cost of conflict. *Nursing Economics, 15*(3), 199-123.

Gardner, D. B., & Cary, A. (1999). Collaboration, conflict, and power: Lessons for case managers. *Family Community Health, 22*(3), 64-77.

Heim, P., & Murphy, S. (2001). *In the company of women: Turning workplace conflict into powerful alliances.* New York: Putnam.

Hurst, J. (1996). Building hospital TQM teams. *The HealthCare Supervisor, 15*(1), 68-75.

Johnson, S., & Blanchard, K. H. (1998). *Who moved my cheese?* New York: G. P. Putnam's Sons.

Key, M. K. (2000). A method for mediating conflict among different mindsets. *Journal for Healthcare Quality, 22*(6), 4-8.

Kramer, M., & Schmalenberg, C. (1993). Learning from success: Autonomy and empowerment. *Nursing Management, 2*(5), 58-64.

Kusbell, E., & Rub, S. (1996). Dealing with conflict: The Margaret Chapman case. *Journal of Nursing Administration, 26*(2), 34-40.

Lee, D. (2001). Confrontation equals conflict management. *Tennessee Nurse, 62*(2), 21-25.

Levine, S. (2000). *Getting to resolution: Turning conflict into collaboration.* San Francisco: Berett-Koehler.

Martin, K., Wimberly, D., & O'Keefe, K. (1993). Resolving conflict in a multicultural nursing department. *Nursing Management, 25*(1), 49-51.

McClure, L. F. (2000). *Anger and conflict in the workplace: Spot the signs, avoid the trauma.* Manassas Park, VA: Impact.

O'Mara, K. (1999). Communication and conflict resolution in emergency medicine. *Ethical Issues in Clinical Emergency Medicine, 17*(2), 451-459.

Schmidt, W. H. (2001). *Is it always right to be right? A tale of transforming workplace conflict into creativity and collaboration.* New York: Amacom.

Sessa, V. I. (1998). Using conflict to improve effectiveness of nurse teams. *Orthopaedic Nursing, 17*(3), 41-48.

Sochalski, J., Estabrooks, C. A., & Humphrey, C. K. (1999). Nurse staffing and patient outcomes: Evolution of an international study. *Canadian Journal of Nursing Research, 31*(3), 69-88.

Stone, F. M. (1999). *How to resolve conflicts at work.* New York: American Management Association.

Tomajan, K. (1999). Resolving workplace concerns/conflicts. *The Oklahoma Nurse, 44*(4), 10.

Vilardo, L. E. (1993). Linking collaborative governance with job satisfaction. *Nursing Management, 24*(6), 75.

Volkema, R. E., & Bergman, T. J. (1996). Conflict styles as indicators of behavioral patterns in interpersonal conflicts. *Journal of Social Psychology, 135*(1), 5-15.

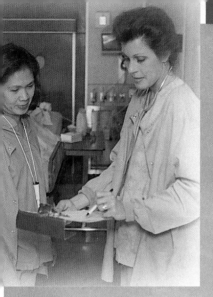

Delegation: An Art of Professional Practice

Patricia S. Yoder-Wise

*D*elegation is a complex process that can be quite effective in accomplishing work. This chapter defines various aspects of delegation, including legal perspectives and how to make delegation decisions. The emphasis is on the role of the nurse as delegator, irrespective of the formal position an individual may hold.

Objectives

- Define *delegation* and its component parts.
- Describe how tasks and relationships influence delegation to a specific individual.
- Comprehend the legal authority for a registered nurse to delegate.
- Value the complexity of decision making related to delegation.

Questions to Consider

- How does a registered nurse make delegation decisions?
- How complex is delegation?
- When is it appropriate to delegate?
- To whom can tasks be delegated?
- What can be delegated?

The Challenge

Molly Patteson, RN, BSN
Weekend Supervisor, Rollins Brook Community Hospital, Lampasas, Texas

Weekend staffing is a challenge. As a supervisor, I had a dilemma. The census (16) was rising and the 7-3 staff on Sunday did not have sufficient personnel. I had depleted my call list and reassured my 1-year-out-of-school RN that I would find a solution. We had a seasoned LVN and an aide. We also had one RN assigned to the emergency room. Normally, this sounds good, but our hospital has eight new beds on one unit and the rest of the beds in the older part of the hospital. There is no way of communicating between the two except by phone. A 3-11 RN volunteered to come in at 11 AM. I chose to go home at 9 PM Saturday night and pray for returned calls from the staff I could not reach previously.

 What do you think you would do if you were this nurse?

INTRODUCTION

Delegation is a complex, loophole-ridden, work-enhancing strategy. It can make the difference between caring for a group of patients and experiencing great anxiety and caring for that same group with a controlled expectation of what can be achieved. Used properly, it can enlarge the effect you have on patient care; used improperly, it can be frustrating and scary. Delegation is an art and a skill that can be developed and honed into one of the most effective professional management strategies. Each of the following sections is designed to foster the best of delegation.

HISTORICAL PERSPECTIVE

Until the early 1970s, registered nurses (RNs) were quite familiar with the art of delegation. Most care occurred in acute care hospitals, which were staffed by RNs (mostly diploma graduates, frequently prepared in the hospital in which they worked), licensed practical/vocational nurses (LPNs/LVNs), and nurse aides (commonly called *unlicensed assistive personnel* today). Team nursing was used, and staffing ratios were such that it was not uncommon for relatively few RNs to be present on a nursing unit. Direct care was provided primarily by LPNs/LVNs and the aides. Of course, because there were few complex procedures, the direct care provided was related primarily to physical comfort and to what today would be termed *simple treatments*.

As care became far more intricate and the monitoring demands and expectations placed on nursing increased, moving to a higher ratio of RNs was logical. Thus, during the 1970s and 1980s, many nurses entered the profession with relatively limited experience or knowledge about the details of delegation—there was no one in the clinical area to whom one could delegate anything related to patient care except the basic physical care. Sometimes the professional staff even dealt with that. In a study by Standing, Anthony, and Hertz (2001), most nurses identified that they were prepared for delegation mainly by experience rather than by education.

In the mid-1990s a dramatic shift from primary nursing (an all-professional staff concept) to a multilevel nursing staff occurred. As a result, addressing the topic of delegation in some detail became critical to safe care. This return, however, is not to delegation as it was known earlier. In part, the difference today is based on the sophisticated demand for cost containment and reduction and the new complexities that are present in healthcare. As the healthcare industry emphasizes community-based care, the challenge of delegation and the resultant supervision become even more difficult. The increase, especially in unlicensed assistive personnel (UAPs), related in the past to a shortage of nurses. Although a shortage exists now, an even more dramatic one is predicted through 2010 (Division of Nursing, 2001). So, in addition to the supply of nurses and healthcare cost control measures, the role of the RN will change to meet the increasing demands for care. Nursing's flexibility to alter how we function based on the changes we find has allowed nursing to survive and sometimes thrive. Whether or not UAPs are part of the system, nurses really just want to give good patient care (M. Foley, personal communication, March 12, 2001).

DEFINITION

Delegate, or *delegation,* is defined in multiple ways. However, consistent elements can be found in each definition. Each definition calls for at least two people (a **delegator** and a **delegatee**), work, and some kind of transfer of authority to perform the work. No definition suggests it is an abdication of **responsibility** for the overall outcomes or performance or the abdication of the need to be involved. This is an important point because remaining in touch with others who are completing work on behalf of a manager is sometimes difficult.

A definition of *delegation* then might be as follows: achieving performance of care outcomes for which you are accountable and responsible by sharing activities with other individuals who have the appropriate authority to accomplish the work. Acceptance of the delegated work must occur, either passively (i.e., no protest occurs) or actively (i.e., communication indicates acceptance). Thus delegation can occur only when two people are involved in a mutual work situation and one of the persons has **accountability** and the other has some authority for performing specific tasks. When two RNs work together sharing activities, delegation does not occur. On the other hand, if one RN has specific accountability for an outcome and that nurse asks another RN to perform a specific component of the overall function, that is delegation (see Assignment versus Delegation, p. 375, for further clarity.)

Delegation also occurs when an RN assigns an LPN/LVN or UAP to perform a specific function or aspect of care. The American Nurses Association (ANA, 1994) defines *UAPs* as unlicensed people "trained to function in an assistive role to the registered professional nurse in the patient/client activities as delegated by and under the supervision of the registered professional nurse" (p. 2). Authority is a critical component. It may be designated by law, such as the nursing practice act, or it may be designated by educational preparation/certification. Typically, a position description further defines what the nature of the authority is for a specific position.

A word of caution, however: There is great variance among training programs for UAPs; therefore understanding the qualifications and abilities of the person to whom you are delegating something is critical. The Institute of Medicine (1996) reported that only 20% of the hospitals surveyed required a high school diploma for people seeking training as UAPs. Couple that factor with the length of the program (some were as minimal as a few hours), and it becomes obvious that knowing someone's preparation to receive a delegated task is critical.

Two of the numerous recommendations Fagin (2001) made that relate to delegating are (1) being certain that delegation is made only to those properly qualified to perform whatever the assignment is and (2) requiring that all staff be properly identified. The first recommendation is evident from the previous discussion in this chapter; the second is designed to help patient, families, and others know the type of personnel providing care to an individual or group. Finally, Standing, Anthony, and Hertz (2001) found in a study about delegation the two most common errors associated with poor patient outcomes related to (1) giving improper directions and (2) providing improper follow-through of agency protocol. These findings suggest that communication and agency protocols are crucial to achieving positive performance outcomes.

Achieving Performance Outcomes

Achieving performance outcomes is the driving force of all healthcare. If what anyone does has little or no benefit in improving the delivery of care, it is, of course, ineffective. Therefore all care is based on attaining expected outcomes, whether that care is provided directly by an individual or group of professionals or whether that care was shared between professionals and assistants. Performance of care outcomes relates to the profession's keeping its trust with the public, that is, to perform safely and competently. The Research Perspective identifies that negative outcomes seem more related to delegation situations in which the nurse is less experienced in practice and the UAP is less experienced in a specific setting. In ever-changing healthcare settings, it is critical to know that you must delegate to achieve all that is expected of you. In essence, this means that if you cannot trust others or if you are frustrated because you cannot do it all yourself, you will be very frustrated with the way in which healthcare is delivered and your career opportunities will be fairly limited.

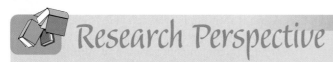

Research Perspective

Anthony, M. K., Standing, T., & Hertz, J. E. (2000). Factors influencing outcomes after delegation to unlicensed assistive personnel. *Journal of Nursing Administration, 30,* 474-481.

This national study about delegation and patient outcomes included both RNs and LPN/LVNs, although there were relatively few of the latter. The conceptual framework for this exploratory, cross-sectional survey was the five rights of delegation; a five-stage modified Dillman technique involving a questionnaire produced results of importance to nurses.

Only 148 of the 516 mailed questionnaires produced usable data. All types of settings were represented in the targeted sample. Nurses were asked to write about two situations involving UAPs: one with a positive outcome and one with a negative. Although this was a small convenience sample, there were some specific factors related to negative outcomes that were not true for positive outcomes. Those associated with negative outcomes included the nurse having less than 5 years' experience and the UAP having less than 1 year of experience in the specific setting.

IMPLICATIONS FOR PRACTICE

This research suggests that support and resources for nurses with less than 5 years' experience might reduce the number and intensity of negative outcomes.

Accountability and Responsibility

The terms *accountability* and *responsibility* refer to the legal expectation the state has vested in persons with the designation of RN. *Accountability* means that someone must be able to explain actions and results. Legally, the RN is accountable for nursing care. *Responsibility* refers to reliability, dependability, and obligation to accomplish work. It also refers to each person's obligation to perform at an acceptable level. Thus assistants, whether UAPs or LPNs/LVNs, are obligated to perform that which they can at acceptable quality levels. Those individuals are also responsible for informing the delegator what limitations, if any, would prevent the accomplishment of expected outcomes.

Sharing Activities

Sharing activities may sound simplistic; however, when someone with the legal accountability for a role shares elements, that individual is not giving away role elements. That individual is sharing activities or functions to ensure total outcomes. Therefore the delegation definition here emphasizes that care itself is not delegated—only elements (activities) are. Thus responsibility rests with the delegator. Sharing may consist of many strategies ranging from asking an assistant to perform a specific task to expecting the same performance as the day before. For delegation to be effective, the RN must accept that sharing activities is important and provides benefits to patient care.

The professional, technical, and amenity (PTA) model (Hansten & Washburn, 1998) is a useful framework for determining which activities may be shared. Amenity (hotel-like service factors) may almost always be delegated. Certain technical tasks may be delegated if the delegatee is appropriately qualified and the circumstances do not warrant a different approach. Professional aspects may never be delegated. Each aspect is important in the total care, and each can be measured. For example, patient surveys often address amenity factors, flow sheets frequently document technical factors (or specific reports note deviations), and broader responses such as patient behavior are reflective of the professional aspects.

Other Individuals

Other individuals may include persons with no formal preparation or recognition (e.g., UAPs), those with dependent status (e.g., LPNs/LVNs who function under the direction of a physician or RN), or others who are designated as being accountable to the delegator (e.g., other RNs or healthcare providers who report to a designated delegator such as a nurse manager).

Span of control is an important concept to keep in mind when interacting with others to achieve care. This term refers to how many people you have responsibility for. For example, if a nurse has responsibility for 5 staff members, each of whom cares for 10 patients, the nurse has responsibility for 5 staff and 50 patients. This may not be as overwhelming as it may seem at first if the patients are in stable condition and their needs are predictable, if the staff are well-prepared, experienced providers of routine care, and if the geographic area is restricted. On the other hand, if any of these factors is not true of a situation, this responsibility may be overwhelming, even if each staff member provides care for only five patients. Thus, if others render elements of care, multiple factors must be assessed to determine how manageable the situation is.

Appropriate Authority

Appropriate authority to perform certain functions stems from various sources. For example, the practice of LPNs/LVNs is defined by state titling or practice acts, as well as by institutional policies. UAPs, such as certified nursing assistants, are prepared to meet a specific set of functions. As mentioned, considerable variation exists in the preparation of UAPs. That preparation, coupled with institutional policies, defines what UAPs may do. Position descriptions may provide more specific insight about the authority designated in certain positions. In essence, the term *appropriate authority*, as used in the previous definition, refers to a baseline indicator that an individual is expected to be able to perform certain aspects of care and therefore may receive an assignment to execute those aspects.

Notably, the ANA (1995) differentiates between direct and indirect delegation. The difference relates to whether the RN is actively deciding what to delegate (direct) or whether the decision is based on organizational protocols that designate certain tasks as appropriate for others to perform (indirect). Even when organizational protocols indicate someone else may perform a task on behalf of the RN, the employee must be competent to perform the tasks. This expectation suggests that the delegator will make initial and ongoing assessments related to the delegatees' performance. Three elements of nursing may not be delegated (ANA, 1995). They are initial and subsequent nursing assessments requiring professional judgment; determination of nursing diagnoses, care goals, care plans, and progress; and interventions that require professional knowledge and skill.

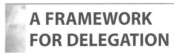

A FRAMEWORK FOR DELEGATION

One way to consider the concept of delegation can be found in Hersey and Blanchard's original work about leadership style (1988). (See the Theory Box.) Although the terms have changed in subsequent revisions, the key concepts have not. These researchers explained followership behavior in the context of two factors: ability and willingness. Both factors relate to specific situations. *Ability* relates to knowledge and skills; *willingness* relates to attitude. Thus, if a delegatee indicates reluctance to perform some work, the delegator assumes more control of the situation to determine whether knowledge is lacking; whether there is some psychomotor interference with performing the work; or whether the delegatee is bored, anxious, or upset and thus unwilling to meet the expectations of the situation. The less able or willing the delegatee is in a situation, the more involvement is needed from the delegator. Concomitantly, the more able and willing the delegatee is, the less involved is the delegator. At no time, however, is the delegator not involved with the situation or the delegatee.

So, what strategy does the delegator use to interact with a delegatee? By inserting a vertical line from the follower readiness box to intersect the bell-shaped curve in Figure 21-1, you find the best strategy. In essence, the greater the ability and willingness of the delegatees are, the more likely it is that the delegator could use delegation as the strategy for interacting with that person in a specific situation. In other words, both the amount of guidance (task behavior) and the amount of support (relationship behavior) would be relatively low. This seems logical for established work relationships. However, not all situations are established. For example, a delegatee may have limited knowledge and ability to perform a task. Such a situation would require more guidance. If the relationship is limited (i.e., these two people are unlikely to work together again), the delegator would likely simply tell the individual what to do and how to perform. Hersey and Blanchard call this "tell." In another instance, however, there may be only a new task (i.e., the relationship is an ongoing one or the relationship will become such). In this case researchers found that the best strategy is to explain what to do and how to do it. This option is labeled "sell." Logically, if producing outcomes in a given situation is the driving force, delegators are much less

Theory Box

SITUATIONAL THEORY

THEORY/CONTRIBUTOR	KEY IDEAS	APPLICATION TO PRACTICE
Hersey and Blanchard (1988) created this theory to explain how leader/managers need to behave differently.	A wise leader analyzes how an individual interacts in a specific situation. The analysis consists of the sophistication of the employee and the task itself and the need for interaction. A leader then responds differently based on this analysis.	Treating people equally is unfair. Before delegating, an RN must know what a specific employee needs in a specific situation.

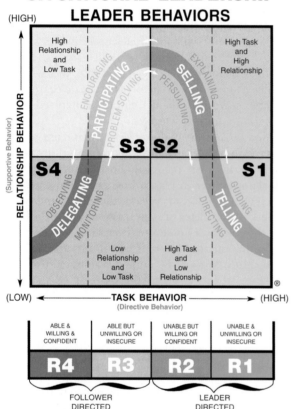

Figure 21-1   Situational leadership. (© 1998. The Situational Leadership model is the registered trademark of The Center for Leadership Studies, Escondido, Calif. All rights reserved. Used with permission.)

likely to expend additional time and effort investing in a casual, limited relationship than they are in one that will be repeated. A third behavior described by these researchers is called "participate." This behavior is appropriate for situations in which the delegatee has abilities and willingness but the relationship is relatively new (see Figure 21-1). In other words, in such situations both the delegator and the delegatee must determine mutual expectations and conditions of performance. The final behavior is called "delegate" and is best used with established relationships and expertise.

Each of these behavior styles is evident in real work situations. For example, when a new team begins to work together, the first thing the delegator needs to evaluate is the ability and willingness of the delegatee, and this must be based on trust. If those factors (ability and willingness) are low, the delegator has two ways to interact with the delegatee: tell or sell. If the nature of the relationship is limited, for example, the delegatee has been reassigned from one service to another for this day only, telling is probably the appropriate strategy. Little, if any, time is lost on interaction, and a fair amount of guidance is provided. On the other hand, if the relationship is an ongoing or developing one, the delegatee will need to gain the necessary ability and/or comprehend the motivation related to the situation. Thus selling or explaining is the appropriate strategy. Although this strategy is more time consuming, the interaction leads to a more supportive relationship.

When the delegatee has a high degree of ability and willingness and the expected task is familiar, little guidance is needed. If the relationship is new or developing, more support is needed, so the delegator and delegatee need to interact in a participating mode. This approach helps each learn more about the other and contributes to advancing to the most developed relationship, at which true delegation is possible: The delegatee is willing and able, needs little guidance, and needs relatively little support to accomplish work. Such behavior is evident when people work together in the same situations for some time. The delegatee knows what needs to be done, what needs to be reported, how to prioritize, and when to ask for help.

Delegation can be viewed as a spectrum of behaviors based on the context and needs in a specific situation. Knowing how to interact with a given delegatee is one of the key challenges of a delegator if effective outcomes are desired.

Another way to think about delegation is described in Hansten and Washburn's work (1998). These authors suggest a "big picture" view that has seven key elements. Knowing your world (the environment in which you practice) provides a context. Knowing yourself and what needs to be done leads to the complex process of knowing the delegatee, communicating, resolving conflict, and providing feedback and evaluating. This should be considered a cyclic process: As you gain various experiences you might have a different understanding of your world and yourself, which leads to new abilities in the other elements of the process.

ASSIGNMENT VERSUS DELEGATION

Assignment transfers both responsibility and accountability. This strategy is most common when one RN assigns a patient to another. Although nurses typically refer to the way work is distributed as an assignment, in reality, some portions of the work distribution are delegated care, not assigned. Thus UAPs receive delegated activities, whereas RNs receive assigned care/assignments. When an RN assigns care to another RN, both accountability and responsibility are transferred. When an RN delegates care to someone, such as a UAP, responsibility is transferred; accountability is not. Table 21-1 depicts the differences.

IMPORTANCE OF DELEGATING

"We accomplish all we do through delegation—either to time or to other people. If we delegate to

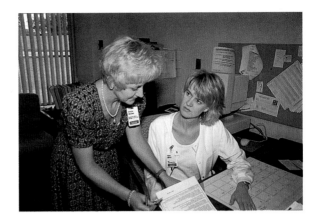

Nursing managers face complex decisions with delegation involving patients and staff.

Table 21-1	DELEGATION VERSUS ASSIGNMENT	
Aspect	**Responsibility**	**Accountability**
Delegation	Yes	No
Assignment	Yes	Yes

time, we think efficiency. If we delegate to other people, we think effectiveness" (Covey, September 29, 1995).

Delegation is a critical skill for accomplishing care in a timely manner. It usually saves time in the long run and, when effective, is cost effective. At its worst, however, it is exceedingly costly. Therefore making the best decisions about care is imperative. One of the misperceptions about the profession of nursing that has been a plague is to think of nursing care in terms of psychomotor tasks. Therefore professional nurses must convey the consistent message that doing a task is one component of care. Although the performance of a psychomotor task is critical, the critical analyses "behind the scenes" are clearly the precipitator of the actions.

Hansten and Washburn (1998) identify five advantages of delegating. Patients receive more attention because more staff are available. Because all of the RN's time is not consumed with direct care activities, more time is available for what might be viewed as the professional components, such as managing and teaching. An increased sense of belonging develops. Overtime is reduced because the team is efficient and productive. Finally, nurses report that they feel less pressure because they do not have to do everything alone. These advantages suggest that delegation has direct patient and professional benefits.

Seldom should a decision to delegate be based on timesaving considerations alone, but the truth is that in an effective team, delegation can be an effective time conservation technique.

■ *Exercise 21–1*
Ask a staff nurse and a nurse manager about their individual perspectives of the pros and cons of delegation. Now ask a UAP employee the same questions.

LEGAL AUTHORITY TO DELEGATE

Most state practice acts address the concept of delegation; some explicate rules and regulations governing what may be delegated and when. State boards of nursing are vested with protecting the public; therefore they regulate practice and the educational preparation required to practice nursing. The expectation that specific knowledge about nursing and delegation is needed to perform safely makes the nurse legally accountable and thus liable. Because nursing roles evolve over time, thinking about the scope of liability for the RN is valuable.

Legally, the concept of delegation is complex. First, the individual doing the delegation is personally responsible for prudent action. If delegation is not performed within acceptable standards, malpractice may be the outcome. In addition, according to Guido (1999), failure to delegate and supervise within acceptable standards may extend to direct corporate liability for the institution. Furthermore, whenever care is provided by other than a registered nurse, the accountability for care remains with the manager [of care]/delegator even though others provide various aspects of care. This view of professional liability is consistent with the idea that licensure conveys both privilege and expectations.

■ *Exercise 21–2*
Review your state nursing practice act, rules, and regulations. Discuss with two or more classmates what your state provides as direction about delegation. What conclusions can you reach?

Habgood (2000) further suggests that nurses (in the author's case, perioperative nurses) have the right and responsibility to address issues with the state board, to understand the law and rules and regulations, gain clarification from the state board, and request rule changes when necessary to assure delegation occurs in a positive manner.

SELECTING THE DELEGATEE

In many settings, you are one of a group of professional staff members who have the authority to delegate; therefore you probably will not be able to select the person with whom you will work. On the other hand, a few opportunities may occur in your career when you have a chance to select your own assistant. Several aspects of selecting an assistant are important. For example, knowing that you can communicate readily is important. If an LPN/LVN who has functioned in a physician's office for some time and is not familiar with working under the directions of an RN or having nursing care supervised is concerned about your supervision, talking about it can eliminate or diminish feelings of concern.

Appreciating and valuing each other's cultural perspectives can help with communication and with care itself. For example, an assistant who does not concur with you about the goals of hospice might actually work at counter purposes to the organizational philosophy. In addition, if the assistant is like you in terms of strengths, you will both want to do the same things, possibly leaving gaps in care. So, selecting someone with strengths that are different from yours enhances the work the two of you can accomplish together. This approach is consistent with strengths theory (Buckingham & Clifton, 2001), which suggests that we all should focus on building our strengths rather than "fixing" our weaknesses to be more effective at what we do.

SUPERVISING THE DELEGATEE

Because the registered nurse is always accountable for assessment, diagnosis, planning, and evaluation, it is important that UAPs understand what elements of implementation they may carry out and why the registered nurse is responsible for analyzing data gathered. "Supervision in its broadest context is the active process of directing, guiding, and influencing the outcome of an individual's performance of an activity or task" (ANA, 1994, p. 9). Supervision consists of the initial direction (the delegation) and periodic inspection (reassessment and evaluation) (Hansten & Washburn, 1998). Both elements must be present to ensure effectiveness in entrusting an element of care to someone else.

DELEGATION DECISION MAKING

Sometimes we fail to delegate to others. We may think it is too time or energy consuming. Sometimes we frankly believe we can do a better job ourselves or we seek the recognition for specific care. Yet, when delegation is done well, we have leveraged our contributions to care.

Considering how much information must be processed to make a sound decision about delegation, a specific matrix has been devised to make the process consistent. Although the original work was performed in critical care settings, several factors can clearly drive all decisions. Deciding to delegate, what to delegate, and to whom to delegate requires an active decision-making process.

In 1990 the American Association of Critical Care Nurses (AACN) identified the factors in the following list as ones that require active decision making before delegating a component of care:

- Potential for harm
- Complexity of task
- Need for problem solving and innovation
- Unpredictability of outcome
- Level of interaction with patient

These factors are accompanied by a rating scale of 0 (better outcome of delegation) to 3 (less desirable outcome). In essence, when no risks are likely, each of the preceding five factors would be rated with zeros. When risks are great, however, a score approaching 15 would be likely. Realistically, the experienced RN may take only a few minutes or less to reach a conclusion about what can be delegated. On the other hand, RNs in beginning competence levels may need to carry a reminder to be sure to consider all factors, and therefore the decision may take longer. When new staff are incorporated or when the RN changes practice settings, the thought process may be more deliberate.

Potential for Harm

Potential for harm refers to the possibility that in the performance of a task or function something might negatively affect the patient. Thus the more unstable the patient's condition is, the more potential there is for harm. As a result, when the potential for harm is greater, either the desirability to delegate care elements is lessened or the amount of close supervision is increased.

Complexity of Care

Complexity of care is a similar factor; that is, if care is less complex, someone with less preparation can safely provide care. On the other hand, if the care is complex, greater risk is involved in delegation. As a result, an RN may want to delegate only a few elements of care—those that are the least complex. In addition, the delegation may be more specific; the delegatee would have less individual determination of how to perform the delegated care. An example might be when several tasks need to occur in sequence and some of them are very detailed and others are relatively simple. The RN might specify exactly when some task must be done and how.

Need for Problem Solving and Innovation

The need for problem solving and innovation relates to whether the delegatee will need to determine how to modify care or find new strategies for performing the functions. This factor is important in any situation, but it is critical when supervision is less direct. Such is the case with most community-based care. If being able to establish (invent) individualized care is important, the RN may determine that only a professional staff member may deliver care until the care pattern is established. The more experienced the assistant, the more likely that individual also has significant experience in innovating aspects of care.

Unpredictability of Outcome

Unpredictability of outcome refers to how like the "textbook picture" this particular care situation is. When predictable outcomes are fairly certain, for example, with established treatments for a given patient population, safe delegation of care elements is more likely. On the other hand, new treatments may have undetermined nursing outcome. Therefore delegation may not be the best option.

Level of Interaction

Level of interaction with the patient refers to such aspects as the need for psychosocial interactions and educational strategies. Again, although many delegatees can provide both, establishing the expected interactions may be necessary or it may be possible to delegate only a component of the interaction.

■ *Exercise 21–3*

Select three patient records from a clinical setting in which delegation occurs. On the basis of the documentation only, describe the previously described AACN factors for those three patients. Next make a determination about the PTA elements (see Sharing Activities, p. 372). If you are familiar with any UAPs in the setting, use Figure 21-1 to identify how you would work with prospective delegates to accomplish the care. You may choose to create two grids (one for the AACN factors, a second for the PTA model). Finally, in one or two sentences, state the rationale for your conclusions about delegation.

Integrating Factors

Combining these factors into an integrated whole for making decisions is valuable. One factor may be the overriding element. For example, when the potential for harm is great, the other factors may be relatively less influential. Thus reaching decisions about to whom to delegate, what to delegate, and when to delegate is a complex process.

Providing specific feedback about performance is the best strategy for shaping future behavior. Therefore statements such as "You performed that procedure with ease" are more effective than saying "Nice job." Equally important is the feedback from the person performing the tasks. Was the work completed? How did the patient respond? What changes were noted? These are examples of what the RN must know from the person who performed the delegated portion of care.

When possible, provide positive feedback; however, it undermines your credibility to convey satisfaction when the performance is less than desirable. Therefore being honest about feedback is the best strategy. Being honest about the circumstances and performance and what we can do to change them helps the delegatee develop for the future. Attacking the person or personal characteristics not only has little, if any, positive effect on care but also has the potential to undermine a long-term relationship. The Literature Perspective identifies that communication is critical to positive teamwork.

Finally, keep in mind that some individuals occupy positions for which they are not qualified. One strategy for dealing with this is to lower your expectations so that the individual can be successful. *Before doing that, however, think about the effect on others.* For example, why is one employee held to the standard and another is not? Who becomes responsible for accomplishing the work the one person cannot achieve? Is it fair to compensate for someone who cannot meet performance expectations? What are the potential liabilities of altering the standards of performance? Reaching decisions about delegating elements of care is a complex process. When the professional nurse knows the individual is incapable

 ## Literature Perspective

Anthony, M. K., Casey, D., Chau, T., & Brennan, P. F. (2000). Congruence between registered nurses and unlicensed assistive personnel perception of nursing practice. *Nursing Economics, 18,* 285-293.

Questionnaires were given to 647 RNs and 241 non-RN staff in three acute care hospitals. Both RNs and UAPs were asked for their perception about various aspects of nursing practice. There were considerable differences of agreement on various aspects. Especially important to RNs and UAPs working together is communication. Although there was 100% agreement that nurses and UAPs speak throughout the shift, there was only 25% agreement on the nature of that communication. RNs believed that they commonly were asking for help, whereas UAPs perceived the conversation to be about observations of patients (as opposed to a request for help, work management or personal issues).

IMPLICATIONS FOR PRACTICE

Being clear about communication is especially important when working with others.

of appropriate performance and does not intervene, the potential for liability increases. Even eliminating the legal questions, ethical considerations should influence the nurse (ANA, 1976).

The National Council of State Boards of Nursing (1995) proposed five rights of delegation as follows: (1) the right task, (2) the right circumstances, (3) the right person, (4) the right direction/communication, and (5) the right supervision. Keeping these in mind enhances success when delegation occurs. Table 21-2 poses some appropriate questions to reach the right decision about delegation.

DELEGATION PROCESS

Unless you are well established at delegation or you work consistently with only persons you know well, you will need to plan how to delegate to be effective. Parsons (1998) suggests that specific preparation for the role is important for RNs. Figure 21-2 provides a decision tree for delegation. The first step involves professional accountability. If an RN has not assessed the patient, delegation should not occur. This step ensures that an RN has determined baseline data and needs. Only if the delegatee is properly prepared to accept a specific delegation should the RN proceed to delegate.

In settings other than those of confined geography, such as hospitals, long-term care facilities, and clinics, one of the greatest challenges of delegation relates to supervision. In such situations, it is especially important to be very clear about what is expected of the delegatee. Box 21-1 presents a communication template to use when delegating. The more that is understood between the delegator and the delegatee about a particular delegation situation, the greater the chances are of being effective in patient care.

Exercise 21–4

Think about what you could delegate, then use the delegation communication template found in Box 21-1 to practice with a classmate the transfer of specific responsibilities for care.

PRACTICALITIES OF DELEGATION

Delegation clearly is complex, but there are some ways to simplify the process. For example, when possible, selecting the delegatee whose talents match the task is better than merely selecting a competent individual. In large organizations, having a choice about who the delegatee is is more likely to occur than in smaller facilities. In rural settings the delegatees tend to be more predictable, long-term employees; thus delegation is made easier because more is known about them and their abilities.

Delegation may be difficult early in careers and in specific circumstances. In those situations it may be helpful to initiate working together with an oral acknowledgment that the delegatee's abilities are

Table 21-2 GETTING TO THE RIGHT ANSWERS FOR THE FIVE RIGHTS	
The Rights	**Questions You Might Ask Yourself**
The right task	Is it appropriate to delegate (based on legal and institutional factors)? Is the person able and willing to do this specific task?
The right circumstances	Would the AACN factors suggest that the circumstances are right? Is staffing such that the circumstances demand delegation strategies?
The right person	Is the prospective delegatee a willing and able employee? Is the patient the right person to pair with the delegatee?
The right direction/communication	Do you and the delegatee have "common language"? (Do words, such as time frames, needs, and critical, mean the same to both of you?) Does the delegatee know what and when to report? Is your communication based on a "fit" with the situation and culture?
The right supervision	Do you know how and when you will interact about patient care with the delegatee? How often will you need to provide direct observation?

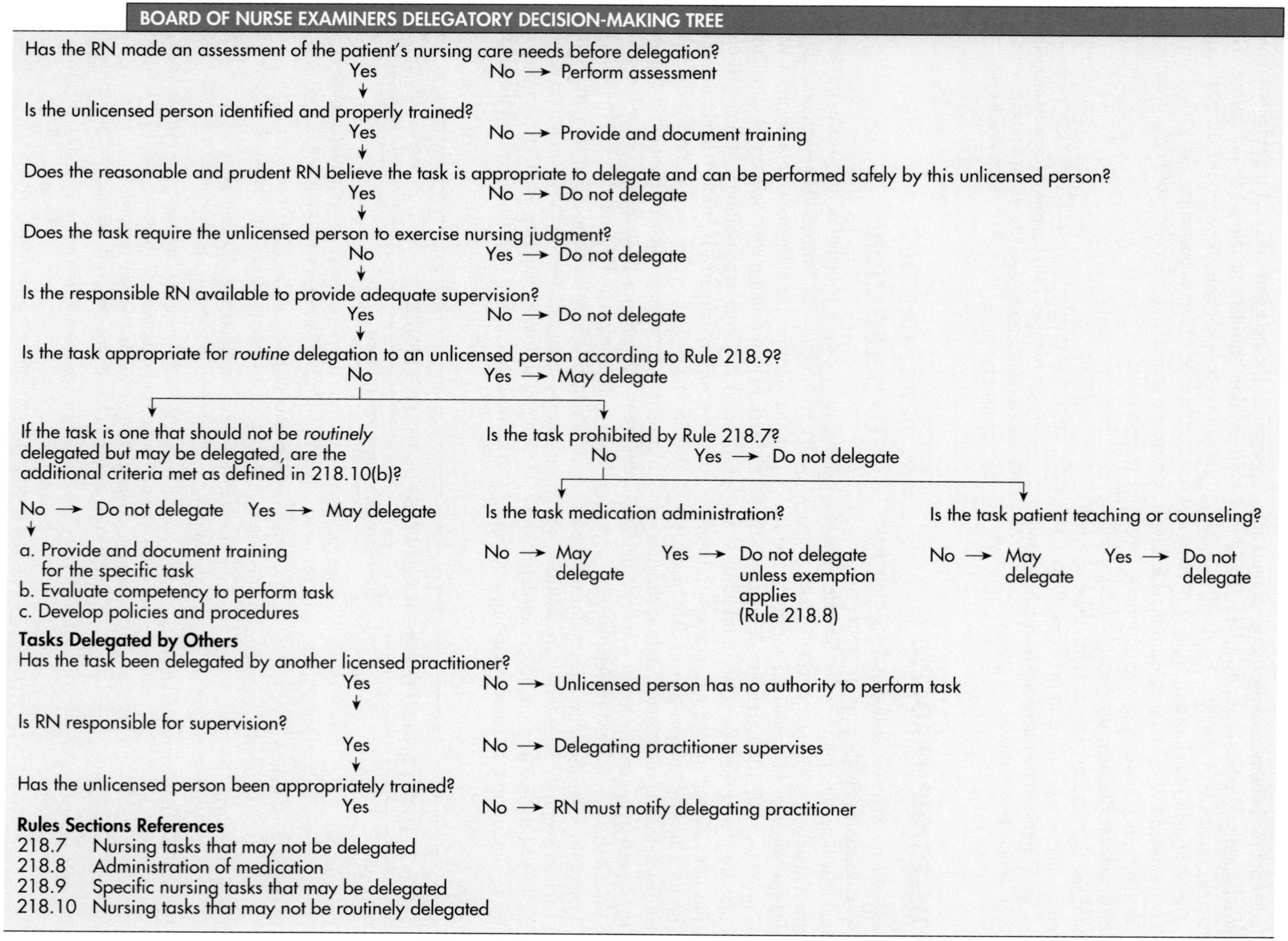

BOARD OF NURSE EXAMINERS DELEGATORY DECISION-MAKING TREE

Has the RN made an assessment of the patient's nursing care needs before delegation?
Yes ↓   No → Perform assessment

Is the unlicensed person identified and properly trained?
Yes ↓   No → Provide and document training

Does the reasonable and prudent RN believe the task is appropriate to delegate and can be performed safely by this unlicensed person?
Yes ↓   No → Do not delegate

Does the task require the unlicensed person to exercise nursing judgment?
No ↓   Yes → Do not delegate

Is the responsible RN available to provide adequate supervision?
Yes ↓   No → Do not delegate

Is the task appropriate for *routine* delegation to an unlicensed person according to Rule 218.9?
No →   Yes → May delegate

If the task is one that should not be routinely delegated but may be delegated, are the additional criteria met as defined in 218.10(b)?
No → Do not delegate   Yes → May delegate
a. Provide and document training for the specific task
b. Evaluate competency to perform task
c. Develop policies and procedures

Is the task prohibited by Rule 218.7?
No →   Yes → Do not delegate

Is the task medication administration?
No → May delegate   Yes → Do not delegate unless exemption applies (Rule 218.8)

Is the task patient teaching or counseling?
No → May delegate   Yes → Do not delegate

Tasks Delegated by Others
Has the task been delegated by another licensed practitioner?
Yes ↓   No → Unlicensed person has no authority to perform task

Is RN responsible for supervision?
Yes ↓   No → Delegating practitioner supervises

Has the unlicensed person been appropriately trained?
Yes ↓   No → RN must notify delegating practitioner

Rules Sections References
218.7   Nursing tasks that may not be delegated
218.8   Administration of medication
218.9   Specific nursing tasks that may be delegated
218.10   Nursing tasks that may not be routinely delegated

Figure 21-2   Board of Nurse Examiners Delegatory Decision-Making Tree. (From Board of Nurse Examiners for the State of Texas, August 1993. Reproduced with permission.)

BOX 21-1

Delegation Communication Template

- State exactly what is being delegated and what the expected outcome is.
- Convey recognition of the authority to perform what is expected.
- Identify priorities.
- Acknowledge monitoring activities you may perform.
- Specify any performance limitations, such as time limits on performing a procedure.
- Specify deadline, including exact timing if that is important.
- Specify report time lines and data expected.
- Specify parameter deviations, including when immediate action must be taken.
- Identify appropriate resources, including people who may be consulted.
- Be clear about what may not be delegated.

Exercise 21–5

Using the assignments made by a nurse manager or charge nurse where you have a clinical experience, answer the following questions: Was it clear what was delegated? Why or why not? Were delegation decisions logical? Why or why not? From what you know about your nursing practice act and professional standards, did the assignments make sense legally and ethically? What is your rationale?

unknown but that together this team is committed to providing the best care for its patients. Stating up front that offense or insult are not intended and then seeking feedback later makes the delegatee more receptive to hearing messages. The key is to specifically seek feedback so that messages that are offensive can be changed. The goal, however, remains the same: to focus on the outcomes of patient care.

Letting the delegatee implement the task in his or her own way can be a challenge. Someone else will be unlikely to do a task just as the delegator would. However, assuming no safety or ethical discrepancies are likely, delegation really is a matter of trust. If the delegator intervenes, the delegatee loses confidence or becomes frustrated and the delegator has lost the benefits of delegating.

Having deadlines helps keep the delegatee on target without oversupervising. Being clear about the need to check quality and effectiveness ensures that monitoring will be ongoing.

Finally, situations may occur in which you see issues associated with delegation but you have no authority. Fisher and Sharp (1998) suggest that influencing positive outcomes is still possible. Assuming no negative patient outcomes or safety issues are involved, you can help other delegators achieve positive outcomes by doing three things: asking, offering, and doing. Begin by asking questions related to the problem/issue/mission. This in itself may help the delegator see a situation differently. Making an offer such as an idea to move the process ahead toward a favorable outcome may be necessary or desirable. Finally, whatever you advocate is best valued if you can demonstrate the behavior you propose (doing).

INTEGRATED CARE

In the late 1990s care moved from multidisciplinary, coordinated care to an integrated approach. Again, this move provides an impetus for a multi-skilled worker. Having someone who performs "what is needed now" for the patient or the professional staff is the focus rather than the "me and my assistants" approach. However, as McCloskey, Bulechek, Moorhead, and Daly (1996) suggest, the nurse will continue to provide the important "glue role" so that care achieves positive outcomes. In other words, in many settings, nursing's presence on a regular basis predisposes nurses to the "glue" role (holding patient care together) for logical reasons.

The Solution

Sunday morning came. I arrived at 6:30 AM, took report, and sent the unseasoned RN and the seasoned LVN to the eight patients on the older side, where they were assigned the day before. The aide and I went to the eight patients on the new side. We teamed up room to room doing vital signs, passing trays, and conducting quick assessments. At 8:00 AM, the emergency room RN came to that unit to pass the morning medications. Although I do not support such fragmented care, I knew to whom I could delegate what, I knew the abilities of the various people I work with, I knew I could prioritize care and seek additional resources for

short periods, I knew that I may not be timely in everything I got done, and I knew my own abilities. Because we truly work as a whole, I had others volunteering to answer phones and call lights. Is this ideal? Absolutely not! Is it sometimes the reality? Absolutely.

— Molly Patteson

 Would this be a suitable approach for you? Why?

CHAPTER CHECKLIST

Delegation obviously is a complex issue. It has many facets, each of which by itself is complex. One of the critical roles of RNs is that of the "glue factor," by which the RN coordinates care across the spectrum of providers and affects the quality of care. Current research suggests that many indirect care interventions are not delegated by RNs because of the complexities and quality implications.

- Delegation involves achieving outcomes and sharing activities with other individuals who have the authority to accomplish work for which the delegator is accountable and responsible.
- The ways in which delegation can actually be enacted can be based on a situational leadership model.
- Nursing practice acts, rules, and regulations provide the legal structure for delegation; the *Code of Ethics for Nurses* provides the ethical structure.
- Knowing the skills and abilities of the delegatees is critical to feeling comfortable and confident in delegation.
- The AACN framework for making decisions about delegation is comprehensive.

TIPS FOR DELEGATING

- Be familiar with your nursing practice act and the corresponding rules and regulations.
- Ascertain the skills of unlicensed assistive personnel to whom you may delegate tasks.
- Assess your patients with the perspective that some of their care will be provided by others.
- Use the communication template to enhance successful delegating.
- Use a decision-making framework, such as the one developed by the AACN for critical care patients, to screen what can be delegated to unlicensed assistive personnel.
- Evaluate on a regular basis your effectiveness in delegating to others.

TERMS TO KNOW

accountability	delegator
delegatee	responsibility
delegation	

REFERENCES

American Association of Critical Care Nurses. (1990). *Delegation of nursing and non-nursing activities in critical care: A framework for decision making.* Laguna Viquel, CA: American Association of Critical Care Nurses.

American Nurses Association. (1976). *Code for nurses.* Kansas City, MO: Author.

American Nurses Association. (1994). *Registered professional nurses and unlicensed assistive personnel.* Washington, DC: Author.

American Nurses Association. (1995). *The ANA basic guide to safe delegation*. Washington, DC: Author.

Anthony, M. K., Casey, D., Chau, T., & Brennan, P. F. (2000). Congruence between registered nurses and unlicensed assistive personnel perception of nursing practice. *Nursing Economics, 18*, 285-293.

Anthony, M. K., Standing, T., & Hertz, J. E. (2000). Factors influencing outcomes after delegation to unlicensed assistive personnel. *Journal of Nursing Administration, 30*, 474-481.

Buckingham, M., & Clifton, D. O. (2001). *Now, discover your strengths*. New York: The Free Press.

Covey, S. (1995). *The Covey calendar*. Provo, UT: FranklinCovey.

Division of Nursing. (2001). *The registered nurse population: National sample survey of registered nurses—March 2000. Preliminary Findings. February 2001.* Washington, DC: US Department of Health and Human Services: Health Resources and Services Administration, Bureau of Health Professions.

Fagin, C. M. (2001). *When care becomes a burden: Diminishing access to adequate nursing*. New York: Milbank Memorial Fund.

Fisher, R., & Sharp, A. (1998). *Getting it done: How to lead when you're not in charge*. New York: HarperPerrenial.

Guido, G. W. (1999). Legal and ethical issues. In P. S. Yoder-Wise (Ed.), *Leading and managing in nursing* (2nd ed.). St. Louis: Mosby.

Habgood, C. M. (2000). Ensuring proper delegation to unlicensed assistive personnel. *AORN Journal, 71*, 1058-1060.

Hansten, R. I., & Washburn, M. J. (1998). *Clinical delegation skills: A handbook for nurses*. Gaithersburg, MD: Aspen.

Hersey, P., & Blanchard, K. H. (1988). *Management organizational behavior* (5th ed.). Englewood Cliffs, NJ: Prentice Hall.

Institute of Medicine. (1996). *Nursing staff in hospitals and nursing homes: Is it adequate?* Washington, DC: National Academy Press.

McCloskey, J. C., Bulechek, G. M., Moorhead, S., & Daly, J. (1996). Nurses' use and delegation of indirect care interventions. *Nursing Economics, 14*, 22-33.

National Council of State Boards of Nursing. (1995). Delegation: Concepts and decision-making process. *Issues, 16*(4), 1-4.

Parsons, L. C. (1998). Delegation skills and nurse job satisfaction. *Nursing Economics, 16*, 18-26.

Standing, T., Anthony, M. K., & Hertz, J. E. (2001). Nurses' narratives of outcomes after delegation to unlicensed assistive personnel. *Outcomes Management for Nursing Practice, 5*(1), 18-23.

SUGGESTED READINGS

Badovinac, C. C., Wilson, S., & Woodhouse, D. (1999). The use of unlicensed assistive personnel and selected outcome indicators. *Nursing Economics, 17*, 190-200.

Barter, M., McLaughlin, F. E., & Thomas, S. A. (1997). Registered nurse role changes and satisfaction with unlicensed assistive personnel. *JONA, 27*(1), 29-38.

Bernreuter, M. E., & Cardona, S. (1997). Survey and critique of studies related to unlicensed assistive personnel from 1975-1997, Part 1. *Journal of Nursing Administration, 27*(6), 24-29.

Bernreuter, M. E., & Cardona, S. (1997). Survey and critique of studies related to unlicensed assistive personnel from 1975-1997, Part 2. *Journal of Nursing Administration, 27*(7/8), 49-55.

Heller, R. (1998). *How to delegate*. New York: DK Publishing.

Huston, C. L. (1996). Unlicensed assistive personnel: A solution to dwindling health care resources or the precursor to the apocalypse of registered nursing? *Nursing Outlook, 44*(2), 67-73.

Kany, K. (1999). Workplace protections: Working with UAPs. *American Journal of Nursing, 99*(10), 71.

Parsons, L. C. (1999). Building RN confidence for delegation decision-making skills in practice. *Journal for Nurses in Staff Development, 15*, 263-269.

Sullivan, E. J., & Decker, P. J. (1992). *Effective management in nursing* (3rd ed.). Redwood City, CA: Addison-Wesley.

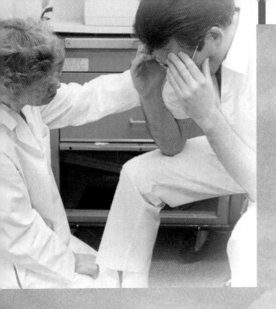

Chapter

22

Managing Personal/Personnel Problems

Cynthia Whittig Roach

The purpose of this chapter is to discuss various personal and personnel problems that a manager must face in all nursing settings. Some specific tips and tools are provided as ways to intervene, coach, correct, and document problem behaviors. Emphasis is placed on effective communication, both written and verbal.

Objectives

- Differentiate common personal/personnel problems.
- Relate role concepts to clarification of personnel problems.
- Examine strategies useful for approaching specific personnel problems.
- Prepare specific guidelines for documenting performance problems.

Questions to Consider

- How do you react when you see that an employee is absent often and you or others seem to have a heavier workload as a result?
- Have you ever been in a position in which you were not really sure what was expected of you? How did you feel?
- What would you do if you observed clinical incompetence in a co-worker or peer?
- What is the best approach to deal with someone you believe is chemically dependent or impaired at work?

The Challenge

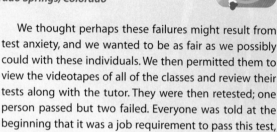

Cherie Gorby, RN, MSN
Senior Administrator Patient Services, Memorial Hospital, Colorado Springs, Colorado

New monitoring equipment was installed on the pediatric unit in an acute care hospital. This necessitated the instigation of several new standards of care. Everyone who worked in this area had to demonstrate competency in these standards.

The clinical manager and I determined that one competency could be demonstrated through a basic ECG take-home test. Of the 42 nurses who took this test, 7 failed with a score of less than 70%. These seven who failed were required to take an 8-hour class focusing on a review of pediatric arrhythmias. This class consisted of a pretest and posttest, along with hands-on didactic exercises. Six of the seven failed the posttest and/or the didactic. These six people were then required to do a 6-week basic ECG class. We also provided a tutor who was a clinical nurse specialist to help them with their homework when necessary. Three of these six failed the basic ECG class.

We thought perhaps these failures might result from test anxiety, and we wanted to be as fair as we possibly could with these individuals. We then permitted them to view the videotapes of all of the classes and review their tests along with the tutor. They were then retested; one person passed but two failed. Everyone was told at the beginning that it was a job requirement to pass this test, which indicated mastery of the standard of care for this pediatric unit.

How can a manager deal fairly with employees who fail to meet established standards of care despite numerous efforts on the manager's part to assist the employee in meeting these standards?

What do you think you would do if you were this nurse?

INTRODUCTION

In managing nursing personnel, much of the satisfaction that a manager receives comes from working with people. On the other hand, working with people presents some of the greatest challenges with which a manager must cope. Problems such as **absenteeism**, uncooperative or unproductive employees, clinical incompetence, employees with emotional problems, and **chemically dependent** employees are only a few of the issues that challenge a manager. If a manager wants to be successful, these problems must be dealt with in ways to minimize their effects on patient care and on staff morale. Documentation of performance problems and documentation for termination are critical. Overall goals are to assist the employee in the improvement of performance, to maintain the highest standards for the delivery of patient care, and to provide a supportive environment in which all employees might deliver the best care and attain work satisfaction.

PERSONAL/PERSONNEL PROBLEMS

Absenteeism

One of the most vexing personal/personnel problems to the nurse manager is that of absenteeism because inadequate staffing adversely affects patient care both directly and indirectly. When an absent caregiver is replaced by another who is unfamiliar with the routines, employee morale suffers and the care may not meet established standards. Working short-staffed or working overtime to cover for absent workers creates physical and mental stress. Replacement personnel usually need more supervision, which not only is costly but also may decrease productivity and the quality of patient care. Indirectly, co-workers may become resentful about being forced to assume heavier workloads and/or may be pressured to work extra hours. Chronic absenteeism may lead to increased staff conflicts and eventually to an increase in absenteeism among the entire staff.

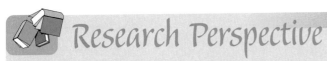

Research Perspective

Barnes, B., Leis, S., Brammer, J. M., Gustin, T. J., & Lupo, T. C. (1999). A developmental evaluation process for nurses: Enhancing professional excellence. *Journal of Nursing Administration, 29*(4), 25-32.

Challenged with dissatisfaction of the evaluation process, a project for redesign was implemented over a 2-year period in one Midwestern hospital. Focus groups of middle managers, shift managers, and clinical staff nurses met to identify problems with the current performance appraisal system and define behaviors to "exceed standards." Essential components were divided into five categories: professional practice development, citizenship, research/performance improvement, customer relations, and clinical practice/continuum of care. Benefits of this process enabled the staff to collaborate, plan future projects, develop a self-assessment tool, and improve work satisfaction. This process of redesign encouraged a significant change throughout the institution.

IMPLICATIONS FOR PRACTICE

Dissatisfactions in the work setting are likely to exist. Securing the input of various individuals, representative of affected groups, can produce positive outcomes.

Absenteeism also has a deleterious effect on the financial management of a nursing unit. Replacement of absent personnel by temporary personnel or overtime paid to other employees is very costly, and the cost of fringe benefits used by absent workers is very high. Also, as our care delivery systems become more complex and technically oriented, the successful nurse manager must realize that technology is not a replacement for human caregivers. Absent caregivers cannot be replaced with machines.

Absenteeism cannot be totally eliminated. There are always unplanned illnesses, accidents, bad weather, sick family members, a death in the family, and even jury duty, which are legitimate reasons for missing work and beyond the control of management. However, some portion of absenteeism is voluntary and preventable; thus the manager must identify the cause so that it may be addressed. Absenteeism may also indicate poor work satisfaction. If the manager believes that the issue is based in work satisfaction, focus groups might lead to insight about the sources (see Research Perspective). If the underlying cause can be identified, there may a way to prevent the loss of the employee, should retention of the employee be the goal. Some employees who convey they are never happy with their job may continually disrupt the overall unit with their absenteeism and should be terminated.

With role theory as a framework, absenteeism has been linked to **role stress** and **role strain** (see Theory Box). Absence from work is a way of withdrawing from an undesirable situation short of actually leaving, and many employees increase their absenteeism just before submitting their resignation. If the healthcare worker is experiencing some form of role stress, leading to role strain, it might be manifested through absenteeism. Hardy and Conway (1988) state that role strain may be reflected by (1) withdrawal from interaction, (2) reduced involvement with colleagues and organizations, and (3) job dissatisfaction. All of these could be manifested through absenteeism. With this framework, management of absenteeism is based on the belief that competent role performance requires interpersonal competence. "Role competence is the ability of a person in an interdependent position, which is ongoing in time, to carry out lines of action that are task and interpersonally effective" (Hardy & Conway, 1988, p. 195). Hardy and Conway further explain that role competence is (1) learned through socialization processes, (2) necessary for adequate role performance, and (3) accountable for individual and social progress. In other words, to engage successfully in roles, people need role-specific skills, but they also need interpersonal competence to guide their behaviors. Role behavior occurs in a social context rather than in isolation. Therefore the nurse manager needs to know the existing situation, when it has changed, when it needs to be changed, and how to change it. Because people who are more satisfied in their work usually

Theory Box

ROLE THEORY

THEORY/CONTRIBUTOR	KEY IDEA	APPLICATION TO PRACTICE
Role theory is not considered a true scientific theory but more of a perspective or framework to understand individual behavior as it applies to specific roles (Hardy & Conway, 1988).	Professional socialization is a learned behavior and clarifies specific role prescriptions or sets of rules that are inherent within a given profession.	Within each area of practice or within each organization, there are specific rules, behaviors, and expectations that are prescribed and that will direct practice. Each professional nurse has the responsibility to completely understand his or her role. When this does not occur, role ambiguity or role strain may result. Absence of role clarity can also lead to decreased work satisfaction.

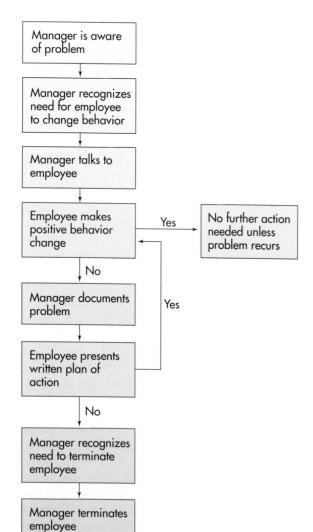

Figure 22-1 Model for behavioral change.

commit to "be there" for their team, enhancing job satisfaction may be an effective strategy toward reducing absenteeism.

An adaptation from Haddock's (1989) model of **nonpunitive discipline** is also useful in addressing absenteeism behavior, as the example in the next paragraph illustrates. This model demonstrates how undesirable behaviors, such as absenteeism, can be successfully changed. Figure 22-1 illustrates how changing undesirable behaviors can be accomplished.

When an employee demonstrates an unacceptable level of absenteeism, the manager should take specific steps. Box 22-1 identifies those steps.

This model of nonpunitive discipline allows employees to free themselves from some role stress by clarification of role expectations. Employees can receive satisfaction from the realization that a problem is not inadequate performance attributed to personal faults, but rather a lack of clarification of role expectations within the organization.

Exercise 22-1

Review the policy manual at a local healthcare organization. Determine what constitutes excessive absenteeism. What are the consequences?

Uncooperative or Unproductive Employees

The problem of uncooperative or unproductive employees is another area of frustration for the nurse manager. Hersey, Blanchard, and Johnson (1996) identify two major dimensions of job performance that relate to this problem: motivation

BOX 22-1

Steps to Clarify Role Expectations

Step 1: Remind the employee of the employment policies and procedures of the agency. Sometimes an employee does not know, or has forgotten, the existing standards, and a reminder with no threats or discipline is all that is needed. The employee must remain ultimately accountable to the organization's policies and procedures.

Step 2: When the oral reminder does not result in a behavior change, put the reminder in writing for the employee. These oral and written reminders are simply statements of the problem and the goals to which both the manager and the employee agree. The employee must voluntarily agree with the manager that the behavior in question is not acceptable and must agree to change.

Step 3: If the written reminder fails, only then grant the employee a day of decision, which is a day off with pay to arrive at a decision about future action. Pay is given for this day so that it is not interpreted as punishment. The employee must return to work with a written decision as to whether or not to accept the standards for work attendance. Remember that this is a voluntary decision on the employee's part. Emphasize to the employee that it is the employee's decision to adhere to the standards.

Step 4: If the employee decides not to adhere to standards, termination results. On the other hand, if the employee agrees to adhere to the standards, and in the future does not, the employee in essence has terminated employment. Keep a copy of the written agreements and also give the employee a copy. The manager should be clearly aware of the organization's policy for termination and request assistance from the human resources department as deemed necessary.

---

and ability. The type and intensity of motivation vary among employees because of differing needs and goals that employees express. The manager can best handle employees with motivation problems by attempting to determine the cause of the problem and by trying to provide an environment that is conducive to increased motivation for the employee. If the employee is uncooperative or unproductive because of a lack of ability, education and training are appropriate interventions.

The manager can determine lack of ability on the part of an employee in various ways. Frequent errors in judgment or techniques are often an indication of lack of knowledge, skill, or critical thinking. This illustrates the need for the nurse manager to carefully document all variances or untoward events. When the nurse manager does thorough documentation, trends may be discovered that in turn suggest that a specific employee is having problems. The nurse manager can cite problem behaviors and perhaps even trends to the employee. Corrective action is easier to pursue and resolution is more effective with this strategy. When the problem is determined to result from a need for more education or training, the manager can work with the education department or the clinical specialist for the involved unit to help the employee improve his or her skills. Most employees are extremely co-operative in situations such as this because they want to do a good job but sometimes do not know how. Employees may deny they need help or may be too embarrassed to ask for help. When the manager can show an employee concrete evidence of a problem area, cooperation is enhanced.

Immature Employees

Sometimes an unproductive employee simply lacks maturity. This lack of maturity may be described as *emotional intelligence underdevelopment* that results in such problems as being socially inept or unable to control one's impulses (Strickland, 2000). Immaturity in an employee may not be readily apparent to the manager but may be manifested in any of the following actions: defiance, testing of workplace guidelines, passivity or hostility, or little appreciation for any management decisions. The challenge for the nurse manager is not to react in kind, but rather to relate to this employee in a positive and mature manner. First, however, the manager needs to determine whether these behaviors are reflecting a state of being uncomfortable or incompetent (LaDuke, 2000). For example, if an employee states, "Administration is always making decisions to make our jobs harder," rather than making a hostile or defensive comment in reply, the manager could take the employee aside and say,

"I notice that you seem to be angry about this new policy. Let's talk about it some more." Immature employees either act immaturely all of the time or regress to an immature level when stressed. The nurse manager must recognize immaturity in an employee and react calmly and without anger. The manager must keep in mind that this employee may be displaying dynamics rooted in unresolved areas of personality development and that the behavior is not a personal attack on the manager. The best way to deal with this behavior is to confront the employee with the specific problem and define realistic limits of acceptable behavior with consequences for nonadherence. Generally, employees comply with specific limits but will test management in other areas. As this testing occurs, the manager must continue the same limit-setting technique. Remember that the immature employee usually has problems because of a lack of self-worth, power, and self-control. Praise and affirmation are valuable tools that the manager can use to help these employees feel better about themselves. For information on addressing generational issues, see Chapter 2.

Exercise 22-2

A nurse comes to you, the nurse manager, and states that one of the other nurses is tying a knot in the air vent (pigtail) of nasogastric tubes. This nurse does not know how to approach the employee to discuss the problem. What would you do?

Clinical Incompetence

Clinical incompetence is possibly one of the most frustrating problems that the nurse manager faces, although it may be entirely correctable. The problem may surface immediately in a new employee. At other times, clinical incompetence comes as a surprise to a nurse manager if co-workers "cover" for another employee. Some nurses are unwilling to report instances of clinical incompetence because they do not want to feel responsible for getting one of their peers in trouble. When other employees are engaged in enabling behavior by covering for the mistakes of one of their peers, the nurse manager may be surprised to discover that the employee does not know or cannot do what is expected of him or her at work. Sadly, the employee in question has been able to cover incompetence by hiding behind the performance of another employee. The nurse manager must remind employees that part of professional responsibility is to maintain quality care and thus they are obligated to report instances of clinical incompetence, even when it means reporting a co-worker. Ignoring violations of a safety rule or poor practice is unprofessional and cannot be tolerated. As the following Research Perspective illustrates, however, there may be differing perceptions about competencies and standards.

Most healthcare agencies use skills checklists or a competency evaluation program to ascertain that their employees have and maintain essential skills for the job they are expected to do. A skills checklist is one way to determine basic clinical competency (Table 22-1). This checklist typically contains

 Research Perspective

Osborne, J., Blais, K., & Hayes, J. S. (1999). Nurses' perceptions: When is it a medication error? *Journal of Nursing Administration,* 29(4), 33-38.

This descriptive, comparative survey of registered nurses working on medical surgical units of a 700-bed community hospital addressed several issues related to medication administration and their related errors. The responses were anonymous. Ninety-two surveys were distributed, and fifty-seven were returned. The percentage of medication errors actually reported was estimated to be 25% (43.9% stated this percentage). When scenarios were presented, differing opinions arose about whether the event was reportable as an error. The respondents also identified that they believed other nurses did not report errors because of fear of reactions by the manager and peers.

IMPLICATIONS FOR PRACTICE

This study suggests that there needs to be a consensus about what constitutes a medication error and that the negative consequences may prevent or at least limit accurate reporting. Potentially, many issues may need consensus.

Table 22-1 EXAMPLE OF A SKILLS CHECKLIST

Purpose

1. The clinical skills inventory is a three-phase tool to enable the newly hired RN and the nurse manager to determine individual learning needs, verify competency, and plan performance goals.
2. The RN will complete the self-assessment of clinical skills during the first week of employment. The RN will use the appropriate scale to document current knowledge of clinical skills.
3. The nurse manager will document observed competency of the orientee or delegate this to a peer. All columns must be completed on the inventory level.
4. At the end of orientation, the new RN and the manager will use the inventory to identify performance goals on the plan sheet. The skills inventory will be in a specified place on the nursing unit so that it is available to the manager and other RNs. It should be updated at appropriate intervals as specified by the manager.

Scale for Self-Assessment

1 = Unfamiliar/never done
2 = Able to perform with assistance
3 = Can perform with minimal supervision
4 = Independent performance/proficient

Score for Validation of Competency

1 = Unable to perform at present
2 = Able to perform with assistance
3 = Progressing/repeat performance necessary
4 = Able to perform independently

Clinical Skills	Self Assessment		Comment	Validation			Comment
	Scale	Date		Score	Date	Initials	
Epidural catheter care							
NG/Dobbhoff							
Insertion							
Management							
Preoperative care/teaching							
Postoperative care/teaching							

Plans Sheet for Skills Inventory

Name _____

Date _____

Goals   **Date to be Completed** _____

_____

_____

_____

_____

_____

_____

_____

Orientee's Signature _____

Manager's Signature _____

Date _____

Skills Inventory modified from one used at Memorial Hospital, Colorado Springs, CO.

a number of basic skills along with ones that are essential for safe functioning in the area of employment. Any type of skills review should be directly linked to quality improvement indicators. Completion of a checklist of skills that is not based on problems is essentially a waste of time and may take away from areas that have been found to be problems. The employee may be asked to do a self-assessment of the listed skills and then have performance of the skills validated by a peer or co-worker. This is a very effective method for the manager to assess the skill level of employees and to determine where additional education and training may be necessary. In addition, if the manager discovers that an employee is unable to adequately perform a skill, the manager can easily check the skills list, directly observe behaviors to see at what level this employee is functioning, and recommend a specific plan for remediation. Sometimes an employee may be able to perform all of the tasks on a skills checklist but is still unable to effectively manage overall patient care. If in questioning the employee, or in evaluating the employee's performance, the manager determines that there is a lack of knowledge or that there are problems with time management, formal education may be the proper course of action. In either event, the manager must establish a written contract containing a plan of action that sets time limits within which certain expectations must be achieved. This ensures compliance on the part of the employee. A more comprehensive program for competency evaluation might include not only the skills checklist but also unit-specific objectives, an overall framework for evaluation, and critical thinking exercises that are interactive in nature (Johnson, Opfer, VanCura, & Williams, 2000).

Emotional Problems

Emotional problems among nursing personnel may affect not only the involved individual but also co-workers and ultimately the delivery of patient care. The nurse manager must be aware that certain behaviors, such as poor judgment, increased errors, increased absenteeism, decreased productivity, and a negative attitude, may be manifestations of emotional problems in employees.

Example
A nurse manager began hearing complaints from patients about a nurse named Nancy. Patients were saying that Nancy was abrupt and uncaring with them. The manager had not received any complaints about

Nancy before this time, so she questioned Nancy about why this was occurring. Nancy reported that her mother was very ill and she was so worried about her and was so upset that she could not sleep and was tired all of the time. She went on to say that she was having trouble being sympathetic with complaining patients when they did not seem to be as sick as her mother.

When a new trend of these behaviors is evident, a problem that an employee is unable to handle may be the cause. The nurse manager is not and should not be a therapist but must intercede, not only to help the individual with the problems but also to maintain proper functioning of the unit. In dealing with the employee who exhibits behaviors that indicate emotional problems, the manager, after identifying the problem, should assist the individual to obtain professional help to cope with the problem. The manager may have to make some adjustments in the individual's work setting and schedule if this is deemed necessary and does not have a negative effect on patient care. The manager acknowledges that an employee is experiencing emotional difficulties, but the standards of patient care cannot be compromised. If standards are lowered to help an individual, the effect will be deleterious to everyone involved. The most important approach that the manager can take with an emotionally troubled employee is to provide support and encouragement and to assist the individual to obtain appropriate help. Many agencies have some kind of employee assistance program (EAP) to which the manager should refer any troubled employee. During this process, the manager must remember to check with the human resources department about any implications that may occur because of the Americans with Disabilities Act (ADA). If an employee has a documented mental illness, the employing agency may be under certain legal constraints as specified in the ADA. The nurse manager should always remember that many resources are available to assist with personnel problems. The manager should never feel required to know all of the legal implications regarding employment policies. Rather, the manager must know that help is available and how to access it.

Exercise 22-3

As a nurse manager in a community health agency, you have just had a meeting that was called by several of your staff nurses. They expressed concern regarding another nurse colleague who has come to work tearful several times during the past week. They state she often goes into the break room when she is in the agency and appears as if she has been crying when she comes out. She has refused to discuss her distress with her colleagues. These nurses express concern and want you to help her. What is your response? What would you do?

Chemical Dependency

Chemical dependency among nursing personnel places patients and the organization at risk. Such an employee adversely affects staff morale by increasing stress on other staff members when they have to assume heavier workloads to cover for the chemically dependent employee who is not performing at full capacity or who is often absent. As a result, patient care may be jeopardized because staff are focusing more on the problems of a co-worker than on those of the patients they are assigned to care for.

The manager is responsible for early recognition of chemical dependency and referral for treatment when appropriate (McAndrew & McAndrew, 2000). State laws vary as to the reportability of chemical dependency. As is true of all nurses, a nurse manager is responsible for upholding the nurse practice act and should be familiar with the legal aspects of chemical dependency in the state in which he or she is employed. As with the employee with emotional problems, the nurse manager should be aware of ADA issues and check with the human resource department for help with how to handle the employment of a chemically dependent

employee. Most states and agencies have reporting requirements regarding substance abuse. The state board of nursing is a key place to determine specific details required by a given state. All nurse managers should familiarize themselves with the nurse practice act in the state in which they reside and with the personnel policies relating to substance abuse in their employing agency. Furthermore, nurse managers should make certain that staff are familiar with legal requirements.

In the present social climate, there is more interest in helping affected individuals than in punishing them, and there is also more empathy and understanding toward them. Identification of an employee with a chemical dependency is usually difficult, especially because one of the primary symptoms is denial. The primary clue to which a manager should be alert when there is a suspicion of chemical dependency is any behavioral change in an employee. This change could be any deviation from the behaviors the employee normally exhibits. Some specific behaviors to note might be mood swings, a change from a tidy appearance to an untidy one, an unusual interest in patients' pain control, frequent changes in jobs and shifts, or an increase in absenteeism and tardiness.

When a manager suspects that an employee may be chemically dependent, the manager must intervene because patient care may be jeopardized. A manager facing a problem with an impaired nurse must be compassionate yet therapeutic. Knowing that denial may be one of the primary signs of substance abuse, the manager must focus on performance problems that the nurse is exhibiting and urge the nurse to voluntarily seek counseling or treatment. EAPs always protect the employee's privacy and are usually available free or at a minimal charge to the employee. The manager should strive to refer any troubled employee to the EAP whenever possible. This removes the manager from the counseling role and helps employees get the professional help they need without fear of a breach in confidentiality. If a nurse refuses to seek help voluntarily for a substance abuse problem, the manager is responsible for following the established policy for such employees. The manager must remember that if the substance-abusing employee is terminated and not reported, the manager not only may be violating a law but also may be enabling this employee to obtain employment in another agency and potentially be in a position to harm patients and co-workers.

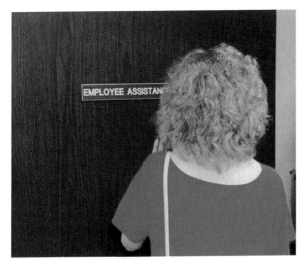

Many agencies have an employee assistance program to which the manager can refer the troubled employee.

Many states have rehabilitation programs for chemically impaired nurses so that they may return to nursing if rehabilitated. Nurse managers are sometimes asked to assist with monitoring the progress of a chemically impaired nurse. Specific guidelines are established through the rehabilitation program with the cooperation of the employee, the agency, and the manager. The manager is typically asked to provide feedback about the employee's progress to the employee and to the state or rehabilitation program involved. These programs vary, but, for example, a nurse who has been an admitted abuser of meperidine may be allowed to work in a setting in which this drug is never used, or the nurse may not be permitted to administer any controlled substances to patients. This, of course, puts an added burden on other staff members, but it can be a positive experience for all because nurses face some of their professional responsibility by helping another nurse while upholding patient care. Often, as a part of their therapy, these nurses are required to openly share with other staff members what their problem is and what they are doing to control it. When handled in a positive, professional way, the nurse manager can turn a potentially destructive situation into a positive, constructive one.

Regardless of the type of personnel issue, the manager needs to have a plan in place for ongoing monitoring and follow-up of issues/problems.

Exercise 22-4

Review your state's nurse practice act and rules and regulations. What are you required to do if you believe a nurse has a problem with chemical dependency?

DOCUMENTATION

Documentation of personnel problems is unquestionably one of the most important, but also one of the most onerous, aspects of the nurse manager's job. As much as some managers may wish they would, personnel problems probably will not "disappear," and therefore will eventually have to be dealt with. Through careful ongoing documentation of problems, the manager makes the task of identifying and correcting problems much less burdensome.

Documentation cannot be left to memory! When an employee is involved in a problem situation or if an employee receives a compliment or does something extremely well, a brief notation to

this effect should be placed in the personnel file. This entry should include the date, time, and a brief description of the incident. Adding a small notation as to what was done about a problem when it occurred is also helpful. Along with this, the nurse manager should keep a log or summary sheet of all reported errors, unusual incidents, and accidents. These extremely important data should include the date, time, and names of involved individuals and should be tallied at monthly intervals for analysis by the manager. The few extra minutes each day that the manager spends tracking these data provides invaluable information to the manager about organizational and individual functioning. This tracking can then be used to pinpoint an individual's problem areas, areas of excellence in individual performance, and overall organizational problem areas. The manager who keeps careful records about organizational functioning has greater control in the management of personal and personnel problems. Box 22-2 describes content and format for such documentation and provides an example as an illustration.

PROGRESSIVE DISCIPLINE

When an employee's performance falls below the acceptable standard, despite corrective measures that have been taken, some form of discipline must be enacted. Most organizations use some form of **progressive discipline** to correct problem behaviors. Progressive discipline consists of evaluating performance and providing feedback with steps of increasing sanctions. These sanctions progress from least severe to most severe, as described in Box 22-3. One example of the kind of workplace behavior that usually involves progressive discipline but that could result in immediate termination is harassment (Brennan, 1999).

TERMINATION

At times, even though the manager has done everything possible to gain the cooperation of a problem employee, the problems may persist. In such cases, there is no choice but to terminate the employee. Because termination is one of the most difficult things a manager does, the following guidelines should be adhered to: First, the manager must be confident that everything possible has

BOX 22-2

Documentation of Problems

- Description of incident—an objective statement of the facts related to the incident
- Actions—statement(s) describing the plan to correct and/or prevent future problems
- Follow-up—dates and times that the plan is to be carried out, including required meeting with the employee
  Example:

  Several patients reported to the nurse manager that Becky, one of the night shift registered nurses, was "curt" and "gruff" and seemed uncaring with them. The manager called Becky into her office and reiterated the complaints that she had received. The nurse manager was specific as to times and incidents. The manager then reminded Becky about what her expectations were relating to patient care, emphasizing the importance of a caring attitude with all patients. She discussed with Becky what the possible cause of Becky's behavior might be, such as problems at home or lack of sleep. Becky denied being curt or gruff, but agreed that some of her mannerisms might be misinterpreted. The manager suggested to Becky that perhaps she needed to be particularly aware of her body language and to soften her tone of voice. After discussing this incident and reminding Becky of the importance of caring in nursing, the manager told Becky that this behavior would not be tolerated. The manager told Becky she wanted to meet with her every Friday morning at the end of Becky's shift to discuss how the week had gone and to determine how she was interacting with the patients assigned to her. The manager also told Becky that she would be checking with patients to see what they had thought of Becky. The manager routinely asked patients about their nursing care as she made rounds, so this was not an unusual thing for her to do. These weekly meetings were to be conducted for 6 weeks, followed by monthly meetings for a 3-month period. If there was no recurrence of problems, the meetings would be discontinued after this time.

been done to help the employee correct the problem behaviors. Second, the manager must recognize that if employment continues, this employee will have a deleterious effect on overall organizational functioning and, more important, on nursing care. Third, the employee must have been made fully aware of the problem performance and of the fact that all of the correct disciplinary steps have been followed. Finally, a nurse manager should check with the human resources and legal departments before proceeding to ensure that termination is justifiable legally and that proper steps have been followed. The nurse manager needs to be confident in the knowledge that all policies regarding termination have been followed before having an actual termination meeting with the employee. It is always preferable to err on the side of caution when proceeding with termination of an employee. Remember that termination is something that the employee has caused as a result of persistent problem behaviors or certain behaviors for which the organization has zero tolerance. Termination is not done at the whim of management; it results from failure on the part of the employee to change a problem behavior.

Situations that may warrant immediate dismissal include theft, violence in the workplace, and willful

BOX 22-3

Steps in Progressive Discipline

1. Counsel the employee regarding the problem.
2. Reprimand the employee. A verbal reprimand usually precedes a written one, but some organizations issue both a verbal and a written reprimand simultaneously. When the documentation is written, the employee must sign to verify that the problem was discussed. This does not mean that the employee agrees with the reprimand. It means only that the employee is aware of a written reprimand that is to be placed in the employee's personnel file. The employee always receives a copy of a written reprimand.
3. Suspend the employee if the problem persists. The employee will be suspended without pay for a specified period, usually several days or longer according to the agency policy. During this time the employee may realize the seriousness of the problem based on the resulting discipline.
4. Allow the employee to return to work with written stipulations regarding problem behavior.
5. Terminate the employee if the problem recurs.

abuse of the patient, to name a few. Again, the manager should use the assistance of the human resource department to ensure that all of the organization's policies are being upheld correctly. The following example illustrates that a manager needs to anticipate a termination to ensure ongoing standards:

Example

Linda has gone through all of the steps in the progressive discipline process as a result of her abusive behavior toward her co-workers. She returned to work and seemed to be doing well until about 6 weeks later, when she slammed down her clipboard during report and angrily accused the charge nurse of always giving her the worst assignments. The nurse manager was present and asked Linda to come into her office. At this point, she told Linda she was relieving her of her assignment that day and asked her to go home to cool off. The manager told her that she would call her the following day about what would be done. Linda went home, and the manager reviewed the incident with her nurse administrator. They both agreed that Linda's behavior not only was intolerable but also violated the terms of her probation and therefore she should be terminated. The manager called Linda the following day as she had agreed to do and asked Linda to come and meet with her. The manager and administrator met with Linda and reviewed the incidents and the disciplinary measures leading up to this incident. The nurse manager asked the administrator to be present at the scheduled meeting because it is a good practice to have a witness in a confrontative situation such as termination. The manager stated to Linda that she regretted it had come to this, but pointed out to her that her behavior had violated all of the agreed-upon stipulations, and as a result she would be terminated immediately. Linda was tearful and had numerous excuses, but the manager remained firm and merely repeated that Linda, in not fulfilling the agreement, had chosen to end her employment.

■ Exercise 22–5

Review a healthcare organization's policies regarding termination. What are the conditions, such as stealing or violence, that are described as cause for immediate dismissal? Is abusing substances at work one of those conditions?

CONCLUSION

All employees share a role with managers to prevent and control personal/personnel problems in their work setting. Everyone must be willing to refuse to allow unethical behavior from co-workers and to speak out and act appropriately when problems occur.

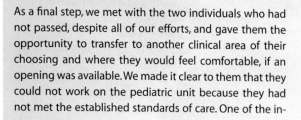

The Solution

As a final step, we met with the two individuals who had not passed, despite all of our efforts, and gave them the opportunity to transfer to another clinical area of their choosing and where they would feel comfortable, if an opening was available. We made it clear to them that they could not work on the pediatric unit because they had not met the established standards of care. One of the individuals chose to resign from the organization, and the other one transferred to another area.

— Cherie Gorby

 Would this be a suitable approach for you? Why?

CHAPTER CHECKLIST

To obtain satisfaction from working with people, a nurse manager must be knowledgeable about personal and personnel issues that are likely to occur in the work setting. The nurse manager must be able to detect, prevent, and correct problems that affect nursing care and staff morale in a nursing agency. Proper documentation and follow-up are key elements in the successful management of all personnel issues.

- ■ Absenteeism's detrimental effects are as follows:
  - • Patient care may be below standard.
  - • Replacement personnel require additional supervision.
  - • Absenteeism may increase among the entire staff.

- Financial management of the unit suffers adverse effects.
- Effective strategies to reduce absenteeism include the following:
  - Enhancing nurses' job satisfaction
  - Using Haddock's model of nonpunitive discipline:
    - Remind the employee of the problem orally.
    - Follow up with a written reminder if the oral one fails.
    - Grant the employee a day of decision if the written reminder fails.
    - Terminate if the employee decides not to adhere to standards.
- Uncooperative or unproductive employees may lack motivation, ability, or maturity.
  - The nurse manager can try to provide an environment that is more conducive to motivation.
  - Education and training are appropriate interventions for lack of ability.
  - Praise and affirmation are often the most effective strategies for an employee who lacks maturity.
- Clinical incompetence is a highly correctable problem for nurse managers.
  - Clinical incompetence may be masked by coworkers' enabling behavior.
  - A skills checklist helps determine basic clinical competency and pinpoint the need for additional training and education.
  - A comprehensive competency program may include not only a skills checklist but also a means for evaluating critical-thinking ability of the employee.
- When emotional problems are evident, the nurse manager should assist the employee in getting professional help. The nurse manager is responsible for early recognition of chemical dependency and referral for treatment when appropriate.
  - The manager must do the following:
    - Uphold the state's nurse practice act.
    - Be familiar with state laws on chemical dependency.
    - Know the healthcare organization's personnel policy on chemical dependency.

- Some warning signs of possible chemical dependency are as follows:
  - Behavioral changes such as mood swings
  - Sudden and unusual neglect for personal appearance
  - Unusual interest in patients' pain control
  - Increased absenteeism and tardiness
- Documentation of problems should include the following:
  - A description of the incident
  - A description of the manager's actions
  - A plan to correct/prevent future occurrences
  - Dates and times of follow-up measures
- Progressive discipline may be used when other corrective measures have failed. Steps in progressive discipline are as follows:
  - Counsel the employee regarding the problem.
  - Reprimand the employee (first verbally, then in writing).
  - Suspend the employee if the problem persists.
  - Allow the employee to return to work, with written stipulations regarding problem behavior.
  - Terminate the employee if the problem recurs.

TIPS IN THE DOCUMENTATION OF PROBLEMS

- Identify the incident and related facts.
- Describe actions taken by the manager when the problem was identified.
- Develop an action plan for everyone involved.
- Schedule a follow-up meeting to evaluate progress of the action plan.
- Remember to document everything objectively and completely!

TERMS TO KNOW

absenteeism	progressive discipline
chemically dependent	role strain
nonpunitive discipline	role stress

REFERENCES

Barnes, B., Leis, S., Brammer, I. M., Gustin, T. J., & Lupo, T. C. (1999). A developmental evaluation process for nurses. Enhancing professional excellence. *Journal of Nursing Administration, 29*(4), 25-32.

Brennan, W. (1999). Bully off! *Nursing Standard, 13*(18), 27-28.

Haddock, C. (1989). Transformation leadership and the employee discipline process. *Hospital Health Service Administration, 34*(2), 185-194.

Hardy, M. E., & Conway, M. E. (1988). *Role theory: Perspectives for health professionals* (2nd ed.). Norwalk, CT: Appleton & Lange.

Hersey, P., Blanchard, K., & Johnson, D. E. (1996). *Management of organizational behavior: Utilizing human resources* (7th ed.). Englewood Cliffs, NJ: Prentice Hall.

Johnson, T., Opfer, K., VanCura, B., & Williams, L. (2000). A comprehensive interactive competency program. Part I: Development and framework. *MedSurg Nursing, 9*(5), 265-268.

LaDuke, S. (2000). Nurses' perceptions: Is your nurse uncomfortable or incompetent? *Journal of Nursing Administration, 30*(4), 163-165.

McAndrew, K. G., & McAndrew, S. J. (2000). Workplace substance abuse impairment: The occupational health care provider's role. *AAOHN Journal, 48*(1), 32-47.

Osborne, J., Blais, K., & Hayes, J. S. (1999). Nurses' perceptions: When is it a medication error? *Journal of Nursing Administration, 29*(4), 33-38.

Strickland, D. (2000). Emotional intelligence: The most potent factor in the success equation. *JONA, 30*(3), 112-117.

SUGGESTED READINGS

Quinn, C., & Barton, A. (1999). The implications of drug treatment and testing orders. *Nursing Standard, 14*(27), 38-41.

Wright, D. (1998). *The ultimate guide to competency assessment in health care.* Eau Claire, WI: PESI HealthCare, LLC.

Yoder, L. H. (1995). Staff nurses' career development relationships and self-reports of professionalism, job satisfaction, and intent to stay. *Nursing Research, 44*(5), 290-297.

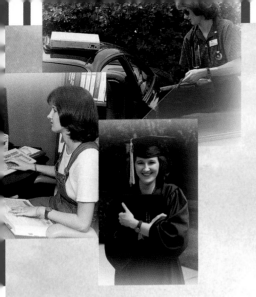

Chapter 23

Role Transition

Jennifer Jackson Gray

This chapter provides information about role transition, the process of moving from a clinically focused position to a supervisory position with increased responsibility. A basic overview of management roles illustrates the complexity of managing work done by others and provides a foundation for understanding role transition. The exercises offer opportunities to recognize one's own expectations, resources, and management potential.

Objectives

- Construct a nonnursing role using responsibilities, opportunities, lines of communication, expectations, and support (ROLES).
- Analyze specific examples of role transitions as a leader, manager, and follower.
- Hypothesize the phases of role transition using comparisons to the phases in developing an intimate relationship.
- Compare the phases of an unexpected role transition to the grieving process.
- Compare the strategies used during a previous transition: strengthening internal resources, negotiating a role, growing with mentors, or learning necessary skills.

Questions to Consider

- *What do I need to know about a management position before accepting it?*
- *How can I quickly make the transition from clinical nurse to nurse manager?*
- *Am I currently in a role transition?*

The Challenge

Robin E. Keene, RNC
ICU Nurse Manager, Central Texas Veterans Health Care Services, Temple, Texas

I was a staff nurse for 6 years before becoming nurse manager, the last 4 of which were in the intensive care unit (ICU), where I am now manager. I was motivated to join the management team because I believed I could help to improve working conditions for staff nurses at this facility. I always thought that the nurse managers forgot where they came from and what it is like to be a staff nurse. The management team at my facility is composed of mainly older female registered nurses (RNs). I envisioned that by being the youngest and most energetic member of the team, I would be able to motivate them and facilitate a more progressive and positive management team.

My role changed dramatically and quickly once I was put in the management role. I went from caring for patients to writing reports, proficiencies, and time schedules and dealing with personnel conflicts and problems overnight. I had no prior training for this and felt totally lost. My workday quickly became one of policy/procedure and the Joint Commission on Accreditation of Healthcare Organizations rather than providing patient care.

The most difficult part of the transition for me was making the change from patient care provider to management. The second most difficult part of this transition was making the move from staff nurse to administration in the same unit. My former friends could no longer be my friends and my co-workers became my employees. I already knew their good and bad habits, who I wanted to work for me and who I didn't. Everyone looked at me differently immediately (even though I was still the same person). Some of my staff members brought up the word *favoritism* anytime I gave one of my former friends time off. The last part of the transition that has been so difficult is the realization that I cannot make changes at this facility without a struggle. Because I manage in a government facility, making change is extremely difficult and I was not prepared for that. How could I be comfortable in this new role?

 What do you think you would do if you were this nurse?

INTRODUCTION

Role transition involves transforming one's professional identity. A new graduate makes a transition from the student role to the nurse role. Expectations of students are clearly specified in course and clinical objectives. Expectations for a new nurse as an employee may not be so clear. The new graduate nurse faces the first of several professional transitions.

Consider the staff nurse who becomes a nurse manager. The staff nurse performs tasks related to the care of patients. As a follower, the staff nurse has accountability and responsibility for the work that is accomplished. A staff nurse who becomes a nurse manager must transition into the new role as a generalist, orchestrating diverse tasks and getting work done through others.

A staff nurse who moves from an acute care setting to a home health agency must also undergo a role transition. Instead of balancing the needs of multiple patients, the home health nurse can focus on one client at a time. Yet, when a collegial opinion is needed during a visit, there are no readily available peers with whom to consult.

Role stress affects the organization's outcomes (Conley & Woosley, 2000) such as quality of patient care and customer satisfaction. Role stress is especially high for persons who span the organization's boundary and serve as the front-line link between the consumer and the organization (Flaherty, Dahlstrom, & Skinner, 1999). Whether the reason is moving to a new management position, assuming a different clinical role, or changing from one setting to another, a new professional identity must be forged through the process of role transition, or the nurse may become dissatisfied and unable to function in the new role (Jost, 2000).

Knowing what to expect during the transformation can reduce the stress of accepting and transitioning into a new role and result in quality outcomes. Following an overview of the roles of leader,

Table 23-1 LEADER, MANAGER, AND FOLLOWER ROLES: PEOPLE WITH WHOM YOU INTERACT AND PROCESSES INVOLVED IN EACH ROLE

Role	People With Whom Interactions Occur	Processes Involved in the Role
Leader	Persons being led Peers	Listening Encouraging Motivating Organizing Problem solving Developing Supporting
Manager	Persons being supervised Administrators Supervisors Regulating agencies	Organizing Budgeting Hiring Evaluating Reporting Disseminating
Follower	Supervisor Peers	Conforming Implementing Contributing Completing assignments

manager, and follower, this chapter describes the process of role transition, with an emphasis on strategies that can be used to ease the transition.

TYPES OF ROLES

Accepting a management position dictates accepting three roles that involve complex processes. The roles of leader, manager, and follower are complex because they involve working through and with unique individuals in a rapidly changing environment. Examples of the people with whom you interact and the processes involved in each role are shown in Table 23-1. In nursing, each of these roles relates to patients and clients.

The leader role involves being willing to take risks and look for new ways of doing things (Kerfoot, 1999b). The nurse leader brings employees together to discuss concerns, solve problems, and dream about possibilities. The nurse leader listens to employees and cares about them as people and vesting themselves in the development of others (Vargo, 2000). The nurse leader encourages employees to develop relationships with each other so that they can function as a team (Dixon, 1999).

Changes in the processes of delivering patient care and organizing healthcare agencies have led to

transformation in the roles and responsibilities of managers (Porter-O'Grady, 1999). Multiskilled, interdisciplinary teams require managers who provide resources and information in "rapid-throughput, high-intensity environments" (Fralic, 2000, p. 340) and maintain stability in the context of instability (Dixon, 1999). The nurse manager interprets information and makes it available to those making patient care decisions (Antrobus & Kitson, 1999). Organizational outcomes are communicated to the group, and team outcomes are developed.

The role of follower involves respecting the authority of others and working within the system to contribute to the organizational outcomes. Managers as followers recognize their accountability to the persons above them on the organizational chart. Within a team, the manager recognizes the leadership being provided by others and supports decisions made by the group.

In the evolving healthcare environment, the nurse providing direct patient care also must function as a leader, manager, and follower. As leader, the nurse recognizes the uniqueness of each patient and provides feedback on clinical progress. As manager, the nurse links the patient to the resources to achieve clinical outcomes. Medical information is translated into a format that the patient can use to make informed decisions about treatment and self-care. Through referrals, the nurse facilitates continuity of care within the larger system. As a follower, the nurse is accountable to the team and the supervisor for completing the work that is assigned. The nurse as a follower practices within the policies and procedures of the organization and the standards of the profession.

Learning the leader, manager, and follower aspects of any new role can be overwhelming. Another approach to the complexity of role transition is the acronym **ROLES**, in which each letter represents a component common to all roles.

ROLES: THE ABCS OF UNDERSTANDING ROLES

Acronyms help us retain and organize information. "ROLES" (Box 23-1) is an acronym useful in role transition.

R stands for responsibilities. What are the specified duties in the position description for the new position? What tasks are to be completed? What decisions must the person in this position make? For example, the job description for a nurse practitioner would include medical diagnosis and prescribing medications (Mick & Ackerman, 2000), whereas the job description for a clinic manager would include responsibilities for staff morale and cost effectiveness of clinic routines (Henry, 2000). Each position has specific tasks for which the position holder is responsible.

O stands for opportunities, which are untapped aspects of the position. In the employment interview the nurse executive may have said that the previous manager did not encourage the staff nurses to participate in continuing education. Or while touring the unit, a manager observes that the report room is lacking in amenities. Maybe there is a new method of delivering patient care appropriate for the unit. These possibilities represent opportunities for a manager to influence organizational and unit goals.

L represents lines of communication. All roles involve relationships with other people (Dixon, 1999; Porter-O'Grady, 1999). Some of these people are above the manager on the organizational chart; others are below. Still others are peers. Roles incorporate patterns of structured interactions between the manager and people in these groups. The nurse manager receives and sends messages. Being a skillful listener can be more important than being skill-

---

BOX 23-1

"ROLES" Acronym

Responsibilities
Opportunities
Lines of communication
Expectations
Support

---

ful in sending messages. Skill is required to effectively communicate both the content and the intent of the message; only through practice can one develop skill. Chapter 19 describes techniques of effective communication that are extremely important to a new manager in building the team.

E stands for expectations. Expectations vary depending on your goals. Colleagues may expect a new nurse anesthetist to be on call every weekend. Staff nurses have specific expectations of their manager and particularly want the manager to be a facilitator and a leader. The nursing executive or administrator will likely have expectations about how managers spend their time on the job—even about how much time they spend at work. Nurse executives' expectations evolve from their perspective of the manager's accountability and duties.

Finding out in advance what the explicit and implicit expectations are of the people involved can facilitate a smoother role transition by decreasing role ambiguity (Hardy, 1978). Hardy's work with role theory suggests a strong relationship between role ambiguity (one type of role stress) and **role strain.** The major concepts of role theory are presented in the theory box.

There are also personal expectations related to performance as a manager. You have a mental image of the role of a manager or person in this position. The process of role transition unfolds as a new manager identifies expectations, recognizes the similarities and differences, and develops the roles of leader, manager, and follower.

S stands for support, which is closely tied to expectations about performance. All roles are shaped to some degree by the support and services others provide. The acute care nurse has peers readily available when a second opinion is needed. The same nurse may feel lost when confronted with questionable findings during a home visit. The nurse manager who must develop the unit's budget

Theory Box

HARDY'S ROLE THEORY

THEORY/CONTRIBUTOR	KEY IDEAS	APPLICATION TO PRACTICE
Hardy (1978) is credited with applying role theory to healthcare professionals. *Role* is the expected and actual behaviors associated with a position. *Role expectations* are the attitudes and behaviors others anticipate a person in the role will possess or demonstrate. *Role stress* is a social condition in which role demands are conflicting, irritating, difficult, or impossible to fulfill. *Role strain* is the subjective feeling of discomfort experienced as the result of role stress.	Role stress is a precursor to role strain. Role stress is associated with low productivity and performance. Role stress and role strain can lead to the person psychologically withdrawing from the role. Clear, realistic role expectations can decrease the role stress for a new nurse manager.	Clear, realistic role expectations can increase productivity.

 Research Perspective

Godinez, G., Schweiger, J., Gruver, J., & Ryan, P. (1999). Role transition from graduate to staff nurse: A qualitative analysis. *Journal of Nurses in Staff Development, 15*(3), 97-110.

Orientees (*n* = 27) and preceptors in an acute care hospital completed daily feedback logs to evaluate the clinical experiences of the graduate nurses and plan opportunities to meet their learning needs. The researchers analyzed qualitative data from 299 logs to identify themes related to role transition. The transitional process from graduate to staff nurse was composed of balancing learning opportunities, having organizational abilities, and providing care for a larger number of patients. The dynamic interaction between the graduate and the preceptor was the context for experiencing "real nurse work." The graduate nurses described real nurse work as learning assessment, teaching, medication administration, and organizational skills necessary to survive as a staff nurse. Another theme was the guidance provided by the preceptor to the graduate learning the specific work systems of the assigned unit. The theme of interpersonal dynamics linked all the themes together.

IMPLICATIONS FOR PRACTICE

Graduate nurses are able to make a smoother transition to staff nurse when preceptors provide guidance, feedback, and learning opportunities. Preceptors need to be educated and supported to promote the role transition from student and graduate to staff nurse.

in a skilled care facility may have no accounting department to provide services such as a detailed analysis of the facility's expenditures. Each role has some support available. When a new position is being considered, it is important to evaluate whether support is available in areas in which a manager may lack knowledge or skill. When implementing changes in roles, the organization needs to develop support services to facilitate role transition. The two Research Perspectives describe the support needed by new graduates who are transitioning to the role of staff nurse.

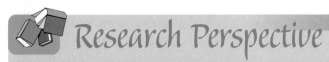
Research Perspective

Gerrish, K. (2000). Still fumbling along? A comparative study of the newly qualified nurse's perception of the transition from student to qualified nurse. *Journal of Advanced Nursing, 32*(2), 473-480.

The researcher interviewed newly qualified British nurses in 1985 and again in 1998. The transcripts from these interviews were submitted to grounded theory and constant comparative analyses. The purpose of the study was to examine the transitional perceptions of the 1998 sample of newly qualified nurses and to compare these perceptions with the 1985 sample. The major theme was "fumbling along," defined as the haphazard way in which nurses learned to perform their new role. They believed the reasons for this fumbling were inadequate educational preparation and transition support. The 1998 sample did feel their support was greater, but still viewed the transition as stressful because of their heightened awareness of their individual accountability. Assuming managerial responsibilities and performing technical skills were also perceived as stressful aspects of the role.

IMPLICATIONS FOR PRACTICE
Anticipatory guidance for graduate nurses needs to include preparation for transitioning to the role of staff nurse. The nurse who is equipped with active learning strategies will bridge more quickly to the new role. Preceptors and managers working with new nurses need to acknowledge the stressful transition and support nurses through the process.

Exercise 23-1
ROLES Assessment
Answer these questions for a position in management that you are considering.
Responsibilities
1. From the position description, what are the responsibilities?

2. For what decisions are you responsible?

3. Consider information about the management position that you learned during the interview (this may be role-played). Also consider the responsibilities of managers you have observed. Are there other responsibilities to add to your list?

Opportunities
4. What would you like to do differently from the previous manager?

5. How could your strengths or expertise benefit the people or nursing unit you would manage?

6. Dream a little (or a lot). If a person who had been a patient on the unit was describing the nursing care to another potential patient, what would you want the first patient to say? Describe the unit as you want it to be known.

Lines of Communication
7. Draw yourself in the middle of a separate piece of paper. Now fill in the people above you and below you with whom you would communicate. Draw lines from you to each person or group. On the line, identify the form of communication. For example, if you communicate with the director of nursing through a weekly report, write on the line, "Written report."

Expectations
8. This may be the most difficult part to assess. List in short sentences or phrases the expectations each person or group may have for you in relation to your management position.

SELF	FAMILY
ADMINISTRATION	IMMEDIATE SUPERVISOR

PEOPLE YOU WILL MANAGE

Now compare the lists. Place a star next to those expectations that are held by more than one person or group. For example, you want to handle the budget of the unit efficiently, an expectation shared with nursing administration. Circle those items that could cause conflicts. Read the strategies section in the chapter for ideas on how to resolve these conflicts.

Support

9. What people do you know in the organization who could provide information that you will need to do your job?

10. What departments provide services that you could access for assistance?

Save your responses to these questions to review in 3 months. You may be surprised how your own perception of your ROLES may change over time.

ROLE TRANSITION

Unlearning old roles while learning new roles requires an identity adjustment over time. The persons involved must invest themselves in the process. In this way, role transition can be compared with developing a relationship. The process of developing an intimate relationship with another person provides a familiar framework for considering role transition. Relationships typically move through the phases of dating, commitment, honeymoon, disillusionment, resolution, and maturity.

During the dating phase the interested persons spend structured time together. Both parties present their best characteristics and dedicate a lot of energy to developing the relationship. Although both parties present their best characteristics, both are also alert to clues that the other party cannot meet their expectations. For example, one may consider the financial and emotional resources that the other person would bring to the relationship. The individuals might spend time with each other's families to get a feel for the emotional climate in which the other person grew up.

Interviewing for a management position is similar to dating. An interview involves touring the unit, visiting with people, and attempting to make a good impression. The potential employer is also attempting to make a favorable impression. The interviewee wants to find out whether this is an organization that will support his or her growth as he or she supports the growth of the organization (Kerfoot, 2000). Questions are asked about the role of the manager, and the potential manager mentally evaluates whether the described role matches personal expectations about management. Both of these examples represent the phase "role preview."

Through the dating process, two people may decide that they want to spend the rest of their lives together and commit to the relationship. Sometimes, one or both of the people decide that they do not want to establish a long-term relationship. In a similar way, following the role preview of the interview process, both parties may agree to establish a relationship as employee and employer. Or one or more of the parties may decide not to establish the relationship. In dating, the public decision to leave other similar relationships and establish this new relationship represents a formal commitment. In role transition the formal commitment of the employment contract implies acceptance of the management role, or "role acceptance."

In new relationships a time of dating and commitment is usually followed by a honeymoon. More than a trip to a vacation spot, the honeymoon has become synonymous with excitement, happiness, and confidence. In a new work role, people also experience a honeymoon phase. The new graduate may be relieved the educational program was successfully completed and now a salary can be earned. When a new manager is hired, the employer is excited that the search is over. The staff is happy to have a leader, especially if staff members had input into the hiring decision. The new manager is happy, excited, and, most of all, confident in exploring the new roles involved in the management position.

Whether by a gradual process or as the result of a particular event that serves as the turning point, eventually the honeymoon is over and disillusionment about the relationship occurs. For example, one person may make an expensive purchase without consulting the partner. An argument is followed by a period of painful silence. Similarly, the honeymoon phase in a new employment position can be followed by a period of disillusionment.

Role discrepancy, a gap between **role expectations** and role performance, causes discomfort and frustration. Role discrepancy can be resolved by either dissolving the relationship or by changing expectations and performance. The importance of the relationship and the perceived differences between performance and expectations, the basis of role discrepancy, must be considered in light of personal values. When the relationship is valued and the differences are seen as correctable, the decision is made to stay in the relationship. This decision requires the couple or the manager to develop the role.

Choosing to change either role expectations or role performance or to change both is the process of

role development. In an intimate relationship, open communication can clarify expectations. Negotiation may result in reasonable expectations. Certain behaviors may be changed to improve role performance. For example, one person in the relationship learns to call home to let the other know about the possibility of being late.

To reduce role discrepancy in a new management position, the same open communication and negotiation must occur. Expectations need to be clarified and stipulated by both parties. New managers evaluate management styles and techniques to determine which ones best fit them and the situation. The personal management style evolves as the individuals develop the management roles in their own unique ways. If role discrepancy can be reduced and the role developed to be satisfactory to both parties, the new manager can focus on developing the roles of the position and proceed to the phase of **role internalization.**

Role internalization occurs in relationships as they mature. No longer do the persons in the relationship consciously consider their roles. They have learned the behaviors that maintain and nurture the relationship. The behaviors become second nature. The energy spent on establishing and developing the relationship can be redirected toward achieving mutual goals. In the same way, managers who have been in management positions for several years have internalized their roles. Most of the time they do not consciously consider their roles. Managers know they have reached the stage of role internalization when they focus on accomplishing mutual goals instead of contemplating whether their role performance matches their role expectations. Managers who have internalized their roles have developed their own unique personal style of management. Table 23-2 summarizes the comparison between the phases of developing an intimate relationship and the phases of role transition to a nurse manager.

UNEXPECTED ROLE TRANSITION

Not every relationship is successful. Some relationships end in an argument, divorce, or death. When a relationship ends unexpectedly, a person goes through a grieving process. In a similar way, when a person is fired, a position is eliminated, or a job description changes dramatically, the person may have to grieve before being able to engage in role transition. The manager has the role of supporting

---

Table 23-2 COMPARISON OF PHASES IN DEVELOPING AN INTIMATE RELATIONSHIP AND IN UNDERGOING ROLE TRANSITION AS A NURSE MANAGER

Phase in Developing an Intimate Relationship	Phase in Role Transition as a Nurse Manager	Characteristics of Phase
Dating	Role preview	Presentation of best characteristics to make favorable impression; both parties evaluate each other to determine likelihood of the other being able to fulfill one's expectations
Commitment to relationship	Role acceptance	Public announcement of mutual decision to initiate contract
Honeymoon	Role exploration	Experience of excitement, confidence, and mutual appreciation
Disillusionment	Role discrepancy	Awareness of difference between role expectations and role performance; reconsideration of whether to continue with contract
Resolution	Role development	Negotiation of role expectations; adjustment of role performance to approximate expectations and to find own unique style
Maturation of relationship	Role internalization	Performance of role congruent with own beliefs and individual style; achievement of mutual goals

others through the trauma and transformation that accompany transitions (Porter-O'Grady, 1999). To be successful, workplace restructuring must be undertaken with the same sensitivity afforded a person who has lost a relationship through death or divorce. Role transition takes time, even in reverse.

The initial response to a change in role can be shock and disbelief. The person may feel numb and unable to function. As the numbness wears off, the person may become angry. The anger fuels resistance to the change and may be directed toward those who initiated the role change. The anger may be directed internally, leading to depression. If the person is unable to acknowledge and talk about the loss, the period of grief may be extended or emotional baggage may be created that is carried into the next role. Grieving can eventually resolve in acceptance. Lessons learned from the experience are identified and internalized. A new role is sought, and the "dating" begins again.

When a relationship is dissolved in the case of death or divorce, a legal document is prepared to formally dissolve the financial and social obligations between the persons involved. The loss of a position as a result of restructuring or a buyout should involve a similar process. The employer may offer the nurse a severance package that includes financial compensation and outplacement services. If the employer does not offer a written agreement, the nurse should formally request and negotiate reasonable compensation and assistance. Similar to signing a prenuptial agreement, a nurse may have signed a contract with the employer when hired. The terms of that agreement may require the employer to buy out (pay the salary and benefits) for the time remaining on the contract.

STRATEGIES TO PROMOTE ROLE TRANSITION

Becoming a manager or assuming a new role requires a transformation—a profound change in identity. Such a transformation invokes stress as the person unlearns old roles and learns the management role. Several strategies can be helpful in easing the strain and speeding the process of role transition (Box 23-2).

Internal Resources

A key strategy in promoting role transition is to recognize, use, and strengthen the internal resources of commitment, character, self-respect, and flexibility. Work commitment is a function of the fit between the role and the person's professional goals and commitments in other areas of life, such as family or church.

The role of manager is not for everyone. One must consider whether personal goals and professional fulfillment can best be achieved through management. One's commitment to the challenges of managing can provide the desire to persevere during the process of role transition.

Another internal resource is character. Character is the essence of the person—the values, beliefs, and habits of a person. Centering one's character on correct principles creates power to realize dreams (Covey, 1990). Persons whose characters are based on principles continue to be educated by their experiences and are service-oriented. Principle-centered people believe in others, creating a climate that promotes growth and opportunity. A manager with a principle-centered character can be trusted. A person with character can maintain grace even in difficult, stressful circumstances (Kerfoot, 1999a).

Closely related to character is another internal resource—self-respect. Self-respect allows managers to weather the difficult times when there may be little external recognition. A person's value does not depend on the quality or quickness of the adjustment to the management role. Knowing what you believe in is especially important during a transition period. Writing down short statements of belief or self-affirmations and posting this information may be helpful as a visual reminder.

Flexibility is needed as you adjust to a new role in an environment of accelerating change (Kerfoot, 1999a). Survival as a leader demands that you be able to learn and master new skills, translate information for staff, adapt your role to the needs of the situation, and be open to innovation (Kerfoot, 1999b).

BOX 23-2

Strategies to Promote Role Transition

- Strengthen internal resources
- Assess the organization's resources, culture, and group dynamics
- Negotiate the role
- Grow with a mentor
- Develop management knowledge and skills

Organizational Assessment

A new manager is much like an immigrant in a new country. An immigrant learns how to access the available resources to acclimate to the new environment. Cultural practices of the new country may seem strange or odd. Such differences can be analyzed and decisions made about which aspects to incorporate into one's own culture. More subtle differences in communication patterns or group dynamics can also be identified. Understanding the nuances of social interactions is often the most difficult aspect of acclimating to a new country. The transition is smoother for the immigrant who understands himself or herself, assesses the new environment, and learns how to communicate within groups.

The new manager must also learn how to access resources in the organization. Approaching the organization as a foreign culture, the new manager can keenly observe the rituals, accepted practices, and patterns of communication within the organization. This ongoing assessment promotes a speedier transition into the role of manager. The immigrant who spends energy bemoaning the difficulties of the new country may fail to enjoy the advantages that drew the individual to the country in the first place. In the same way, the manager who focuses on the weaknesses of the organization may lack the energy to internalize the new role, a step that is critical to being an effective leader.

Role Negotiation

A strategy that is helpful during conflicting role expectations is **role negotiation.** The ROLES assessment (see Box 23-1) may have identified areas of significant conflict. Writing the expectations down provides the first step in resolving areas of conflict. It is important to review the expectations listed to determine whether they are realistic. Unrealistic expectations strongly held by others may require diplomatic reeducation so that their expectations can become more realistic.

The priority of different role expectations may also require role negotiation with the person above you in the line of command. Ask for input as to which expectations have the highest priorities. Explain personal and family expectations and clearly state the priority that meeting those expectations has. The process may have to be repeated several times before agreement on the expectations related to roles and the priority of each expectation is found. Rewriting the unrealistic expectations to be achievable can reduce three common sources of role stress—ambiguity, overload, and conflict. For example, patient care vice presidents in a newly merged healthcare system met over 14 months to clarify their roles. The change in structure required role changes, which they worked together to clarify (Formella & Bahner, 1999).

Mentors

In Greek mythology, Mentor was an advisor and counselor (Parsloe, 1992). The word **mentor** refers to a more experienced person who helps a less experienced person navigate the world. Mentors are often experts in their field who provide guidance to new members of the profession (Meigs, 1999). Mentors are an important component of a nurturing environment that promotes staff retention.

Mentors can be a tremendous source of guidance and support for staff nurses and managers, serving both career functions and psychosocial functions (Box 23-3). Career functions are possible because the mentor has sufficient professional experience and organizational authority to facilitate the career of the "mentee." Psychosocial functions are possible because of a connection between the mentor and mentee (Olson, 1999/2000). Modeling desirable behaviors, the mentor allows the mentee to learn through observation (Murray, 1999).

Sponsorship involves volunteering or nominating the mentee for additional responsibilities. A mentor can be a sponsor by creating opportunities for individual achievement and providing encouragement (Olson, 1999/2000). The mentor may suggest the mentee be appointed to a key nursing committee or volunteer for a special assignment. Sponsorship leads to exposure or opportunities for the mentee to build

---

BOX 23-3

Functions of a Mentor

Career functions	Sponsorship
	Exposure/protection
	Coaching
	Challenging assignments
Psychosocial functions	Role modeling
	Mutual positive regard
	Counseling
	Social interaction

Modified from Kram, K. E. (1985). *Mentoring at work: Development relationships in organizational life.* Glenview, IL: Scott, Foresman.

a reputation of competence. With exposure, the mentor provides protection by absorbing negative feedback, sharing responsibility for controversial decisions, and teaching the unwritten rules about "how things are done around here." These unwritten rules may be more important to job success than the written rules.

Coaches provide information about how to improve performance, including feedback on current performance. Coaching requires frequent contact and willingness on the part of the mentee to accept feedback. Challenging assignments are given to the mentee that will stretch the limits of knowledge and skill. The mentor helps the mentee learn the technical and management skills necessary to accomplish the task, such as which numbers on the budget printout are added to achieve the total expenditures.

The interpersonal relationship between the mentor and the mentee involves mutual positive regard. Because the mentee respects the career accomplishments of the mentor, the mentee identifies with the mentor's example. This role modeling is both conscious and unconscious. The mentee with character and self-respect will evaluate the behaviors of the mentor and select those behaviors worthy of being emulated.

Counseling, as another psychosocial function of the mentor, allows the mentee to explore personal concerns. Confidentiality is a prerequisite to sharing personal information. Because the opinion of the mentor is respected, the mentor may provide guidance to the mentee. The best mentors can provide guidance while recognizing that the mentee may choose to disregard the advice.

Being mentored is a learning process. Admiration for a mentor and a recognition of the mentor's commitment to self-success can provide an environment of trust in which a mentor-mentee relationship begins. Both persons develop positive expectations of the relationship, and both take the initiative to nurture the new relationship. A mentee needs to be open to receiving support and guidance so that the mentor can stimulate problem solving by asking challenging questions (Murray, 1999). As more of the mentor functions are experienced, the bond between the mentor and mentee grows stronger.

Relationships between mentors and mentees vary because of individual characteristics and the career phase of each. During the early phases of a career, a nurse manager is concerned about competence and a mentor can provide valuable coaching.

As the nurse manager develops, sponsorship by a mentor can prepare the manager for a promotion. A mentor nearing the end of the work career can find fulfillment in sharing knowledge with new managers and at the same time benefit from the counsel of a recently retired colleague.

Management Education

Management performance can be hindered by a specific knowledge deficit. For example, the manager may lack business skills or knowledge about legal aspects of supervision. Most healthcare organizations have little or no management orientation. Instead of depending on others for management development, a manager should identify areas where competence will require new information and actively pursue acquiring this information through educational programs, workshops, books, professional journals, and electronic sources. Graduate education in nursing administration or business is a valuable professional investment. Membership in the American Organization of Nurse Executives is another avenue for networking with more experienced managers and learning through continuing education programs.

Experience and education provide a firm basis for seeking additional credentials. A nursing administrator with a baccalaureate degree and 24 months of experience at a middle management level can take an examination to become a certified nursing administrator. Nursing administrators with master's degrees and experience at the executive level can take an examination to become a certified nursing administrator, advanced. The website of the

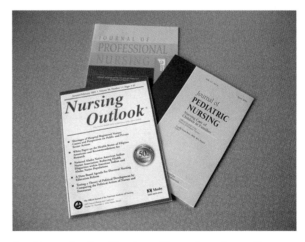

Reading professional books and journals and attending conferences are effective management education strategies.

American Nurses Credentialing Center has more detailed information about certification examinations (http://www.nursingworld.org/ancc).

FROM ROLE TRANSITION TO ROLE TRIUMPH

Developing an intimate relationship can be a difficult process, but most people still value relationships enough to make the effort. Making the transition and transformation into a management role is also worth the effort. Leading lives of integrity and commitment, nurse managers set examples, bringing out the best in staff nurses and thereby multiplying their influence on quality patient care.

■ *Exercise 23—2*
Self-Assessment
Respond to each item using the scale. Add up your score.

1 = Strongly disagree
2 = Disagree
3 = Unsure
4 = Agree
5 = Strongly agree

1. I am responsible for my own professional development.
2. I feel confident about my ability to learn the skills I need to be an effective manager.
3. I am able to balance multiple priorities and activities.
4. I have a strong psychological desire to influence others.
5. I can develop a personal network of support.

There is no magical score that indicates your readiness for management. If you are unsure in every category, your score will be 15. A score of 20 or above indicates that you are confident you can master the management role. If you currently have a mentor, ask that person to respond to each item to analyze your abilities. Compare those responses with your own. Do you have a realistic view of yourself?

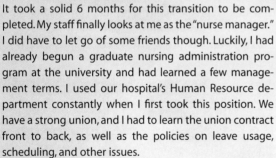

The Solution

It took a solid 6 months for this transition to be completed. My staff finally looks at me as the "nurse manager." I did have to let go of some friends though. Luckily, I had already begun a graduate nursing administration program at the university and had learned a few management terms. I used our hospital's Human Resource department constantly when I first took this position. We have a strong union, and I had to learn the union contract front to back, as well as the policies on leave usage, scheduling, and other issues.

I have always loved providing care for our sick veterans, and it was so difficult to give that up. Even now when the code pager goes off, it is difficult not to run. To balance this, I wear scrubs once a week and work side by side with my staff. It reminds me of what their day is like and keeps up my competencies, and I love it.

I also had two role models who I relied on heavily. One was the former nurse manager of the ICU, who took the nursing operations coordinator position. She showed me how to conduct the "official" business of running a unit. My mentor is the nurse manager of the operating room.

She taught me how to run the ICU while "loving" my staff. I go to her when I have a difficult day, and she reminds me just how great my staff is (I already know that I am lucky to have them) and how much I have grown and where I am headed. I always feel better when I talk with her. She has taught me how to deal with difficult physicians, and we are allies. She has been my lifesaver this first year.

Taking this management position has been a life-changing experience for me. Now that I have adjusted to the role, what I enjoy most is the work I do with new graduates. I like taking young graduate nurses into the internship I created for the ICU and watching them grow into fully functioning ICU nurses. I was told it was not a good idea to take new graduates into the unit, but I have been so pleased. They are our future and it is so exciting to watch their enthusiasm and growth!

— Robin E. Keene

 Would this be a suitable approach for you? Why?

CHAPTER CHECKLIST

Role transition is a process that takes time and energy—two scarce resources for nurse managers. Knowing what to expect and how to facilitate the process can speed role transition and minimize the expenditure of energy as the nurse manager negotiates new roles.

- Responsibilities, opportunities, lines of communication, expectations, and support are aspects common to all roles. When considering a management role, gather information about each of these aspects.
- Managers are also leaders and followers.
- Role transition is a process of unlearning old roles and learning new roles.
- The phases of role transition are as follows:
  - Role preview
  - Role acceptance
  - Role exploration
  - Role discrepancy
  - Role development
  - Role internalization
- Unexpected role transitions involve a grieving process. Financial and social obligations of the manager and the employer may need to be formally dissolved with appropriate compensation and outplacement services.
- The phase of role preview is similar to dating in that both parties present their best characteristics to make a favorable impression.
- Commitment to a relationship is analogous to role acceptance, a public announcement of a mutual decision to initiate a contract.
- Role exploration is similar to the honeymoon phase of an intimate relationship.
- Role discrepancy has its roots in the disillusionment experienced when role expectations do not match role performance.

- Role development is a time of resolution, when role expectations are negotiated and performance is adjusted to approximate expectations.
- A maturing relationship is similar to role internalization; during role internalization the performance of the role is congruent with one's own beliefs.
- Commitment, character, self-respect, and flexibility are internal resources that can facilitate the process of role transition.
- Role negotiation involves communicating with your supervisor to come to an agreement as to role expectations.
- Mentors can provide career and psychosocial functions enhancing the career development of the manager.
- Educational programs provide information needed by nurses to fulfill management roles.

TIPS IN ROLE TRANSITIONING

- Role transition is a normal process. Anticipate and prepare for role changes.
- Identify the responsibilities, opportunities, lines of communication, expectations, and support for the role.
- Use your internal resources to negotiate a role consistent with your values and life commitments.

TERMS TO KNOW

mentor	role negotiation
role development	ROLES
role discrepancy	role strain
role expectations	role stress
role internalization	role transition

REFERENCES

Antrobus, S., & Kitson, A. (1999). Nursing leadership: Influencing and shaping health and nursing practice. *Journal of Advanced Nursing, 29*(3), 746-753.

Conley, S., & Woosley, S. A. (2000). Teacher role stress, higher order needs, and work outcomes. *Journal of Educational Administration, 38*(2), 179-201.

Covey, S. R. (1990). *Principle-centered leadership.* New York: Simon & Schuster.

Dixon, D. L. (1999). Achieving results through transformational leadership. *Journal of Nursing Administration, 29*(12), 17-21.

Flaherty, T. B., Dahlstrom, R., & Skinner, S. J. (1999). Organizational values and role stress as determinants of customer-oriented selling performance. *Journal of Personal Selling & Sales Management, 19*(2), 1-18.

Formella, N. M., & Bahner, J. (1999). Role transition for patient care vice presidents: From a single entity to a system focus. *Journal of Nursing Administration, 29*(4), 11-17.

Fralic, M. A. (2000). What is leadership? *Journal of Nursing Administration, 30*(7/8), 340-341.

Gerrish, K. (2000). Still fumbling along? A comparative study of the newly qualified nurse's perception of the transition from student to qualified nurse. *Journal of Advanced Nursing, 32*(2), 473-480.

Godinez, G., Schweiger, J., Gruver, J., & Ryan, P. (1999). Role transition from graduate to staff nurse: A qualitative analysis. *Journal for Nurses in Staff Development, 15*(3), 97-110.

Hardy, M. E. (1978). Role stress and role strain. In M. E. Hardy & M. E. Conway (Eds.), *Role theory: Perspectives for health professionals.* New York: Appleton-Century-Crofts.

Henry, B. (2000). Leadership is about quality, cost, access, and morale. *Journal of Advanced Nursing, 31*(6), 1275-1276.

Jost, S. G. (2000). An assessment and intervention strategy for managing staff needs during change. *Journal of Nursing Administration, 30*(1), 34-40.

Kerfoot, K. (1999a). The art of leading with grace. *Dermatology Nursing, 11*(3), 222-223.

Kerfoot, K. (1999b). The new millennium and leadership: Evolution and entropy? *Dermatology Nursing, 11*(6), 459-460.

Kerfoot, K. (2000). Leadership: Creating a shared destiny. *Dermatology Nursing, 12*(5), 363-364.

Kram, K. E. (1985). *Mentoring at work: Development relationships in organizational life.* Glenview, IL: Scott, Foresman.

Meigs, J. (1999). Mentoring: Building nursing's future now. *AWHONN Lifelines, 3*(1), 55-56.

Mick, D. J., & Ackerman, M. H. (2000). Advanced practice nursing role delineation in acute and clinical care: Application of the strong model of advanced practice. *Heart & Lung: Journal of Acute & Critical Care, 29*(3), 210-221.

Murray, T. A. (1999). Implications for staff development of perceived self efficacy in nurses who changed to home care practice. *Journal for Nurses in Staff Development, 15*(2), 78-82.

Olson, K. (1999/2000). Time spent in a mentor's garden: Sowing the seeds of promise and future in nursing. *AWHONN Lifelines, 3*(6), 10.

Parsloe, E. (1992). *Coaching, mentoring, and assessing.* London: Kogan Page Limited.

Porter-O'Grady, T. (1999). Quantum leadership: New roles for a new age. *Journal of Nursing Administration, 29*(10), 37-42.

Vargo, N. (2000). Empowering leadership. *Dermatology Nursing, 12*(2), 81, 123.

SUGGESTED READINGS

Campbell, P. T., & Rudisill, P. T. (1999). Nursing in the new millennium: Leadership skills for surviving and thriving. *AWHONN Lifelines, 3*(5), 56-58.

Glen, S. (1998). Role transition from staff nurse to clinical nurse specialist: A case study. *Journal of Clinical Nursing, 7*(3), 283-290.

Morgenstern, J. (2000). *Time management from the inside out.* New York: Henry Holt.

Winter-Collins, A., & McDaniel, A. (2000). Sense of belonging and new graduate job satisfaction. *Journal of Nurses in Staff Development, 16*(3), 103-111.

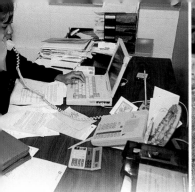
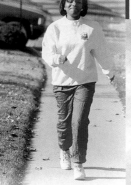

Chapter

24

Self-Management: Stress and Time

Amy C. Pettigrew

This chapter examines the concept of self-management—the ability of individuals to manage themselves. Four components of self-management are explored: stress management, time management, meeting management, and delegation. Methods for managing stress and organizing one's time are introduced. Practical exercises and suggestions for stress and time management are presented that can be used for personal and professional situations to reduce stress and enhance efficiency.

Objectives

- Define self-management.
- Explore personal and professional stressors.
- Analyze selected strategies to decrease stress.
- Assess the manager's role in helping staff to manage stress.
- Evaluate common barriers to effective time management.

- Critique the strengths and weaknesses of selected time management strategies.

- Evaluate selected strategies to manage time more effectively.

Questions to Consider

- Are you currently using self-management strategies?
- What types of activities cause stress for you?
- Can you identify ways to handle stress more effectively?
- What are your highest-priority personal and professional goals?
- Does the way you spend your time reflect your priorities?
- Are you drowning in information and paperwork?
- How does a nurse manager successfully use time to attain work goals?

The Challenge

Kathleen Slat, RN, BSN, LMT
Staff Nurse, Mercy Hospital Fairfield, MSN student at the University of Cincinnati, Cincinnati, Ohio

After a devastating divorce, I made the decision to return to school and start a new career. I knew that I did not want to stop at an entry-level position and needed to make long-range plans for my future. I planned on continuing until I reached the educational and professional level that I wanted. I also had to work to support myself financially during this time. I realized that I would have to plan very carefully, make many changes in my life, and not lose sight of my goal.

What do you think you would do if you were this nurse?

INTRODUCTION

How many times have you gone to bed at night feeling guilty about not having accomplished anything during the day? How many times have you stopped to wonder what you really want to be when you grow up? **Self-management** is about deciding what you want for your personal and professional self, setting life goals, developing objectives and short-term outcomes to reach the goals, and finally organizing the time and activities you undertake to reach them. Self-management is also about finding a balance among and between career, family, social activities, and self. Drucker (2000) suggests that understanding one's own strengths, articulating personal values, and knowing where one's self belongs are also important components of self-management.

To find this balance within ourselves, we must actively engage in taking control of our lives—no one else is going to! The two key strategies introduced in this chapter—stress management and **time management**—constantly interplay with our life goals. We can move in a straight line toward our personal and professional goals if stress or distractions do not interfere. When stress becomes overwhelming or others rob us of our time, the path suddenly becomes unclear. Time and stress are somewhat of a "chicken and egg" phenomenon—not enough time creates stress, and stress can erode efficiency and thus decrease time on task. The key lies in our ability to manage both time and stress, not only personally but also professionally. The outcome of self-management is the ability to accomplish one's high-priority professional and personal goals.

MANAGEMENT OF STRESS

Nurses have learned about the effect of stress on patients and how to manage its consequences. Nurses also need to recognize the stressors in their own lives. Everyone experiences stress—the exhilaration of a joyous event and the negative feelings and unpleasant physical symptoms that may be associated with a difficult life situation or even the anticipation of difficulty. Nurses are not immune to the effects of stress. Learning what stress is, its dynamics, and some strategies to manage the distress should be part of the personal and professional maturation of nurses.

Definition

In this chapter *stress* and *distress* are used interchangeably, although some writers regard stress as neutral and refer to the positive and negative attributes of eustress and distress, respectively. Stress management does not necessarily mean stress reduction. Rather, stress management is finding the right mix of stress and distress.

SOURCES OF JOB STRESS

Job stress is pandemic. Smith (2000) reports that approximately 20% of a random sample of 17,000 British citizens reported that they had high or extremely high levels of stress at work. Fischer, Calame, Deetling, Zeier, and Fanconi (2000) report that stress-related cortisol surges occur frequently in neonatal and pediatric critical care staff and are independent of the subjective stress perception. Professional experience did not decrease the endocrine reaction to stress. As more is learned about

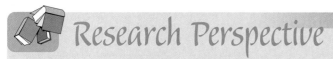
Research Perspective

Maurier, W., & Northcutt, H. (2000). Job uncertainty and health status for nurses during restructuring of health care in Alberta. *Western Journal of Nursing Research, 22*(5), 623-641.

This study examined the relationship between job uncertainty, working conditions, cognitive appraisal, and coping strategies and the health of nurses during a period of healthcare restructuring. A sample of 271 registered nurses working in a large urban hospital completed self-administered questionnaires. The study found that high levels of threat (being placed on recall, having co-workers lose their positions, and perceiving job insecurity) were associated with high levels of depression and poor physical health.

IMPLICATIONS FOR PRACTICE
The uncertainty and layoffs affected not only those nurses who have left but also those nurses left behind. Fewer co-workers may mean more work for fewer nurses. Working conditions such as understaffing can result in poor health for the remaining nurses. Even the cognitive appraisal of job insecurity can result in depression and poorer health status.

the relationship of stress to physiological changes, stressors will become even easier to identify. When one looks at job-related stressors, the stressors fall into one of two categories: external and internal.

External Sources

Occupational stress in nursing has been well defined and documented. Work-related stressors such as workload, rotating shifts, high patient acuity, ethical conflicts, dealing with death and acute illness, role ambiguity, and job insecurity have all been associated with increased stress and **burnout** (Maurier & Northcutt, 2000) (see Research Perspective).

Change

Restructuring, rightsizing, workforce redesign, and similar terms encapsulated the dramatic shift in healthcare practices, management, and values in the 1990s. Nurses, as well as other healthcare providers, are still recovering from the effects of changes in healthcare financing and care delivery systems. Although the distress that results from change takes many forms, two underlying patterns appear to be constant. First, nurses feel trapped by conflicting expectations. They expect to furnish care, to meet patients' needs, and to be nurturing. However, organizations require nurses to be managers of patient care and of systems and value their contribution to efficiency and cost-effectiveness while simultaneously preserving quality of care. Because nurses cannot comply with both expectations, they experience considerable role conflict, frustration, and distress.

Second, the rapid required changes in work design implemented in the 1990s were changes made by managers, often with little input from the nursing staff. Loss of autonomy, together with increases in rules and regulations, resulted in distress for nurses and for other clinicians. They felt powerless and devalued. Nurses in some institutions have become empowered by models of shared governance. However, the processes necessary to develop such models are stressful in and of themselves, and many nurses still find themselves in systems where they have little input to change processes.

Social

Interpersonal relations can buffer stressors or can become stressors. Outside the work setting, home can be a refuge for harried nurses; however, stresses at home, when severe, can impair work performance and relationships among staff or even result in violence that may invade the workplace.

Changes in healthcare delivery systems, as well as the current nursing shortage, have reduced the number of professional nurses to a minimum. Consequently, some nurses lose supportive, collegial relationships that may have been established over many years. Many institutions now depend on supplemental staffing with agency or "traveling" nurses, thus creating a very transient nursing staff. In other situations, nurses are reassigned or they "float" to various patient care units, which requires that they work with unfamiliar staff. Thus they may feel isolated or become unwillingly involved in dysfunctional politics on the unit. Such situations may also necessitate that nurses work with patients whose requirements for care may be unfamiliar, resulting in further stress related to patient safety concerns.

Persons in corporate-level positions may also become stressors. Communication may come from the top down, with little opportunity for nurses to participate in decisions that affect them directly or that they may need to implement without proper training or support. Nurses may experience distress from feelings of frustration and helplessness with this lack of opportunity for input to decisions.

The Position

Most nurses expect that caring for patients who are chronically or critically ill and for families who have experienced tragedy will be stressful. The current environment in many healthcare agencies, however, is more complex and is often characterized by **overwork,** as well as by the stresses inherent in nursing practice.

According the to American Nurses Association (2000), many healthcare organizations, in the midst of a nursing shortage and steadily increasing acuity levels, have become dependent on the use of mandated overtime to solve staffing problems. Nurses are expected to stay for extra shifts with little or no notice, with managers using threats of dismissal or peer pressure to ensure cooperation. Nurses, aware of and concerned about inadequate staffing, are resentful that they are now carrying the stress and burden of the staffing problems that resulted from earlier changes in skill mix and care delivery models.

Additional Roles

The vast majority of nurses are women and many go home to gender-related responsibilities that may include household management, children, and aging parents. When added to the already stressful workday of the nurse, the additional responsibilities often contribute to the level of distress felt by the nurse. Erdwins, Buffardi, Casper, and O'Brien (2001) report that effectiveness in work role is directly related to a woman's perception of fewer conflicts between work and home. They also report that the less support a woman perceives from her spouse and her direct supervisor, the more she is likely to experience work/family conflict and role strain. Kirkcaldy and Martin (2000) also found that nursing professionals perceive the home/work conflict a major stressor. Home/work conflict was a significant predictor of decreased work satisfaction,

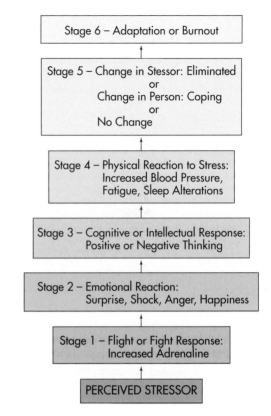

Figure 24-1 The stress diagram. (Modified from Selye, H. [1991]. History and present status of the stress concept. In A. Monat & R. Lazarus [Eds.], *Stress and coping: An anthology* [pp. 21-36]. New York: Columbia University Press.)

physical health, and mental health. Age was significantly related to total stress, with older nurses reporting additional family commitments and domestic responsibility.

Internal Sources

Lifestyle choices such as the use of caffeine, lack of exercise, poor diet, and cigarette smoking have a direct effect on increasing stress. Personality traits such as perfectionism and the workaholic trait place additional stressful demands on an individual. Another internal source of stress can be negative self-talk, such as pessimistic thinking; self-criticism; and overanalysis of situations.

Dynamics of Stress

Stress may be the consequence of unrealistic or conflicting expectations, the pace and magnitude of change, human behavior, individual personality characteristics, the characteristics of the position itself, or the culture of the organization. Other stres-

Theory Box

THEORIES APPLICABLE TO SELF-MANAGEMENT

KEY CONTRIBUTORS	KEY IDEAS	APPLICATION TO PRACTICE
General adaptation syndrome. Selye (1956) is credited with developing this theory.	The "stress response" is an adrenocortical reaction to stressors that is accompanied by psychological changes and physiological alterations that follow a pattern of fight or flight. The general adaptation syndrome includes an alarm, resistance, and adaptation or exhaustion.	Change, lack of control, and excessive workload are common stressors that evoke psychological and physiological distress among nurses.
The Pareto principle Hafner, A. W. (2001)	The "Pareto principle" refers to a universal observation of "vital few, trivial many." Pareto (1848-1923) studied distribution of personal incomes in Italy and observed that 80% of the wealth was controlled by 20% of the population. This concept of disproportion often holds in many areas. Although the exact values of 20 and 80 are not significant, the observation of considerable disproportion is important to remember.	The 80-20 rule can be applied to many aspects of healthcare today. For example, 80% of healthcare expenditures are on 20% of the population, and 80% of personnel problems come from 20% of the staff. In quality improvement, 80% of improvement can be expected by removing 20% of the causes of unacceptable quality or performance. A nurse can also expect that 80% of patient care time will be spent working with 20% of her patient assignment.

sors may be unique to certain environments, situations, and persons or groups. Initially, increased stress produces increased performance. However, once peak performance has been reached, additional stress results in decreased performance (Epstein, 2000).

Although some stress may be motivating and make employees more effective (eustress), distress is more often a problem that results in decreased position performance, unpleasant feelings, and illness (Rabin, 1999). Hans Selye's midcentury investigations of the nature of and reactions to stress have been very influential. In his classic theory, Selye (1991) described the concept of stress, identified the **general adaptation syndrome (GAS)** and detailed a predictable pattern of response (Figure 24-1 and the Theory box). More recent investigations of the relationship among the brain, the immune system, and health have found that psychological and physical stressors do indeed alter both humoral and immune function. Stress has also been associated with the deterioration of immune-related health out-

comes, including decreased host resistance to infection and the development or exacerbation of autoimmune disorders (Cohen & Manuck, 1999).

Most nurses can easily recognize the origins of stress and its symptoms. For example, a healthcare agency may make demands on nurses, such as excessive work, that the nurses regard as beyond their capacity to perform. When they are unable to resolve the problem through overwork, with more staff, or by looking at the situation in another way, the nurses may feel threatened or depressed. They may also experience headache, fatigue, or other physical symptoms. If the stress persists, such symptoms may increase; nurses may attempt to cope by becoming apathetic or by resigning their positions. Table 24-1 gives physical, mental, and spiritual/emotional signs of overstress in individuals.

Managing Stress

Individuals respond to stress by eliciting **coping** strategies that are a means of dealing with stress to maintain or achieve well-being. These strategies

Table 24–1 SIGNS OF OVERSTRESS IN INDIVIDUALS

Physical	Mental	Spiritual/Emotional
Physical signs of ill health:	Dread going to work every day	Sense of being a failure; disappointed in work performance

a. Increase in flu, colds, accidents
  b. Change in sleeping habits
  c. Fatigue
	Rigid thinking and a desire to go by all the rules in all cases; inability to tolerate any changes	Anger and resentment toward patients, colleagues, and managers; overall irritable attitude

Chronic signs of decreased ability to manage stress:	Forgetfulness and anxiety about work to be done; more frequent errors and incidents	Lack of positive feelings toward others

a. Headaches
  b. Hypertension
  c. Backaches
  d. Gastrointestinal problems
	Returning home exhausted and unable to participate in enjoyable activities	Cynicism toward patients, blaming them for their problems

Use of unhealthy coping activities:	Confusion about duties and roles	Excessive worry; insecurity; lowered self-esteem
a. Increased use of drugs and alcohol b. Increased weight		Increased family and friend conflict

may be ineffective and rely on methods such as withdrawal or substance abuse, or they may be effective in helping restore a greater sense of well-being and effectiveness. Some of these strategies are discussed here.

Primary Prevention

One effective way to deal with stress is to determine and eliminate its source. Discovering the origin of stress in patient care may be difficult because some environments have changed so rapidly that the nursing staff is overwhelmed trying to balance bureaucratic rules and limited resources with the demands of vulnerable human beings. In their distress, nurses may need to step back and look at the "big picture." By identifying daily stressors, the nurse can then develop a plan of action for management of the stress. This plan may include elimination of the stressor, modification of the stressor, or changing perceptions of the stressor (e.g., viewing mistakes as opportunities for new learning). Analyze your stress experiences by completing Exercise 24-1.

■ *Exercise 24-1*

Evaluation of Experienced Stress
Identify what stress you experience and how you usually manage it. Create and complete the following log at the end of every day for 1 week. Review the log and note what situ-

ations (e.g., people, technology, value conflict) were the most common. Also identify how you most often react to stress: physically, mentally, and emotionally/spiritually. Keeping this diary for a week is helpful to determine what causes you stress and learn about your reactions.
DATE _____
SITUATION _____
YOUR RESPONSE _____
ACTION _____
EVALUATION _____

Secondary Prevention

Unpredictable and uncontrollable changes, together with immense responsibility and little control over the work environment, produce stress for nurses and other healthcare professionals. Consequently, nurses may develop emotional symptoms such as anxiety, depression, or anger; physical alterations such as fatigue, headache, and insomnia; mental changes such as a decrease in concentration and memory; and behavioral changes such as smoking, drinking, crying, and swearing. The important factor is not the stressor, but rather how the individual perceives the stressor and what coping mechanisms are available to mediate the hormonal response to the stressor. This perception of the stressor is modulated by the baseline physiology of the individual and by earlier life experiences with stress (Rabin, 1999).

Multiple "stress-buffering" behaviors can be elicited to reduce the detrimental effects of stress. The stressor-induced changes in the hormonal and immune systems can be modulated by an individual's behavioral coping responses. These coping responses include positive social support, a strong belief system, a sense of humor, exercise, and use of the relaxation response.

Meditation to elicit the relaxation response can be beneficial. The benefits of practicing relaxation techniques for 20 minutes daily include a feeling of well-being, the ability to learn how tension makes the body feel, and the sense that tension can be controlled. In cases of some stress-related disorders (e.g., hypertension), biofeedback may be used to monitor physiological relaxation processes. This technique enables some individuals to better relax and to gain control over selected physiological processes (Kuhn, 1999). Exercise 24-2 outlines one systematic relaxation technique.

Exercise 24–2

Relaxation Response

This exercise can be used in the middle of a working day, the last thing at night, or at any time you feel tense or anxious.

1. Find a place away from interruption for 10 minutes.
2. Loosen tight clothes; lie on the floor, a mat, a towel, or a couch, if possible. Close your eyes, and let your body go slack.
3. Starting from the top of your body, work steadily through all your muscles, tightening and then relaxing them.
4. Lift up your head and pull it forward as far as you can, then let it fall back gently.
5. Continuing downward, press your shoulders down hard, then slowly relax them.
6. Open your fingers wide, stretch your arms out to your side, and hold them as tight and hard as you can. Then slowly let them go.
7. With your arms lying at your side, tighten your abdominal muscles as hard as you can, then relax them.
8. Lift your buttocks, tightening them as they go, and then gently let them fall back. Relax the buttocks and spine muscles, thinking consciously of the areas you are working on.
9. Do a mental check to make sure other muscles have not tightened up. Put your heels together and stretch your legs and toes as far as you can, then slowly relax them.
10. Turn on your side and lie that way for 2 to 3 minutes. Sit up slowly and recognize how you are feeling; try to keep that feeling as you go back to your activities.

(Modified from Wilson [1990].)

Social support, in the form of positive work relationships, as well as nurturing family and friends, may be an important way to buffer the negative effects of a stressful work environment (Erdwins et al., 2001). Although friendships may be formed with colleagues, the workload and the shifting of staff from one unit to another often make it difficult to establish and maintain close relationships with peers. However, managers and co-workers who are supportive may improve morale in the workplace (Erdwins et al., 2001). Nurses in a new position or in an unfamiliar geographic area must anticipate that they will benefit from the security of being part of a group that can furnish emotional support. Without easily accessible family and friends, nurses need to be intentional about seeking new, supportive personal relationships. Such efforts may help nurses cope with workplace demands that seem to exceed their capabilities. Positive coping strategies may also make nurses less likely to adopt such potentially negative coping strategies as withdrawal, lowering their standards of care, and abusing alcohol or other substances.

Tertiary Prevention

Sometimes individuals are unable to manage stress successfully through their own efforts and require assistance. Examples of behavior related to stress that feels overwhelming are found in Table 24-1. Coping strategies, such as those described previously, may furnish temporary relief or none at all. With this level of distress, one can feel overwhelmed or helpless and may be at greater risk for mental or physical illness. This constellation of emotions is commonly called *burnout*.

Burnout has been defined as a "prolonged response to chronic emotional and interpersonal stressors on the job" (Maslach, Schaufeli, & Leiter, 2000, p. 398). The sources of the stressors may exist in the environment, in the individual, or in the interaction between the individual and the environment. Some stressors, such as employment termination, appear to be universal, whereas other stressors, such as meeting deadlines, are more personal. For example, some nurses thrive on goals and timetables, whereas others feel constrained and frustrated and thereby experience distress. Burnout is not an objective phenomenon, as if it were the accumulation of a certain number and type of stressors. How the stressors are perceived and how they are mediated by an individual's ability to adapt are important variables in determining levels of distress.

Nurses who are burned out feel as if their resources are depleted to the point that their well-being is at risk. A self-analysis usually uncovers the characteristics of burnout. First, a feeling of emotional exhaustion can be recognized. Greenglass, Burke, and Fiksenbaum (2001) found that emotional exhaustion was directly related to workload. For example, recent graduates may value total, detailed care for individuals and may have little experience in caring for more than two patients simultaneously. When confronted with the responsibility of caring for a group of eight acutely ill patients, they may have difficulty adapting to the realities of the workplace, and emotional exhaustion ensues.

Emotional exhaustion in turn has a direct positive effect on cynicism and somatization. A second characteristic of burnout is **depersonalization** or cynicism, a state characterized by distancing oneself from the work itself and developing negative attitudes toward work in general (Greenglass et al., 2001). Nurses pushed to do too much in too little time may distance themselves from patients as a means of dealing with emotional exhaustion.

A decreased sense of effectiveness (professional accomplishment and competence) is the third hallmark of burnout. Low professional efficacy has been found to be a function of higher levels of cynicism (Greenglass et al., 2001). Via complex mechanisms not yet fully understood, prolonged stress and burnout are also related to physiological problems. Some studies have demonstrated a link between the nature of the workplace and illness; however, the field of psychoneuroimmunology, the study of how psychological factors influence the immune system and illness, is still in its infancy (Rabin, 1999).

Resolving High Levels of Stress

Resolution of stress in its early stages can be accomplished through a variety of techniques. Table 24-2 summarizes physical, mental, and emotional/spiritual strategies.

Social Support

Peers and followers can be supportive and help reduce stress by providing assistance with problem solving and by developing new perspectives. Family and friends can provide a safe haven and a vacation from stress. Social isolation increases stress.

Counseling

Persistent unpleasant feelings, problem behavior, and helplessness during prolonged stress may suggest the need for assistance from a mental health professional. Examples of problem behaviors include tearfulness or angry outbursts over seemingly minor incidents, major changes in eating and/or sleeping patterns, frequent unwillingness to go to work, and substance abuse. In such cases the aforementioned coping strategies afford only temporary

Table 24–2 STRESS MANAGEMENT STRATEGIES

Physical	Mental	Emotional/Spiritual
Accept physical limitations Modify nutrition: high carbohydrate, low caffeine, low sugar Exercise: participate in an enjoyable activity three times a week for 30 minutes Make your physical health a priority Nurture yourself by taking time for breaks and lunch Sleep: get enough in quantity and quality Relax: use meditation, massage, yoga, or biofeedback	Learn to say no! Use cognitive restructuring and self-talk Use imagery Develop hobbies or activities Plan vacations Learn about the system and how problems are handled Learn communication, conflict resolution, and time management skills Take continuing education courses	Use meditation Seek solace in prayer Seek professional counseling Participate in support groups Participate in networking Communicate feelings Identify and acquire a mentor Ask for feedback and clarification

relief; nurses with this level of distress feel overwhelmed and believe that their well-being cannot be maintained. In these stressful situations nurses may feel helpless and must seek professional assistance from a clinical psychologist, psychiatrist, or other mental health worker.

In some organizations, **employee assistance programs** (EAPs) provide counseling and other services for employees either via in-house staff or by contract with a mental health agency. This type of counseling can be effective because the counselors may already be aware of organizational stressors. Some nurses may have confidentiality concerns when using employer-recommended or employer-provided counseling services. Mental health professionals are bound by their professional standards of confidentiality. Nonetheless, there may be times when it is in the nurse's best interest to sign a release of information, such as when seeking employer accommodation for a certain physical or emotional problem.

Those who seek counseling outside of the workplace may be guided in their selection of mental health professionals by a personal physician, a knowledgeable colleague, or such publications as the most recent edition of *Directory of Medical Specialists,* which is available in many hospital libraries. When the problem underlying the distress is ethical or moral, a trained pastoral counselor may be helpful. Some clergy are certified in pastoral care or have earned a degree in another discipline such as psychology. Referrals can be obtained from hospital pastoral-care departments or churches that sponsor regional centers where certified counselors are available. When private counseling is being arranged, the health insurance contract should be checked to determine mental health benefits and the payment limitations and types of providers eligible for reimbursement.

Leadership and Management

Although social support and counseling can alter how stressors are perceived, time management and good leadership can modify or remove stressors. Perhaps the most important stress modifier is enhancing the control of nursing staff over their environment. First-line nurse managers have limited formal authority as individuals in most organizations, although managerial groups may be able to influence policy and resource allocation. Nurse managers can, however, control some environmental stressors on their units. First, managers can ex-

amine their own behavior as a source of subordinates' stress. A review of selected literature (Offermann & Hellmann, 1996) reveals that some leaders underestimate the influence of their behavior on subordinates' stress level and that they may attribute observed stress to the environment rather than their own behavior. This review also reported that lower performance and position satisfaction among subordinates was associated with nonparticipative, autocratic leadership styles.

In some cases a controlling style of management is appropriate, such as in emergency situations and when working with a large percentage of new and inexperienced employees. For the most part, however, professional nurses need and want the latitude to direct their activities within their sphere of competence. "Letting go," or delegating, means that the nurse leader trusts the personal integrity and professional competence of subordinates. It does not mean abdicating responsibility for achieving accepted standards of patient care and agreed-on outcomes.

Assistance with problem solving is an additional way to reduce environmental stressors. Nurse leaders may provide technical advice, direct staff to appropriate resources, or mediate conflicts. Often, nurse leaders enable staff to meet the demands of their work more independently by providing time for continuing education and professional meetings to enhance competence.

Another way in which nurse leaders can reduce stress is to be supportive of staff. Support is not equated with being a friend, but rather with helping one's peers accomplish good care, develop professionally, and feel valued personally. Encouraging innovation and experimentation, for example, can motivate staff and give them a sense of greater control over their environment. Affirming a good idea or finding resources to study or implement a promising new procedure or proposal by a staff nurse is supportive. In contrast, when staff members struggle with overwork and other stressors, support is recognizing the condition and helping the nurses avoid such passive coping strategies as feeling helpless or lowering standards of care in favor of active problem solving. Nurse leaders must be sensitive to the distress of the nursing staff and recognize it verbally without becoming counselors, which is in conflict with their role. Support may involve making nursing staff aware of resources that furnish counseling while being careful to avoid diagnostic labels and to maintain strict confidentiality.

When distress relates to the personal life of subordinates, managers should focus on the effect of such situations on workplace performance, not on the events that have produced the stress.

Finally, leaders can enhance the workplace by dealing effectively with their own stressors. Maintaining a sense of perspective and even a sense of humor is important. Some stressors, in fact, can be ignored or minimized by posing three questions:

1. "Is this event or situation important?" Stressors are not all equally significant. Do not waste energy on little stressors.
2. "Does this stressor affect me or my unit?" Although some situations that produce distress are institutionwide and need group action, others target specific units or activities. Do not borrow stressors.
3. "Can I change this situation?" If not, then find a way to cope with it or, if the situation is intolerable, make plans to change positions or employers. This decision may require gaining added credentials that may produce long-term career benefits.

Keeping stressful situations in perspective can enable nurses to conserve their energies to cope with stressful situations that are important, that are within their domain, or that can be changed or modified.

MANAGEMENT OF TIME

There is a very close relationship between stress management and time management. Time management is one method of stress prevention or reduction. Stress can decrease productivity and lead to poor use of time, but time management can be considered a preventive action to help reduce the elements of stress in a nurse's life.

Everyone has two choices when it comes to managing time: organize or "go with the flow." There are only 24 hours in every day, and it is clear that some people make better use of time than others. It is how people use time that makes some people more successful than others. The current status of healthcare organizations, trying to do more with less, has led to more demands (stressors) being placed on care providers and care managers. The effective use of time management skills thus becomes an even more important tool to achieve personal and professional goals. *Time management* is the use of tools, techniques, and principles to control time spent on low-priority needs and to ensure that time is invested in activities leading toward achieving desired, high-priority goals. More simply, time management is the ability to spend your time on the things that matter to you and your organization.

Where Does Your Time Go?

Have you ever wasted time? Time, although a cheap commodity, is our most valuable resource. There are some commonly identified time wasters, and individuals must recognize them to guard against them.

Doing Too Much

Do you try to do too much at once? At work, do you have three or four major projects going simultaneously? Are you a member of more than one organizational committee? Do you have to worry about what will be on the table for dinner while you are hanging an IV and planning a staff meeting? Have you ever completed a nursing intervention and realized that your mind was really somewhere else, and the patient had been ignored? If you *think* you have too much to do, you probably do! Learn to have fewer projects running simultaneously and to concentrate your efforts on one thing at a time. The first step is to realistically limit major commitments and then give each activity your full and undivided attention. Sometimes completing one task before starting another is the most efficient method of getting everything done. Prioritization of goals and activities each day is very helpful.

Inability to Say "No"

If you are suffering from overload, you probably have gotten there by not being able to say "no." Learning to say "no" to requests is difficult, and in the process others may be displeased. If you do not say "no," however, you may end up spending a great deal of time on projects that are uninteresting or have no relationship to your personal goals and priorities. When someone asks you to do something, you need to stop and consider the request. Do you want to do the task now or sometime in the future? If not, then say so. If you wish to do the task but simply do not have the time, consider **delegation**. However, be honest with the requester—if you simply do not have the time, say so as politely as possible. If you wish to take on the task but at a later date, negotiate. Remember, accepting an assignment you will never be able to complete does not shed a favorable light on you.

Procrastination

Do you put off important tasks because they are not enjoyable? Do you find excuses for not starting or completing tasks? Are you a procrastinator? By engaging in **procrastination,** or doing one thing when you should be doing something else, you give up time to complete your task and therefore limit the quality of the work you produce. There are techniques to help deal with procrastination. First, identify the reason for procrastinating. Then make that task your highest priority the next day. Reward yourself after you finish the task. Some people find that they procrastinate when the task ahead is very large. The solution is to break the task down into manageable pieces and plan rewards for accomplishing each of the smaller tasks. Another technique is to select the least attractive element of the task to do first, and the rest will seem easy. Exercise 24-3 is one way to manage procrastination.

Exercise 24-3

What tasks have you been putting off? Identify three tasks (1-3) that you really need to do—tasks that you labeled high priority, yet still have not done. For each task, write down two reasons why you have been avoiding the work (R1 and R2). Prioritize the tasks. Now break each task down into three or more manageable pieces (A, B, and C). Plan a reward to follow completion of each task.

TASKS I HAVE PROCRASTINATED ON: PRIORITY

1. _____   _____
   R1 _____
   R2 _____
   A. _____
   B. _____
   C. _____
2. _____   _____
   R1 _____
   R2 _____
   A. _____
   B. _____
   C. _____
3. _____   _____
   R1 _____
   R2 _____
   A. _____
   B. _____
   C. _____

Complaining

Often, the time nurses spend complaining about a task or a particular situation is greater than the time needed to solve the problem. If you find yourself complaining, stop and ask yourself what would be the ideal solution to the problem, and then take the risk to act on it. If the problem is another person, either take the time to talk with the person and get the problem out in the open, or sit down and write a letter to the person discussing your point of view (even if you do not mail it). If there is a problem within the workplace, take the time to think about the problem and generate some possible solutions, then talk to your manager. Go prepared to discuss solutions, not just problems. In this way your manager will see you as interested in contributing to the goals of the organization.

Perfectionism

Perfectionism is the tendency to never finish anything because it is not yet perfect. This approach tends to consume a great deal of time when your expected outcome is not attainable. Overcoming perfectionism takes considerable effort. However, this does not mean that you should do less than your best. Being aware of perfectionism means that you occasionally need to give yourself permission to do slightly less than a perfect job, such as buying a carryout dinner rather than preparing a four-course meal after a day at work.

Interruptions

One common distraction from priority activities is interruptions. Some interruptions are integral to the positions that you hold, but others can be controlled. A home care nurse with a large caseload can expect to be paged at any time. More common, however, are the numerous small interruptions by individuals who want just a "minute of your time" and take 2 minutes getting to the point! Box 24-1 identifies some specific strategies to prevent and control interruptions. The two keys to dealing with interruptions are to resume "doing it now" so that an interruption does not destroy your schedule and to maintain the attitude that whatever the interruption, it is a part of your responsibility. When you make a conscious decision not to worry about the things you cannot control, you have more energy to maintain a positive perspective and to move projects forward.

Disorganization

One of the most serious time wasters of all is disorganization. How many times have you had to spend 5 minutes trying to find something you have misplaced or misfiled? Organization can be a great time saver. Remember that the guiding principle is that organization is a process rather than the product.

BOX 24-1

Tips to Avoid Interruptions and Work More Effectively

- Chart somewhere other than in the place you will be most accessible to others.
- Ask people to put their comments in writing—do not let them catch you "on the run."
- Let the office/unit secretary know what information you need immediately.
- Conduct a conversation in the hall to help keep it short or in a separate room to keep from being interrupted.
- Be comfortable saying "no."
- When involved in a long procedure or home visit, ask someone else to cover your other responsibilities.
- Break projects into small, manageable pieces.
- Get yourself organized.
- Minimize interruptions—for example, allow voice mail to pick up the phone; shut the door.
- Keep your manager informed of your goals.
- Plan to accomplish high-priority or difficult tasks early in the day.
- Develop a plan for the day and stick to it. Remember to schedule in some time for interruptions.
- Schedule time to meet regularly throughout the shift with staff for whom you are responsible.
- Recognize that crises and interruptions are part of the position.
- Be cognizant of your personal time-waster habits, and try to avoid them.

You can spend so much time organizing that you will never get to the task at hand (procrastination). Simple organizing guidelines include eliminating clutter, keeping everything in its place, and doing similar tasks together.

Too Much Information

The newest time waster to evolve is data proliferation. We are now in the midst of a paradigm shift to the Information Age. The technology within our workplace forces us to receive huge amounts of data and to transform these data into useful information. The computer workstation, once touted as a time-saving device, has become the driving force behind care delivery. Nurses can view the computer either as a stress-producing slave driver or as a simple tool to assist them in their daily activities.

Information overload, or "data smog," occurs when you are overwhelmed by too much informa-

tion, too fast, and too often and do not have the skills to interpret the data into useful information. Symptoms of information overload may include a sense of inability to keep up with everything; a feeling that data keep you from accomplishing your "real job"; an inability to proceed from the question or problem to fact finding; interference with sleep; a decreased ability to concentrate; irritability; and physical distress, including indigestion, heart problems, and hypertension (Murray, 2001).

Developing data and information receiving and sending skills can greatly reduce stress and improve efficiency and productivity. Gaining a new appreciation for information is important. Information is simply a tool to use to plan action or make decisions. By learning what information is important, you can learn to use it to your advantage.

Time Management Concepts

Table 24-3 presents a classification scheme for time management techniques. The unifying theme is that each activity undertaken should lead to goal attainment and that goal should be the number one priority at that time.

Time Management Strategies

Goal Setting

The first step in time management is setting goals and developing a plan to reach the goals. If determining long-term goals is difficult for you, consider setting more short-term goals—steps along the way to the long-term goal. Set goals that are reasonable and achievable. Do not expect to reach long-term goals overnight—long-term means just that. Give yourself time to meet the goals. Set many short-term goals to reach the long-term goal to give yourself a frequent sense of goal achievement. Annual goals should be broken down into monthly goals, monthly goals broken down into weekly goals, and weekly goals broken down into daily goals. Give yourself flexibility. If the path you chose last year is no longer appropriate, change it. Write your goals on paper, date the page, keep it handy, and refer to it often to give yourself a progress report.

Setting Priorities

Once goals are known, priorities are set. They may, however, shift throughout a given period in terms of goal attainment. For example, working on a budget may take precedence at certain times of the year, whereas new staff orientation is high priority at other times. Knowing what your goals and priorities

Table 24–3 CLASSIFICATION OF TIME MANAGEMENT TECHNIQUES

Level of Technique	Purpose	Actions
Primary	Designed to promote efficiency and productivity	Organize and systematize things, tasks, and people Use basic time management skills
Secondary	Focuses on goal achievement	Assemble a prioritized "to do" list based on goals daily
	Uses the right tool for planning and preparation	Use tools such as the PalmPilot
Tertiary	Helps to refocus, to gain control, and to use information	Develop a personal time management plan appropriately

are helps shape the "to do" list. On a nursing unit or as you work in a community setting, you must know your personal goals and current priorities. How you organize work may depend on geographic considerations, patient acuity, or some other schema. Covey, Merrill, and Merrill (1994) identify a particular strategy to assist in prioritization. They state that people generally focus on those things that are important and urgent. By placing the elements of importance and urgency in a grid as shown in Figure 24-2, all activities can be classified, as shown.

Typically, we tend to focus on those items in cell A because they are both important and urgent and therefore command our attention. Making shift assignments is an A task because it is both important to the work to be accomplished and commonly urgent because there is a time frame during which data about patients and qualifications of staff can be matched. Conversely, if something is neither important nor urgent (cell D), it may be considered a waste of time, at least in terms of personal goals. An example of a D activity might be reading "junk" email. Even if something is urgent but not important (cell C), it contributes minimally to productivity and goal achievement. An example of a C activity might be responding to a memo that has a specific time line but is not important to goal attainment. The real key to setting priorities is to attend to the B tasks, those that are important but not urgent. Examples of B activities are reviewing the organization's strategic plan or participating on organizational committees.

Organization

A number of simple routines for organization can save many minutes over a day and enhance your ef-

Figure 24-2   Classification of priorities. (Modified from Covey, S. R., Merrill, A. R., & Merrill, R. R. [1994]. *First things first: To love, to learn, to leave a legacy.* New York: Simon & Schuster.)

ficiency. Keeping a workspace neat or arranging things in an orderly fashion may be a powerful time management tool. Rather than a system of "pile management," use file management. The adage "there is a place for everything, and everything in its place" makes for a successful workspace. A few hints include (1) planning ahead where things should go (frequently used items should be more accessible), (2) not using the top of your desk (table, computer station) for storage, (3) creating a "to do" folder, (4) creating a "to be filed" folder, and (5) having a regularly scheduled time to work your way through the folders. Everyone accumulates a pile of papers that becomes a problem over time. Take the time to sort the piles, perhaps tossing a page or two, acting on those things that are urgent, or if all else fails, filing it! The easiest way to keep a desk neat is to clean off the desk at the end of every day. After cleaning the desk, determine your priority goals for the next day and have the materials ready to work on when you start the next morning.

Time Tools

Sometimes the real problem is that the events of the day become the driving force, rather than a planned schedule. Days may become so tightly scheduled that any little interruption can become a crisis. If you do not plan the day, you may find yourself responding to events rather than prioritized goals. If you think you are a reactor rather than a proactive time user, use a time log to list work-related activities for several days. One reason you may not be able to plan well is that you really do not have a good estimate of how long a particular activity actually takes, or you do not know how many activities can be accomplished in a given time frame.

As the nurse's role in care management increases in complexity, the need for organizational tools increases. Tracking the care of groups of patients, either as the member of a care team or in a leadership capacity, can be overwhelming. Each nurse must devise a method for tracking care and organizing time, as well as delegating and monitoring care provided by others. Although some nurses depend on a shift flow sheet or a Kardex system, others are enjoying the benefit of computerized information tracking systems. The use of handheld computer devices such as personal digital assistants (PDAs) like the PalmPilot or bar code scanners for medication administration are other methods to track information and increase safety and efficiency.

Dealing With Information

The first step in managing information is to assess the source. Once you have identified the sources of your data, you have a better idea of how to deal with the information. Track incoming information for a few days. Patterns will begin to emerge and will give clues as to how to deal with it. You can generally predict that, using the Pareto principle, 80% of your incoming data comes from approxi-

mately 20% of your sources and that 80% of useful information comes from 20% of information received.

By developing information-receiving skills, you can quickly interpret the data and convert them to useful information, discarding that which is not needed. Initially, you should reduce or eliminate that which is useless. Delete the email or toss the memo in the trash. Next, monitor the information flow and decide what to do with incoming data. Find and focus on the most important pieces and then quickly narrow down the specific details you need. Identify resources that are most helpful and have them readily available. Be able to build the "big picture" from the masses of data you receive. Finally, recognize when you have enough information to act.

Once you have mastered the receiving end of information, concentrate on information-sending skills. Remember, your information is simply another person's data! Try to keep your outflow short; make it a synthesis of the information. Finally, select the most appropriate mode of communication for your message from the technology available. You may be sending your information in written (memo or report) or verbal form (face-to-face or presentation) or via telephone, voice mail, email, or fax. Remember, the most important skill is to know when you have said enough. Exercise 24-4 will help you consider how you have dealt with information.

Exercise 24-4

Think of the last time you were in the clinical area. How often did you record the same piece of data (e.g., a finding in your assessment of the patient)? Remember to include all steps, from your jotting down notes on a piece of paper to the final report of the day. What information processing tools could decrease the number of steps?

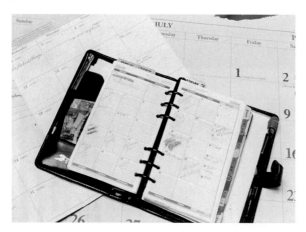

Systems for organizing time include calendars, organizers, and appointment books.

MEETING MANAGEMENT AND DELEGATION

Two key time management strategies critical to success are managing meetings and delegation, which are discussed in the next two sections of this chapter. Even nurses who may not have extensive management responsibilities usually are in the position of delegating tasks to less skilled workers and can benefit from learning to make the most of meetings, either as the leader or as a group member.

Managing Meetings

Unfocused, poorly managed meetings can waste valuable time and can frustrate busy staff members. Meetings serve various purposes ranging from creating social networks to setting formal policy. They may be designed to solve problems, disseminate information, seek input, inspire the group, delegate work or authority, or create/maintain a formal power base. Unless the purpose of a meeting is to socialize, the meeting is unlikely to be effective if it is poorly managed. The following is a list of several popular techniques and strategies to enhance the productivity and effectiveness of meetings.

Tips for Managing Meetings Effectively

Before scheduling a meeting ask yourself several questions:

- Is this meeting really necessary? What would happen if the meeting never happened?
- Could a phone call or one-on-one meeting better achieve the goal?
- Is this meeting simply informational? If so, would written communication better meet the need? Would a memo or posting an announcement suffice?
- Are the people who really need to attend available to meet?

Schedule meetings right before lunch or at the end of the day. Participants will have an incentive to stick to the schedule. Set a start and stop time and reward prompt members by starting on schedule. Most of the work of the meeting is accomplished in the first hour. Try to avoid meetings lasting longer than 1.5 to 2 hours. Select an appropriate setting, where the participants are not readily accessible to interruptions. If necessary, plan the seating arrangement to prevent inappropriate behaviors such as whispering or other interruptions. If the group meets over a period of time, have group members set rules for conduct and behavior.

Distribute an **agenda.** Whenever possible, provide a written agenda to each member in advance of the meeting. Establish and make known the goal of the meeting. Attach all needed preparation reading to the agenda. The more advanced the reading or preparation that is required, the earlier members should receive agendas. Different types of agendas can be used for different purposes:

Structured agendas: If a topic is particularly controversial, consider setting a rule that requires any negative comment to be preceded by a positive one.

Timed agendas: Consider setting a specific amount of time to be dedicated to each item on the agenda. If you stick to the schedule, discussion will stay focused and you will be more likely to make it through the agenda.

Action agendas: Consider submitting an agenda with a description of the needed/desired action, such as review proposals, approve minutes, or establish outcomes.

Keep the group on task. Use rules of order to facilitate meetings. Robert's Rules of Order (Robert, Evans, & Balch, 2000) may seem overly structured; however, this structure is particularly helpful when diversity of opinion is likely or important. Specifically, these rules help the person chairing the meeting by setting limits on discussion and using a specific order of priorities to deal with concerns.

Keep minutes and distribute them to participants. The minutes provide a record to refer back to if needed and also serve to convey contents to persons unable to attend.

Planning ahead for the meeting is a group leader's best strategy for a satisfactory experience. Participants must also prepare for meetings. Reviewing the agenda (or requesting one in advance if not provided), reviewing preparatory materials, and thinking through agenda items are ways that group members may assist in accomplishing the meeting goals. Meeting participants should be on time for all meetings or communicate that they will be late or unable to attend. Participants should be prepared to leave on time as well. When a meeting is poorly chaired, a committee member could volunteer to be sure that the meeting agendas and minutes are distributed. It is important to recognize that some people deliberately avoid preparing agendas and distributing minutes in an attempt to control the meeting. Exercise 24-5 will help you understand the importance of well-run meetings.

Exercise 24-5

Have you ever sat in a meeting and wondered why you were there? Perhaps you were unclear about the purpose of the meeting or where the meeting was heading, or even who was in charge! Write down the three things about the meeting that were most annoying, and then analyze how the situation could have been handled better.

Delegating

Delegation is a critical component of self-management for nurse managers and care managers. Appropriate delegation not only increases time efficiency but also serves as a means of reducing stress. Delegation is discussed in depth in Chapter 21, but it is also appropriate to discuss briefly as a time management strategy. Delegation works only when the delegator trusts the delegatee to accomplish the task and to report findings back to the nurse. It does not save time for the nurse to go back and check or redo everything someone else has done. Delegation requires empowerment of the delegatee to accomplish the task. If the nurse does not delegate appropriately, with clear expectations, the delegatee will constantly be asking for assistance or direction. Delegation can also be a means of reducing stress if used appropriately. If the nurse does not understand delegation and does not use it appropriately, it can be a major source of stress as the nurse assumes accountability and responsibility for care administered by others.

SUMMARY

Self-management is a means to achieve a balance between work and personal life, as well as a way of life developed to achieve personal goals within self-imposed priorities and deadlines. Time management is clock-oriented, and stress management is the control of external and internal stressors.

To achieve a balance in life and minimize stressors, nurses must learn to sit back and see their own personal "big picture" and examine their personal and professional goals. Personal priorities also must be established. Stressors and coping strategies need to be identified and used. By developing these techniques, nurses can gain a sense of control and become far better nurses in the process.

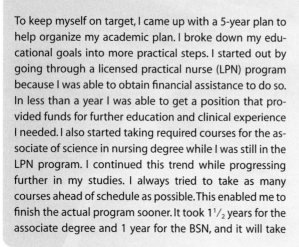

The Solution

To keep myself on target, I came up with a 5-year plan to help organize my academic plan. I broke down my educational goals into more practical steps. I started out by going through a licensed practical nurse (LPN) program because I was able to obtain financial assistance to do so. In less than a year I was able to get a position that provided funds for further education and clinical experience I needed. I also started taking required courses for the associate of science in nursing degree while I was still in the LPN program. I continued this trend while progressing further in my studies. I always tried to take as many courses ahead of schedule as possible. This enabled me to finish the actual program sooner. It took 1 $\frac{1}{2}$ years for the associate degree and 1 year for the BSN, and it will take another year for the MSN degree. I also lowered my standard of living and worked part-time as a registered nurse. It was enough to support myself without compromising my health or my educational goals.

Multitasking became second nature for me throughout school. Time management has become a very useful tool for me as a nurse, as well as a student. It can be crucial if you have many objectives to achieve.

— Kathleen Slat

 Would this be a suitable approach for you? Why?

CHAPTER CHECKLIST

Stress management and time management are two strategies for self-management. Balancing stress means caring for your emotional, physical, and mental needs. Effective delegation, using schedules and calendars and other planners, using time management principles, and managing meetings are key strategies to be integrated into the nurse leader role. By accomplishing self-management, managers, leaders, and followers will find themselves in control of work time and stressors, as well as more confident in achieving both personal and work-related goals.

Stress and overwork are inherent in the nursing profession, and nurses can adapt and cope with stress and time pressures by learning effective ways to care for themselves and to manage time. By assessing and reducing specific stressors and time wasters, nurses can thrive within the healthcare challenges before them. Increasing skills in coping, organization, delegation, and effective time management are vital components of effective leadership. A nurse manager who can be a role model and support his or her staff in turbulent times is a true leader.

- Stress management includes using cognitive and psychosocial activities to decrease the stress or enhance the ability to handle stress.
- Time management includes using tools and strategies to ensure that priority goals are achieved.
- Signs of excess stress must be heeded to prevent burnout or chronic health problems.
- Strategies to reduce stress include the following:
  - Physical
    - Accept physical limitations.
    - Plan physical activity.
    - Maintain adequate physical health, including adequate nutrition.
    - Schedule time for breaks and relaxation.
  - Mental/emotional
    - Use problem-identification and problem-solving strategies.
    - Differentiate between perceived and objective stressors.
    - Evoke the relaxation response via meditation.
    - Recognize stress-induced behavioral changes.
    - Seek social support.
  - Management
    - Maintain awareness of the effect of behavior on others.
    - Develop a participative management style.
    - Practice a systems perspective.
    - Retain a sense of distance from stress.
- Strategies to improve time management include the following:
  - Identification of potential time wasters
    - Too much work
    - Inability to say "no"
    - Procrastination
    - Complaining
    - Perfectionism
    - Interruptions
    - Disorganization
    - Too much information

- Use of time management strategies
  - Setting priorities
  - Being organized
  - Using time tools such as time logs, Kardex, shift flow sheets, and PDAs
  - Devising a personal time management system
  - Effectively dealing with data and information
- Appropriate delegation
  - Being willing to delegate/be delegated to
  - Giving the delegatee sufficient responsibility and authority
  - Conveying expectations clearly
  - Requiring the delegatee to be accountable
- Strategies to improve meeting management include the following:
  - Distribute meeting agendas and minutes.
  - Schedule meetings appropriately.
  - Use rules of order to facilitate meetings.

TIPS FOR SELF-MANAGEMENT

- Know what your high-priority goals are and use them to filter decisions.
- Know your personal response to stress and self-evaluate frequently.
- Make your health a priority and use strategies that keep yourself in control.
- Use organizational systems that meet your needs; the simpler, the better.
- Simplify.
- Refocus on your priorities whenever you begin to feel overwhelmed.

TERMS TO KNOW

agenda	information overload
burnout	overwork
coping	perfectionism
delegation	procrastination
depersonalization	self-management
employee assistance programs	time management
general adaptation syndrome (GAS)	

REFERENCES

American Nurses Association. (2000). *Opposing the use of mandatory overtime as a staffing solution (action report)*. Retrieved from www.nursingworld.org/about/summary/sum00/overtme.htm

Cohen, S., & Manuck, S. (1999). Preface. In B. Rabin. *Stress, immune function and health* (pp. xi-xii). New York: Wiley-Liss.

Covey, S. R., Merrill, A. R., & Merrill, R. R. (1994). *First things first: To love, to learn, to leave a legacy*. New York: Simon & Schuster.

Drucker, P. F. (2000, Spring). Managing knowledge means managing one's self. *Leader to Leader, 16*, 8-10.

Epstein, R. (2000). *The big book of stress relief games*. New York: McGraw-Hill.

Erdwins, C. J., Buffardi, L. C., Casper, W. J., & O'Brien, A. S. (2001). The relationship of women's role strain to social support, role satisfaction, and self-efficacy. *Family Relations, 50*(3), 230-238.

Fischer, J., Calame, A., Dettling, A., Zeier, H., & Fanconi, S. (2000). Experience and endocrine stress responses in neonatal and pediatric critical care nurses and physicians. *Critical Care Medicine, 28*(9), 3281-3288.

Greenglass, E., Burke, R., & Fiksenbaum, L. (2001). Workload and burnout in nurses. *Journal of Community and Applied Social Psychology, 11*, 211-215.

Hafner, A. W. (2001). *Pareto's principle: The 80-20 rule*. Retrieved from http://library.shu.edu/HafnerAW/awh-th-math-pareto.html. Accessed July 2002.

Kirkcaldy, B., & Martin, T. (2000). Job stress and satisfaction among nurses. *Stress Medicine, 16*, 77-89.

Kuhn, M. A. (1999). *Complementary therapies for health care providers*. Philadelphia: Lippincott Williams & Wilkins.

Maslach, C., Schaufeli, W., Leiter, M. (2000). Job burnout. *Annual Review of Psychology, 52*, 397-422.

Maurier, W., & Northcutt, H. (2000). Job uncertainty and health status for nurses during restructuring of health care in Alberta. *Western Journal of Nursing Research, 22*(5), 623-641.

Murray, B. (2001). *Data smog: Newest culprit in brain drain*. Retrieved from http://pespmc1.vub.ac.be/CHINNEG.html

Offermann, L. R., & Hellmann, P. (1996). Leadership behavior and subordinate stress: A 360° view. *Journal of Occupational Health Psychology, 1*(4), 382-390.

Rabin, B.(1999). *Stress, immune function and health*. New York: Wiley-Liss.

Robert, H., Evans, W., & Balch, J. (Eds.). (2000). *Robert's rules of order newly revised*. Cambridge, MA: Perseus Book Group.

Selye, H. (1956). *The stress of life*. New York: McGraw-Hill.

Selye, H. (1991). History and present status of the stress concept. In A. Monat & R. Lazarus (Eds.), *Stress and coping: An anthology* (pp. 21-36). New York: Columbia University Press.

Smith, A. (2000). The scale of perceived occupational stress. *Occupational Medicine, 50*(5), 294-298.

Wilson, J. (1990). *Woman: Your body, your health*. New York: Harcourt, Brace, Jovanovich.

SUGGESTED READINGS

Drucker, R. (1999). *Management challenges for the 21st century*. New York: HarperCollins.

Field, T., Quintino, O., Henteleff, T., Wells-Keife, L., & Delvecchio-Feinberg, G. (1997). Job stress reduction therapies. *Alternative Therapies in Health & Medicine, 3*(4): 54-56.

Lee, R., & Ashforth, B. (1996). A meta-analytic examination of the correlates of the three dimensions of job burnout. *Journal of Applied Psychology, 81*(2), 123-133.

Lyon, B. (2000). Conquering stress. *Reflections on Nursing Leadership, 26*(1), 22-23, 43.

Oncken, W., & Wass, D. (1999, November/December). Management time: Who's got the monkey? *Harvard Business Review*, Reprint 99609.

Schwartz, J. E., Pickering, T., & Landsbergis, P. (1996). Work-related stress and blood pressure: Current theoretical models and considerations from a behavioral medicine perspective. *Journal of Occupational Health Psychology, 1*(3), 287-310.

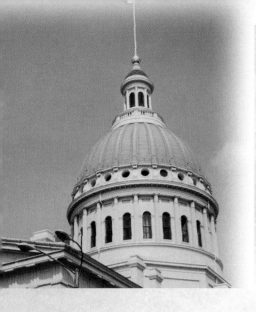

Chapter

25

Power, Politics, and Influence

Karen Kelly

This chapter describes how power and politics influence the roles of leaders and managers. It focuses on contemporary concepts of power, empowerment, types of power exercised by nurses, key factors in developing a powerful image, personal and organizational strategies for exercising power, and the power of nurses to shape health policy and take action in the political arena of legislative politics. Having the opportunity to relate to politics in the workplace is critical for effective leadership and management.

Objectives

- Apply the concept of power to leadership and management in nursing.
- Use different types of power in the exercise of nursing leadership.
- Develop a power image for effective nursing leadership.
- Choose appropriate strategies for exercising power to influence the politics of the work setting, professional organizations, legislators, and the development of health policy.

Questions to Consider

- *What does the phrase* a powerful nurse *mean to you?*
- *Do you ever think of yourself as a powerful nurse?*
- *What factors, persons, and events have influenced your development as a nurse?*
- *What kinds of behaviors do you observe in people that tell you whether they are powerful? Which are socially desirable? Which are undesirable? What are your behaviors?*
- *What are your beliefs and values about power and politics in organizations?*
- *How can you shape health policy and legislative politics?*

The Challenge

Gail Haller, MSN, RN
Former Chairperson, Illinois Nurses Association Political Action Committee, Illinois

The chairperson of the state nurses' association political action committee (PAC) was involved in working with the state nurses association's (SNA) nurse-lobbyist on an amendment to the nurse practice act (NPA) to recognize certified registered nurse anesthetists (CRNAs) among advanced practice nurses. A hostile amendment to allow one anesthesia technician, with a bachelor's degree in anesthesia technology from a university in another state, was being offered by a legislator from the northern part of the state. The hostile amendment was a threat to the entire system of nursing licensure because it would legitimize the practice of a nonnurse as a CRNA.

The technician, on whose behalf the hostile amendment was offered, lived in the southern part of the state and was employed by an anesthesiology practice. The practice wanted her to work beyond the usual scope of practice of an anesthesia technician because of her prior work experience in another state where she was licensed and worked much like a CRNA. The hospital and anesthe-

sia group had been unable to convince any local legislators in the area where she lived to sponsor this amendment; the legislators had a close working relationship with the district nurses' association and did not want to oppose their supporters' interests. The legislator from the northern part of the state was reported to have offered the amendment because of contacts with the family of the technician.

The key issue here focused on the hospital's willingness to credential this unlicensed individual. If the hospital's credentialing policy was allowed to override the state's licensure laws, the licensure system would be in chaos and the door could be opened to institutional licensure. A hearing was scheduled before the Senate Licensed Activities Committee to determine support for the hostile amendment.

What do you think you would do if you were this nurse?

INTRODUCTION

The profession of nursing developed in the United States at a time when women had limited legal rights (e.g., most were prohibited from voting, and many could not own property). Women were viewed as neither powerful nor political; in the late nineteenth century, *feminine* and *powerful* were practically contradictory terms. During the twentieth century, as the status and role of women changed, so did the status and role of nurses. As the economic and social **power** of women evolved, so did the power of nurses. This is significant because nursing historically has been, and continues to be, a discipline comprised primarily of women.

As the healthcare environment continues to change in the twenty-first century, the exercise of power by nurses is essential to a strong voice for nursing in shaping these changes. In an era of rapid and often unplanned change and of a developing nursing shortage like none before, nurses must exercise their power and flex their political muscles to create a preferred future for the health-

care system, healthcare consumers, and the profession of nursing.

HISTORY

Power was once considered almost a taboo in nursing. In the profession's earliest years, the exercise of power was considered inappropriate, unladylike, and unprofessional. Many decisions about nursing education and practice were often made by persons outside of nursing (Ashley, 1976). Nurses began to exercise their collective power with the rise of nursing leaders such as Lillian Wald, Isabel Stewart, Annie Goodrich, Lavinia Dock, M. Adelaide Nutting, and Isabel Hampton Robb and the development of organizations that evolved into the American Nurses Association and the National League for Nursing.

Many social, technological, scientific, and economic trends have shaped nursing and nurses and our ability to exercise power during the twentieth century. When the American Medical Association (AMA), in

1988, proposed a new category of healthcare worker (the Registered Care Technologist or RCT) to replace nurses during a time of nursing shortage, nurses and nursing organizations responded powerfully. Leaders of nursing organizations came together in "summit meetings" to formulate powerful responses to the AMA and implemented a range of actions, including public education and the education of legislators. The new healthcare worker did not materialize from this proposal. In this new century, nurses must be skilled and confident in exercising power to ensure the continuing development of the profession and that the voice of nurses will be heard in shaping the future of the healthcare system.

The media, politicians, organized medicine, and some healthcare executives have traditionally viewed nurses and nursing as powerless. That view began to change radically in the 1990s as nurses began to appear frequently on local (Lukas, 2001) and national news and talk shows as experts on the changes occurring in the healthcare system and the effect of these changes on the public. As nurses have become increasingly visible in political campaigns on the local, state, and national levels, both as candidates and as political influentials, nurses and nursing have gained new respect in the political arena.

Sadly, even today, as we enter a new and different era of nursing shortage, there are a few nurses who see themselves as powerless and oppressed, demonstrating aspects of oppressed group behavior. Like many politically and economically oppressed people, some nurses still persist in engaging in intragroup conflicts (e.g., "infighting"), and they distance themselves from other nurses (e.g., the failure of many nurses to join professional organizations) (Roberts, 1983). All nurses need to continue to expand their understanding of the concept of power and to develop their skills in exercising power. Avoiding involvement in the **politics** of nursing, in the workplace, in the profession at large, or in the area of public **policy** limits the power of the individual nurse and the profession as a collective whole.

Some nurses are still uncomfortable about politics, treating *politics* as if it is a dirty word. Politics can be defined in many ways (e.g., the science of government or a process of formal human interactions) (Kalisch & Kalisch, 1982). One simple definition of politics that I use when teaching a course on politics in nursing is "a process of human interaction within organizations." Politics permeates all organizations, including workplaces, legislatures, professions, and even families. Young children of-

ten learn that one parent is more likely than the other to give permission for special activities and more likely to buy toys and other desired items. They quickly learn to ask permission or ask for a desired item from that parent before asking the other. This is an unwritten political rule in many families. One source (Anderson, Anderson, & Glanze, 1998) defines *political nursing* as "the use of knowledge about power processes and strategies to influence the nature and direction of health care and professional nursing" (p. 1287).

Like an earlier model by Kalisch and Kalisch (1982), Cohen, Mason, Kovner, Leavitt, Pulcini, and Sochalski (1996) have identified four stages of political development for the profession of nursing:

1. *Buy-in:* recognizing the importance of activism
2. *Self-interest:* developing and using political expertise to further the profession's self-interests
3. *Political sophistication:* moving beyond self-interests, recognizing the need for activism on behalf of the public
4. *Leading the way:* providing true leadership on broad healthcare interests

Cohen et al. contend that the fourth stage represents nursing's current level of political evolution, with the possibility of further stage development.

With the addition of an initial stage identified by Kalisch and Kalisch (1982), this model can also be applied to the political development and activism of individual nurses related to both professional and legislative political arenas:

1. *Apathy:* no membership in professional organizations; little or no interest in legislative politics as they relate to nursing and healthcare
2. *Buy-in:* recognition of the importance of activism within professional organizations (without active participation) and legislative politics related to critical nursing issues
3. *Self-interest:* involvement in professional organizations to further one's own career; the development and use of political expertise to further the profession's self-interests
4. *Political sophistication:* high level of professional organization activism (e.g., holding office at the local and state level) moving beyond self-interests; recognition of the need for activism on behalf of the public
5. *Leading the way:* serving in elected or appointed positions in professional organizations at the state

and national levels; providing true leadership on broad healthcare interests within legislative politics, including seeking appointment to policy-making bodies and election to political positions

FOCUS ON POWER

Power comes from the Latin word *potere*, meaning "to be able." Simply defined, *power* is the ability to **influence** others in the effort to achieve goals. Nurses have sometimes viewed power as if it were something immoral, corrupting, and totally contradictory to the caring nature of nursing. However, the preceding definition demonstrates the essential nature of power to nursing. Nurses regularly influence patients in an effort to improve their health status as an essential element of nursing practice. When nurses are providing health teaching to patients and their families, their goal is to provide needed information and to change behavior to promote optimal health. That is an exercise of power in nursing practice. Changing a colleague's behavior by instructing him or her about a new policy being implemented on the nursing unit is another example of how a nurse can exercise power. Coaching a nurse to improve his or her performance is an exercise of power.

> ### Exercise 25–1
>
> Recall a recent opportunity you had to observe the work of an expert nurse. Think about that nurse's interactions with patients, family members, nursing colleagues, and other professionals. What kinds of power did you observe this nurse exercise? What did the nurse do that suggested to you, "this is a powerful person?"

Social scientists have studied the use and abuse of power in human organizations. They have analyzed and categorized the sources and applications of power in human experience. Hersey, Blanchard, and Natemeyer (1979) offer a classic formulation on the bases of social power. They identified seven bases of power, which are most easily understood as sources or types of social power that apply readily to the power exercised by nurses (see Theory box). These types of power are not mutually exclusive. They are often used in concert to exert influence on individuals or groups.

Nurses commonly use all of these types of power in a range of nursing activities. Nurses who teach parents about the care of their newborn use expert and information power by virtue of the information they share with parents; they also exercise legitimate power because they are registered nurses and thus are accorded a certain status by society. Members of a state nurses' association who lobby their members of the house and senate use expert power when trying to gain legislators' support for a piece of healthcare legislation. New graduates are employed on probationary status until they successfully meet and demonstrate the initial clinical competencies of a position. They may view the nurse manager as exercising both coercive and reward power related to their evaluation for continued employment. Nursing faculty and skilled clinicians often serve as role models to nursing students. The faculty and clinicians exercise referent power as students emulate their behavior. Examples of connection power are evident at any kind of social gathering in the workplace. People of high status (e.g., vice presidents, directors) within an organization may be sought for conversation by managers who want to move up the organizational hierarchy. Congresswoman Lois Capps (D-CA) is a former school nurse who took her husband's seat in Congress when he died unexpectedly. Recognized on her own as an effective member of Congress, she was reelected to office on her own merits. She uses expert, informational, and legitimate power as she promotes children's health issues in Washington (Cunningham, 2000).

These types of power describe the potential for power. Having a high-status position in an organization immediately provides stature, but power depends on the ability to accomplish goals from that position. Although some may think that "knowledge is power," acting on that knowledge is where the real power lies. Sharing knowledge expands one's power and, in turn, empowers our colleagues by giving them information or skills that they need to take action in a situation.

Nursing's early history in the United States was marked by powerlessness (Ashley, 1976; Schwirian, 1998). Nurses were absent from the decision-making processes about their education, practice, and employment. As the social, political, and economic status of women and nurses changed, so did the exercise of power by nursing as a profession and nurses as individuals. We recognize today that powerlessness results in apathy, anger, and indifference (Ferguson, 1993). This can result in a workplace culture that is marked by conflict, anger, and other dysfunctional behaviors. Sharing power and facilitating the em-

Theory Box

THEORY OF TYPES OR BASES OF SOCIAL POWER

KEY CONTRIBUTORS	KEY IDEAS	APPLICATION TO PRACTICE
Types or bases of social power were formulated by Hersey, Blanchard, and Natemeyer (1979) to explain the use of power within the human experience.	• Coercive power: Based on fear, coercion, and the ability to punish. *A nurse manager may be viewed as exercising coercive power by an employee who performs poorly and does not respond to efforts by the nurse to educate the staff person and improve that individual's performance. The nurse manager informs the employee that suspension or termination may result from the unsatisfactory performance.* • Reward power: Based on the ability to grant rewards and favors. *A nurse manager is viewed as exercising reward power during performance evaluations for employees earning merit pay increases based on the quality of their job performances.* • Expert power: Results from the knowledge and skills one possesses that are needed by others. *An advanced practice nurse is viewed as the clinical expert on a nursing unit and as a relatively powerful person.* • Legitimate power: Possessed by virtue of one's position within an organization or status within a group. *The President of the United States is viewed around the world as a powerful person as a result of election to this office.* • Referent power: Results from followers' desire to identify with a powerful person. *A nursing student completing a leadership and management practicum experience with an expert nurse manager sets a professional goal to emulate the behavior of this nurse manager.* • Information power: Stems from one's possession of selected information that is needed by others. *A staff nurse demonstrates great skill in teaching patients difficult self-care activities and is sought out by colleagues to help them teach their patients.* • Connection power: Gained by association with people who are perceived as powerful. *At a Nurses' Week celebration, nurses take advantage of the opportunity to have extended, informal conversations with the chief nurse executive.*	These categories help explain how we use power to influence others. The categories are not mutually exclusive and usually are used in concert with one another.

powerment of colleagues are strong forces in creating revitalized workplace cultures.

Influence is the process of using power. Influence can range from the punitive power of coercion to the interactive power of collaboration. Coaching a new graduate nurse in orientation to complete a complicated nursing procedure successfully vividly demonstrates the ability of the experienced nurse to influence that orientee. The coach uses reward, expert, legitimate, referent, and information power to influence the orientee not only at that moment but also perhaps over the span of a career. A nurse who testifies before a legislative committee uses expert, information, and legitimate power to encourage support for a bill to expand healthcare services to the children of the working poor. Nurses can use reward power by working on the campaigns of legislators who support nursing and healthcare issues; they also use coercive power by avoiding the campaigns of those legislators who are not supportive of such issues.

EMPOWERMENT

Empowerment is a term that has come into common usage in nursing in recent years. It has been used extensively in the nursing literature related to administration and management; it is also highly relevant to the domain of clinical practice. Empowerment is the process by which we facilitate the participation of others in decision making and taking action within an environment where there is an equitable distribution of power. Empowerment is consistent with the contemporary view of leadership, a paradigm that is exemplified by behaviors characteristic of nurses: facilitator, coach, teacher, and collaborator. These leadership skills are an essential component of professional nursing practice, whether a nurse is a clinician, an educator, a researcher, or an administrator/ manager. Nursing leaders, whether in the employment setting or in professional organizations, exercise power in making professional judgments as they do their daily work.

These leadership skills are essential to effective followers, too. Powerful nurse managers empower their staffs, influencing them to grow professionally. Powerful nurses empower their patients and the families in their care. Hence these leadership skills can be viewed as an essential component of professional nursing practice whether one is a clinician, an educator, a researcher, or an executive/manager.

Empowerment is the process by which power is shared with colleagues and patients as part of the nurse's exercise of power. This is in sharp contrast to traditional conceptualizations of power, a patriarchal model of power, which relies on coercion, hierarchy, authority, control, and force. Empowerment, by embracing a feminist conceptualization of power, emphasizes cooperation as a vital element for the exercise of power (Chinn, 2001). Nurses have too often viewed power as a finite quantity: "If I give you some of my power, I will have less." Empowerment emphasizes the notion that power grows when shared. I have observed the following:

- Nurses who view power as finite will avoid cooperation with their colleagues and refuse to share their expertise.

- Nurses who conceptualize power as infinite are strong collaborators who gain satisfaction by helping their colleagues expand their expertise and their power base.

The empowerment of nurses makes truly professional practice possible, the kind of professional practice that is satisfying to all nurses. Empowered clinicians are essential for effective nursing management, just as empowered managers set the stage for excellence in clinical practice. Encouraging a reticent colleague to be an active participant in committee meetings serves to empower that nurse and to shape practice policy with the institution. Guiding a novice nurse in exercising professional judgment empowers both the senior nurse and the novice clinician. Coaching a patient on how to be more assertive with a physician who is reluctant to answer the patient's questions is another form of empowerment.

Exercise 25-2

Think about a recent clinical experience when you empowered a patient. What did you do for and/or with the patient (and family) that was empowering? How did you feel about your own actions in this situation? How did the patient respond?

Strategies for Developing a Powerful Image

As Margaret Thatcher, former prime minister of Great Britain, said, "Being powerful is like being a lady. If you have to tell people you are, you aren't."

The most basic power strategy is the development of a powerful image. Lady Thatcher's statement emphasizes the importance of this powerful image. If nurses think they are powerful, others will view them as powerful; if they view themselves as powerless, so will others. A sense of self-confidence is a strong foundation in developing one's "power image," and it is essential for successful political efforts in the workplace, within the profession, and within the public policy arena. Several key factors contribute to one's power image:

- *Self-image:* thinking of one's self as powerful and effective
- *Grooming and dress:* ensuring that clothing, hair, and general appearance are neat, clean, and appropriate to the situation

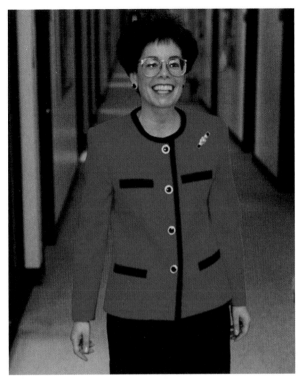

A powerful image is needed when representing the profession of nursing.

- *Good manners:* treating people with courtesy and respect
- *Body language:* maintaining good posture, using gestures that avoid too much drama, maintaining good eye contact, and being confident in your movement
- *Speech:* using a firm, confident voice; good grammar and diction; an appropriate vocabulary; and strong communication skills

Exercise 25-3

Think about a powerful public figure whom you admire. What key factors contribute to this person's powerful image? Think about a powerful nurse you have met. Identify this person's key image factors.

Concern about a powerful image may seem superficial. However, the impressions we make on people influence the way they view us now and in the future and how they value what we do and say. First impressions are important; we do not get a second chance to make a first impression. Given similar educational and experiential backgrounds, who is more likely to be hired for a nursing position: the candidate who comes dressed in a suit or the candidate who arrives in jeans and sandals? Who will be seen as the more competent professional by a patient: the nurse in wrinkled scrubs or the nurse in neat street clothes and a freshly laundered laboratory coat? Who will have a greater positive impact on a member of the state legislature: the nurse who visits in a sweatshirt and shorts or the nurse in a suit? A powerful image signals to others that you are professionally competent, influential, powerful, and capable of exercising appropriate judgments.

Attitudes and beliefs are another important aspect of a powerful image; they reflect one's values. Believing that power is a positive force in nursing is essential to one's powerful image. A firm belief in nursing's value to society and the centrality of nursing's contribution to the healthcare delivery system is also important. Powerful nurses do not allow the phrase "I'm just a nurse" in their vocabulary. Behavior reflects one's pride in the profession of nursing. This not only increases a nurse's own power but also helps empower nursing colleagues.

Make a Commitment to Nursing as a Career. Nursing is a profession; professions offer careers, not just a series of jobs. For a long time, nursing marketed itself to recruits as the perfect preparation for marriage and family. Even some contemporary job advertisements hint at romance as an outcome of employment at the agency featured. Some people still view nurses only as members of an occupation who drop in and out of employment, not as members of a profession with a long-term career commitment. Having a career commitment does not preclude leaving employment temporarily for family, education, or other demands. Having a career commitment implies that a nurse views himself or herself first and foremost as a member of the discipline of nursing with an obligation to make a contribution to the profession. Status as an employee of a particular hospital, home health agency, long-term-care facility, or other venue is secondary to the person's status as a member of the profession of nursing.

Value Continuing Education in Nursing. Valuing education is one of the hallmarks of a profession. The continuing development of one's professional skills and knowledge is an empowering experience, preparing the nurse to make decisions with the support of an expanding body of knowledge. Seminars, workshops, and conferences offer opportunities for continued professional growth and empowerment. Returning to school for advanced degrees is also a powerful growth experience and reflects commitment to the profession of nursing. For several decades some nurses thought the best way to get ahead in nursing was to seek education outside of nursing at the baccalaureate and graduate level. To develop expertise in the science and art of nursing, one needs to be educated in the discipline of nursing.

Change will continue in the healthcare system, necessitating continuing education to empower nurses to be proactive, not just reactive. A well-educated nursing workforce is essential if nursing is to have a strong voice in shaping the changes in healthcare. An additional advantage of participating in educational experiences is that it creates opportunities for networking, a strategy that is discussed later in this chapter.

PERSONAL POWER STRATEGIES

Developing a collection of power strategies, or power tools, is an important aspect of personal empowerment. These strategies should be used in situations that demand the exercise of leadership. Such strategies are techniques for building a professional power base and for developing political skills within an organization (Boxes 25-1 and 25-2). They also indicate to others that one is a powerful nurse and a leader. These boxes identify personal power strategies beyond those discussed in this section. These "power tools" have been developed and collected by this author during nearly 30 years of nursing experience and observation of successful, effective, powerful nurses.

Communication Skills

The most basic tool is effective verbal communication skills, which help define a power image. These are the same communication skills nurses learn to ensure effective interaction with patients and families. Listening skills are essential leadership skills. Just as the clinician listens to the patient to collect assessment data, the manager uses listening skills to assess and evaluate. Managers who are good listeners develop reputations for being fair and consistent. Listening to recurring themes related to minor issues of staff dissatisfaction in informal conversations can enable the manager to take action before a staff crisis occurs.

Verbal and nonverbal skills are important personal power strategies; the ability to assess these messages is a critical power strategy. Experts in communication estimate that 90% of the messages we communicate to others are nonverbal. When nonverbal and verbal messages conflict, the nonverbal message is more powerful. The basic lessons on the power of nonverbal communication most nurses learn in an introductory psychiatric course are relevant in all nursing arenas!

BOX 25-1

Strategies for Developing a Powerful Image

- Self-image
- Grooming and dress
- Speech
- Body language
- Belief in power as a positive force
- Belief in value of nursing to society
- Career commitment
- Continuing professional education

BOX 25-2

Additional Personal Power Strategies

- Be honest.
- Always be courteous; it makes other people feel good!
- Smile when appropriate; it puts people at ease.
- Accept responsibility for your own mistakes and learn from them.
- Be a risk taker.
- Win and lose gracefully.
- Learn to be comfortable with conflict and ambiguity; they are both normal states of the human condition.
- Give credit to others where credit is due.
- Develop the ability to take constructive criticism gracefully; learn to let destructive criticism "roll off your back."
- Use business cards when introducing yourself to new contacts and collect the business cards of those you meet when networking.
- Always follow through on promises.

■ *Exercise 25–4*

You encounter an old friend in a restaurant. You greet one another warmly, each stating how good it is to see the other. Yet your friend visibly backs away when you extend your arms to embrace. What is your immediate reaction? Despite the warm words of greeting, do you question your old friend's sincerity because of the strong nonverbal message regarding physical contact? Consider other situations you have experienced recently when words and actions contradict one another. Which message, the verbal or the nonverbal, did you accept as the person's "real" communication to you? Practice with a friend: Pretend you are greeting a visitor to your home, a colleague, or a patient. In the first trial, state your greeting warmly, extend your hand to shake the other person's hand, smile, and make eye contact. In the second trial, use the same words of greeting, but use an angry tone of voice, avoid eye contact, and fold your arms across your chest while moving one step back from the other person. Observe the physical actions and listen carefully, especially to the tone of voice. Repeat the exercise, switching roles. Discuss your response to these interactions.

Networking

Networking is an important power strategy and political skill. A **network** is a system of contacts that is developed, nurtured, and maintained as sources of information, advice, and moral support (Schutzenhofer, 1995). Networking supports the empowerment of participants through interaction and the refinement of their interpersonal skills. Most nurses have relatively limited networks within the organizations where they are employed. They tend to have lunch or coffee with those people with whom they work most closely. One strategy to expand a workplace network is to have lunch or coffee with someone from another department, including managers from nonnursing departments, at least two or three times a month.

Active participation in nursing organizations is the most effective method of establishing a professional network outside one's place of employment. Participation in professional organizations can propel a nurse into the politics of nursing, including involvement in shaping public policy. State and district nurses' associations offer an excellent opportunity to develop a network that includes nurses from various clinical and functional areas. Membership in specialty organizations, especially organizations for nurse managers and executives, provides the opportunity to network with nurses with similar expertise and interests. In addition, membership in civic, volunteer, and special interest groups and participation in educational programs (e.g., formal academic programs and conferences) also provide networking opportunities.

The successful networker identifies a core of networking partners who are particularly skilled, insightful, and eager to support the development of colleagues. These partners need to be nurtured. The following represent ways partners can be nurtured (Schutzenhofer, 1995):

- Send them articles on topics of interest to them.
- Call them to keep in touch if face-to-face contact is sporadic or infrequent.
- Never argue the merit of advice given by a networking partner; consider its value later.
- Be reasonable in making requests for help or information; ask for only one thing at a time and be specific about what is wanted.
- Most important, be prepared to reciprocate with networking partners.

Mentoring

In recent years mentoring has become a driving force in nursing. *Mentors* are competent, experienced professionals who develop a relationship with a novice for the purpose of providing advice, support, information, and feedback to encourage the development of another individual. Mentoring has been an important element in the career development of men in business, academia, and selected professions. Mentoring has become a significant power strategy for women in general and for nurses in particular during the last 20 years. Mentoring provides novices with expanded access to information, power, and career opportunities. Mentors have historically been a critical asset to novices trying to negotiate workplace and professional politics. Effective mentoring in nursing can be characterized by certain attributes (Stewart & Kruger, 1996):

1. Mentoring is a teaching-learning process for both the mentor and the mentee.
2. Mentoring is a reciprocal relationship for the mentor and mentee, a give-and-take situation for both parties.
3. A knowledge or competence differential exists between participants.
4. The focus of the relationship is on career development.
5. The relationship will endure over several years.
6. Mentees will in turn become mentors to others.

Mentoring is an empowering experience for both mentors and novices. The process of seeking out mentors is an exercise in growth for novices or protégés. Mentors often come from one's professional networks. Some mentors select their protégés; other times the reverse is true. Novices may attract mentors by implementing the following strategies (Schutzenhofer, 1995):

- Demonstrating a developing expertise
- Developing a sensitivity to the attention of powerful people within the organization
- Volunteering to serve on committees and doing the work well
- Discussing openly professional goals and personal desire to grow
- Asking experienced and talented people within the network for advice and help

Novices learn new skills from influential mentors and gain self-confidence. Mentors gain stature within their peer groups, extend their scope of influence through relationships with novices, refine their professional skills, and gain self-confidence through the satisfaction experienced in observing the development of novices.

Goal Setting

Goal setting is another power strategy. Every nurse knows about setting goals. Students learn to devise patient care goals or patient outcomes as part of the care planning process. Nurses may be expected to write annual goals for performance reviews at work. Even a project at home (e.g., painting rooms) may necessitate setting goals (e.g., painting a room each day of one's vacation). Goals help one to know if what was planned was actually accomplished. Likewise, a successful nursing career needs goals to define what one wants to achieve as a nurse. Without such goals, one can wander endlessly through a series of jobs without a real sense of satisfaction. To paraphrase what the Cheshire Cat told Alice during her trip through Wonderland, any road will take you there if you don't know where you are going.

Well-defined, long-term goals may be hard to formulate early in a career. For example, few new graduates know specifically that they want to be chief nurse executives, deans, managers, or researchers, yet, eventually, some will choose those career paths. However, developing such a vision early in a career is an important personal power strategy. Once this career vision is developed, one

must create opportunities to move toward that vision. Such planning is empowering; it puts the nurse in charge, rather than letting a career unfold by chance. Having this sense of vision is consistent with the commitment to a career in nursing that is part of developing a power image. This vision is always subject to change as new opportunities are experienced, and new interests, knowledge, and skills are gained. Education and work experiences are tools for achieving the vision of one's career.

Developing Expertise

As noted earlier in this chapter, expertise is one of the bases of power. Developing expertise in nursing is an important power strategy. Expertise must not be limited to clinical knowledge. Leadership and communication skills, for example, are essential to the effective exercise of power in a range of nursing roles. Education and practice provide the means for developing such expertise in any of the domains of nursing: clinical practice, education, research, and management. Developing expertise expands one's power among nursing colleagues, other professional colleagues, and patients. A high level of expertise can make one nearly indispensable within an organization. This is a powerful position to have within any organization, whether it is the workplace or a professional association. A high level of expertise can also lead to a high level of visibility within an organization.

High Visibility

The strategy of high visibility within an organization also requires volunteering to serve as a member or the chairperson of committees and task forces. High visibility can be nurtured by attending the open meetings of committees and other groups of which you are not a member in the workplace, professional associations, or the community. Review the agendas of such meetings if they are circulated ahead of the meeting. Use opportunities both before and after meetings to share your expertise, providing valuable information and ideas to members and leaders of such groups. Share this expertise at open meetings when appropriate. Speak up confidently, but have something relevant to say. Be concise and precise; members of the committee will ask for more information if they need it. Create your own business cards using a computer and sheets of business card stock (this can be purchased at any office supply store). Give members of these committees your personal card so that they can contact you later for information.

EXERCISING POWER AND INFLUENCE IN THE WORKPLACE AND OTHER ORGANIZATIONS: SHAPING POLICY

To use influence effectively in any organization, one must understand how the system works and develop organizational strategies. Developing organizational savvy includes identifying the real decision makers and those persons who have a high level of influence with the decision makers. Recognize the informal leaders within any organization. In the workplace an influential senior staff nurse may have more decision-making power than the nurse manager on significant aspects of the nursing unit's operations. The senior staff nurse may have more clinical expertise and a greater wealth of knowledge about the history of the unit and its personnel than a nurse manager with excellent management and leadership skills who is new to the unit.

Secretaries of chief nurse executives (CNEs), for example, are usually very powerful people, although they are not always recognized as such. The CNE's secretary has a great deal of control over information, making decisions about who gets to meet with the nurse executive and when, screening incoming and outgoing mail, letting the CNE know when a letter or memo needs immediate attention, or placing a memo on the bottom of the stack of mail for review at a later time.

Collegiality and Collaboration

Nursing does not exist in a vacuum, nor do nurses work in isolation from one another, other professionals, and support personnel. Nurses function within a wide range of organizations, such as schools, hospitals, community health organizations, government agencies, professional associations, and universities. Nursing's historic lack of unity on important issues, such as basic educational preparation for entry into professional practice, has weakened our power base and political clout in the healthcare and educational systems (Barter & McFarland, 2001). Developing a sense of unity requires each nurse to act collaboratively and collegially in the workplace and in other organizations (e.g., professional associations). Collegiality demands that nurses value the accomplishments of nursing colleagues and express a sincere interest in their efforts. Turning to nursing colleagues for advice and support empowers them and expands one's

own power base at the same time. Unity of purpose does not contradict diversity of thought. One does not have to be a friend to everyone who is a colleague. Collegiality demands mutual respect, not friendship.

Collaboration and collegiality require that nurses work collectively to ensure that the voice of nursing is heard in the workplace and the legislature. Volunteer to serve on committees and task forces in the workplace, not only within the nursing department but also on organizationwide committees. Become an active member of nursing organizations, especially those that are represented by lobbyists in your state capital and in Washington. Get involved in the politics of the organization, whether in the workplace or through a professional association. If workplace organization uses shared governance or continuous quality improvement models, get involved in these councils, committees, task forces, and work groups to share your energy, ideas, and expertise. Many organizations have instituted joint practice committees that bring together nurses and physicians to improve the quality of interdisciplinary collaboration and, in turn, the quality of patient care. Become an active, productive member of such groups within the workplace and in the professional associations and community groups dealing with healthcare issues and problems. As illustrated in the Research Perspective, nurses can be very effective when working together on broad issues.

An Empowering Attitude

Demonstrate a positive and professional attitude about being a nurse to nursing colleagues, patients and their families, other colleagues in the workplace, and the public, including legislators. This attitude is very contagious and can empower colleagues while educating others about nurses and nursing. A power image is an important aspect of demonstrating this positive professional attitude. The current practice of nurses to identify themselves by first name only may decrease their power image in the eyes of physicians, patients, and others. Physicians are always addressed as "Doctor"; when they address others by their first names, inequality of power and status is evident. The use of first names among colleagues is not inappropriate, as long as everyone is playing by the same rules. Managers may want to enhance the empowerment of their staffs by encouraging them to introduce themselves as "Dr.," "Ms.," or "Mr." Arriving at work, appointments, or meetings on time; looking neat and appropriately attired for the work setting

Research Perspective

Gebbie, K. M., Wakefield, M., & Kerfoot, K. (2000). Nursing and health policy. *Journal of Nursing Scholarship, 32,* 307-315.

Nursing literature is filled with articles on the importance of nurses' involvement in public policy and political processes. For some nurses who participate in policy development, this is their nursing practice. Policy development may take many forms, including speaking publicly for patients, families, and communities where these people have little or no voice.

This study looked at what factors influenced nurses to make policy development their arena of practice. A sample of 27 nurses participated in telephone interviews that lasted from 20 minutes to 3 hours, with a mean length of 40 minutes. The participants had government positions (elected or appointed) or nongovernment, organizational positions (e.g., state nurses' association). Twenty-four were female. Twenty were older than 50 years of age. Twenty-four were white/Caucasian. Ten held an MSN. Sixteen held a doctoral degree.

Participants viewed policy development as another way nurses change people's lives. For some, involvement resulted from experiences with a key mentor or role model or a passion for a cause. For others, experiences shaped their activity as they assumed positions of increasing responsibility or as they became more aware of opportunities for involvement in policy development.

KEY FACTORS IN CREATING A PASSION FOR POLICY DEVELOPMENT

- *Family:* Parents or other family members who were politically active were cited as strong influences. One nurse cited her experiences as the parent of a hospitalized child.
- *Education:* Parochial school education was noted by many participants as a key factor, especially the influence of nuns who expected high levels of achievement. Nursing school experiences on activist campuses and exposure to courses in sociology, economics, or political science were also cited. Advanced education, including special mentorships and programs such as the Robert Wood Johnson Health Policy Fellowship, were also cited as factors.
- *Professional experience:* These nurses had experienced professional practice that demon-

strated to them how policy affects people's lives on a daily basis. Frustration with the failure of "the system" to meet the needs of people was another influence.
- *Organizations:* Involvement in various professional or health-related groups, working in political campaigns, and activity on political action committees (PACs) were also key influences.

RECOMMENDATIONS FOR IMPROVING AND EXPANDING NURSES' INVOLVEMENT IN POLICY DEVELOPMENT

The authors recommend three categories of activities for improving and expanding nurses' involvement in policy development based on their interviews with a sample of nursing activists in policy development.

1. Individual activity:
   - Educating self on policy and politics
   - Networking with individuals and groups related to policy
   - Joining nursing organizations
   - Linking research to politics and policy
   - Being visible at public forums on policy matters
2. Organizational activity:
   - Working through coalitions on policy matters
   - Articulating policy to bodies such as legislative committees based on nursing expertise
   - Setting agendas for meetings of organizations so that there is sufficient time to discuss policy strategies/activities
   - Working with the media
3. Educational activity:
   - Developing health policy course work and courses in nursing education programs
   - Encouraging students to join the student nurses association
   - Emphasizing opportunities for interdisciplinary work that focuses on policy development

IMPLICATIONS FOR PRACTICE

Taking time to commit to involvement in policy development can yield personal and professional benefits as well as public benefits.

or other professional situation; and speaking positively about one's work are examples of how easy it is to demonstrate a positive, powerful, and professional attitude.

▌ *Exercise 25–5*

How do you routinely introduce yourself to patients, families, physicians, and other colleagues? A powerful and positive approach involves making eye contact with each individual, shaking hands, and introducing yourself by saying, "I'm Terry Jones, a registered nurse [or nursing student]." If you do not currently use this technique, try it out. Note any difference in the responses of people whom you meet using this technique in comparison with your usual approach.

Developing Coalitions

The exercise of power is often directed at creating change. Although an individual can often be effective at exercising power and creating change, creating certain changes within most organizations requires collective action. Coalition building is an effective political strategy for collective action. **Coalitions** are groups of individuals or organizations that join together temporarily around a common goal. This goal often focuses on an effort to effect change. The networking between organizations that results in coalition building requires members of one group to reach out to members of other groups. This often occurs at the leadership level and may come through formal mechanisms, such as letters that identify an issue or problem—a shared interest—around which a coalition could be built. For example, a state nurses' association may invite the leaders of organizations interested in child health (e.g., organizations of pediatric nurses, public health nurses and physicians, elementary school teachers, day-care providers) and consumers (e.g., parents) to discuss collaborative support for a legislative initiative to improve access to immunization programs in urban and rural areas. Such coalitions of professionals and consumers are powerful in influencing public policy related to healthcare.

Enlisting the support of others who share the same goal or interest often results in greater success in effecting change and exercising power in the workplace and within other organizations, including legislative bodies (Stanhope, 1999; Wakefield, 1999). Expanding networks in the workplace, as suggested earlier in this chapter, facilitates creating a coalition by developing a pool of candidates for coalition building before they are needed. Invite people with common goals to lunch or coffee. Discuss this shared interest and gain the commitment of the individual. Meet over lunch or coffee with members of the committee or task force that is working on this issue. Attend the open meetings of professional groups that share the same interests as the organization to which you belong. Share ideas on how to create the desired change most effectively.

Coalition building is an important skill for involvement in legislative politics. Nursing organizations often use coalition building when dealing with state legislatures and Congress. Changes in nurse practice acts to expand opportunities for advanced nursing practice have been accomplished in many states through coalition building. Such changes are often opposed by state medical societies or the state agencies that license physicians. Efforts by a single nursing organization (e.g., a state nurses' association or a nurse practitioners' organization), representing a limited nursing constituency, often lack the clout to overcome opposition by the unified voice of the state's physicians. However, the unified effort of a coalition of nursing organizations, other healthcare organizations, and consumer groups can be powerful in effecting change through legislation.

Negotiating

Kritek (2002) points out nursing's vulnerability in the title of her book *Negotiating at an Uneven Table*. **Negotiating,** or bargaining, is a critically important skill for organizational and political power. It is a process of making trade-offs. Children are natural negotiators. Often, they will initially ask their parents for more than what they are willing to accept in the way of privileges, toys, or activities. The logic is simple to children: Ask for more than is reasonable and negotiate down to what you really want!

Negotiating often works the same way within organizations. People will sometimes ask for more than what they want and be willing to accept less. In other situations, both sides will enter a negotiation asking for radically different things, but each may be willing to settle for a position that differs significantly from their original positions. In the simplest forms of bargaining, each participant has something that the other party values: goods, services, or information. At the "bargaining table" each party presents an opening position, and the process moves on until they reach a mutually agreeable result or until one or both parties walk away from the unsuccessful process.

Bargaining may take many forms. Individuals may negotiate with a supervisor for a more desirable work schedule or with a peer to effect a schedule change so that the nurse can attend an out-of-town conference. A nurse manager may sit at the bargaining table with the department director during budget planning to expand training hours for the nursing unit in the next year's budget. A group of nurses may bargain with nursing and hospital administration over wages, staffing levels, other working conditions, and the conditions and policies that govern clinical practice. This is called *collective bargaining*, a specific type of negotiating that is regulated by both state and federal labor laws and that usually involves representation by a state nurses' association or a nursing or nonnursing labor union (see Chapter 10). Representatives of a coalition of nursing organizations meeting with a legislator may negotiate with the legislator over sections of a proposed healthcare-related bill in an effort to eliminate or modify those sections not viewed by the nursing coalition as in the best interests of nurses, patients, or the healthcare system.

Successful negotiators are well informed about not only their own positions but also those of the opposing side. Successful negotiators must be able to discuss the pros and cons of both positions. They are able to assist the other party in recognizing the costs versus the benefits of each position. These skills are also essential to exercising power effectively with the arenas of professional and legislative politics. When lobbying a member of the legislature to support a bill that is desired by nurses, one must understand the position of those opposed to the bill to respond effectively to questions that the legislator may ask.

■ *Exercise 25–6*

Consider a situation in which you engaged in bargaining or negotiating. Have you ever bought a car? Negotiating the price of the car is a great American tradition. Few people enter into the purchase of a car intending to pay the sticker price. Most sticker prices are set by the manufacturer at a level that gives the dealer room to negotiate the price down. Have you ever negotiated a schedule change at work or school? Have you ever negotiated a raise in your salary? What was the trade-off you made in the process? How far did the other person move from his or her original position? What factors led to your success or failure in this negotiation?

Taking Political Action to Influence Policy

In the 1990s Carolyn McCarthy was a licensed practical nurse (LPN) from New York when a tragedy turned her life around. Her husband was killed and her son injured by a gunman on the Long Island Railroad. She sought the support of her congressman on gun control legislation as a result of her personal tragedy. He refused to support such legislation. She took extraordinary action, changing her party affiliation from Republican to Democrat and then running against the incumbent for his seat in Congress. Today she is still an LPN, but she is also Congresswoman Carolyn McCarthy (D-NY). Taking action may include such simple acts as working in a legislative campaign or volunteering to work on a church committee to establish a parish health ministry. Extraordinary actions like those taken by Carolyn McCarthy are also essential for nursing's voice to be heard loudly and clearly in the uncertain future.

Meier (1999) recommends some basic strategies for political action:

- Join political organizations.
- Build a working relationship with a single legislator.
- Invite a legislator to a professional organization meeting.
- Invite a legislator or staff person from the legislator's office to spend a day with you at work.

Additional political action strategies include the following:

- Register to vote and vote in every election.
- Join your state nurses' association and get involved with the association's government relations or legislative committee and political action committee (PAC).
- Be in touch with your federal and state legislators on nursing and healthcare issues, especially related to specific bills, by letter writing, telephone calls, or emails.
- Participate in nurse lobby day and meet with your state legislators.
- Work on a federal or state legislative campaign.
- Visit your U.S. senators and member of Congress if visiting in the Washington, DC, area to discuss federal legislation related to nursing and healthcare.
- Get involved in the local group of your political party.
- Run for office at the local, county, state, or congressional level.

Brendtro and Schwerin (2000) offer additional strategies for political action to shape policy, some of which have been noted elsewhere in this chapter:

- Use power effectively.
- Always appear self-confident.
- Empower others to work on policy issues.
- Build your visibility.
- Build relationships through coalitions and networks.
- Identify resources, human and physical, that can support your efforts.

- Enhance the image of nursing in all your policy efforts.
- Communicate your message effectively and clearly.
- Develop your expertise in shaping policy.
- Seek appointive positions or elective office to shape policy more effectively.

The Political Astuteness Inventory (Goldwater & Zusy, 1990) is a helpful tool in determining how well prepared you are to influence legislative politics and public policy, especially public policy related to healthcare (Box 25-3).

BOX 25-3

Political Astuteness Inventory

Place a check mark (√) next to those items for which your answer is yes. Then give yourself one point for each yes. After completing the inventory, compare your total score with the scoring criteria at the end of the inventory.

1. I am registered to vote.
2. I know where my voting precinct is located.
3. I voted in the last general election.
4. I voted in the last two elections.
5. I recognized the names of the majority of the candidates on the ballot and was acquainted with the majority of issues in the last election.
6. I stay abreast of current health issues.
7. I belong to the state professional or student nurse organization.
8. I participate (e.g., as a committee member, officer) in this organization.
9. I attended the most recent meeting of my district nurses' association.
10. I attended the last state or national convention held by my organization.
11. I am aware of at least two issues discussed and the stands taken at this convention.
12. I read literature published by my state nurses' association, a professional journal/magazine/newsletter, or other literature on a regular basis to stay abreast of current health issues.
13. I know the names of my senators in Washington.
14. I know the name of my representative in Washington.
15. I know the name of the state senator from my district.
16. I know the name of the state representative from my district.
17. I am acquainted with the voting record of at least one of the above in relation to a specific health issue.
18. I am aware of the stand taken by at least one of the above in relation to a specific health issue.
19. I know whom to contact for information about health-related issues at the state or federal level.
20. I know whether my professional organization employs lobbyists at the state or federal level.
21. I know how to contact these lobbyists.
22. I contribute financially to my state and national professional organization's political action committee (PAC).
23. I give information about effectiveness of elected officials to assist the PAC's endorsement process.
24. I actively supported a senator or representative during the last election.
25. I have written to one of my state or national representatives in the last year regarding a health issue.
26. I am personally acquainted with a senator or representative or member of his or her staff.
27. I serve as a resource person for one of my representatives or his or her staff.

From Goldwater, M., & Zusy, M. J. L. (1990). *Prescription for nurses: Effective political action.* St. Louis: Mosby.

Continued

BOX 25-3

Political Astuteness Inventory—*cont'd*

28. I know the process by which a bill is introduced in my state legislature.
29. I know which senators or representatives are supportive of nursing.
30. I know which House and Senate committees usually deal with health-related issues.
31. I know the committees of which my representatives are members.
32. I know of at least two health issues related to my profession that are currently under discussion.
33. I know of at least two health-related issues that are currently under discussion at the state or national level.
34. I am aware of the composition of the state board that regulates my profession.
35. I know the process whereby one becomes a member of the state board that regulates my profession.
36. I know what DHHS stands for.
37. I have at least a vague notion of the purpose of the DHHS.
38. I am a member of a health board or advisory group to a health organization or agency.
39. I attend public hearings related to health issues.
40. I find myself more interested in political issues now than in the past.

Scoring:
0-9	Totally unaware politically/apathetic
10-19	Slightly more aware of the implications of the politics of nursing/buy-in
20-29	Beginning political astuteness/self-interest to political sophistication
30-40	Politically astute, an asset to nursing/leading the way

From Goldwater, M., & Zusy, M. J. L. (1990). *Prescription for nurses: Effective political action.* St. Louis: Mosby.

The Solution

The PAC chairperson and the SNA lobbyist put out an action alert by mail, email, and telephone to alert members to this situation. This alert resulted in hundreds of calls to members of the senate committee from SNA members, other registered nurses, and student nurses. The members of the committee were overwhelmed with calls in opposition to the hostile amendment. In addition, the executive director of the SNA testified at the hearing about the disastrous results this hostile amendment would hold for quality healthcare in the state. By using their collective power, nurses were successful in defeating this amendment, thus shaping public policy related to the integrity of the state's nursing practice act and other licensing laws.

— Gail Haller

 Would this be a suitable approach for you? Why?

CHAPTER CHECKLIST

Power was once a taboo issue in nursing. The exercise of power in nursing conflicted sharply with the historic feminine stereotypes that surrounded nursing. The evolving social and political status of women has also opened nursing to the exercise of power. Power is essential to the effective implementation of both the clinical and the managerial roles of nurses.

■ Contemporary concepts of power focus on power as influence and a force for collaboration rather than coercion, an infinite quality rather than a finite quantity.
■ Empowerment is a feminine-feminist process of power sharing and leadership.

- Contemporary views of leadership in social systems are consistent with the concept of empowerment.
- Seven types of power exercised by nurses include the following:
  - Coercive
  - Reward
  - Expert
  - Legitimate
  - Referent
  - Information
  - Connection
- Key factors in developing a powerful image include the following:
  - Self-confidence
  - Body language
  - Self-image
  - Career commitment
  - Grooming and dress
  - Speech
  - Attitudes, beliefs, and values
  - Continuing professional education
- Key personal and organizational strategies for exercising power include the following:
  - Communication skills
  - Career goal setting
  - High visibility
  - A sense of unity
  - Coalition building
  - Networking
  - Expertise
  - Organizational savvy
  - Collaboration and collegiality
- Negotiation skills
- Mentoring
- An empowering attitude

TIPS ON POWER AND POLITICS

- Remember that power is not a "dirty word," nor is it an undesirable professional characteristic for nurses; it is the ability to influence others effectively.
- By exercising power in the workplace and other professional activities, you empower patients, families, and colleagues to accomplish their goals.
- Believing in your own ability to create change (i.e., exercise power), valuing the exercise of power, and projecting a powerful image (e.g., grooming, manners, body language, verbal communication skills) are essential to functioning as an influential professional nurse.
- Participating in networking and mentoring, setting clear career goals, and developing your expertise are key power strategies.
- Shaping policy is an extension of nursing practice, part of the nurse's advocacy role.

TERMS TO KNOW

coalitions	network
empowerment	policy
influence	politics
negotiating	power

REFERENCES

Anderson, K. N., Anderson, L. E., & Glanze, W. D. (1998). *Mosby's medical, nursing, & allied health dictionary* (5th ed.). St. Louis: Mosby.

Ashley, J. A. (1976). *Hospitals, paternalism, and the role of the nurse.* New York: Teachers College Press.

Barter, M., & McFarland, P. L. (2001). BSN by 2010: A California initiative. *Journal of Nursing Administration, 31,* 141-144.

Brendto, M., & Schwerin, J. (2000, June). *Influencing nursing practice through participation in the public policy process.* Paper presented at American Nurses Association 2000 Biennial Convention, Indianapolis.

Chinn, P. L. (2001). *Peace and power: Building communities for the future* (5th ed.). Sudbury, MA: Jones and Bartlett.

Cohen, S. S., Mason, D. J., Kovner, C., Leavitt, J. K., Pulcini, J., & Sochalski, J. (1996). Stages of nursing political development: Where we've been and where we ought to go. *Nursing Outlook, 44,* 259-266.

Cunningham, M. P. (2000). Breaking the mold: The many legacies of nurses in progressive movements. *American Journal of Nursing, 100*(10), 121, 123-124, 126, 129, 131, 133, 135-136.

Ferguson, V. (1993). Perspectives on power. In D. J. Mason, S. W. Talbott, & J. K. Leavitt (Eds.), *Policy and politics for nurses* (2nd ed.). Philadelphia: WB Saunders.

Gebbie, K. M., Wakefield, M., & Kerfoot, K. (2000). Nursing and health policy. *Journal of Nursing Scholarship, 32,* 307-315.

Goldwater, M., & Zusy, M. J. L. (1990). *Prescription for nurses: Effective political action*. St. Louis: Mosby.

Hersey, P., Blanchard, K., & Natemeyer, W. (1979). Situational leadership, perception and impact of power. *Group and Organizational Studies, 4*, 418-428.

Kalisch, B. J., & Kalisch, P. A. (1982). *Politics of nursing*. Philadelphia: JB Lippincott.

Kritek, P. B. (2002). *Negotiating at an uneven table: A practical approach to working with differences and diversity* (2nd ed.). San Francisco: Jossey-Bass.

Lukas, K. M. (2001). Use the media: Seek the spotlight. *American Journal of Nursing, 101*(3), 65-66.

Meier, E. (1999). Political activities for rainy days. *Nurse Educator, 17*(3), 181-182.

Roberts, S. J. (1983). Oppressed group behavior: Implications for nursing. *Advances in Nursing Sciences, 5*, 21-30.

Schutzenhofer, K. K. (1995). Networking and professionalism. In M. Strader & P. J. Decker (Eds.), *Role transition to patient care management*. Norwalk, CT: Appleton & Lange.

Schwirian, P. M. (1998). *Professionalization of nursing*. Philadelphia: Lippincott.

Stanhope, M. (1999). Health policy: Strategies for analysis and influence. In J. Lancaster (Ed.), *Nursing issues in leading and managing change*. St. Louis: Mosby.

Stewart, B. M., & Kruger, L. E. (1996). An evolutionary concept of mentoring in nursing. *Journal of Professional Nursing, 12*, 311-321.

Wakefield, M. (1999). Nursing future in health care policy. In E. J. Sullivan (Ed.), *Creating nursing's future: Issues, opportunities, and challenges*. St. Louis: Mosby.

SUGGESTED READINGS

Ashley, J. A. (1980). Power in structured misogyny: Implications for the politics of care. *Advances in Nursing Science, 2*, 3-22.

Borman, J., & Biordi, D. (1992). Female nurse executive: Finally, at an advantage? *Journal of Nursing Administration, 22*(9), 37-41.

Campbell-Heider, N., & Hart, C. A. (1993). Updating the nurse's bedside manner. *Image: Journal of Nursing Scholarship, 25*, 133-139.

del Bueno, D. (1986). Power and policy in organizations. *Nursing Outlook, 34*, 124-128.

Dobos, C. (1997). Understanding personal risk taking among staff nurses: Critical information for nurse administrators. *Journal of Nursing Administration, 27*(1), 12-13.

Fisher, R., Ury, W., & Patton, B. (1991). *Getting to yes: Negotiating agreement without giving in* (2nd ed.). New York: Penguin.

Heim, P., & Goliant, S. K. (1993). *Hardball for women: Winning at the game of business*. Los Angeles: Plume Books.

Holloran, S. D. (1993). Mentoring: The experience of nursing service executives. *Journal of Nursing Administration, 23*(2), 49-54.

Kippenbrock, T. A. (1992). Power at meetings: Strategies to move people. *Nursing Economics, 10*, 282-286.

Laschinger, H. K. S., & Havens, D. S. (1996). Staff nurse work empowerment and perceived control over nursing practice: Conditions for work effectiveness. *Journal of Nursing Administration, 26*(9), 27-35.

Schutzenhofer, K. K. (1992). Essential for the year 2000. *Nursing Connections, 5*(1), 15-26.

Schutzenhofer, K. K., Shelley, S. R., & Pontious, S. L. (1992). Communication systems. In P. J. Decker & E. J. Sullivan (Eds.), *Nursing administration: A micro/macro approach for effective nurse executives*. Norwalk, CT: Appleton & Lange.

Vance, C. N. (1985). Political influence: Building effective interpersonal skills. In D. J. Mason & S. W. Talbott (Eds.), *Political action handbook for nurses: Changing the workplace, government, and organizations, and community*. Menlo Park, CA: Addison-Wesley.

Wolf, G. A. (1989). The effective use of influence. *Journal of Nursing Administration, 19*(11), 8-9.

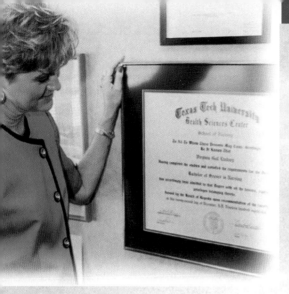

26

Career Management: Putting Yourself in Charge

Karen A. Dadich

This chapter focuses on planning and developing a professional career. These elements include identifying a career style and developing the tools needed to create career opportunities. Career development is linked to ongoing professional development. The concept of continuous lifelong learning and elements of the process of professional certification are introduced.

Objectives

- Differentiate between career styles and how they influence career options.
- Analyze person-position fit.
- Evaluate the relevance of a cover letter, curriculum vitae, and résumé as entries to interviews.
- Use critical elements of the cover letter, résumé or curriculum vitae to develop each.
- Analyze critical elements of an interview.

- Compare and contrast different types of professional learning opportunities.

- Value professional expectations.

Questions to Consider

- *What excites you about nursing?*
- *What clinical nursing experience has been most stimulating and challenging? Why?*
- *What excites you about leadership and management options?*
- *What do you want to be doing in 3 years?*

The Challenge

Rebecca A. Brawley, RN, BSN
Public Health Coordinator/Prevention Manager, City of Lubbock Health Department, Lubbock, Texas

I began my nursing career as a licensed vocational nurse. My peers and I worked in a very relaxed environment with very effective communication among ourselves. Most of the time, the nurse manager was not included in our activities. Nor did we share information about our lives with her. With the encouragement of my husband and a close nursing colleague, I decided to return to school to complete a baccalaureate in nursing.

Following graduation, I returned to the unit where I had worked as an licensed vocational nurse (LVN) for more than 8 years and assumed the position of charge nurse on the day shift. Although I was confident that I was educationally prepared to assume this role, it never entered my mind that I would be making assignments and directing the care of my former peers. I asked myself, "How do I handle this? Do I remain a peer and a friend?

How do I keep my staff from abusing me? Will they see me as their peer and friend, or a manager? Will they do the work I assign or take it as an insult if I assign too much work?" My worst fears about each of these questions came true.

Initially, I tried to remain the friend and peer I had been before becoming the charge nurse. Clearly, that was not going to work. Quickly I discovered I was being used and abused not only by the staff who were my friends but also by staff who were new to the unit. I had to get the management of the day shift under control before it controlled me. How should I solve this problem?

 What do you think you would do if you were this nurse?

 ## INTRODUCTION

Although taking advantage of opportunities as they develop during a **career** is important, making decisions about what you want to do in nursing and how you can go about doing it is also important. Because a nursing career can extend across a lifetime and is not institutionally based (i.e., not defined by the institution but rather by law), the options for careers in nursing are vast. Some options build primarily on experience, others build primarily on educational background, and still others require a mix of education and experience. In general, you can assume that you must continue to learn and to develop your expertise to meet the challenges of this diverse profession. How you reach a career goal, however, depends on what goals you set and how you manage your own development.

 ## CAREER DEVELOPMENT

When you chose nursing as the focus of your professional career, you probably had no idea about the opportunities the profession would hold. The beginning of the twenty-first century reflected changes in the healthcare environment occurring at a fast and frantic pace. Solutions that resolve today's problems may not work for tomorrow's challenges. Throughout a nursing career, consumers, insurers, legislators, regulatory agencies, and professional peers will demand demonstration of competence in the areas of knowledge, judgment, and technical/interpersonal skills relevant to the position held (McCann, 1999).

A career can be defined as progress throughout an individual's professional life. A career can be developed in several ways. Some people, including professional nurses, have a series of positions with no connection among them. Others can have divergent positions that are connected in some way. Regardless of how careers develop, the real focus is continued competence.

There are several ways to develop a career. Basing career decisions on goals is a useful beginning. Some of the most notable work about careers has been conducted by Friss (1989), who identified four career styles (Box 26-1). One career pathway is not better than another; rather, each is different. For example, the types of positions sought differ. *Steady state* and *linear* are the traditional career styles. The first remains at a positional plateau and

BOX 26-1

Career Styles

	EXAMPLE	DESCRIPTION	MOTIVATION AND CHARACTERISTICS	MANAGERIAL COMPLICATIONS
Steady State	Staff nurses	Constancy in position with increasing professional skill	Increasing expertise High professional identity Obligation to serve Maintenance of standards Autonomy in performance of care Preference for action Personal accountability The work itself Stability	Hold work in high esteem Decentralize Use and recognize abilities Provide feedback about patient outcomes Reward competence and tenure Provide continuing education Provide permanent assignment
Linear	Nursing service administrator	Hierarchical orientation with steady climb	Requisite authority and power Had a challenging first job Guided by internalized norms Money Recognition Opportunities for self-development	Provide management development Reward and value both education and competence Modify management selection and development systems Provide decreasing supervision
Entrepreneurial and Transient	Nurses in private practice; temporary assignments	Desire to create new service; meeting own priorities	Limited organizational commitment Opportunists Novelty/creativity Other people Achievement	Use flexibility to organization's benefit Avoid burdening them with organizational and practice decisions Provide immediate feedback
Spiral	Nurse who returns after raising a family	Rational, independent responsibility for shaping career	Novelty Prestige Intense period of employment followed by nonemployment or a different employment Care for others Opportunities for self-development Typically well paid, service-oriented recognition	Configure specific job that needs doing Be flexible about terms and length of commitment Find challenging initial assignment Negotiate Encourage creativity

Modified from Friss, L. (1989). *Strategic management of nurses: A policy oriented approach.* Owings Mills, MD: AUPHA Press.

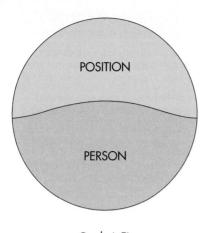

Goal: A Fit

Figure 26-1   Person-position fit.

becomes increasingly competent; the second moves up the hierarchy of the organization and becomes more diversified. The *entrepreneurial and transient style* is one that has fostered many nurses' creative bent. For a great deal of flexibility, and in a time of rapid changes in healthcare, this style can permit creative solutions to traditional problems. Finally, the *spiral* style is one seen in situations in which nurses move in and out of active practice and in situations in which nurses move in and out of a subspecialty focus, such as general pediatrics and neonatal nursing.

Several strategies can be used to elicit appropriate information before selecting a position to achieve a good person-position fit. A good fit is built on strong similar goals and tolerable (or growth-producing) differences. Figure 26-1 suggests that the whole of any work situation is composed of two elements interacting in an environment with other elements. That whole is symbolized by blending a person's talents with the position's expectations to create a productive whole.

In today's rapidly changing society, a position that was once "a fit" may no longer work. The position is as likely to change as is the person. In this situation a promotion may result from the expansion of a designated position. As a result, a new title/position description is created. Another nontraditional approach to promotions occurs when a major reorganization occurs and creates different positions to meet the redefined demands. Although neither of these promotion approaches may have been a part of an individual's career plan, both are likely to happen as healthcare continuously reshapes itself.

Irrespective of career style, core career development strategies are important. Selecting professional peers and mentors to share your development is important. Even the steady-state nurse who is not typically seeking a new position needs to develop a **curriculum vitae** (CV) or **résumé** that can document continued development of expertise. Interviewing, a two-way process, is also an important strategy to develop.

Few nurses have achieved a significant nursing career without assistance from peers and mentors. Heeding the "nay-sayers" can dampen career prospects. Having a few well-chosen peers and mentors who can respond openly with various perspectives to help with career decisions is important. For example, a nurse who seeks a career as a direct-care provider in an acute care setting could seek support from a mentor such as a charge nurse, nurse manager, or advanced practice nurse. The mentor provides honest appraisals of an individual's career development, suggests specific strategies to enhance development, and helps with meeting the leaders in an organization. Being in a relationship with a strong role model is also valuable.

CAREER MARKETING STRATEGIES

Although professional data can be recorded in numerous ways, the fact remains that most people do not do so in a systematic manner. Therefore, when information about one's career is needed, it is often difficult to recall. A goal of this chapter is to develop a systematic strategy for developing marketing documents that you can use throughout your professional career.

Data Collection

Depending on your unique background, the time spent on this activity varies considerably. The first step is to collect all previous professional information about yourself. If you are fairly new in the profession, analyze anything special you did in school, such as electives, offices held, and special assignments, and honors or special recognition that you received. If you have an employment history, start with your nursing positions. Keep in mind that you will need to include other relevant information. For example, serving as a volunteer at a rape crisis center may augment a brief professional history; serving as an officer of your student organization or on

Table 26-1 DATA COLLECTION

Topics	Facts Needed
1. Education	Name of school, address, telephone number, years of attendance, date of graduation, name of degree(s) received, minor earned, honors received (e.g., Dean's list), name of dean, faculty advisor, registrar's phone number
2. Continuing education	Date attended, places, topics and any special outcomes, type and amount of credit earned
3. Experience	Dates of employment, title of position, name of employing agency, location and phone number, name of chief executive officer, chief nursing officer, immediate supervisor, salary range, typical duties (role description)
4. Community/institutional service	Dates of service, name of committee/task force and the parent organization (e.g., name of hospital or professional organization), your role on the committee (e.g., chairperson, secretary, member), general description of committee's functions, any unique accomplishments
5. Publications	Articles: author(s) name(s), year of publication, title, journal, volume, issue, pages; books: author(s), year of publication, title, location, and name of publisher
6. Honors	Date, description of award, special factors related to award (e.g., competitive, communitywide, national)
7. Research	Date, title of research, role in research (e.g., principal investigator, co-investigator, team member), funded/unfunded
8. Speeches/presentations given	Date, title of speech presented, place, name of sponsoring organization, nature of the presentation (e.g., keynote, concurrent session), your honorarium
9. Workshops/conferences presented	Date, title of workshop/conference presented, place, name of sponsoring group and nature of the presentation, brief description of the activity, your honorarium
10. Certification	Initial date of certification, expiration date, certifying body, area/type of certification

the board of a voluntary association may be useful to secure a position with similar responsibilities. In addition, each of the aforementioned examples conveys a professional commitment to community life.

To begin data collection, it may be useful to start where you are and think back. If you have limited "thinking back" to do, you are in great shape for starting a systematic plan. If, however, you have been practicing nursing for a long time or had "another life" before your nursing career, you may have more difficulty compiling the information. In fact, some information may be irretrievable—do not dwell on that aspect, just record as much as you can recall. In either case, the important thing is to begin the process.

Using the categories identified in Table 26-1, compile as many facts for each category as you can recall. If you do not have information for a specific topic heading, for example, publications, create the topic heading anyway. When you publish your first article, you will have a place to record the pertinent details. Remember, the information you compile today will not have to be remembered tomorrow.

It is most useful to do this data entry on your computer. A table with headings will facilitate the process. If you do not have access to a computer, the data collection process can be done using file cards with dividers for the separate categories. One card with all the required information for *each* item in a heading will make this file useful. Whether you use a computer or a file box for organizing these topic headings and all the pertinent data about yourself, this compilation of facts is for your use only. This data bank serves as your professional career memory.

Draft an entry for your data bank. If you have sufficient time, draft a CV and résumé now. The Merlin website for this text contains an example of each. As a checkpoint for yourself, make a list of four to five professional facts/qualities that you want others to know about. You can use this list in checking your CV or résumé and in interviewing. Keep in mind that a CV or résumé serves one primary purpose—letting others know enough about you that they want to meet you, advance your career, or gain more information.

Curriculum Vitae

A CV is a listing of professional life activities. It is designed to be all-inclusive but not detailed. This document lists all your professional accomplishments without elaboration on the details of your career. It is an effective tool for listing all the facts of your professional life.

To develop a CV, simply select a logical flow of information and assemble. Information should be presented in reverse chronological order. In this way, attention is drawn to your latest contributions and is a better presentation than a historic chronological sequence. Include your name, credentials, degrees, address, phone number, fax number, and email address in the heading of the document. This set of information should be distinct so that you are easy to contact.

Arranging the information facts by category, assemble a CV that reflects all professional involvement. The CV contains profile data about each entry; no lengthy descriptions are required. The document must be typed and appear organized. The use of subheadings for each topic facilitates development.

Résumé

A résumé is a customized document developed to highlight your accomplishments and tailored to describe the way in which you can fulfill a role or meet the needs of a specific organization. Unlike the CV, the résumé is detailed. A résumé sells the individual for the specific position being sought and illustrates the fit of an individual for a specific position. For the steady-state nurse, a résumé could be used to reflect increasing skills and abilities; for others, a résumé can create specific messages about an individual's unique experiences, education, and abilities in relation to a new opportunity.

To sell yourself, you need to provide more than the facts. You need to include details. Although the information needs to be brief and to the point, it should be meaningful and reflect your experience and your accomplishments. The ideal résumé is one page, although two pages are acceptable. When detailing your accomplishments, use action words that describe your experiences. For example, if you were a volunteer for the American Diabetes Association annual "Walk for America," describing your role as a "volunteer fundraiser" is more meaningful than saying a "volunteer." Consider use of action words that typify activities of your career. Words such as *developed, created,* and *initiated* convey a powerful message in a résumé. It is important to "quantify for the organization the economic value you can potentially deliver" (Fox, 2001, p. 30).

The résumé is the best choice for selling your abilities to a potential employer. It is designed to focus on an individual's special abilities in relation to the organizational need as described in the position description. When developing a résumé, avoid fads, buzz words, and automated formats for résumé building. Using an automated format for résumé building may seem like a "quick fix," but the end product will look like all the other résumés developed in this fashion. Because your résumé will look like many others, it will be less likely to be read critically. In our world of rapid change, fads and buzz words are soon outdated. Posting a résumé on the Internet is an example of a fad whose popularity is questionable. Although many have posted their résumé on the numerous Internet sites available, few employers even look at the posted documents (Bolles, 2001).

Your customized résumé should be error free and grammatically correct, present an accurate and articulate portrayal of your accomplishments, and be printed on high-quality paper, preferably 100% cotton bond.

There are basically two ways to develop a résumé: a conventional or a functional approach. In either case the document should include your name, address, phone number, fax number, and email address at the top of the page. The conventional approach provides an optional career summary and includes position title, name and address (city and state only), inclusive dates, and a succinct description of responsibilities and achievements. Education and other categories of special meaning that relate to the position sought should be included. (This information will be in your database of facts about yourself.)

The functional approach provides a career summary and identifies role functions that you have filled during your career. Those functions might include staff nurse, manager, and educator, to name a few. A functional approach is best if you are planning a sharp departure from your present position. The focus is on your experience in diverse roles, not on the specific positions held. Education and other categories of special meaning may be added.

Professional Letters

During your career you will develop a series of letters to meet specific needs as you market yourself. These include a cover letter, a thank-you letter, and a resignation letter. Typically, these letters have common elements and individual characteristics that make each one unique.

All of these letters should include your name, address, phone number, fax number, and email address as they appear on your résumé or CV. Designating both daytime and evening telephone numbers may be helpful. Placing this information in a format similar to that used on your résumé or CV will make an effective package when you present your documents. Quality-bond paper reflects the image you wish to portray.

Each of these letters should be no longer than one page. The date and an inside address should be included. An inside address includes the name (with credentials) of the addressee, the person's title, the name of the organization, street address, city, state, and zip code. The inside address is followed by the salutation. Usually, first names are not used. The typical salutation, "Dear Ms. Smith," for example, is followed by a colon.

Each of these professional letters usually contains three paragraphs, which are described in the following sections. The closing follows the text of the letter; the closing is followed by your name. The usual spacing between the closing (e.g., "Sincerely") and your name is four lines. Include your full name with credentials and degrees. Sign your name as it is typed using black or blue ink. Proof all letters for layout, typographical errors, spelling, and content.

Cover Letter

The cover letter is the key to getting your résumé read. It is a brief but carefully written document that is a vital source of information. The cover letter includes a statement that indicates why you are writing, why you "fit" the organization and a specific position or type of position, and how you will follow up.

Numerous positions may be advertised by an organization simultaneously. In addition, an organization may use a variety of vehicles to issue a call for applicants. Thus immediately stating why you are writing is crucial. It is often helpful to identify how you learned of the position.

Once you have stated your reason for writing, you should address the issue of "why you." The second paragraph should indicate why someone should take time to read your attached résumé. This section should state what you know about the organization and how you will fit in. Examples of competencies can be included to clarify your strengths. Reference to the enclosed résumé or CV is appropriate. Fox (2001) calls a cover letter an "impact letter" and states "a good impact letter demonstrates your potential to make an impact" (p. 49).

The closing paragraph should convey optimism— that is, you anticipate being interviewed. If you want to assure yourself of having an additional opportunity to sell yourself, you should indicate when you will follow up with a phone call.

> ■ *Exercise 26–2*
>
> Write a cover letter that highlights information from at least two items from your data bank. Select items that best market you and that will entice the reader to call you for an interview.

Thank-You Letter

Once again, the business format described earlier is used in a formal thank-you letter. Written and sent within 24 hours of the interview, the thank-you letter may be the last chance to "sell" yourself. For this reason, careful thought should be given to what you need to say in this document.

The lead paragraph should recall the interview date and purpose so that the reader can place you. If you discussed more than one position, list your preference first and follow it with "as well as other positions."

To help the interviewer remember you, the body of the letter should focus on elements of the interview. If a key point was described as crucial, focus your comments about your ability on that point. Use action words in describing your fit in this organization.

The closing paragraph should reference specific times identified in the interview. These times may include when you expect to hear about a position offer or when you are available. In addition, this section includes a statement of what you will do and when you will do it if you do not hear from the interviewer. This action indicates to the prospective employer that you expect to maintain control of your career.

Resignation Letter

When you secure a new position, it is essential to resign effectively from your current position. A letter slipped under a manager's office door should not be the initial mechanism for notifying an organization of your intent to leave. A face-to-face meeting between you and your manager is most effective. Your resignation should be given with adequate notice. Conditions of employment will define adequate notice.

The face-to-face meeting is followed by a formal letter of resignation. Again, the business format is used. The introductory paragraph references the meeting at which you stated your intent to resign. Your date of resignation is identified and indication of whether this date is negotiable is included.

BOX 26-2

Checklist for Constructing Marketing Documents

Data Collection
_____ 1. Data sets are used for information development.
_____ 2. Information is assembled in categorical manner.

Data Assembly
_____ 1. Discrete categories are used.
_____ 2. Assembly addresses specific position.
_____ 3. Current name, address, telephone number, voice mail, and email address are prominent (use as many as are appropriate for you).
_____ 4. Career summary (if used) (or cover letter) is prominent.
_____ 5. Key points about positions/experiences are evident.
_____ 6. A logical flow is evident.
_____ 7. Grammar, spelling, and syntax are correct.
_____ 8. Writing style is positive and direct, but not terse.
_____ 9. Action verbs are evident.
_____ 10. If writing in full sentences, third person and passive voice are avoided (i.e., write in the active voice).
_____ 11. "Canned" résumé language is avoided (e.g., "distinguished" and "all phases of...").
_____ 12. Emphasis is on competence, not years (cover letter).
_____ 13. Specific examples of key competences are cited (cover letter).
_____ 14. The format is consistent throughout.
_____ 15. Personal information (e.g., health, marital status) is absent.

Appearance and Format
_____ 1. There are no typographical errors.
_____ 2. The product is "clean" (e.g., no smudges, no discrepant margins).
_____ 3. The product is readable (e.g., layout design is pleasing: white space, capitalization).
_____ 4. The paper is high-quality bond (100% cotton), white or cream.
_____ 5. The type is businesslike (no script); text is at least 10 to 12 points, and fonts are limited to one or two.
_____ 6. Emphasis is evident (e.g., centering and bold print or underlining).
_____ 7. The product is only one or two pages in length (not applicable for a CV).

Overview
_____ 1. It is attractive, interesting, quick reading, and competency based.
_____ 2. The package sells you.
_____ 3. You are pleased to have it precede you.
_____ 4. Additional items are enclosed or they are assembled for personal handling at an interview.
_____ 5. If you were receiving this CV or résumé, you would want to interview this person.

The second paragraph highlights aspects of the employment setting that enhanced your career development. Do not use your resignation letter to off-load negative feelings you may have about your current position. Keep in mind that you can always say something positive about any position you hold.

The closing paragraph concludes by asking for an exit evaluation. As you leave an organization, it is important to learn your final standing within the organization. Requesting a copy of this appraisal for your own records is also wise.

DATA ASSEMBLY CHECKLIST FOR PROFESSIONAL PORTFOLIOS

The checklist in Box 26-2 will help you keep track of your data and assemble the facts attractively. Inclusion of these elements ensures a comprehensive view of your professional contributions and comprises a portfolio.

THE INTERVIEW

Assuming you have used your career marketing strategies effectively, the next logical step is partici-

pating in an interview. Interviewing is a two-way proposition; the interviewee should be gathering as much information as the interviewer is. Both should be making judgments throughout the process so that if a position is offered, the interviewee will be prepared to accept, decline, or explore further. Interviews may take place with one or more individuals and may include a range of activities. To be at ease, the interviewee should wear comfortable but professional clothing. Rehearsing specific questions to ask and points to make can create comfort for these somewhat challenging situations. Be prepared to cite challenges and dilemmas you have faced and what you did and why because these types of questions may be posed to you.

Do not be deluded into thinking that because you are a nurse and there is a vacancy that you will automatically secure the position. Even in times of a nursing shortage, employers are using behavioral interviewing techniques to identify the most appropriate applicant for the vacant position. Rather than being asked, "What are your weaknesses?" you may be asked, "Tell me how you handled the last mistake you made" or "How did a baccalaureate program prepare you for critical care nursing?" Applicants in some organizations are also being screened and interviewed by a panel and being asked to participate in a series of interviews. This allows more participants to have a say in the hiring

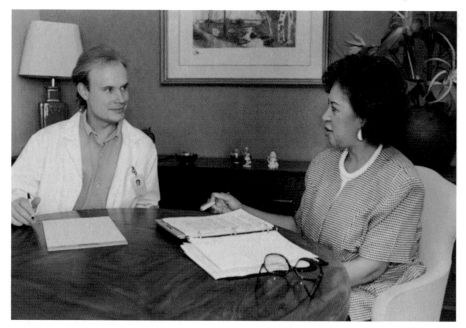

Interviewing is a two-way proposition in which both participants gather as much information as possible.

process. In the business setting, more than 40% of prospective employers are administering basic skills tests (Armour, 2001). You may see this practice in some healthcare settings as well.

Interview Topics and Questions of Concern

During interviews, employers should ask all applicants for a given position the same questions. In addition to providing comparable information as the basis for a decision, the applicant's expectation for equal treatment is upheld. Only questions related to the position and its description are legitimate. Employers should not ask other questions (Box 26-3), and applicants should express appropriate concern if asked such inappropriate questions.

If the interviewer asks an inappropriate question, the applicant can choose not to answer the direct question by addressing the content area. For example, if asked about your spouse's employment, you might say, "I believe what you are asking is how long I will be able to be in this position. Let me assure you that I intend to be here for at least 2 years."

Each of the content areas in Box 26-3 may be acceptable, but the question is phrased inappropriately. The following examples are ways to verify/secure the information as an employer, in a manner that is both appropriate and legal.

1. Do you know that this position requires someone at least 21 years old?
2. This position requires that no one in your immediate family be in the healthcare field or own interest/shares in any healthcare facility. Does this pose a problem for you?
3. Attendance is important. Are you able to meet this expectation?
4. What are your short- and long-term goals?
5. Is there anything that would prevent you from performing this work as described?
6. This position requires U.S. citizenship. May I assume you meet this criterion?
7. What professional organizations do you belong to?
8. As you have read in our philosophy, we subscribe to a Christian philosophy. Do you understand that all employees are expected to promote that philosophy?

The key to ensuring a fair interviewing process is being prepared ahead of time and knowing what can be asked legitimately and what a reasonable answer is.

BOX 26-3

Sample of Inappropriate Questions

1. How old are you?
2. What does your husband (wife) do?
3. Who takes care of your children?
4. Are you working "just to help out"?
5. Do you have any disabilities?
5. Where were you born?
6. What are the names of all organizations to which you belong?
8. What is your religious preference?

Exercise 26-3

Select a partner and role play an interview for a professional nursing position. The potential employer (manager) should focus on competencies of the prospective employee. Include questions and scenarios about common conflicts and challenges seen in the clinical setting. The interviewee (prospective employee) should highlight competencies, decision-making abilities, and critical-thinking abilities when responding to the situationally based questions.

If you have prepared well, you will know what the organization's stated beliefs are and whether they are compatible with yours. The challenge in an interview is to determine whether those beliefs are lived or merely printed words. If numerous people can relate how the mission actually is translated in a specific role, the beliefs are likely lived ones.

This chapter includes two tools designed to be used in preparing for an interview: "Checklist for Interviewing" (Box 26-4), and "Interview Goals and Content" (Table 26-2). Using the thank-you letter described earlier in this chapter is an additional opportunity to market yourself, especially if you wish to correct or expand on an answer you provided during the interview.

The interrelationship of these strategies allows people to emphasize specialization or diversity. Each strategy leads to the next so that the potential for attaining a preferred position is enhanced. As careers progress, factors other than the specific nursing school or in-school activities take precedence in influencing career development and how an individual is seen by others. Thus updating a CV or résumé is important. Keeping a passion alive must be evident.

The Career Tips (p. 466) will help to keep your career vibrant.

BOX 26-4

Checklist for Interviewing

1. Check interviewing guides, such as *What Color Is Your Parachute?*
2. Check out the new organization.
   a. Review the organization's mission, vision, and values statements before the interview (via the web or hard copy).
   b. Obtain statistics and facts.
   c. Ask about new directions.
3. Recheck your résumé or curriculum vitae for the following:
   a. Emphasis
   b. New information
4. Practice using "action" words.
5. Decide about the following:
   a. Appearance
   b. Key points
      i. To make
      ii. To learn
   c. Tool for quick check (e.g., a file card with key points)
6. Arrive on time and alone.
7. Make a memorable entrance.
   a. Make eye contact.
   b. Shake hands.
   c. Smile.
   d. Say, "Hello, I'm [name]."
8. Position yourself with the interviewer (e.g., decide to sit at an angle).
9. Keep in mind your key points.
10. Appear interested—project competence, confidence, and energy.
11. Accentuate the positive!
12. Answer questions directly but know when not to.
13. Ask for more information.
14. Say only positive things about your present employer.
15. Secure a time frame for notification of a position offer.
16. Thank interviewer personally.
17. Write a thank-you letter.
18. Let interviewer know your decision.
19. Put commitments in writing.

Table 26-2 INTERVIEW GOALS AND CONTENT

Interview Goals	Content
1. Personal characteristics	• Describe the kind of person you are, including personality traits. Be expected to cite examples of when these traits helped or hindered you in previous situations. • List situations that characterize your energy, initiative, drive, ambition, and enthusiasm.
2. Can you do the work?	• What makes you stand out among the rest? How did your education and experience prepare you for this position? • Describe your team skills: ability to manage, motivate, and persuade. • Prepare to address hypothetical situations that display your problem solving, reasoning, self-confidence, knowledge, and critical thinking. (Creates opportunity to evaluate you in action and under some stress.) • Ask intelligent questions.
3. Organizational fit	• Why this organization versus another? • Articulate your "fit" with the organization's philosophy, mission, and vision.

Data from Adler, L. (1998). *Hire with your head.* New York: John Wiley & Sons; Bolles, R. N. (2001). *What color is your parachute?* Berkley: Ten Speed Press; and Fox, J. J. (2001). *Don't send a résumé.* New York: Hyperion.

PROFESSIONAL DEVELOPMENT

Today's employees have to manage and understand themselves, choosing work settings in which they make the greatest contributions and learning how and when to change what is done while staying mentally fit and youthful for a 50-year career (P. F. Drucker in Rosenstein, 2001). One of the keys to maintaining competence and versatility is continued learning. Learning occurs in various ways. It can occur in a conversation with colleagues, by reading an article in the general literature, or sometimes in an "ah hah" experience that provides sudden enlightenment. Although nurses could share these experiences with others, the continued learning that the profession, healthcare employers, boards of nursing, and **professional associations** are most concerned with is formal study.

"Nursing professional development begins within the basic nursing education program, continues throughout the career of the nurse and encompasses the educational concepts of continuing education, staff development, and academic preparation" (American Nurses Association, 2000, p. 1).

A graduate degree opens numerous career opportunities and leads to new levels or areas of expertise. A graduate education may focus on a clinical area, a functional area, or a combination of both. Admission to graduate programs typically requires taking a test (often the Graduate Record Examination [GRE]), having an above-average grade point average (GPA), and graduating from a professionally accredited school of nursing.

Graduate education consists of both master's- and doctorate-level study. In some employment situations or career specialties, graduate education is required. For example, expectations for nurse practitioner preparation are centered on graduate-level preparation as opposed to the earlier certificate programs. As healthcare becomes more complex, persons licensed as individual practitioners, such as nurses, necessarily need more education to continue to meet the healthcare system's demands.

Deciding to pursue graduate education may be very simple. Some applicants to baccalaureate programs already have a specific career focus in mind and the required graduate preparation is a given. New graduates are sometimes encouraged (or even required) to gain experience before seeking a master's degree or doctorate. Although experience enriches previous learning, it may not be relevant to specific graduate programs such as those entailing a major career redirection. Working while attending a graduate program may be difficult, but it is common among graduate students in nursing. Box 26-5 lists some factors to consider in selecting a graduate program.

If you are geographically bound, your fields of study may be limited. If you are not and you know what general area you want to pursue, consider the following illustration:

Example
You know you want to work with elderly patients. Your library subscribes to *The Journal of Gerontological Nursing* and *Geriatric Nursing*. You review the most recent year's issues of both. You scan the masthead (e.g., the page with the editors, board members). Where are these individuals affiliated? Now you scan the articles. Are there some that are particularly intriguing? Where are the authors affiliated? Finally, you look back over your lists. Are there any places emerging where the leaders in the field may be? You now have a good starting place.

Distance education provides an additional option for earning an advanced degree. Although the concept of distance learning is not new (think of correspondence courses), the complex technologies used to deliver distance education is new. Distance educational opportunities increase access for many. Flexible scheduling and convenience permit many individuals to participate. Students may find that the increased costs (a computer with faster speed and increased memory, higher academic fees, and the potential unavailability of financial aid) associated with distance learning and the lack of face-to-face interaction are obstacles to overcome.

Exercise 26-4

Analyze the academic and clinical preparation you received in your nursing program. Do you feel confident in your knowledge base and clinical skill? Can you effectively manage multiple roles? Based on these answers, determine whether you should pursue graduate education immediately or wait until you have gained additional work experience.

Exercise 26-5

Assume you are interested in graduate education.
• Talk with your local financial aid official to determine how you can learn more about financial assistance for graduate education.
• Using the internet or the library, locate information about graduate education.

- What specialties exist at the master's level?
- What programs are near you?
- What programs stimulate clinical interest?
- Do you know about the diverse roles of the advanced practice nurse?
- What about doctoral programs? Can you enter a doctoral program with a baccalaureate degree?

Continuing education also contributes to professional growth. *Continuing education* is defined as "systematic professional learning experiences designed to augment the knowledge, skill, and attitudes of nurses and therefore enrich the nurses' contributions to quality health care and their pursuit of professional career goals" (American Nurses Association, 2000, p. 5).

Numerous opportunities for continuing education exist at local, state, regional, and broader levels. Selecting which opportunities to pursue may be a difficult choice. Box 26-6 lists several factors to consider in selecting any offering, but depending on your particular goal, certain factors may be more influential than others. For example, if cost is a ma-

jor factor, length and speaker may be less influential factors.

In addition to increasing your knowledge base, continuing education provides professional networking opportunities, contributes to meeting certification and licensure requirements, and documents additional pursuits in maintaining or developing clinical expertise. Sponsors of continuing education include employers, professional associations, schools of nursing, and private entrepreneurial groups.

Both types of formal professional development, graduate education and continuing education, are valuable to your professional development, and both can contribute to a specific area of career development—certification.

Exercise 26-6

Like an organization, you will develop a strategic plan for yourself. Imagine you have decided to earn a master's degree in nursing. This decision can be enhanced by a strategic plan.
- What values do you have that influence your plan?
- Are your interests in primary care, administration, or education?

Continued

BOX 26-5

Factors to Consider in Selecting a Graduate Program

Accreditation	• Does the program have national nursing accreditation (master's level)? • Is the institution regionally accredited (e.g., North Central Association of Colleges and Schools)?	Faculty	• What credentials do faculty hold? • Are they in leadership positions in the state/national/international scenes? • Are they competent in your field of interest? • What is their reputation?
Clinical/ functional role	• How closely do the descriptions of clinical/functional courses of study meet career goals?	Current research	• What are the current research strengths of the institution?
Credits	• How many graduate credits are minimally required to complete the degree? • How many are devoted to gaining experience? • How many relate to classroom experiences?	Flexibility	• Do these strengths fit with your interests or is there flexibility to create your own direction? • Is flexibility present in scheduling and progress through the program?
		Admission	• What is required? • Is the GRE used? • What is the minimum undergraduate GPA expected? • Is experience required? What kind? How much?
Thesis/research	• Is a thesis required? • If not, what opportunities exist for research development? • What support is available for graduate students?	Costs	• What are the total projected costs? • What financial aid is available?

BOX 26-6

Factors to Consider in Selecting a Continuing Education Course

Accreditation/ approval	• Is the course accredited/approved? If so, by whom? • Is that recognition accepted by a certification entity and by the board of nursing (if continuing education is required for reregistration of licensure)?	Content	• Is the content reflective of the objectives? • Is the content at an appropriate level?
Credit	• Is the amount of credit appropriate in terms of the expected outcomes?	Audience	• Is the audience designed as a general or target one (e.g., all registered nurses or experienced nurses in state health positions)?
Course title	• Does it suggest the type of learner to be involved (e.g., advanced)? • Does it reflect the expected outcomes?	Cost	• Is it equitable with what similar nursing conferences cost? • Is travel required? • What is the actual direct expense for an individual to attend? Is it affordable?
Speaker(s)	• Is the instructor known as an expert in the field? • Is the instructor experienced in the field?	Length	• Is the total time frame logical in terms of objectives, personal needs, and time away from work? • Does the time frame permit breaks from intense learning?
Objectives	• Are the objectives logical and attainable? • Do they reflect knowledge, skills, attitudes, or a combination of these? • Do they fit a learner's needs?	Provider	• Does the provider have an established reputation?

■ *Exercise 26-6—cont'd*
- What is your target date for completion of the master's program?
- What are other factors that would interfere with your strategic plan?
- Do you have specific short-term goals or operational plans that must be attained before enrollment?

CERTIFICATION

Numerous opportunities exist for nurses to become certified (see Research Perspective). "Board certification signifies those nurses who have met requirements for clinical or functional practice in a specialized field, pursued education beyond basic nursing preparation, and received endorsement of their peers" (American Nurses Credentialing Center, 2000, p. 2). It is an expectation in some employment settings for career advancement; in the field of advanced practice nursing, it is viewed as a requirement for practice and reimbursement. In some states, certification in advanced practice is the mechanism to achieve recognition as an advance practice nurse from the board of nursing.

Obtaining certification may require testing and continuing education or documented time in practice in the specialty area in addition to testing and continuing education. Recertification is a process of continued recognition of competence within a defined practice area. Many certifications require an expectation for participation in continuing education, as reported annually in the January-February issue of *The Journal of Continuing Education in Nursing*.

Certification plays an important part in the advancement of a career and the profession. In some fields, more than one examination exists; in others, there is an examination in the broad field and numerous options for very defined subspecialties. The American Nurses Credentialing Center offers numerous certification examinations for nurse generalists, nurse practitioners, clinical specialists, nurse administrators, nurse case managers, ambulatory nurses, and informatics nurses. In addition, other

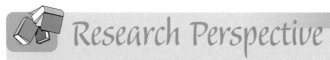

Research Perspective

Cary, A. H. (2001). Certified registered nurses: Results of the study of the certified workforce. *American Journal of Nursing,* *101*(1), 44-52.

The work of this author reflects the outcome of the third part of the *International Study of the Certified Nurse Workforce*. A previous study indicates that registered nurses hold more than 410,000 certifications, in 134 specialties, from 67 certifying organizations, with 95 different credentials designating those certifications. This research study is the largest study of certified nurses to date. A random sample of 19,452 nurses from the registries of the 23 certifying organizations in the United States, Canada, and U.S. territories were studied to determine the certified nurses' demographic characteristics, the nature of their practice, and the benefits they attribute to certification.

Respondents came from all 50 states, the District of Columbia, Puerto Rico, the Virgin Islands, and all 12 Canadian provinces. The mean age of certified nurses was 47.2 years, with more than 39% of certified nurses age 50 or older. Thirty-five percent held a baccalaureate degree. Ninety-five percent of respondents were working in nursing at the time of the survey, with hospitals being the most common practice site (50%), fol-

lowed by community settings (17%). Forty-four percent reported working more than 40 hours per week; forty-one percent earned $50,000 to $75,000 annually.

Registered Nurse, Certified (RN,C) was the most common credential (20%). Participants had been registered nurses for an average of 22 years and credentialed for an average of 7.8 years. Ninety-four percent practiced in the field in which they were certified; forty-seven percent provided medical-surgical nursing care.

Almost all participants (95%) reported that certification brought about at least one change in their practice; 72% reported one or more benefits.

IMPLICATIONS FOR PRACTICE

The findings of this work suggest that professional certification may provide opportunities for professional and personal growth and financial rewards. Increased confidence, competence, credibility, and control were reported. Certification has the potential for improving patient care outcomes.

---

certifications are offered by nursing specialty organizations. The websites of these specialty organizations provide specific certification requirements. Certification recognizes the competence of the nurse in a specialized area.

PROFESSIONAL EXPECTATIONS

Being a professional holds both privileges and obligations. The legal privileges and expectations are codified in the state nursing practice acts, rules, and regulations. Because licensure is designed to provide the baseline (i.e., the minimum expectation), it does not identify or obligate any practitioner to function in a professional manner as defined by the profession itself. For example, no practice act identifies membership in a professional association as an ex-

pectation. Nor is there an expectation for community service or scholarship. Yet the profession, through various professional organizations, holds the expectation that nurses will belong to professional associations and provide leadership in improving communities. How to incorporate these activities in a busy, committed life can at times seem difficult.

The key is to use a concept known as **reintegration** (Langford, 1990), which refers to the process of returning to a whole of nursing. It designates an incorporation of four role aspects into the role of professional nursing: education, scholarship, practice, and service. For example, the nurse who is expert in geriatric nursing might provide guest lectures at a nearby university in problems related to aging (education). This same nurse might help explain the latest research related to dementia, a common concern

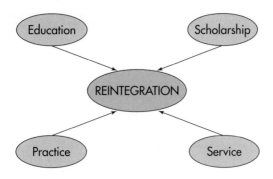

Figure 26-2   Reintegrated nursing.

of institutionalized elderly patients, to the staff of a nursing facility (scholarship). This individual might also be certified as a gerontological nurse through the American Nurses Credentialing Center. This is an example of expertise in a specialized area of practice (practice). In addition, this nurse might provide community blood pressure screenings at a senior citizens center and belong to the Gerontological Nurses Association (service). Thus each of the four elements of reintegration capitalizes on all other areas to contribute to this nurse's expertise in caring for the elderly. Figure 26-2 reflects the reintegration model. Each element could stand alone as a major role; instead the synthesis of these functional elements in an area of expertise contributes to the totality of professional competence.

Belonging to a professional association not only demonstrates professional leadership but also provides numerous opportunities to meet other leaders, participate in policy formation, continue specialized education, and shape the future of the profession. To learn more about an association, write to the national association and ask for information or access the website. Each April all state boards of nursing and professional associations are listed in the *American Journal of Nursing*, with the relevant demographic data to secure additional information. Requesting information should provide insight into both direct and indirect benefits of organizational membership. For example, a direct benefit may be receiving a publication or attending a meeting at reduced or no cost. An indirect benefit is knowing that your association actively lobbies on behalf of professional nurses. Numerous organizations can also be contacted through the American Nurses Association's website (http://www.nursingworld.org).

Depending on the type of career you want to have, belonging to a specific association may be very important because it is synonymous with leadership in the field. In nursing, the American Academy of Nursing and Sigma Theta Tau International are examples of such organizations.

Determining a logical level of involvement in an organization at the local, state, regional, or national level is important. When a bright, articulate, committed member is discovered, that individual is often asked to fulfill other expectations of the organization's work. Once again, knowing what is important to do to meet your professional goals can help you decide what level of involvement is desirable and acceptable.

Because the public places its trust in any licensed profession, there are numerous other obligations and privileges to being a professional. Some are exciting, for instance, providing testimony related to healthcare concerns. Others are troublesome, such as reporting a colleague to the state nursing board for incompetent practice. These are opportunities to improve the profession and the resultant care the general public can expect.

CAREER POTENTIAL

Traditionally, nursing has been perceived by the public as hospital based, but that has changed dramatically. There are numerous other nursing careers, such as teacher, administrator, manager, clinical specialist, researcher, organizational executive, entrepreneur, and practitioner. These roles occur in hospitals, community and professional organizations, and the business setting. In addition, the number of clinical specialties continues to increase. Some have been a part of nursing for a long time and are experiencing major growth and recognition because of the financial impact on healthcare. These include such foci as occupational health, school health, and public health. Concomitantly, the traditional hospital careers are simultaneously focusing and expanding. Nurses with these focused, expert skills need to be able to function with more than one clinical population. This ability to increase expertise and flexibility will continue to be in demand. Positioning within the profession to achieve this flexibility and expertise requires career commitment, continuous self-development, a passion for nursing, and a strong foundation as a leader.

The Solution

Although I was a recent graduate and thought I knew what I needed to know, I returned to my textbooks looking for a strategy. Information on professionalism and how to handle difficult people provided a solution to my problem.

Initially, I began to pull myself away from my peers who were my friends. Long, lonely workdays were the outcome of this solution. My next strategy proved more effective. I would not assign anything to anyone that I myself would not or could not do. I became available to assist with any task including those of the nurse aide, LVN, and other registered nurses. My knowledge and professionalism enabled the staff to begin seeing me as an integral part of the staff. Soon they began to be more open to accepting more challenging assignments.

As the days, weeks, and months passed, my relationship with the nursing staff (some of whom were my friends) blossomed into a wonderful professional relationship. Each day, I found it easier to make assignments without fear of upsetting a co-worker or a friend. We all knew what work had to be done. I recognized that I needed to treat my staff with dignity and professionalism; valuing the contribution each staff member makes was an integral part of my career development.

— Rebecca A. Brawley

 Would this be a suitable approach for you? Why?

CHAPTER CHECKLIST

Nurses must make decisions about career goals and career development. Managing a career requires a set of planned strategies designed to lead systematically toward the desired goal. The use of each strategy should be geared toward finding a good person-position fit. Career planning and development is a lifelong process focused on continual competence. Continued professional development, whether via graduate education or continuing education, is a crucial component of success as a nurse.

- Career styles contribute to the diversity of the nursing profession and reflect different ways of achieving success.
- The four career styles are as follows:
  - Steady state: characterized by constancy with increasing professional skill
  - Linear: a hierarchical orientation with a steady climb
  - Entrepreneurial/transient: focused on new services and personal priorities
  - Spiral: rational, independent responsibility for shaping the career
- Certain career control strategies are effective with every career style:
  - Selecting professional peers, mentors, and role models help shape professional development.

- Designing personal/professional documents that open doors for further action includes:
  - The CV (a listing of facts) (quantitative)
  - The résumé (a sampling of the most relevant facts, with details) (qualitative)
  - Appropriate business letters that effectively market
- Interviewing at its best is a two-way interaction that enables both people to determine whether there is a good person-position fit.
- Both graduate education and continuing education contribute to a nurse's ability to provide competent care.
- Graduate education (master's- or doctorate-level study) may focus on the following:
  - A clinical area
  - A functional area
  - A combination of both
- Factors to consider in selecting a graduate program include the following:
  - Accreditation
  - Clinical/functional role
  - Credits
  - Thesis/research requirements
  - Faculty
  - Current research
  - Flexibility
  - Admission policy
  - Cost

Continued

CHAPTER CHECKLIST—cont'd

- Continuing-education opportunities exist at local, state, regional, national, and international levels.
- Certification is the designation of special knowledge beyond the basic licensure and is a requirement in some employment settings. Being a professional carries additional obligations and privileges to ensure that the nurse remains competent, advances the profession, and improves healthcare.

CAREER TIPS

- Use an expanding file to organize hard copies of your accomplishments, such as continuing-education certificates, by year so that you can report accurate data for licensure or certification.
- Update your CV at least once a year (6 months is better and 3 months is ideal) so that you always have an accurate, current set of data to share with someone should a special opportunity appear.
- Keep connected with people.
- Find a mentor; be a mentor; self-mentor.
- Review the most difficult events of the day immediately and determine how to improve yourself (Kane, 1996).

- Improve your abilities, especially those you use all of the time—get better at being better (Kane, 1996).
- Think about the future and what you need to be employable.
- Join two professional organizations—such as the American Nurses Association (broad professional) and the American Association of Critical Care Nurses (a specialty).
- Read professional journals and, on a regular basis, at least one other journal external to nursing to keep current with the world.
- Attend at least one professional meeting each year, especially outside of your geographic area, to network.
- Volunteer in your profession and your community.

TERMS TO KNOW

career	licensure
certification	professional association
continuing education	reintegration
curriculum vitae	résumé

REFERENCES

Adler, L. (1998). *Hire with your head*. New York: John Wiley & Sons.

American Nurses Association. (2000). *Scopes and standards of practice for nursing professional development*. Washington, DC: Author.

American Nurses Credentialing Center. (2000). *Credentialing catalog*. Washington, DC: Author.

Armour, S. (2001, August 17). Job seekers get put through the wringer. *USA Today*, p. 1B.

Bolles, R. N. (2001). *What color is your parachute?* Berkley: Ten Speed Press.

Cary, A. H. (2001). Certified registered nurses: Results of the study of the certified workforce. *American Journal of Nursing, 101*(1), 44-52.

Fox, J. J. (2001). *Don't send a résumé*. New York: Hyperion.

Friss, L. (1989). *Strategic management of nurses: A policy oriented approach*. Owings Mills, MD: AUPHA Press.

Kane, K. A. (1996, June/July). Do it yourself mentoring. *Fast Company, 133*.

Langford, T. L. (1990). *Managing and being managed: Preparation for reintegrated professional nursing practice*. Lubbock, TX: Landover Publishing.

McCann, S. (1999). Competency in the 21st century. *Dermatology Nursing, 11*(6), 407, 454.

Rosenstein, B. (2001, August 20). 91-year-old legend shares advice. *USA Today*, p. 6B.

SUGGESTED READINGS

Fox, J. J. (2001). *Don't send a resume and other contrarian rules to help land a great job*. New York: Hyperion.

Hawley, C. (2001). *100+ winning answers to the toughest interview questions*. Hauppauge, NY: Barrons.

Leider, D. J., & Shapiro, D. A. (2001). *Whistle while you work: Heeding your life's calling*. San Francisco: Berrett-Koehler.

Moses, B. (1998). *Career intelligence: The 12 new rules for work and life success*. San Francisco: Berrett-Koehler.

Peters, T. (1999). *Reinventing work: The brand you.* New York: Alfred A. Knopf.

ADDITIONAL RESOURCES

American Nurses Association website: www.nursingworld.org

American Nurses Credentialing Center website: www.nursingworld.org/ancc

Sigma Theta Tau International Honor Society website: www.nursingsociety.org

ADDITIONAL WEBSITES

BestjobsUSA.com

Careermosaic.com

Monster.com

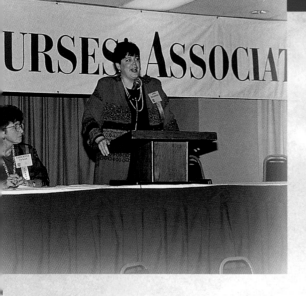

Chapter

27

Leading Through Professional Associations

Sharon A. Brigner

*T*his chapter describes professional organizations and association concepts, as well as values obtained through leadership and participation in organizations. The primary focus is on the variety of opportunities and advantages that can be gained through a relationship with preprofessional and professional nursing organizations. In today's changing healthcare environment, it is more important than ever for the nurse to be connected and unified with other nursing colleagues who are prepared to confront challenges and who are equipped with solutions.

Objectives

- Define organizations and associations.
- Identify the need for involvement.
- Explain various structures within organizations.
- Describe organizational concepts, such as mission statements and goals.
- Define different roles within an association.
- Explore individual personal strengths and weaknesses.

- Describe what kind of contributions you can make to the organization.

- Decide on benefits that you want to derive from involvement in the organization.

Questions to Consider

- *What are your strengths and weaknesses?*
- *How will they be used within an organization?*
- *What is your motivation to join and/or participate?*
- *What do you want to get out of your experience with an association?*
- *How much time do you have to devote to involvement with the organization?*

The Challenge

Howard Holsinger, RN, BSN, CNRN
National Institutes of Health Clinical Center, Bethesda, Maryland

Nurse Jane, an experienced charge nurse on the medical-surgical floor, had a reputation of constantly delegating her own work to new staff members, justifying her actions by saying she needed fewer patients because she must focus on her charge nurse duties. She claimed that being a charge nurse was stressful and that we could use the experience anyway. I had been working on this medical-surgical floor for almost a year and felt confident working with my patients and the nurses, even though I was one of the youngest and least experienced nurses on the staff. Being a team player, I rarely turned Nurse Jane down when she asked me for something, whether it was simply to page a physician, change her patient's IV bags, call the pharmacy for a medication, or so forth. I thought that she must by busy with discharge planning and would not have asked me if she did not really need the help. However, I quickly realized that she was taking advantage of her position, as well as my helpful attitude. I began to resent her when I would take her chores and she would then sit in the lounge and use that time for social phone calls, which were obviously not essential charge nurse duties.

Before our morning shift one day, she made out the assignments and again gave herself a light assignment that consisted of two early-morning discharges, whereas the other nurse and I were given more challenging patient assignments. As the day proceeded, I was able to handle my assignment without asking for help. Nurse Jane's patients left before 11 am without complications. After they left, she did not pick up any of our patients, and she did not have any unusual charge responsibilities on this day. I noticed that Jane seemed to take a long break after her patients were discharged, and the other nurse and I had not even stopped for lunch. Neither of her discharge patients' rooms had been cleared for housekeeping; it is the nurses' responsibility to clear before housekeeping can enter the room to prepare for more admissions.

A few hours before the shift was over, Nurse Jane came into my patient's room while I was in the middle of patient care and interrupted by saying, "Can you do me a favor?" Of course, I replied that I could. "What can I do?" Her request: "Can you clear the rooms of my discharged patients?" Frustrated, I began to think about how I would respond. How should I follow-up with Nurse Jane? Do I have to complete every task delegated from her because she is in charge? I told her that I would be out in a few minutes and she turned around and left the room.

 What do you think you would do if you were this nurse?

INTRODUCTION

People have always been in search of others who share common interests. Associations exist to provide this opportunity, as well as to serve a purpose, such as working to improve the environment or to promote medical research, advocacy for seniors, and more. Professional associations, or organizations, have been defined as groups of people who share a set of professional **values** who decide to join their colleagues to affect change. Many nursing associations set standards and objectives to guide the profession and specialty practice. Standards can also serve as critical measurements for the profession and its practitioners. In today's changing healthcare environment, increasing numbers of associations are serving unique healthcare interests in society. Healthcare professionals have a plethora of associations from which to choose. Although associations have very different agendas and goals, many of the nursing organizations share the same motivation and long-term goal of uniting and advancing the profession.

Nursing students have the opportunity to become involved with the **preprofessional** nursing organization, the National Student Nurses Association (NSNA). NSNA provides a wonderful training ground for future professionals. For example, nursing students can join the national association, which automatically makes them a member of the state and local associations. Through their local school chapter, nursing students can become involved, learn about policy issues, participate in leadership opportunities, and explore ways to influence the profession at an early stage in their career. For many students, NSNA has had a major impact on the direction of their careers because of the exposure to the variety of career paths and introduction to nursing leaders throughout the country. For example, an NSNA convention holds a variety of events that might include focus sessions on specific clinical or career development topics, a panel of nurses with different jobs in nursing, and exhibitors from research institutions and educational facilities. Needless to say, students are not typically exposed to this kind of environment in the classroom or clinical area. Clearly, there is a great assortment of organizations from which to choose, irrespective of your role, clinical area, education, and experience. There are more than 75 specialty nurse organizations that represent nurses in particular areas of the profession, such as the American Association of Critical Care Nurses, the Oncology Nurses Association, and the American Association of Neuroscience Nurses (Shinn, 1998) (Box 27-1). To attract future members, many specialty organizations offer reduced membership rates to students and new graduates, which include discounted meeting and convention rates, discounts on insurance, networking opportunities, and informative publications and mailings about the association. This reduced student membership is a wonderful opportunity to learn more about the specific fields of nursing.

With more than 75 organizations, it can be overwhelming for an individual to decipher their differences. The "umbrella organization" that represents all nurses is the American Nurses Association (ANA), which is a full-service professional organization that represents more than 2.6 million registered nurses through its 54 constituent associations and 13 organizational affiliate members (www.ana.org). The ANA advances the nursing profession by fostering high standards of nursing practice. Some functions of the ANA include promoting the economic and general welfare of nurses in the workplace, projecting a positive and realistic view of nursing, and lobbying Congress and regulatory agencies on healthcare issues affecting nurses and the public (www.nursingworld.org). When the ANA was formed in 1897 and officially founded in 1901, its purpose was to protect the public from unsafe nursing care and to set standards for practice and education that could be changed and adapted over the years (Kelly & Joel, 1995). Today, the ANA continues to be the voice for nursing, serving as a strong advocate and representative for the profession.

Similar to the American Medical Association for physicians, policy makers look to the ANA for guidance on nursing and health policy issues.

Exercise 27-1

Research the ANA and your state nursing organization on the Internet (www.nursingworld.org). Find the **mission** of the organization and the legislative issues of interest. Obtain association brochures or further information that might help you throughout your education.

STRUCTURE

Structures of organizations can vary greatly, depending on the organization's size and purpose. Many organizations are multitiered, designed to reach out to members in all areas of the country. For instance, the ANA is considered a three-tiered organization, with the headquarters located in the Washington, DC, area; its constituent members are the states and a federal nursing group, and local or district associations allow members to network on a grassroots level. This type of organizational structure allows for effective information dissemination. However, it requires that all parties be communicating and responding to each other on a timely basis, which can be a challenge, particularly if an area is lacking in members (e.g., more rural areas). Clear lines of communication and structure are essential for associations.

The mission gives the direction to the organization and often states the purpose for its existence. Examples of an organization's mission include striving to educate the public on healthcare issues, uniting the profession, affecting international healthcare issues, being an active player in policy and managed care, defining nursing and nursing education, developing requirements and scope of practice, and/or empowering nurses to take control of their own practices. Associations work in the following functional areas to achieve their missions (Shinn, 1998) (Box 27-2).

The organization may develop a **strategic plan,** which is a detailed map of the mission and goals for the association's existence. Strategic plans operationalize how the organization can meet its goals and objectives. These plans are most effective when they are developed with the assistance of an outside consultant who can guide the association in an unbiased manner. The board should revisit and revise

BOX 27-1

List of Nursing Organizations

Academy of Medical-Surgical Nurses
American Academy of Ambulatory Care Nursing
American Academy of Nurse Practitioners
American Academy of Nursing
American Assembly for Men in Nursing
American Association of Colleges of Nursing
American Association of Continuity in Care
American Association of Critical-Care Nurses
American Association of Diabetes Educators
American Association for the History of Nursing
American Association of Legal Nurse Consultants
American Association of Neuroscience Nurses
American Association of Nurse Anesthetists
American Association of Nurse Attorneys
American Association of Occupational Health Nurses
American Association of Office Nurses
American Association of Spinal Cord Injury Nurses
American College of Nurse Midwives
American Community Health Nursing Educators
American Holistic Nurses Association
American Nephrology Nurses Association
American Nurses Association
American Organization of Nurse Executives
American Psychiatric Nurses Association
American Radiological Nurses Association
American Society of Ophthalmic Registered Nurses
American Society of periAnesthesia Nurses
American Society of Plastic and Reconstructive Surgical Nurses
Association of Black Nursing Faculty in Higher Education
Association of Child and Adolescent Psychiatric Nurses
Association of Nurses in AIDS Care
Association of Pediatric Oncology Nurses
Association of periOperative Registered Nurses
Association for Professionals in Infection Control and Epidemiology
Association of Rehabilitation Nurses
Association of Women's Health, Obstetric and Neonatal Nurses

Dermatology Nurses Association
Developmental Disabilities Nurses Association
Drug and Alcohol Nursing Association
Emergency Nurses Association
Endocrine Nurses Society
Hospice Nurse Association
International Association of Forensic Nurses
International Nurses Society on Addictions
International Organization of Multiple Sclerosis Nurses
Intravenous Nurses Society
National Alliance of Nurse Practitioners
National Association of Neonatal Nurses
National Association of Nurse Massage Therapists
National Association of Orthopedic Nurses
National Association of Pediatric Nurse Practitioners and Associates
National Association of School Nurses
National Association of State School Nurses Consultants
National Black Nurses Association
National Federation for Specialty Nurse Organizations
National Flight Nurses Association
National Gerontological Nurses Association
National League for Nursing
National Nurses Society on Addictions
National Organization of the Veterans Administration
National Student Nurses Association
Oncology Nursing Society
Philippine Nurses Association of America
Sigma Theta Tau International
Society of Gastroenterology Nurses and Associates, Inc.
Society of Otorhinolaryngology and Head-Neck Nurses, Inc.
Society of Pediatric Nurses
Society for Peripheral Vascular Nursing
Society of Urology Nurses and Associates
Transcultural Nursing Society
Wound, Ostomy and Continence Nurses Society

the strategic plan as needed. Within the strategic plan, clearly defined goals determine the organization's political agenda.

Associations can be formally structured and are legally incorporated, yet neither is a requirement for the organization to exist. Most organizations have a set of bylaws, which refer to specific rules of order of an organization, such as accountability, authority, composition, governance, mission, and purpose. Bylaws can usually be changed by the House of Delegates through an amendment process. The House of Delegates is a part of the association mem-

BOX 27-2

Programs and Services

Image and identity
Human Resources
    Staff
    Leaders
    Members
    Fiscal Resources
    Dues and nondues revenue
Reserves
Structure and governance

bership that has voting authority, thereby making decisions and electing officers to serve at the helm of the association. Officer positions vary from organization to organization. Most boards include the following: president, vice president, secretary, treasurer, and directors. These positions are examples of roles that officers may perform for the organization. The board functions at its best when the individual officers experience a sense of teamwork. The entire board must collectively work together to be as productive and efficient as possible.

Conduct of Business

Parliamentary Procedure, guided by Robert's Rules of Order (2000), is the method used to conduct most association business for board or House of Delegate meetings. The House of Delegates can pass motions, resolutions, and amendments. It can also create goal or policy statements or alter the bylaws. The board is elected by the membership to carry out the directives of the membership. The board can establish subgroups, or committees, to carry out specific functions and tasks for the associations. Examples of committees may include governmental relations, clinical practices, membership recruitment and retention, and convention planning. Committees encourage participation by members with different levels of interest and passion. The members are the volunteers who pay membership dues and contribute their time, play active roles in the organization, and help carry out the mission of the organization. Collectively, the different entities coordinate efforts to have an extraordinary effect within the professional and personal realm of nursing.

Another important part of the organizational structure is the executive staff, which may consist of an executive director and support staff, who are typically salaried and located at the association headquarters, which is usually based in a large, urban city. The association headquarters and size of the staff will vary according to available financial resources and mission. The staff provides general support and disseminates information to the members through phone calls, mailings, and listservs. They coordinate conventions and meetings while serving as a constant point of information and resource for members. Some organizations hire outside consultants to perform specific tasks, such as membership survey design and analysis, strategic planning, financial or organizational restructuring, and other valuable services. Consultants are typically nonbiased, professional individuals who can offer suggestions that make an association more efficient without getting involved in the politics of the organization. Because many organizations have strong political agendas, registered lobbyists are commonly employed to work closely with the state and/or federal members of Congress.

Connecting With an Organization

The size of an organization can be misleading. Bigger is not necessarily better. The size of the group is not as important as how the group is organized and who is leading it. Therefore it is extremely important to do some research before making a commitment through membership. In today's world of high-speed Internet access, it is easy to access an abundance of information through the computer, rather than spending time calling and requesting membership applications and brochures. In addition, reading about the officer and membership composition of the organization is important. Most associations have a website that lists information regarding leader contact and biographical information, locations of their next meetings or activities, current policy issues and their positions, election information, and other valuable resource links.

Exercise 27-2

Find out when the next local district meeting is being held by calling the association, securing a newsletter, or looking on the Internet. Attend a local district meeting in your association, observe the dynamics, and network with the members.

Expectations of Membership

Upon joining a nursing organization, you may receive information on the history of the organization, future meetings and current activities, officer contact information, and local contacts. One of the most important things that you can do is connect with your local organization so that you can immediately begin networking. Decide how much time you can allocate to the organization. There are several different ways to be involved, all of which carry different time commitments. Do not assume that a certain role or committee position entails a set amount of time. The fact remains that most associations are composed of volunteers, all of whom have very busy schedules and different motivations for becoming involved. Taking time to talk to an officer or attend a local meeting and observe the group and the dynamics before deciding to make commitments will help ensure that you make an informed decision. Some members enter into the organizational experience with unreal expectations and quickly become disenchanted and disappointed with the organization, which results in completely pulling away from the organization. To maximize your experience, you owe it to yourself to do your homework, research the organization, talk to the members, get a feel of the group dynamics, and assess what you want to get out of the experience and how you can contribute to the organization. Look at your strengths and talents and see if there is a need or a fit within the organization. Finally, remember that the organization is composed of humans who are volunteering their time; therefore you should not expect a "perfect" organization. Every organization has its struggles, but you can gain tremendous benefits, both personally and professionally, from your involvement.

Exercise 27-3

While you are at an association meeting, challenge yourself to speak to at least two members and find out about their work setting and their nursing role. Make sure to get contact information or a business card from at least two individuals that you can call in the near future. On the back of the business card, write something about that person that will help you remember them for the future (e.g., long black hair, nurse manager on the neurology unit at Methodist Hospital). You may use these cards in the future when you are looking for a job or need a specific question answered, and they will serve as an invaluable resource.

Joining/Reasons for Involvement

Motivation to join an organization can vary a great deal. Organizational membership has become an integral part of one's career development. The average nurse may hold membership in a variety of social and professional organizations, devoting more time to one particular area of interest. For example, nurses may choose to belong to the ANA, as well as one or more specialty organizations. Some reasons for joining organizations may include a sense of responsibility to the profession or the hope that they are contributing to the greater good of the profession. Other reasons might include the desire to enhance their résumé and marketability purposes. The nurses' employer may encourage membership and even pay for the employees' membership fee. Some nurses may join because they want to promote their profession, have particular legislative interests, or have other social reasons. As illustrated in the Research Perspective, the opportunity to be involved is seen as a positive benefit of valued performance. A common belief among nurses is that their organization of choice can help improve conditions and care for their patients. In addition, there are those who choose to be active participants by joining committee work, running for office, or taking on other leadership roles. Organizations need all types of members, both active and passive participants, so that they can carry out their missions and conduct activities and business. In addition, organizational involvement, like any socialization process, can improve nursing morale. Being around others who take pride and celebrate the nursing profession is contagious, and you will inevitably spread that attitude. Whatever your personal preference for level of involvement, you are contributing greatly to your profession by simply joining and becoming a member, but active involvement within an association can guarantee a world of opportunities.

Some individuals belong because they are required to do so. In some cases employment contracts make it mandatory for the nurse to join a union and pay dues to receive a paycheck, which is referred to as a **closed shop.** Other **collective bargaining** workplaces are referred to as an **open shop,** which means nurses are allowed to join if they so choose. There are several different collective bargaining agents for nursing, but the United American Nurses of the American Nurses Association currently represents the greatest number of nurses. In UAN member states the state nurses association serves as the collective bargaining agent in contract negotiations, conflicts or disputes, salary negotiations, and overall communication with management.

Some states are **right to work** states, which means that the nurse employed in an institution that has a union contract has the option to join the

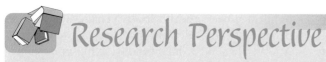
Research Perspective

Cronin, S. N., & Becherer, D. (1999). Recognition of staff nurse job performance and achievements: Staff and manager perceptions. *Journal of Nursing Administration, 29*(1), 26-31.

A convenience sample was used for this comparative descriptive survey of nursing staff in three institutions to determine recognition methods most valued by nurses themselves. Usable questionnaires (*n* = 342) included both staff nurses and nurse managers. A rating-type survey was included with paychecks. Several items emerged as the top contenders for recognizing performance. "Encouraging the nurse to participate in professional activities at the state or national level" was among the top 10 items that were deemed most meaningful to the nurse for recognition of performance. In addition, "recommending the nurse as an expert speaker" was another valued method of recognition.

IMPLICATIONS FOR NURSING PRACTICE
The manager controls various ways in which staff are recognized for performance. Providing opportunities to be involved professionally in an association is among one of those most valued by the participants in this study and could be a valued component of various work settings.

---

organization if so desired. This also implies that the nurse is responsible for direct communication with the employer. Many of these state associations have instituted a workplace advocacy program, which provides the nurse with communication and conflict resolution tools. An example of a valued strategy is shared governance, or self-governance, a concept that was developed in the mid-1980s, where the governance of the organization is shared by those who are directly involved. Groups such as executive management, board members, physicians, nurses, and other interdisciplinary healthcare providers engage in group decision making and professional communication, with the goal of empowerment of the individuals within the system. Often, this involves committee work to discuss issues such as quality assurance and clinical practice. This practice allows nurses to contribute and have input on issues that affect their practice, profession, and workplace. In this organizational structure, the managers take on more of a consulting, collegial role, which can be difficult for some institutions with a long history of hierarchal decision-making processes.

Historically, unions were first organized because of wage cuts or unfair work practices. In return the organized union has a liaison or representative who will represent the nurse on a variety of issues. According to Marquis and Huston (2000), nurses may believe that the union can help advocate and communicate their aims, feelings, complaints, and ideas to others. Second, the union can work to eliminate discrimination and favoritism. Many issues that unions confront involve pay and benefit issues, overtime requirements, or conflict resolutions. In addition, ensuring that basic patient care issues are addressed is a driving force. Another motivation for a nurse to join might be for social acceptance among peers or families who might have a long history in unionized professions. On the reverse side, nurses have reasons to reject the need to join a union. Some nurses dislike the fact that unions discourage individual relationships with management and prefer that the nurse work through the union representative when dealing with issues such as benefits, pay, workplace issues, and so forth, and some nurses prefer their individualism. In some instances nurses may feel that the union's goals or motives are different from their personal desires.

Exercise 27-4
Think about what motivates you to join or not join the state nurses organization. Make a list of your strengths (communication, organization, treasury skills, legislative interests). Look at positions within the organization that interest you. On a separate list, write out reasons why you would want to be a part of the association.

What You Can Get Out of Participating in an Organization
In today's rapidly changing environment of healthcare delivery and services, nurses must remain active and involved in the decision-making process that affects the nursing profession. Policy makers will proceed with making decisions that affect nursing practice if nurses do not ensure that they are at the table

with input and guidance. Nursing organizations recognize this reality and are taking on a more vital role than ever by participating in discussions that range from local and state to national levels.

Organizations provide members with a variety of ways to lead and relate to others. A common misconception is that you must take on an officer or committee position to be "involved." However, even just paying dues is involvement because it is an investment of money in your future. Participation can occur at a variety of levels; it is important to know just what you want to attain from organizational involvement. Assessing your own motivations and goals before joining and making time commitments within the organization is important. Participation is a personal decision and is guided by one's personal commitment and time limits. Evaluate your passion, expertise, and skills and look for areas within the organization that you can put them to use. If you want to strengthen or develop an attribute, such as public speaking, you should seek out positions and opportunities within the organization that would enable you to develop that skill. Likewise, if you wish to become more politically knowledgeable about current legislation and the political process, you could seek involvement in legislative affairs activities. After you have had time to observe the group structure and its working dynamics, it is extremely important to verbalize your interests to the officers and chairs of committees. Often, the voluntary organizations are eager to receive assistance and may take it upon themselves to make your activity assignments for you. You should not hesitate to reject any assignments and start by communicating effectively from the beginning. Take control by vocalizing your time limitations, interests, and objectives. This proactive action will prevent frustration and miscommunication and ensure that you will have a productive, fulfilling experience.

Personal Benefits

Many associations offer substantial scholarships for nurses who are pursuing higher education and certifications. They might also offer scholarships to attend policy meetings, such as the Nurse In Washington Internship, organized by the National Federation for Specialty Nursing Organizations, or the Annual Health Policy Institute, conducted by the Center for Health Policy, Research, and Ethics of George Mason University. These two internships are examples of wonderful opportunities through which nurses can learn about legislative issues, the

political process, healthcare advocacy, and how to be more effective on local, state, and national levels. Another benefit of membership is the opportunity to travel for conventions and meetings. Most organizations rotate their regular convention meeting sites so that members throughout the country will have an opportunity to attend.

With ever-increasing time demands on individuals today, volunteering for activities outside of work and family has become increasingly difficult. Because volunteers comprise the majority of members within an organization, associations are aware that traditional incentives for member participation may not be enough to draw new members. However, there are benefits that are not advertised. For example, networking and exposure to different opportunities within the nursing profession are two of the most valuable benefits of belonging to an organization. Some nurses may stop working for a time because of family or educational priorities. Organizational membership can help these nurses stay connected to professional issues and colleagues through meetings and publications so that the transition back into practice will not be as difficult. Given these possibilities, membership in nursing organizations can provide a continuous source of professional colleagues for today's nurse to draw upon for invaluable advice and collective support.

With the abundant opportunities in nursing, nurses rarely remain in the same position for an extended period. Chances are that most nurses will work in a variety of settings over the course of their career. Therefore today's nurse needs to socialize with nurses in different career paths within nursing. This socialization can take place through district meetings or state or national conventions. For example, many organizations have conventions at which they might feature a nurse panel comprised of a variety of innovative positions within the field, which will expose the member to new and emerging fields. Such meetings also provide members with a potential contact for nurses who hope to transition into that particular area of nursing.

In addition to networking, the professional organization can serve as an additional training ground through which nurses can build skills and gain wonderful experiences. They also provide opportunities for leadership development through committees or in officer positions, which can provide invaluable skills training (Box 27-3).

Members of nursing associations learn firsthand about diversity among patient populations, as

BOX 27-3

Skills Learned From Organizational Involvement

- Conflict resolution
- Interpersonal communication
- Public speaking
- Mentoring
- Conducting meetings
- Creating agendas
- Facilitation
- Delegation
- Consensus building
- Strategic thinking
- Team building
- Political advocacy
- Legislative work/lobbying
- Problem solving

well as within the profession. Clinical issues that affect practice on local, state, and federal levels are addressed. Opportunities to work as a group to influence and educate policy makers are also evident. The organization and members' ability to influence healthcare in a policy arena is one of the most significant benefits of membership. On the most basic level, nurses can influence legislation for their profession by simply becoming a member and adding strength through numbers. For further involvement, nurses can participate on a legislative committee and become involved in their local, grassroots politics. By being acquainted with the political players in their area, nurses can ensure that they are at the table for discussions on healthcare and policy-making decisions. Nurses' ability to advocate for their patients is not confined to the bedside. Nurses must learn to use advocacy in the political arena as well. Nursing organizations are tremendous advocates and can have great political strength (Mason & Leavitt, 1998). In a June 1999 Harris poll, an overwhelming majority of the public, 92%, said they trust information about healthcare provided by registered nurses (Harris Poll, 1999). This powerful statistic reinforces the fact that nurses must be involved in healthcare discussions and decision-making policies.

Whether you are a new or experienced nurse, you will encounter ethical or professional dilemmas. Members of the nurses association can be nonbiased, safe colleagues to ask for advice about your

situation. They can provide feedback options for your situation, based on their experience, especially when you may not want to discuss it with co-workers who could be directly involved.

Professional Benefits

Associations can serve as a springboard for your career. If you are networking within an organization, you will inevitably meet members who work in your field or even one that you hope to enter. Becoming acquainted with these men and women and working with them on association activities provides potential job opportunities or other benefits. How many times have you said to yourself, "What a small world!" after bumping into someone that you haven't seen in a while or finding out that you have a connection with someone with whom you have been talking? Well, the nursing world is even smaller and you could go into a job interview or board meeting and find an ally on your side by simply previously meeting or working with them in an organization. Coalition building, unification, and advancing of nursing's agenda also offer attractive reasons to belong. Politically, nurses are so much stronger if they have one unified voice that speaks to Congress on the profession's behalf. Members of Congress and their staff have voiced concerns about the inconsistency of nursing's message, specifically if a specialty nursing organization pushes its individual agenda without connecting it into the common message that pertains to all nurses. This occurrence can be prevented if the profession organizes messages in advance. Specialty nursing organizations have an extremely important role that is enhanced when tied to communicating and collaborating with the other nursing entities. The American Medical Association has been masterful at coordinating their general legislative message with the specialty medical associations, as well as stating their membership benefits upfront (Box 27-4).

 ## WORKFORCE SHORTAGE

In 2001 the Health Resources Service Administration (Division of Nursing, 2001) printed new data on the nursing workforce that stated that the country is currently experiencing an unprecedented nursing shortage and made projections for an even greater shortage over the next few years. The nursing shortage has been attributed to a number of factors, such as an aging workforce, decreased applications into

BOX 27-4

Tangible Benefits From Organizational Involvement

- Substantial discounts on continuing education
- Certifications
- Credentialing
- Group insurance plans for professional liability, hospitalization, and disability
- Travel services, such as auto rentals, hotel stays, and restaurant visits
- Quick access to staff experts on practice advocacy
- Legal, legislative, and educational issues
- Professional standards
- Discounts on professional journals

nursing school, and image concerns. Nursing organizations are key to helping solve this workforce shortage. Associations have always advocated for quality patient care and adequate nurse staffing. However, nurses are often confronted with mandatory overtime, increased patient loads, and unsafe nursing environments. Nursing organizations can help improve morale, increase job satisfaction, and attract qualified individuals. Nursing organizations can be instrumental in recruiting and retaining registered nurses. Some organizations might even have a membership committee that focuses on outreach to the community for recruitment into the profession. *Nursing's Agenda for the Future* (2002) represents the work of numerous professional organizations in addressing the shortage.

Exercise 27-5

When did you first think about becoming a registered nurse? What made you consider nursing as a career option?

Members could participate in school career fairs, health education seminars, and college days. Many women and men decide on their career choice in grade school and high school. Nursing organizations can play a big part in helping to shape future career decisions.

CONCLUSION

Professional associations and organizations are powerful influences on the nursing profession and healthcare in general. For the individual nurse, the personal and professional opportunities are endless. You can enhance your career development while seizing the opportunity to make a tremendous impact on the profession. When a nurse invests time, passion, and energy into an association, the individual, patient, and nursing profession will all benefit. You owe it to yourself to learn more about nursing organizations that might interest you and get involved. It can change your life and your career path and take you to unbelievable places. After all, what do you have to lose? If you decide that you are not happy with an organization after joining, you have only benefited by experiencing the people and purpose. You should feel confident in searching for one that is a better fit. Meanwhile, be assured that your membership dues allow other nurses and the association to work behind the scenes for the profession's best interest. That is a comforting thought in today's fast-paced environment. Just knowing that there are nurses who are monitoring the issues, ready to respond on behalf of the profession, is quite an empowering thought! In the words of Henry Ford, "Coming together is a beginning, keeping together is progress, and working together is success." Nurses embrace this teamwork spirit more than any other profession. Choose to make a difference and join your association. It is truly a win-win experience!

The Solution

During the previous week, I had asked an experienced nurse colleague for advice, who had served as a charge nurse for several years. This colleague was also an active leader in his professional nursing organization. He knew that I wanted to keep a professional work environment with Nurse Jane, but I was tired of feeling that she was taking advantage of me. He advised me with specific communication tools that worked for him, which was to

The Solution—cont'd

confront the individual in a nonconfrontational manner while communicating my feelings directly and without emotion. I decided to follow his advice.

After I finished my direct patient care, I took a few minutes to calm down and later approached her, asking to speak with her in private in the lounge. I started the conversation by praising her expertise and telling her I recognized that being charge nurse can be stressful at times. I explained that I respected our professional working relationship and that is why I wanted to address a serious concern. I told her that I did not appreciate being asked to complete tasks for her when she would turn around and use that time for social interaction or by sitting in the lounge. Therefore I was not willing to clear her rooms for her, given that there were 2 more hours on the shift. I was firm with my communication and concluded that I wanted to continue being a team player and being helpful to her, but I would not tolerate being "used" when she would have plenty of time to do those tasks on her own. I explained that I would be setting guidelines for myself, gauging when I felt it would be appropriate to help her, depending on my own individual assignment. I encouraged her to try to complete the tasks independently, but

if it was not possible, I would then be more than happy to help her. I felt she was receptive and she explained that she would try to be more sensitive to me and other co-workers and would make an honest effort to complete the task before requesting my help.

By setting those guidelines and covering the communicating techniques with my nurse colleague beforehand, I felt I was able to handle the situation without destroying our working relationship. In the end, it proved to create a stronger working relationship with Nurse Jane. Shortly thereafter, my co-workers began to see a change in Nurse Jane's efforts to complete her assignment. My communication with Nurse Jane was much easier from that point forward, and eventually Nurse Jane approached me and expressed her appreciation for my honest feedback and appreciated the fact that I went to her directly to resolve the situation without going to the nurse manager.

— Howard Holsinger

 Would this be a suitable approach for you? Why?

CHAPTER CHECKLIST

Professional development can take place in a variety of ways. However, involvement in professional associations can open doors to opportunities that would never have been possible otherwise. Levels of participation in the organization can vary from paying your dues to holding an officer position on the board of directors. Assessing your individual strengths, motivations, and goals before making a commitment to an organization is important. Many nurses find that the membership association can help develop professional skills and provide them with goals that they can achieve. When you are seeking your first job, look to members of the state nurses' association to get acquainted with colleagues and find out about their job and workplace environment. Aside from the networking benefits, the opportunity to get involved in the professional nurses association is a chance to make a dif-

ference in the profession, for your patients and for future nurses.

- Numerous organizations exist in healthcare.
  - The American Nurses Association and numerous specialty organizations focus on improving the profession itself and the care patients receive.
  - Most associations have both volunteers and employed staff to accomplish the organizational goals.
- Connecting with an association produces numerous benefits.
  - Involvement levels vary based on personal situations.
  - Strengths and talents should guide selection of involvement.
  - Some nurses are covered by employment contracts via union activities.
  - Workplace advocacy strategies help nurses interact on an individual or group basis in the employment situation.

Continued

CHAPTER CHECKLIST—cont'd

- Nurses can make various contributions to the profession through association involvement.
  - Networking is facilitated.
  - Associations provide the input to policy makers who determine policies and legislation affecting the practice of nursing and patient rights and benefits.
  - Attendance at meetings provides valuable contacts and different points of view.
  - Work to reverse the workforce shortage in nursing is being led by the professional associations.

TIPS FOR PROFESSIONAL DEVELOPMENT AND ORGANIZATIONAL INVOLVEMENT

- Create an individual mission statement.
- Research and create a file of educational programs of interest.
- Research and create a file of potential future professional opportunities.
- Read nursing journals and attend conventions to keep up on the latest within your profession.
- Participate/volunteer for a grassroots political activity (e.g., city council races, PTA elections).

TERMS TO KNOW

closed shop
collective bargaining
committees
mission
open shop
preprofessional association
professional association (organization)
right-to-work
shared governance
strategic plan
values

REFERENCES

American Medical Association. Web site/membership services. Retrieved from www.ama-assn.org. Accessed July 13, 2002.

American Nurses Publishing. (2002). *Nursing's agenda for the future: A call to the nation.* Washington, DC: ANP.

Cronin, S. N., & Becherer, D. (1999). Recognition of staff nurse job performance and achievements: Staff and manager perceptions. *Journal of Nursing Administration,* 29(1), 26-31.

Division of Nursing, Bureau of Health Professions (2001). *National sample survey of registered nurses.* Washington, DC: Health Resources and Services Administration.

Harris Poll on consumer attitudes toward nursing. (1999, June). Sigma Theta Tau and Nurseweek Publishers.

Kelly, L., & Joel, L. (1995). *Dimensions of professional nursing* (7th ed.). New York: McGraw-Hill.

Marquis, B., & Huston, C. (2000). *Leadership roles and management functions in nursing: Theory and application* (3rd ed.). Philadelphia: Lippincott.

Mason, D., & Leavitt, J. (1998). *Policy and politics in nursing and healthcare* (3rd ed.). Philadelphia: WB Saunders.

Robert, H., Evans, W., & Balch, J. (Eds.). (2000). *Robert's rules of order newly revised.* Cambridge, MA: Perseus Book Group.

Shinn, L. J. (1998). Policy and politics in nursing and health care. In Mason D. & Leavitt J. (Eds.), *Contemporary issues in professional organizations* (3rd ed., pp. 524-535). Philadelphia: WB Saunders.

SUGGESTED READINGS

Andersen, C. A. Fetters. (1999). *Nursing student to nursing leader: The critical path to leadership development.* New York: Delmar.

Covey, S. R. (1991). *Principle-centered leadership.* New York: Fireside.

Feldstein, P. (1996). *The relative success of health associations. The politics of health legislation.* Chicago: Health Administration Press.

Kingdon, J. W. (1995). *Outside of government, but not just looking in. Agendas, alternatives, and public policies.* New York: HarperCollins.

Lindell, A. R. (2000). Insights and inquiry: Why would one want to be president of a major association? *Journal of Professional Nursing,* 16(3), 131.

Longest, B. (1998). *Policymaking outcomes and consequences. Health policymaking in the United States* (2nd ed.). Chicago: Health Administration Press.

Weissert, C., & Weissert, W. (1996). *Interest groups. Governing health: The politics of health policy.* Baltimore: John Hopkins Press.

Epilogue: Thriving in the Future

Leading and managing in nursing constitute a consistent challenge. Even nurses who expect to be followers find that new demands call for sporadic leadership and increased self-management skills. More important, the work of the future is being accomplished in teams, and a strong team does not emerge from weak members. You may have heard President Harry S. Truman's often-quoted phrase, "The buck stops here." But Michael Hammer, author of *Beyond Reengineering*, in the videotape "The Secrets of Shared Leadership," says, "The buck stops everywhere!" The point is we are all accountable for something, and unless our part in the overall scheme is inconsequential, which it usually is not, we must lead when we have the insight, the ability, or the skill that is needed to move a situation forward. Sometimes, merely articulating the problem and posing solutions demonstrates leadership (Fagin, 2000).

Nurse administrators and leaders consistently say that the characteristic they are most seeking in tomorrow's professional nurse is leadership. In probing what that means, we often find themes that relate to activities we currently do that may have serendipitous outcomes. We shape the public's view of the profession, the organization in which we work, and healthcare in general. We influence interdisciplinary views of what it is to be a professional and we create the expectations about what the profession's potential can be.

If we think about the world as a loose web, we know that every element has the potential to influence every other element. This connectivity with each other, whether within our profession or within the team, means that we influence others all of the time.

Six leadership strengths seem to be what are needed for the future (Lipman-Blumen, 2000):

Ethical political savvy: knowing how to effect change and use resources from an ethical, altruistic perspective

Authenticity and accountability: being committed to the group rather than self, which leads to credibility; to be open in decisions

A politics of commonalities: ensuring an environment that allows as many stakeholders as possible to achieve at least a part of their respective agendas

Thinking long term, acting short term: committing to what is best for the future and acting in the present to move toward that goal, including developing the future leadership to succeed current leaders

Leadership through expectation: encouraging others through expectations rather than through micromanagement

A quest for meaning: leaving a legacy through guiding others

These abilities are ones that develop over time, but the key is that the foundation is present. The movement from focusing on the nurse-patient relationship to the big picture of nursing (politics and public or health policy activities) may take several years, but the foundation is there (Fagin, 2000).

Nurses who seek leadership opportunities will find that there are many available—in the employment setting; in professional organizations; and in voluntary, community organizations. Balancing the multiple demands in an era of rapid changes and the resultant new expectations becomes an even greater challenge. Merely being employed is no longer sufficient; we must be employable. This suggests that we must constantly be focused on competence, on learning, and on what the future holds. To be valued in the future, we need to know what the future might encompass. In fact, in 2000 Sigma Theta Tau International identified that one of the eight skills needed for career success was to become a "futures thinker" (Sigma Theta Tau, 2000).

VISIONING

Whether you are a leader, a follower, or a manager, being able to visualize in your mind what the ideal future is becomes a critical strategy. A vision can range from that of an individual to that of a group or to a whole organization. No matter how we engage in this visioning activity, we must be open and honest about what we think for the future. Creating our own circle of advisors or brain trusts (those who do not necessarily think as we do, but who are creative thinkers) allows us to test ideas so that we enhance our own thinking and performance to higher levels. Peter Senge, author of *The Fifth Discipline: The Art and Practice of the Learning Organization* (1990), says that all leadership is really about is people working at their best to create the future.

This epilogue is designed to share some views about the future so that you can think about them in relation to what it means to lead and manage. This "thinking about" the future, like visions, is further enriched through sharing in open dialogues.

Although no one knows the future for certain, there are many entities that engage in formal discussions and predictions. These range from structured groups, such as the World Future Society, to regular reports and books. Although not everyone is a futurist, each of us needs to be aware of trends. Thinking about the future should be mind expanding; it is the most nonstereotypical thinking you can do. The leader of tomorrow, as Porter-O'Grady (1997) says, will be "a gatherer of people and a facilitator of the processes that they might use to come to agreement or to find common ground with regard to an issue or direction" (p. 18).

If the future is about teams and group work (which it is), there are many implications for nursing. For example, how will evaluations and compensation be structured in the future? Will you receive favorable reviews because the group you work with is productive? Will a group receive a bonus or merit salary increase? If you are not a team player, will you be useful to the organization at all? This is one example of how to rethink the future.

SHARED VISIONS

The concept of shared visions suggests that several of us buy into a particular view. If we think of a familiar concept, stress, and what Selye (1976) described as eustress and distress, we have a continuum (see following figure).

Eustress   Distress
$\longleftrightarrow$
Stress

Again, if you think about stress, you recall that each of us views an event differently and that having no stress results in death. Comparably, we can think about how society is evolving currently. Stability and total chaos are the ends of a continuum. Moving in some way between those two ends suggests that we live in a constant state of disequilibrium in which we strive toward stability but recognize we experience chaos. The following figure below suggests that in times of great stability, society makes little progress (but life probably seems serene). In times of great chaos, in contrast, society may transform itself (and life may seem uncontrollable). Thus it is even more important to think about the projections for the future. As one example for most of us, think what we were doing, thinking, believing, and valuing on September 10, 2001. Then think about each in relation to September 11, 2001. We moved from some point on that continuum closer to chaos no matter where we were in the world.

Stability   Chaos
$\longleftrightarrow$
Society

PROJECTIONS FOR THE FUTURE

If you watch future reports on television or read Trend Letter or The Futurist (The World Society publication) or current books, you will find comparable themes about the future. The following are some forecasts for the future that could affect nursing:

- Knowledge will change dramatically, requiring that we all be dedicated learners.
- Technology will continue to revolutionize healthcare.
- Increasing diversity will result in:
  - More people who are older.
  - More people moving to different parts of the country or the world.

- More need for speaking two or three languages.
- People no longer will be satisfied with service—they will want an experience.
- There will be increased violence and simultaneously an increased expectation for civility.
- Stores will be either very small or huge.
- Macromarketing (targeting masses) will be out; micromarketing (targeting specific populations) will be in.
- Job security will be out; career options will be in.
- Competition will be out; cooperation will be in.
- Work will be sporadic.
- More people will be living with chronic diseases.
- Emphasis on prevention will redirect care efforts.
- Work will be accomplished by teams.
- Everyone will need to be a leader.

IMPLICATIONS

So should we be concerned with these forecasts? Are they likely to come true? Cornish (1997) analyzed the predictions from the February 1967 issue of *The Futurist*. Of the 34 forecasts that could be judged, 23 were accurate, and 11 were not. However, some of the 11 were accurate trends that did not meet the targeted date, often because of shifting national priorities such as funding. If this is true historically, we might assume that forecasting, which becomes bet-

ter refined each year, will continue to be a valuable tool for the future. For those who want to thrive, the future forecasts are like the gold ring on the merry-go-round. If you risk and reach far enough, you can grasp it! Lead on . . . ¡Adelánte!

REFERENCES

Cornish, E. (1997, January/February). The Futurist forecasts 30 years later. *The Futurist, 31,* 45-48.

Fagin, C. (2000). *Essays on nursing leadership.* New York: Springer.

Lipman-Blumen, J. (2000, Summer). The age of connective leadership. *Leader to Leader, 17,* 39-45.

Porter-O'Grady, T. (1997). Quantum mechanics and the future of healthcare leadership. *JONA, 27,* 15-20.

Selye, H. (1976). *The stress of life.* New York: McGraw-Hill.

Senge, P. (1990). *The fifth discipline: The art and practice of the learning organization.* New York: Doubleday Currency.

Sigma Theta Tau, International. (2000). Eight skills for a healthy career. *Reflections, 26*(1), 20-21.

SUGGESTED READINGS

Begun, J. W., & White, K. R. (1995). Altering nursing's dominant logic: Guidelines from complex adaptive systems theory. *Complexity and Chaos in Nursing, 2*(1), 5-15.

Rubin, H. (2000, March). Here are the 10 commandments of leadership that I carried down from the mountaintop. *Fast Company,* 276-280.

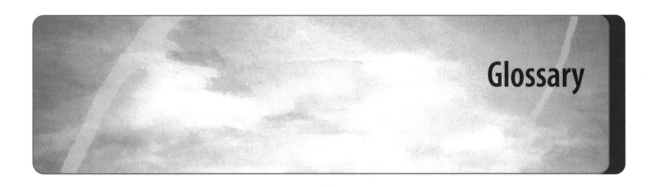

Glossary

Absenteeism The rate at which an individual misses work on an unplanned basis. (Ch. 22)

Accommodation An unassertive, cooperative approach to conflict in which the individual neglects personal needs, goals, and concerns in favor of satisfying those of others. (Ch. 20)

Accountability The expectation of explaining actions and results. (Ch. 21)

Acknowledgment Recognition that an employee is valued and respected for what he or she has to offer to the workplace, team, or group; acknowledgments may be verbal or written, public or private. (Ch. 19)

Active listening Focusing completely on the speaker and listening without judgment to the essence of the conversation; an active listener should be able to repeat accurately at least 95% of the speaker's intended meaning. (Ch. 19)

Activity report A report typically including units of service provided, number of beds, number of occupied beds, number of patients typically cared for per day, and average length of stay. (Ch. 16)

Agenda A written list of items to be covered in a meeting and the related materials that meeting participants should read beforehand or bring along. Types of agendas include structured agendas, timed agendas, and action agendas. (Ch. 24)

Allocation of scarce resources Distribution of resources needed for care but which may exceed budget levels. (Ch. 20)

Apparent agency Doctrine whereby a principal becomes accountable for the actions of his or her agent; created when a person holds himself or herself out as acting on behalf of the principal; also known as *apparent authority*. (Ch. 4)

Associate nurse A licensed nurse in the primary nursing system who provides care to the patient according to the primary nurse's specification when the primary nurse is not working. (Ch. 15)

At-will employee An individual who works without a contract. (Ch. 10)

Autonomy Personal freedom and the right to choose what will happen to one's own person. (Ch. 4)

Average daily census (ADC) Average number of patients cared for per day for a reporting period. (Ch. 16)

Average length of stay The number of patient days in a specific time period divided by the number of discharges in that same time period. (Ch. 16)

Avoiding An unassertive, uncooperative approach to conflict in which the avoider neither pursues his or her own needs, goals, and concerns nor helps others to do so. (Ch. 20)

Barriers Factors, internal or external to the change situation, that interfere with movement toward a desirable outcome. (Ch. 8)

Benchmarking Best practices, processes, or systems identified by a quality improvement team to be compared with the practice, process, or system under review. (Ch. 11)

Beneficence Principle that states that the actions one takes should promote good. (Ch. 4)

Biomedical technology The use of machines and implantable devices to provide physiological monitoring, diagnostic testing, drug administration, and therapeutic treatments in patient care. (Ch. 12)

Budget A detailed financial plan, stated in dollars, for carrying out the activities an organization wants to accomplish within a specific period. (Ch. 13)

Budgeting process An ongoing activity of planning and managing revenues and expenses to meet the goals of the organization. (Ch. 13)

Bureaucratic organization Characterized by formality, low autonomy, a hierarchy of authority, an environment of rules, division of labor, specialization, centralization, and control. (Ch. 9)

Burnout Disengagement from work characterized by emotional exhaustion, depersonalization, and decreased effectiveness. (Ch. 24)

Capital expenditure budget A plan for purchasing major capital items, such as equipment or a physical plant, with a useful life greater than 1 year and exceeding a minimum cost set by the organization. (Ch. 13)

Capitation A reimbursement method in which healthcare providers are paid a per-person-per-year (or per-month) fee for providing specified services over a period of time. (Ch. 13)

Care delivery strategy The method used to provide care to patients. (Ch. 15)

Care MAP An abbreviation for a care Multidisciplinary Action Plan, which combines a nursing care plan with a critical path. The purpose is to expedite patient care by improving the expected outcome during a designated day. (Ch. 15)

Career Progressive achievement throughout a person's professional life. (Ch. 26)

Case management A person-oriented service that reflects multidisciplinary cooperation and coordination. (Ch. 3)

Case management method A method of delivering patient care based on patient outcomes and cost containment. Components of case management are a case manager, critical paths, and unit-based managed care. (Ch. 15)

Case manager A baccalaureate or master's degree–prepared clinical nurse who coordinates patient care from preadmission to and through discharge. (Ch. 15)

Case method A method of care delivery in which one nurse provides total care for one patient during an entire work period. (Ch. 15)

Case mix The volume and type of patients served by a healthcare provider. (Ch. 13)

Cash budget A plan for an organization's cash receipts and disbursements. (Ch. 13)

Centers for Disease Control and Prevention (CDC) The main federal agency protecting the health and safety of people in the United States. (Ch. 10)

Certification Designation of special knowledge beyond basic licensure. (Ch. 26)

Chain of command The hierarchy depicted in vertical dimensions of organizational charts. (Ch. 9)

Change agents Individuals with formal or informal legitimate power whose purpose is to initiate, champion, and direct or guide change. (Ch. 8)

Change management The overall processes and strategies used to moderate and manage the preparation for, effect of, responses to, and outcomes of any condition or circumstance that is new or different from what existed previously. (Ch. 8)

Change outcome The end product of a change process. (Ch. 8)

Change process The series of ongoing efforts applied to managing a change. (Ch. 8)

Change situations The field comprised of various factors and dynamics within which change is occurring. (Ch. 8)

Chaos theory Theoretical construct defining the random-appearing, yet deterministic, characteristics of complex organizations (see *Nonlinear change*). (Ch. 8)

Charge nurse A registered nurse responsible for delegating and coordinating patient care and staff on a specific unit. A resource person for all staff; there is usually one charge nurse each shift per unit. (Ch. 15)

Charges The cost of providing a service plus a markup for profit. (Ch. 13)

Chemically dependent A psychophysiological state in which an individual requires a substance, such as drugs or alcohol, to prevent the onset of symptoms of abstinence. (Ch. 22)

Closed shop A collective bargaining situation that requires membership (or at least dues-equivalent payment) (as opposed to open shop). (Ch. 27)

Coaching The strategy a manager uses to help others learn, think critically, and grow through communications about performance. (Ch. 17)

Coalitions Groups of individuals or organizations that join together temporarily around a common goal. This goal often focuses on an effort to effect change. (Ch. 25)

Collaboration Conjoint, interdisciplinary problem solving from an equal power base on the patient's behalf; also, an assertive, cooperative approach to conflict in which the individual is able to work creatively and openly with others to find the solution that best achieves all important goals. (Ch. 20)

Collective action A mechanism for achieving professional practice through group decision making. (Ch. 10)

Collective bargaining Mechanism for settling labor disputes by negotiation between the employer and representatives of the employees. (Chs. 4, 10, 27)

Commitment A state of being emotionally impelled; feeling passionate about and dedicated to a project or event. (Ch. 19)

Committees A small group of appointed or elected individuals to serve an express function or to accomplish a specific goal for the organization (e.g., advisory committee, policy and agenda committee). (Ch. 27)

Common law System of jurisprudence that is derived from principles rather than rules and regulations and that consists of comprehensive principles based on justice, reason, and common sense. (Ch. 4)

Competing An assertive, uncooperative approach to conflict in which the individual pursues his or her own needs at the expense of others. (Ch. 20)

Compromising A moderately assertive, cooperative approach to conflict in which the individual's ability to negotiate and willingness to "give and take" results in conflict resolution and fulfillment of important priorities for all involved. (Ch. 20)

Computerized patient record (CPR) Technology allowing for immediate and complete access to patient information for clinical decision making, outcome evaluation, and coordination of patient-care resources and patient flow through the healthcare delivery system. (Ch. 12)

Confidentiality Right of privacy to the medical record of a patient; also, a respect for the privacy of information and the ethical use of information for its original purpose. (Ch. 4)

Conflict A perceived difference among people and a four-stage process including frustration, conceptualization, action, and outcomes. (Ch. 20)

Consolidated systems A group of healthcare organizations that are united based on common characteristics of ownership, regional location, or mutual performance objectives for the purpose of optimizing utilization of their resources in achieving their missions. (Ch. 6)

Consumer focus Centering of action or attention on the participant or user as a whole. (Ch. 14)

Continuing education Those learning activities intended to build on the educational and experiential bases of the professional nurse for the enhancement of practice, education, administration, research, or theory development to the end of improving the health of the public (ANCC, 1991, p. 76). (Ch. 26)

Continuous quality improvement A program designed to improve the quality of care. Also, an ongoing process that involves a multidisciplinary team for planning or problem solving. Similar to quality improvement but emphasizes the continuous nature of the process. (Ch. 11)

Contractual allowance A discount from full charges. (Ch. 13)

Coping The immediate response of a person to a threatening situation. (Ch. 24)

Corporate liability The condition of being responsible for corporate loss related to acts performed and not performed in meeting obligations to operate legally and judiciously. (Ch. 4)

Cost The amount spent on something; the national healthcare costs are a function of the price and utilization of healthcare services; a healthcare provider's costs are the expenses involved in providing goods or services. (Ch. 13)

Cost-based reimbursement A retrospective payment method in which all allowable costs are used as the basis for payment. (Ch. 13)

Cost center An organizational unit for which costs can be identified and managed. (Chs. 13, 16)

Creativity Conceptualizing new and innovative approaches to solving problems or making decisions. (Ch. 5)

Critical path A component of a care MAP that is specific to diagnosis-related group reimbursement. The purpose is to ensure patients are discharged before insurance reimbursement is eliminated. (Ch. 15)

Critical thinking A composite of knowledge, attitudes, and skills; an intellectually disciplined process. Also, the ability to assess a situation by asking open-ended questions about the facts and assumptions that underlie it and to use personal judgment and problem-solving ability in deciding how to deal with it. (Ch. 5)

Cultural competence The process in which the healthcare provider continuously strives to achieve the ability to effectively work within the cultural context of a patient (Camphina-Bacote, 1999). This includes attitudes, behaviors, and policies that allow people to work together effectively in cross-cultural situations. (Chs. 14, 18)

Cultural diversity A vast range of cultural differences related to institutional, ethnic, gender, religious, or other variables that convey a set of beliefs or values that have become factors needing attention in living and working together. It is often applied to an organization that seeks to deal with the interface of people who are different from each other (Simons et al., 1993). (Ch. 18)

Culture A way of life. It is developed and communicated by a group of people, consciously or unconsciously, to subsequent generations. It consists of ideas, habits, attitudes, customs, and traditions that help create standards for a group of people to coexist. It makes a group of people unique (Simons et al., 1993). (Chs. 10, 18)

Curriculum vitae A listing of professional life activities. (Ch. 26)

Cybernetic theory Regulation of systems by managing communication and feedback mechanisms. (Ch. 8)

Data Discrete entities that describe or measure something without interpretation. (Ch. 12)

Database A collection of data elements organized and stored together. (Ch. 12)

Decision making Purposeful and goal-directed effort using a systematic process to choose among options. (Ch. 5)

Delegatee The individual who becomes accountable for performing delegated activities. (Ch. 21)

Delegation Achieving performance of care outcomes for which an individual is accountable and responsible by sharing activities with other individuals who have the appropriate authority to accomplish the work. (Chs. 21, 24)

Delegator The individual with authority to share activities with another. (Ch. 21)

Deontological theories From the Greek for "duty," derived norms and rules from the duties that human beings owe one another by virtue of commitments made and roles assumed; sometimes subdivided into situational ethical theories. (Ch. 4)

Depersonalization Inability to become involved in human relationships and interactions. (Ch. 24)

Differentiated nursing practice Recognizing a difference in the level of education and competency of each registered nurse. The differentiation is based on education, position, and clinical expertise. (Ch. 15)

Dualism An "either/or" way of conceptualizing reality in terms of two opposing sides or parts (right or wrong, yes or no), limiting the broad spectrum of possibilities that exists between. (Ch. 19)

Effective communication A process that leads to positive outcomes for senders and receivers in terms of clarity, usefulness, and efficiency. (Ch. 19)

Email A telecommunications system in which a computer user can exchange messages with other computer users via a network. (Ch. 12)

Emancipated minors Persons under the age of adulthood who are no longer under the control and regulation of their parents and who may give valid consent for medical procedures; examples include married teens, underaged parents, and teens in the armed services. (Ch. 4)

Emerging workforce The so-called twenty-something generation that was born between the years of 1965 and 1985. (Ch. 2)

Emotional intelligence Monitoring emotions in a situation to guide actions and inform thought processes. (Ch. 1)

Employee assistance programs Programs designed to provide counseling and other services for employees through either in-house staff or a contracted mental health agency. (Ch. 24)

Empowerment A sharing of power and control with the expectation that people are responsible for themselves; also, the process by which we facilitate the participation of others in decision making within an environment where there is an equitable distribution of power. (Chs. 10, 17, 25)

Entrenched workforce Employed persons over the age of 35 who are thought of as the Baby Boomer generation. (Ch. 2)

Ergonomics Science of fitting the job to the worker. (Ch. 4)

Ethics Science relating to moral actions and moral values; rules of conduct recognized in respect to a particular class of human actions. (Ch. 4)

Ethics committees Groups of persons who provide structure and guidelines for potential healthcare problems, serve as an open forum for discussion, and function as patient advocates. (Ch. 4)

Ethnicity One's migratory status, race, language, and dialect and sense of distinctiveness (Spector, 2000). (Ch. 18)

Ethnocentrism Using the culture of one's own groups as a standard for the judgment of others, or thinking of it as superior to other cultures that are merely different (Simons et al., 1993). (Ch. 18)

Evidence-based practice The integration of individual clinical expertise, built from practice, with the best available clinical evidence from systematic research applied to practice. (Ch. 12)

Expected outcomes The result of patient goals that are achieved through a combination of medical and nursing interventions with patient participation. (Ch. 15)

Expert system A program that mimics the inductive and deductive reasoning of a human expert. (Ch. 12)

Expert witnesses Persons testifying who have special knowledge about a given subject or occupation; knowledge of expert witnesses must generally be such that it is not normally possessed by the average person; contrasts with a lay witness. (Ch. 4)

Facilitators Factors, internal or external to the change situation, that promote movement toward a desired outcome. (Ch. 8)

Factor evaluation system A patient classification system that incorporates specific elements or critical indicators and rates patients on each of these elements. Each indicator is assigned a weight or numerical value. (Ch. 16)

Failure to warn Newer area of potential liability for nurse managers that involves the responsibility to warn subsequent or potential employers of nurses' incompetence or impairment. (Ch. 4)

Fee-for-service A system in which patients have the option of consulting any healthcare provider, subject to reasonable requirements that may include utilization review and prior approval for certain services but does not include a requirement to seek approval through a gatekeeper. (Ch. 6)

Fidelity Keeping one's promises or commitments. (Ch. 4)

Fit The possession of characteristics that are suitable to the work that is to be carried out and the technologies by which the work is to be accomplished. (Ch. 9)

"Five-why" technique Asking the question "Why?" at least five times to attempt to get to the root of a problem. (Ch. 11)

Fixed costs Costs that do not change in total as the volume of patients changes. (Ch. 13)

Fixed FTEs Full-time equivalent roles that do not fluctuate based on patient care demands. (Ch. 16)

Flat organization Characterized by decentralization of decision making to the level of personnel carrying out the work. (Ch. 9)

Followers Persons who contribute to a group's outcomes by implementing activities and providing appropriate feedback. (Ch. 3)

Followership Those with whom a leader interacts; involves the assertive use of personal behaviors in contributing toward organizational outcomes while still acquiescing certain tasks to the leader or other team members. (Chs. 1, 10)

Forecast The process of making decisions about the future based on multiple sources of data. (Ch. 16)

Foreseeability Concept that certain events may reasonably be expected to cause specific consequences; third element of negligence/malpractice. (Ch. 4)

Full-time equivalent (FTE) An employee who works fulltime, 40 hours per week, 2080 hours per year. (Chs. 13, 16)

Functional nursing Care provided by each member providing a specific task for a large group of patients. (Ch. 15)

Gatekeeper Liaison between the consumer and the healthcare market. (Ch. 14)

General adaptation syndrome (GAS) A pattern of response to stress (Selye, 1956). (Ch. 24)

Governance System by which an organization controls and directs formulation and administration of policy. (Ch. 10)

Group A number of individuals assembled together or having a unifying relationship. (Ch. 19)

Halo or recency effect Only positive (halo) or recent (recency) performances are acknowledged. (Ch. 17)

Healthcare consumer Patient/customer who uses healthcare provider resources. (Ch. 14)

Healthcare provider Agencies, insurers, physicians, nurses, and allied health people providing health-related business to consumers. (Chs. 13, 14)

Hierarchy Chain of command that connotes authority and responsibility. (Ch. 9)

High-complexity change A complicated change situation characterized by the interactions of multiple variables of people, technology, and systems. (Ch. 8)

High tech Mechanistic perspective that relates to the use of technology in the diagnosis and treatment of disease. (Ch. 14)

High touch Caring, humanistic perspective that relates to the use of human skills in the care and treatment of patients. (Ch. 14)

Hybrid organization Possessing characteristics from several types of organizational structures. (Ch. 9)

Indemnification Obligation resting on one person to make good any loss or damages another has incurred because of the person's actions or inactions; refers to the total shifting of the economic loss to the party chiefly responsible for that loss. (Ch. 4)

Independent contractor One who makes an agreement with another to perform a service or piece of work and retains in himself or herself control of the means, method, and manner of producing the result to be accomplished; sometimes called an *independent practitioner*. (Ch. 4)

Influence The process of using power; may range from the punitive power of coercion to the interactive power of collaboration. (Ch. 25)

Informal change agent Persons without designated authority who advance the change among a group of people. (Ch. 8)

Informatics The use of knowledge technology. (Ch. 12)

Informatics competencies The integration of knowledge, skills, and attitudes in the performance of various nursing activities that involve data, information, and knowledge within prescribed levels of nursing practice. (Ch. 12)

Information Communication of reception of knowledge, consisting of interpreted, organized, or structured data. (Ch. 12)

Information overload A state of stress brought about by a lack of information-processing skills. (Ch. 24)

Information technology The use of computer hardware and software to process data into information to solve problems. (Ch. 12)

Informed consent Authorization by patient or patient's legal representative to do something to the patient. (Ch. 4)

Internet The worldwide network of computers communicating via an agreed-upon set of protocols. (Ch. 12)

Interpersonal conflict Conflict that occurs between or among people. (Ch. 20)

Intrapersonal conflict Conflict that occurs within an individual. (Ch. 20)

Justice Principle that persons should be treated equally and fairly. (Ch. 4)

Knowledge Information that is combined or synthesized so that interrelationships are identified. (Ch. 12)

Knowledge technology The use of expert and decision support systems to assist in making decisions about patient care delivery. (Ch. 12)

Knowledge worker An individual who performs nonrepetitive, nonroutine work consuming considerable levels of cognitive activity and judgment. (Ch. 12)

Labor cost per unit of service A comparison of budgeted salary costs per budgeted volume of service with actual salary costs per actual volume of service. (Ch. 16)

Labor law Examples of these federal mandates include the 1935 Wagner Act, which established election procedures for collective bargaining representatives, and the 1947 Taft-Hartley Act, which placed curbs on some union activity and excluded employees of not-for-profit hospitals from coverage. (Ch. 10)

Labor unions Associations of workers that exist for the purpose of bargaining, either in whole or in part, on behalf of the workers with management about the terms of employment. (Ch. 4)

Law Sum total of rules and regulations by which a society is governed; rules and regulations established and enforced by authority or custom within a given community, state, or nation. (Ch. 4)

Leaders Persons who demonstrate and exercise influence and power over others. (Ch. 3)

Leadership The use of personal traits to constructively and ethically influence patients, families, and staff through a *process* in which clinical and organizational outcomes are achieved through collective efforts. (Chs. 1, 2)

Learning organization The designation of a type of organization in which continual learning as an expectation permeates all levels to promote adequate responses required by dynamic, accelerated change. (Ch. 8)

Liability Refers to one's responsibility for his or her own conduct; an obligation or duty to be performed; responsibility for an action or outcome. (Ch. 4)

Liable Refers to one's responsibility for his or her actions or inactions. (Ch. 4)

Licensure A right granted that gives the licensee permission to do something that he or she could not legally do absent such permission. Also, the minimum form of credentialing, providing baseline expectations for those in a particular field without identifying or obligating the practitioner to function in a professional manner as defined by the profession itself. (Ch. 26)

Low-complexity change An uncomplicated change situation characterized by the interactions of the limited influences of people, technology, and systems. (Ch. 8)

Magnet Recognition A distinction granted by the American Nurses Credentialing Center for quality nursing services. (Ch. 1)

Malpractice Failure of a professional person to act in accordance with the prevalent professional standards or failure to foresee potential consequences that a professional person, having the necessary skills and expertise to act in a professional manner, should foresee. (Ch. 4)

Managed care Care purchased through a public or private healthcare organization whose goal is to promote quality healthcare outcomes for patients at the lowest cost possible through planning, directing, and coordinating care delivered by healthcare organizations that it may own, have contractual agreements with, or have authority over by virtue of the fact that it reimburses the organization for services provided its patients. This model rewards healthcare providers for low utilization of care that is relatively low in cost; also, a system of care in which a designated person determines the services the patient uses. (Chs. 3, 6, 13)

Management The activities needed to plan, organize, motivate, and control the human and material resources needed to achieve outcomes consistent with the organization's mission and purpose. (Chs. 1, 2)

Management theory The theory related to the activities described in management. (See *Management*) (Ch. 1)

Manager A person who directs a team of workers. (Ch. 3)

Marketing Analysis, planning, implementation, and control of programs for the purpose of meeting organizational objectives. (Ch. 7)

Master staffing plan The overall plan for allocating numbers and types of personnel, taking into consideration numerous factors that predict these factors. (Ch. 16)

Matrix organization An organizational structure influenced by dual authority, such as product line and discipline. (Ch. 9)

Mediation A process using a trained third party to assist with conflict resolution. (Ch. 20)

Mentor An experienced person who helps a less experienced person navigate into expertise. (Chs. 2, 10, 25)

Mission Statement of an organization's reason for being. (Chs. 9, 27)

Modular nursing A modified team nursing approach focused on geographic location of patient rooms and assignment of staff members. (Ch. 15)

MORAL Model An ethical decision-making model consisting of five distinct steps. (Ch. 4)

Motivation The instigation of action based on various factors, both intrinsic and extrinsic. (Ch. 1)

Multicultural Maintaining several different cultures. (Ch. 18)

Negligence Failure to exercise the degree of care that a person of ordinary prudence, based on the reasonable person standard, would exercise under the same or similar circumstances; also known as *ordinary negligence*. (Ch. 4)

Negotiating Conferring with others to bring about a settlement of differences. (Chs. 20, 25)

Networks Resources of colleagues upon whom you can draw for advice; formal systems to provide services. (Chs. 6, 25)

Nonlinear change Change occurring from self-organizing patterns, not human-induced ones, in complex, open system organizations. (Ch. 8)

Nonmaleficence Principle that states that one should do no harm. (Ch. 4)

Nonproductive hours See *Nonproductive time*. (Ch. 13)

Nonproductive time Benefit time such as vacation or sick time. (Ch. 16)

Nonpunitive discipline A disciplinary measure, usually verbal, describing existing standards and goals to which the parties agreed; pay is not withheld; employee either agrees to adhere to the standards in the future or to be terminated. (Ch. 22)

Not-for-profit Organization that has funds redirected to maintenance and growth rather than as dividends to stockholders. (Ch. 6)

Nurse practice act Legal scope of practice allowed by state legislation and authority. (Ch. 4)

Nursing Licensure Compact The mutual recognition model among states that agree to allow a nurse to hold licensure in one state and to practice in other states. (Ch. 3)

Nursing minimum data set (NMDS) Uniform standard for collecting comparable essential patient data. (Ch. 12)

Open shop A contract situation that allows but does not require members to join. (Ch. 27)

Operating budget A financial plan for day-to-day activities of an organization. (Ch. 13)

Optimizing decision Selecting the most ideal solution or option to achieve goals. (Ch. 5)

Organizational chart A chart that defines organizational positions' responsibility for specific functions. (Ch. 9)

Organizational conflict Conflict that occurs when a person confronts an organization's policies and procedures for patient care and personnel and its accepted norms of behavior and communication. (Ch. 20)

Organizational culture The attitudes, behaviors, and policies evident in an organization that create the ambiance and operation of the workplace. (Ch. 3)

Organizational structure A framework that divides work within an organization and delineates points of authority, responsibility, accountability, and non–decision-making support. (Ch. 9)

Organized delivery system (ODS) Networks of healthcare organizations, providers, and payers who provide a comprehensive package of healthcare services at a competitive price. (Ch. 13)

OSHA Occupational Safety and Health Administration. (Ch. 10)

Outcome criteria See *Expected outcomes*. (Ch. 15)

Overwork A situation in which employees are expected to become more productive without additional resources. (Ch. 24)

Partnership model A system of providing patient care when an RN is paired with an LPN or an unlicensed assistive person to provide total care to a number of patients. (Ch. 15)

Paternalism Principle that allows one to make decisions for another; often called *parentalism*. (Ch. 4)

Patient care outcome A measurable end result of patient care. (Ch. 11)

Patient-focused care unit A system in which staff functions become centralized on a unit to reduce the number of staff required; emphasizes quality, cost, and value. (Ch. 15)

Patient outcomes See *Expected outcomes*. (Ch. 15)

Payer mix The volume and type of reimbursement sources for a healthcare provider. (Ch. 13)

Payers Sources of healthcare financing or payment for health services; includes government, private insurance, and individuals (self-pay). (Ch. 13)

Percentage of occupancy The patient census divided by the number of beds on the unit. (Ch. 16)

Perfectionism The tendency to never finish anything because it isn't quite perfect. (Ch. 24)

Performance appraisal Individual evaluation of work performance. (Ch. 17)

Performance improvement (PI) The application of quality improvement principles on an ongoing basis, usually used to assess group or individual activity. (Ch. 11)

Personal liability Serves to make each person responsible at law for his or her own actions. (Ch. 4)

Philosophy Values and beliefs regarding nature of work derived from a mission and the rights/responsibilities of people involved. (Ch. 9)

Planned change Change expected and deliberately prepared beforehand by using systematic directional processes to develop and carry out activities to accomplish a desired outcome. (Ch. 8)

Polarities Situations involving two interdependent opposites between which a shifting of emphasis naturally occurs. (Ch. 20)

Policy A consciously chosen course of action (or inaction) directed toward some end (Kalisch & Kalisch, 1982). (Ch. 25)

Politics A process of human interaction within organizations. (Ch. 25)

Position description A general overall description of the duties and responsibilities of the employee. (Ch. 17)

Power The ability to influence others in the effort to achieve goals. (Ch. 25)

Preprofessional association An alliance of student practitioners within a profession that provides opportunities for its members to meet leaders in the field, hone their own leadership skills, learn about opportunities within the profession, network with mentors and get advice for professional development, participate in policy formation, learn specialized education, and shape the future of the profession. (Ch. 27)

Price See *Charges*. (Ch. 13)

Primary care First access to care. (Ch. 6)

Primary nurse One who is the deliverer of autonomous care. (Ch. 15)

Primary nursing A method of patient care delivery whereby one registered nurse functions autonomously as the patient's main nurse throughout the entire hospital stay. (Ch. 15)

Principlism Emerging theory of ethics that incorporates existing ethical principles and attempts to resolve conflicts by applying one or more of the ethical principles. (Ch. 4)

Privacy The right to protection against unreasonable and unwarranted interference with one's solitude; the right of an individual to be left alone. (Ch. 4)

Private Owned and operated by an individual citizen or group of citizens. (Ch. 6)

Problem solving Using a systematic process to solve a problem. (Ch. 5)

Process of care The desired sequence of steps that have been designed to achieve clinical standardization. (Ch. 1)

Procrastination Doing one thing when one should be doing something else. (Ch. 24)

Productive hours Paid time that is worked. (Ch. 13)

Productive time Time an employee actually works. (Ch. 16)

Productivity The ratio of outputs to inputs or, in nursing terms, of services to resources used to provide services. (Ch. 13)

Professional association (organization) An alliance of practitioners within a profession that provides opportunities for its members to meet leaders in the field, hone their own leadership skills, participate in policy formation, continue specialized education, and shape the future of the profession. (Chs. 26, 27)

Profit An excess of revenues over expenses. (Ch. 13)

Progressive discipline A step-by-step process of increasing disciplinary measures, usually beginning with an oral warning, followed by a written warning, suspension, and termination, if necessary. (Ch. 22)

Prospective reimbursement A method of payment in which the third-party payer decides in advance the flat rate that will be paid for a service or episode of care. (Ch. 13)

Prototype evaluation system System of classifying in broad categories. (Ch. 16)

Providers See *Healthcare provider.* (Ch. 13)

Public Organization providing health services under the support and direction of local, state, or federal government. (Ch. 6)

Quality assurance (QA) A process that focuses on the clinical aspects of a provider's care, often in response to an identified problem. (Ch. 11)

Quality improvement (QI) An ongoing process of innovation, error prevention, and staff development used by an organization that has adopted a quality management philosophy. (Ch. 11)

Quality indicators Quality indicators can be defined as measurable elements of quality that specify the focus of evaluation and documentation. (Ch. 3)

Quality management (QM) A corporate philosophy emphasizing customer satisfaction, innovation, and employee involvement in quality improvement activities. (Ch. 11)

Quantum theory A physics theory stating that energy is not a smooth-flowing continuum, but rather bursts of energy that are related. (Ch. 3)

Reengineering A complete overhaul of an organizational structure. (Hammer & Champy, 1993). (Ch. 9)

Reintegration A concept that focuses on a return to the whole of nursing, incorporating all aspects of the professional nurse's role: education, scholarship, practice, and service. (Ch. 26)

Respect for others The highest ethical principle, respect for others acknowledges the right of individuals to make decisions and to live by those decisions. (Ch. 4)

Respondeat superior A doctrine by which the employer is given accountability and responsibility for an employee's negligent actions incurred during the course and scope of employment. (Ch. 4)

Responsibility The condition of being reliable and dependable and being obligated to accomplish work. (Ch. 21)

Résumé A summary of professional abilities and facts designed for specific opportunities. (Ch. 26)

Revenue Money earned by an organization for providing goods or services. (Ch. 13)

Right-to-work Refers to nonunion workplaces. The employer gives the employee the option to join a union or professional association. The nurse is responsible for direct communication with the employer. (Ch. 27)

Risk management Process of developing and implementing strategies that will minimize the adverse effects of accidental losses on an organization. This includes preventing patient injury, minimizing financial loss after a problem/error occurs, and preserving agency reputation. (Ch. 11)

Role Expected or actual behavior, determined by a person's position or status in a group. (Ch. 3)

Role ambiguity A condition in which individuals do not have a clear understanding about performance and evaluation. (Ch. 17)

ROLES An acronym used to identify the components of a role: *r*esponsibilities, *o*pportunities, *l*ines of communication, *e*xpectations, and *s*upport. (Ch. 23)

Role conflict A condition in which individuals understand the role but are unwilling or unable to meet the requirements. (Ch. 17)

Role development Choosing to change role expectations and/or role performance. (Ch. 23)

Role discrepancy A gap between role expectations and role performance. (Ch. 23)

Role expectations The attitudes and behaviors another anticipates a person in the role will possess or demonstrate. (Ch. 23)

Role internalization The stage at which a person has learned the behaviors that maintain the role so thoroughly that the person performs them without consciously considering them; energy once spent on establishing these behaviors can now be redirected toward other goals. (Ch. 23)

Role model A person who enacts a role, typically in a positive way, so that others can follow the example. (Ch. 10)

Role negotiation Resolving conflicting expectations about personal management performance through communication. (Ch. 23)

Role strain The subjective feeling of discomfort experienced as a result of role stress; may manifest through increased frustration, heightened emotional awareness, or emotional fragility to situations. (Chs. 22, 23)

Role stress A social condition in which role demands are conflicting, irritating, or impossible to fulfill. (Chs. 22, 23)

Role theory A framework used to understand how individuals perform within organizations. (Chs. 3, 17)

Role transition The process of unlearning an old role and learning a new role. Transforming one's identity from being an individual contributor as a staff nurse to being a leader as a nurse manager. (Ch. 23)

Root-cause analysis The process used to identify all possible causes of a sentinel event and all appropriate risk-reduction strategies. (Ch. 11)

Satisficing decision Selecting an option that is acceptable, but not necessarily the best option. (Satisfy + suffice = satisfice) (Ch. 5)

Scheduling The implementation of the staffing plan by assigning unit personnel to work specific hours and days. (Ch. 16)

Secondary care Disease restorative care. (Ch. 6)

Self-management The ability of individuals to actively gain control of their lives; components include stress management, time management, meeting management, and the ability to delegate. (Ch. 24)

Sender-receiver The two required participant roles in the communication process. (Ch. 19)

Sentinel event A serious unexpected occurrence involving death or injury, such as suicide, infant abduction, or surgery on the wrong body part. (Ch. 11)

Service In healthcare context, the interaction between a consumer and the system to the extent needs are addressed. (Ch. 14)

Service lines A functional unit of management in which all related concepts of medical care are grouped. (Ch. 14)

Shared governance A term used to describe a flat type of organizational structure with decision making decentralized. (Chs. 9, 10, 27)

Smart card Credit card–like devices that store data. (Ch. 12)

Staff mix The proportion of RNs to LPNs/LVNs to UAPs in a specific setting. (Ch. 15)

Staffing The function of planning for hiring and deploying qualified personnel to meet the needs of patients for care and services. (Ch. 16)

Staffing model The conceptual approach of accomplishing the work to be done on a given unit. (Ch. 16)

Staffing regulations Licensing regulations required by the state department of health, usually related to the minimum number of professional nurses on a unit at a given time. (Ch. 16)

Standard of care Level or degree of quality considered adequate by a given profession; skills and learning commonly possessed by members of a profession; also written at a minimum level. (Ch. 4)

Statute Rule/regulation created by elected legislative bodies; also known as *statutory law*. (Ch. 4)

Strategic plan The operationalization of an organization's mission, goals, and objectives. (Ch. 27)

Strategic planning A process designed to achieve goals through allocation of resources. (Ch. 7)

Strategies Approaches designed to achieve a specific purpose. (Ch. 8)

Structured nursing language A standardized and organized set of concepts and relationships that nursing informatics research has shown to be useful in representing the nursing domain. (Ch. 12)

Synergy A phenomenon in which teamwork produces extraordinary results that could not have been achieved by any one individual. (Ch. 19)

Teaching institution An academic health center and affiliated hospital. (Ch. 6)

Team A number of people associated together in specific work or activities. (Ch. 19)

Team nursing A small group of licensed and unlicensed personnel, with a team leader, responsible for providing patient care to a group of patients. (Ch. 15)

Technology A method, process, or system for providing services. Also, a scientific method of achieving a practical purpose. (Ch. 9)

Telehealth The use of modern telecommunications and information technologies for the provision of healthcare to individuals at a distance and the transmission of information to provide that care; involves the use of two-way interactive video-conferencing, high-speed phone lines, fiberoptic cable, and satellite transmissions. (Ch. 12)

Teleological theories From the Greek for "end," derived norms and rules for conduct from the consequences of actions. (Ch. 4)

Tertiary care Rehabilitative or long-term care. (Ch. 6)

Third-party payers Private and public agencies that contract with an individual to assume responsibility to pay under defined conditions for specified healthcare services. (Chs. 5, 6)

Time management The use of tools, techniques, strategies, and follow-up systems to control wasted time and to ensure that the time invested in activities leads toward achieving a desired, high-priority goal. (Ch. 24)

Total patient care See *Case method*. (Ch. 15)

Total quality management A combination of quality improvement ideas. (Ch. 11)

Transactional leadership The act of using rewards and punishments as part of daily oversight of employees in seeking to get the group to accomplish a task. (Ch. 2)

Transcultural nursing administration A part of the corporate culture in which nursing administrators are committed to transcultural management, which includes mission statements and policies to reflect the workforce diversity. (Ch. 18)

Transculturalism Bridging significant differences in cultural practices. (Ch. 18)

Transformational leadership An act of encouraging followers to follow the leader's style and change their interests into a group interest with concern for a broader goal. (Ch. 2)

Triangulation A technique used by risk managers and others using multiple data sources and data collection to gather information about unusual occurrences. (Ch. 11)

Unit of service A measure of the work being produced by the organization, such as patient days, patient or home visits, or procedures. (Chs. 13, 16)

Unlicensed assistive personnel Healthcare workers who are not licensed and who are prepared to provide certain elements of care under the supervision of a registered nurse (e.g., technicians, nurse aides, or certified nursing assistants). (Ch. 15)

Utilization The quantity or volume of services provided. (Ch. 13)

Values Inner forces that influence decision making and priority setting. (Chs. 1, 4, 27)

Variable costs Costs that vary in direct proportion to patient volume or acuity. (Ch. 13)

Variable FTEs Those full-time equivalent positions that depend on the demand for care, typically staff positions. (Ch. 16)

Variance Anything that occurs to alter a patient's progress through a normal care path. (Chs. 13, 15)

Variance analysis Budget-control process to determine differences between income and expense, projected and actual costs. (Ch. 13)

Variance report A report defining the difference between the actual and projected staffing or budgeting. (Ch. 16)

Veracity Principle that compels the truth be told completely. (Ch. 4)

Vertical organization A linear structure that describes hierarchal responsibility of positions. (Ch. 9)

Vicarious liability Imputation of accountability upon one person or entity for the actions of another person; substituted liability or imputed liability. (Ch. 4)

Virtual organization An organization that exists in essence or effect, although not in actual fact or form. (Ch. 9)

Vision The desired future state. (Ch. 27)

Voice technology Control of computer by vocal input. (Ch. 12)

Wireless (WL) messaging An extension of an existing wired network that uses radio-based systems to transmit data signals through the air without any physical connections. (Ch. 12)

Whistleblowing Making public a serious wrongdoing or danger concealed within an organization when internal actions have failed to correct or make public a situation. (Ch. 10)

Workload The amount of work distributed to a person or unit for a given time period. (Ch. 16)

Workplace advocacy Multidimensional concept that refers to acting on or in behalf of another who is unable to act for himself or herself to effect change about workplace conditions. (Ch. 10)

World Wide Web A set of standards and communication protocols that allow information to be shared across the Internet regardless of the user's platform. (Ch. 12)

Workbook Activities

Managing, Leading, and Following

INTRODUCTION

Effective managers focus efficiently on objectives, tasks, procedures, and policies. Recently, however, the emphasis has been on leaders who provide vision, inspiration, and empowerment. Exactly what do these terms mean? Who should lead, manage, or follow, and when? The activities in this section are designed to help you recognize the differences between leading, managing, and following and to recognize how and why these behaviors are essential for organizations to move forward.

ACTIVITY 1-1

1. What words come to mind when you think of the word *leader*?

2. What words come to mind when you think of the word *follower*?

3. Analyze the differences between the two lists. Do you think of leaders in different ways than you think of followers?

4. Recall pairs of leaders-followers from politics, science, education, the media, or personal experience. As you recall these pairs of individuals, what made one the "leader" and the other the "follower"? How did the leader contribute to the follower's success? How did the follower contribute to the leader's success? Were there times when the leader functioned more as the follower? Were there times when the follower functioned more as the leader? What does this analysis tell you about the nature of leader-follower relationships?

ACTIVITY 1-2

Write a short analysis of the similarities and differences between managers and leaders on a unit of a hospital with which you are familiar. Discuss these similarities and differences with others (staff nurses, nurse managers, and other students).

ACTIVITY 1-3

1. In the spaces below, write a list of the positive consequences (beneficial outcomes) that occur when one manages well, when one leads well, and when one follows well.

Beneficial Outcomes or Consequences

Managing well	Leading well	Following well
a) Orderly, organized unit	a) Progressive, creative unit	a) Balanced teamwork
b)	b)	b)
c)	c)	c)
d)	d)	d)
e)	e)	e)
f)	f)	f)

2. Write any observations, questions, and/or conclusions you have about the lists you created.

3. Write a list of the negative consequences/outcomes of (or difficulties caused by) overemphasizing managing to the exclusion of leading and then of overemphasizing leading to the exclusion of managing.

Negative Outcomes or Consequences

Overemphasizing managing	**Overemphasizing leading**
a) Limited freedom for staff	a) Out of touch with reality
b)	b)
c)	c)
d)	d)
e)	e)

List negative outcomes of ineffective or passive followership.
a) Waits for others to assume responsibilities

b)

c)

d)

e)

4. Write any questions, observations, and/or conclusions you have about the three lists you have created.

5. Discuss with at least one other person the benefits and negative results (all lists) of leading and managing. List specific ways you could (or have seen others) shift emphasis between leading and managing.
   a) What behaviors, policies, procedures, and so forth, facilitate a shift of emphasis from managing to leading and back again in the institution(s) you have chosen for Activity 1-2?

   b) What behaviors, policies, procedures, and so forth, block this shifting emphasis in the institution(s) you have chosen?

   c) What new behaviors, policies, procedures, and so forth, would produce an effective shifting in the future in the institution(s) you have chosen?

ACTIVITY 1-4

Read at least three articles concerning managing and leading. Notice the degree to which the articles focus on the benefits of either leading or managing and the consequences of the other. When this occurs, the article tends to be a "crusade" for one side of this dilemma as though the author's favored approach is the solution to a particular problem. By overemphasizing the favored side, you could eventually experience its negative consequences, just as walking on top of a seesaw will at some point make it tip downward (refer to the negative consequences you listed). Do any of your articles call for both leading and managing together or mix them into a "superperson" profile? This may lead to clouding the distinctions and ignoring the need to emphasize leading or managing when appropriate.

1. What do the articles recommend about shifting focus?

2. With what level of certainty do the authors speak about the most needed behaviors?

3. What recommendations could you use in your clinical or work setting?

4. Why?

ACTIVITY 1-5

1. Team up with another student in your class. Separately, compile a list of what you each believe are leadership behaviors. Try to list at least 10.

1.   6.

2.   7.

3.   8.

4.   9.

5.   10.

2. Review your lists and mark your initials beside each behavior that you believe describes some of your own behaviors. Do this without input from anyone else. Using the same lists, mark your partner's initials beside those behaviors you have observed in the other student. Do this activity without any input from the other student. When finished, compare lists.

3. What do you both notice about the differences in how you view yourselves and how you view one another?

4. What did you learn about yourself?

5. Do others see you as having more or fewer leadership traits than you believe you have? Why?

Developing the Role of Leader

INTRODUCTION

This section contains three activities that will help you identify your own leadership priorities. Leadership is a privilege that is earned and maintained at the pleasure of followers. Without followers, there is no need for a leader. These exercises should give you an opportunity to explore your own leadership potential.

ACTIVITY 2-1

Fill in the following survey according to the directions.

WHAT NURSES VALUE IN THEIR LEADERS

Directions

For *each* of the four clusters of traits, do the following:
    Circle the three most important traits in the leader you want to follow.
    Then mark each circled trait in order of importance by placing a 1 next to the most important trait in
        your leader, a 2 by the second most important, and a 3 by the third most important.
    Place an "X" next to the least important trait in your leader.

Attitudes

Caring	Optimistic	Supportive	Approachable
Cooperative	Respectful of subordinates	Inspirational	Personable
Hard work ethic	Cheerful	Positive attitude	Flexible
Reasonable	Fair	Calm	

Intrinsic Qualities

Dependable	Dignified	Strong willed	Motivated
Dedicated	Detail oriented	Loyal	Wise
Trustworthy	Nonjudgmental	Understanding	Integrity
Reliable	Creative	Intelligent	Honest

Acquired Skills

Business sense	Professional	Decisive
Good reasoning skills	Risk taker	Available
Advocate	Practical knowledge	Clinical competence
Good people skills	Good communicator	Career experience
Assertive		

Personal

Motivator of others	High energy	Empowering
Interested in quality	Friendly	Visionary
Sense of humor	Communicator	Team player
Responsive to people	Mentoring attitude	Receptive to people and ideas

Now compare your responses with the top 10 responses of more than 100 young nurses and nursing students from throughout the United States.

Top 10 desired traits in a leader:
1. Receptive to people (personal skill)
2. Team player (personal skill)
3. Honest (intrinsic skill)
4. Good communicator (acquired skill)
5. Positive attitude (attitude skill)
6. Good people skills (acquired skill)
7. Approachable (attitude skill)
8. Knowledgeable (acquired skill)
9. Motivates others (personal skill)
10. Competent (acquired skill)

Least desired traits in a nurse manager:
1. Risk taker
2. High energy
3. Cheerful
4. Creative
5. Detail-oriented and Inspirational (tied)

Compare yourself to these young nurses. Notice which of their desired traits are listed in the acquired skills section. Can you think of ways that a leader could improve these skills? How many of your responses were listed in the acquired skills section? What about attitude? Can you change your attitude? The one intrinsic quality listed by the national sample was "honest." What would you do with a leader who was not honest? Do you think that national and global leaders are basically honest? Why is it so important that nursing leaders be seen as honest?

ACTIVITY 2-2

How do you make good followers? Can you be a good leader if you have never been a good follower? Separate into groups of five people. Respond to the following two questions, then regroup and see if you can come to some consensus on these questions.

What are the two most important features of a good follower?

1. _____

2. _____

Which one of each pair of words is more important for an effective follower (Circle the more important word):
Creative or Passive
Steady or Flexible
Trusting or Questioning
Doer or Thinker

Discuss the merits of each word with your group. Now, decide which one word is the most important in describing a follower.

Write the word here:_____

How did you decide on this word? Did you vote? Did someone urge the others to accept his or her word? If it was not your word, did you feel like you lost? A good leader makes even the losers feel like winners. If you followed someone else's lead, did you exhibit the qualities embodied in the word you used to describe a good follower? Sometimes leaders are followers, and sometimes followers are leaders. The key is to do both well to be effective.

ACTIVITY 2-3

Leader Observation Activity or "Watch and Learn"

Attend a professional nursing meeting. Identify the president or chairperson. Watch that person interact with other members.

- Is there anything consistent that he or she does during these interactions?
- Watch the leader's eye contact. What is he or she looking at during the meeting?
- What does the leader do after the meeting?
- Is there someone else at the meeting who seems to be the unofficial leader? What makes you think so?

Questions you might want to ask include the following:
1. What kind of preparation does the president/chairperson have to fulfill this role?
2. What percentage of the membership is present at this meeting?
3. Was this a typical meeting?
4. What kinds of issues does this group deal with? What is the most pressing issue currently?
5. Is this a growing organization or a stable one?
6. How long has the leader been a member?
7. Why does he or she belong?
8. What advice does the leader have for you to become a part of the leadership team?

Developing the Role of Manager

INTRODUCTION

Does the role of nurse manager intrigue you? Do you think you would like to be nurse manager? It is the best of times for nursing because this era of healthcare calls for creativity, flexibility, and tenacity—three attributes that students often possess. The exercises you are about to complete should elevate these attributes to higher peaks of excellence. Try them with your peers, share them with your peers, and most important, learn from them with your peers.

ACTIVITY 3-1

Role-play the following scenario in a group of 9 to 12 peers. Use your experience in clinical settings as the basis for your knowledge.

Roles: Nurse manager of a home health agency
   Staff nurses: 3 to 4
   Home health aides: 5 to 8

Scenario: The agency needs to develop a new care delivery model based on the influence of managed care. Work as a group to develop different roles for this new model—do not limit yourselves to what you currently see in practice. For each new role, identify assets and liabilities, such as costs, inherent in each role (recruitment, education, benefits).

ACTIVITY 3-2

In what ways can technology be used by a home health agency in a home setting? For example, list client data that might be computer based for entry or retrieval at a home site. What teaching aspects for health promotion/disease prevention can be done with your client using computer technology?

ACTIVITY 3-3

You are about to downsize your hospital unit. You have been told that your role as nurse manager will expand to cover more patient care areas and that the staff for each shift on your present unit will be reassigned. How can you prepare yourself and your staff for this change? Consider small staff meetings to let people talk about the new changes; also consider your own and your staff's adaptability traits. Write down a tentative plan for addressing the downsizing and staff relocation.

ACTIVITY 3-4

You have been repeatedly asked to change the quality care program so that it reflects evaluation of outcomes. You have changed the program at least twice, yet your supervisor is not satisfied with the quality outcomes, especially in relation to cost containment. What other strategies can you use to meet management and customer expectations? Write a paragraph that reflects your plan and your ability to maintain objectivity and sustain the demands of the job. Consider research strategies, collaboration with others (in and out of the institution), and patient care standards.

Legal and Ethical Issues

INTRODUCTION

The increasing demands in healthcare for cost containment and quality in patient care services, combined with increasing technology, pose escalating legal and ethical questions. As the healthcare scene changes, so do the questions that are posed to staff nurses and managers. This section presents dilemmas that can assist in heightening your awareness of legal and ethical issues prominent today. The exercises are representative of current examples of common dilemmas that nurses may encounter.

ACTIVITY 4-1

The Required Request law has been enacted in a majority of states. Essentially, this law requires that after all deaths, all families must be made aware of the possibility of donation of organs and tissues. The nurse manager or his or her representative, at the time of death or immediately before the patient's death, may be expected to request the organs.

1. Identify the ethical principles underlying the Required Request law by giving specific examples of how these principles are used by nurses when requesting organs after death.

2. Review the three ethical theories presented in the text. Which theory most guides your position regarding the Required Request law? State three reasons to support your position.

Position:
  a)
  b)
  c)

ACTIVITY 4-2

You are the nurse manager on a busy intermediate coronary care unit. You have just received a request from the admitting department for a bed on your unit, but there are no beds available. You inform the admitting department and request more information on the patient. The information you receive is that the patient is a 73-year-old woman with severe congestive heart failure who needs to receive intravenous (IV) medications. The physician has requested that she be on a monitored bed while receiving the medication. There are no telemetry beds available.

After reviewing all of the patients on the unit, the director decides to transfer a 48-year-old man who had a myocardial infarction 2 days earlier. The patient is transferred, and you receive the woman with congestive heart failure. The next day you find out that during the night the patient who was transferred was found in complete arrest when the nurse on the other unit made rounds at 2 AM. The man was resuscitated but is now in intensive care with brain damage resulting from the anoxia that occurred before he was resuscitated.

1. Was the decision to transfer the patient out of the intermediate care unit appropriate? Given the outcome of the situation, should you have refused to take the elderly female patient and kept the younger male patient in your unit? Provide a rationale for your answer.

2. Use the MORAL model discussed in the text to review this ethical dilemma.
   M   Massage the dilemma; identify and define the issues in the dilemma.
   O   Outline the options.
   R   Resolve the dilemma.
   A   Act by applying the chosen option.
   L   Look back and evaluate the entire process.

ACTIVITY 4-3

As a nurse manager, you are responsible for review of all incidents that occur on your unit to determine whether they were reported according to protocol and if appropriate follow-up has been completed.

On the previous day, one patient received injuries to her hand while ambulating when an IV controller slipped on the IV pole and pinned her hand between the controller and a platform designed to be used as a flat surface to hold equipment while working with the IV. The incident report states: "Patient was ambulating to bathroom at 10:30 PM and used the IV pole to stabilize herself while walking. The controller fell down the pole and pinned her right hand to the small table beneath it. Injury evident to right hand. Hand immediately began to swell, and patient had acute pain. X-ray film revealed a fracture of the third and fourth metacarpal of the right hand. Physician notified, responded, and orthopedic consult ordered."

The nurse's note in the chart states: "Patient ambulating to bathroom using IV pole to stabilize herself. IV controller fell, pinning hand, resulting in injury. This would not have happened if I had been present to help her. She stated that she turned on her light but no one answered because the unit was very busy at the time. Physician notified and responded. Incident report filed."

1. Identify and examine potential liability from this incident.

2. How does the note made in the chart affect the potential liability for (a) the nurse involved, (b) the nurse manager, and (c) the institution?
   a) Nurse

   b) Nurse manager

   c) Institution

3. Rewrite the nurse's note so that you could advise someone in a similar situation about documentation.

Decision Making and Problem Solving

INTRODUCTION

Because proper problem identification is key to effective problem solving and decision making, the exercises in this section provide an opportunity to enhance your skills in this area. Activity 5-1 involves use of a "gap analysis" technique to differentiate a problematic state from the ideal state. Activity 5-2 provides an opportunity to collaborate with a colleague to reflect on the possible causes of a problem and possible remedies to solve it.

ACTIVITY 5-1

Gap Analysis

A gap analysis is another way of envisioning problem solving. Pick a personal or professional problem and describe the elements of the problem under the heading "Description of Present Undesired State/Conditions." Then identify the desired future state/conditions that would ideally solve the problem and list the elements under the heading in the right column.

**Description of Present
Undesired State/Conditions**

**Description of Desired
Future State/Conditions**

ACTIVITY 5-2

Problem Definition

There are many different ways to define a problem, starting with the way different people perceive it. One method is to answer the four questions that follow. Select a problem, choose a partner, and answer the following questions.

1. Who and what are affected in what
   "problematic ways"?
   Who (as you see it):   Who (as your partner sees it):

   What (as you see it):   What (as your partner sees it):

2. Who and/or what is causing it?
   Who (as you see it):   Who (as your partner sees it):

   What (as you see it):   What (as your partner sees it):

3. What type of a problem is being confronted?
   The type of problem (as you see it):   The type of problem (as your partner sees it):

4. What are the intended goals/specific results
   to remedy the situation?
   Specific goals/results (as you see it):   Specific goals/results (as your partner sees it):

Using these four guidelines requires other considerations related to each element of the problem definition. As you formulate and write problem definitions, you can reflect about the following:

1. Who and what are affected in what problematic ways? Consider these possibilities: How many people, and who specifically, are negatively affected? What other things are affected and how?

Modified from Jung, C., Pino, R., & Emory, R. (1973). *Research utilizing problem solving*. Portland, OR: Northwest Regional Educational Library.

2. Who and what are causing this problem? What people are causing this problem, especially in the ways they are interpreting the circumstances and what is happening?

3. What type of problem is being confronted? What is this problem really about: Is it missing resources; a lack of training/skills; power struggles; inaccurate, inadequate, or superfluous communication; a lack of clarity of mission, priorities, roles, or norms; poor performance and results; misunderstandings; unethical actions; poor public relations, etc.?

Is this really a conflict over information, goals, means, or values/standards rather than a problem to solve? Is it a dilemma that has been mismanaged, or treated like a solvable problem?

4. What are the specific goal(s) and intended result(s) to remedy this situation?
Goal(s):

Intended result(s):

How would the situation look if this problem were completely solved? What will be the same and what will be different?

Healthcare Organizations

INTRODUCTION

Changes in the healthcare system, its organizations, and its financing are bringing about rapid developments in the modes and sites of care delivery. As acute care facilities become more focused on the acutely ill, community facilities that focus on people who are less acutely ill are being developed. No longer are people who are ill or who need surgery cared for in acute hospitals. They are in intermediate care agencies, in clinics, and at home. These activities focus on how the community is changing its healthcare facilities, on changes in healthcare delivery that have occurred in the past 5 years, and on the emerging trends.

ACTIVITY 6-1

Community Scavenger Hunt

Form a group with three to five of your classmates who identify themselves as highly committed and productive. Assume that you have been charged with the responsibility to provide the local health planning community with definitive information that they can use for future planning.

1. Scan community publications (e.g., newspapers, magazines, brochures) to develop a scenario of what the healthcare scene in your community was like 3 years ago and how it has changed in yearly increments. Write your description of the agencies and services available in the space below.

    What healthcare was like 3 years ago:

    2 years ago:

    1 year ago:

    Today:

2. Answer the following questions.
   How many new agencies have been established? What are they?

   How have existing agencies been modified by adding programs, redesigning facilities for different services, combining with others, and so forth?

   Describe the patients (clients) served then and now, using the following questions as guidelines:
   How has acuity changed?

   How have census and access changed?

   How has professional nursing staffing changed?

   How have patients' healthcare demands changed?

   How have reimbursement systems (e.g., insurance, HMOs) changed, expanded, declined?

3. Using your answers to the questions in item 2, develop a visual representation (e.g., a form, grid, mindmap, graph, chart, table) to depict the changes in the agencies.

4. Based on the information you have gathered, what are your conclusions? What trends can you identify?

5. Using the information you have gathered and keeping in mind the trends you just described, write a scenario that predicts the future. You already have all the data you need to do so. Keep in mind that nurse-owned and nurse-managed organizations may be essential components of networks in the evaluation. (Use a separate sheet of paper for your forecast.)

ACTIVITY 6-2

Build a Collage

1. Collect news articles, magazine articles, photos, advertisements, brochures, and so forth, regarding local healthcare services or services in some identifiable region. List your article titles below.

2. Organize these items into time frames or developmental stages. Highlight new agencies and services within the time periods you select.

3. Identify geographic areas with the newest developments and expansions, perhaps with a creative visual or map.

4. On a poster board, create a visual collage that displays the historical trends in healthcare delivery in the areas you have selected.

5. Present your collage to others.

Strategic Planning, Goal Setting, and Marketing

INTRODUCTION

In Chapter 7 you learned the importance of planning strategically, developing clear goals and objectives, implementing in a disciplined manner, and marketing concepts in the field of healthcare. You have also considered the critical importance of integrating the planning, targeting, implementing, and marketing functions. This section provides processes to enable you to develop skills in performing these functions.

ACTIVITY 7-1

1. To identify the marketing strategies of a healthcare organization, obtain a copy of at least one marketing brochure or plan for your own organization or one with which you are familiar.

2. Analyze the completeness and effectiveness of your brochure or plan according to the following criteria:
   a) Is the market for each product or service clearly defined?

   b) Are organization resources (capacity to deliver the product or service) quantified for each product or service?

   c) What are the marketing objectives? Are they realistic, specific, measurable, and mutually consistent?

   d) Are specific market segments identified for increased penetration?

   e) Is the planned mix of products and services clearly defined or will the mix be reactive to market requirements?

ACTIVITY 7-2

Select a healthcare organization and assess its current state with regard to the planning, targeting, implementing, and marketing functions. You can conduct this type of assessment by reviewing such relevant documents in the organization as mission statements, strategic plans, tentative budgets, and so forth. In reviewing documents to assess the current state, what would you use as review criteria? List those criteria below. Determine how well each criterion was met by checking one of the columns for meeting each criterion.

Reviewing the Strategic Plan

Review criteria	Not met	Partly met	Fully met
1.			
2.			
3.			

Reviewing Goals and Objectives

Review criteria	Not met	Partly met	Fully met
1.			
2.			
3.			

Reviewing the Marketing Plan

Review criteria	Not met	Partly met	Fully met
1.			
2.			
3.			

ACTIVITY 7-3

Create a small group discussion with students outside of class.

1. The case study in Chapter 7 of the online resources lists four forthcoming changes and develops a strategic planning document that responds to those changes. With your group members, discuss how the plan would have to be altered if the changes included the following, rather than those mentioned in the case:

a) The advisory committee was composed mainly of healthcare professionals.

b) The marketing plan was targeted to lower socioeconomic groups only.

c) The health promotion expectations were divided among existing agencies.

d) Costs and outcomes were the only basis for evaluation.

2. What are the main principles inherent in the concepts of budget reductions and increased regulation?

ACTIVITY 7-4

Planning is a critically important function. Without plans, we cannot sustain long-term initiatives. However, planning must exist within a context of spontaneity, just as spontaneity must exist within a context of planning. To value one and eliminate the other will lead to system dysfunction!

1. List the benefits of planning.

2. List the problems associated with planning. Think about the problems that would occur if everything were planned and people were prohibited from taking any spontaneous action.

3. List the benefits associated with spontaneous action.

4. List the problems associated with spontaneous action. Think about the problems that would occur if no one in the organization did any planning.

ACTIVITY 7-5

Planning requires effective vision, goals, and objectives. The text discusses guidelines for effective goals. Using these guidelines and examples, on a separate sheet of paper, write some specific short-term, medium-range, and long-term goals for a department or team. Discuss them with another student and revise them as needed.

Leading Change

INTRODUCTION

This section contains one application activity, which asks students to propose a plan for an actual or hypothetical change in a nursing situation. Guidelines and a sample plan will guide the development of the plan. The best outcome for this activity is for students to implement their plans in actual healthcare organizations. The ultimate outcome is the development of effective change management skills by further enhancing students' conceptual foundations about roles and approaches in leading change.

ACTIVITY 8-1

The use of planned change models for less complex, low-level change can be effective. Most organizational change, however, takes place in groups, units, and departments responsive to influences outside and inside (open system). Thus managing the influencing factors of a change situation in conjunction with a plan's elements for the change can lead to creative results.

Using the guidelines for planning a change, change planning worksheet, and the sample of a plan for a hypothetical change, develop a plan for a change. Select a change situation, either an actual or a hypothetical one, and follow the problem-solving format of the planning worksheet to (1) assess the change situation, (2) develop an activity plan for implementation supported by sound change theories and principles, and (3) decide on methods to evaluate the change process and outcomes. The activity plan should reflect several potentially feasible outcome scenarios to work toward and specifically identified resources, timelines, responsible parties, and strategies to achieve each outcome. Discuss your proposed plan with your peers, instructors, and individuals in the change situation.

This following worksheet provides a general framework for planning low-level change. The worksheet headings and sections outline essential points to consider. The guidelines explain the completion of the worksheet section by section. A completed sample worksheet is included as a model to follow.

GUIDELINES

Section I: Situational Assessment and Analysis

Developing an appropriate plan for a change requires an accurate assessment of the situation needing the change. Effective assessment results in accurate identification of the key elements operating in the situation, not to be confused with symptoms of the need. The elements may be human, technological, system, or other. The need may be a problem needing resolution, a need requiring innovative action, or a measure improving quality.

Part A
Describe the actual situation needing change, naming and briefly describing the who, what, when, where, why, and how elements.

Part B

Using your initial assessment data in Part A, identify current and anticipated facilitators and barriers operating in the change situation. Using a numerical weighting system, rate each factor's strength or potential to either promote ($+1$ is low and $+5$ is high) or hinder (-1 is low and -5 is high) the change process. Choose strategies that have the most potential to increase the influences of facilitators and reduce or eliminate the effects of barriers.

Part C

Analyze all factors assessed. State whether you will proceed with the plan. If the weight of the barriers outweighs the strength of the facilitators, reconsider the feasibility of initiating the change.

Section II: Implementation Plan

Clearly write acceptable change outcomes/goals and corresponding objectives and evaluation methods. State predictable unexpected occurrences.

Part A

Describe several desired outcomes using specific, concrete terms. Although broad in nature, the outcomes are used to measure change progress throughout and at the end of the change.

Part B

Objectives are specific descriptions of the processes needed to achieve change outcomes. State objectives in terms of needed resources (materials, space, finances, staff) and desired timelines for each outcome/goal. List objectives in the approximate order in which they will occur. Define accountable parties.

Part C

Unexpected occurrences and circumstances will probably affect the change process. Predict these and designate potential strategies to respond to them if they do happen.

Part D

Various methods exist for collecting information throughout and at the end of the change process. Choose appropriate methods as needed to measure attitude, behavior, or knowledge during the change and after the change; the influences or concerns hampering the implementation process; or the degree to which objectives are met and the outcomes achieved.

Section III: Evaluation and Revision

It is important to judge the effectiveness of the plan for change and its implementation. Both the processes and outcomes of the change should be evaluated for effectiveness to project what could be improved in future endeavors.

A. State to what degree outcomes were met.

B. Indicate ways to improve the change process or outcome quality.

Section I: Situational Assessment and Anaylses
A. Describe actual situation in terms of who, what, when, where, how, and why.

B. Complete a force field analysis by identifying the facilitators and barriers in the change situation. Numerically rate their potential strength ($+1$, low; $+5$, high; -1, low; -5, high). For each facilitator or barrier indicate strategies appropriate for managing the influences of the factors. Focus on information, relationships, and possible alterations in the pool of outcome scenarios. Use strategies to reduce the effects of barriers and foster the effects of facilitators.

Facilitators (+/pro)	Strength Rating	Strategies	Barriers (−/anti-)	Strength Rating	Strategies
1.			1.		
2.			2.		
3.			3.		
4.			4.		

C. State how influences of the facilitators and barriers are equal to or different from each other based on your assessment of their strength. State whether you will proceed with plan: _____.

Section II
A. State at least three desirable outcomes/goals for proposed change in specific, measurable terms:
   1.

   2.

   3.
B. State and sequence objectives in terms of specific resources, time frames, strategies, and responsible parties for each outcome.

Outcome 1
a)

C. Identify unexpected occurrences and potential strategies to manage them.
   1.

   2.

D. State methods for measuring the progress and outcome of the change process.

Ongoing/Process   **Outcome/Summative**
1.   1.

2.   2.

3.   3.

Section III
A. State to what degree outcomes/goals were met.

B. Indicate ways to improve the change process or outcome/goal quality.

Sample Worksheet

Section I: Situational Assessment and Analysis

A. Describe actual situation in terms of who, what, when, where, why, and how.

RNs/LPNs [LVNs] hear patient information only on assigned patients at shift change due to unit's 15-month-old policy of nurse-to-nurse shift reports. Frequent complaints exist due to nursing staff's inability to knowledgeably assist other patients, families, and healthcare providers. Miscommunications increase the risk for errors.

B. Identify facilitating and interfering (barrier) factors in the change situation, numerically rate their potential strength, and then indicate strategies appropriate to managing the influences of the factors.

Facilitators (+/pro)	Strength	Strategies	Barriers (−/anti-)	Strength	Strategies
1. Nurse manager supportive	+4	Communication Facilitation	1. Two nurse rejectors	−4	Coercion Co-optation
2. Staff's desire for patient information	+3	Communication Support	2. Perceived late start to provide care	−2	Communication Facilitation
3. Effectiveness of S.O.P. committee	+3	Involvement Support	3. Increased accountability for all patients	−2	Negotiation Support
4. Staff's desire to reduce frustration	+2	Participation Encouragement	4. Possible change in reporting with new information system	−2	Education Support Participation
Total Wt. = +12			Total Wt. = −10		

C. State how influences of the facilitators and barriers are equal to or different from each other based on your assessment of their strength. State whether you will proceed with the plan.

Will proceed with plan as facilitators outweigh barriers by +2. Will carefully monitor during implementation.

Section II: Implementation Plan

A. State desired outcomes for the proposed change in specific, measurable terms.

1. By June 25, all RNs/LPNs [LVNs] will be knowledgeable about all patients on unit due to comprehensive shift report using the patient care Kardex as tool for standardization of information reported.

2. By September 1, all RNs/LPNs [LVNs] will be knowledgeable about all unit patients due to computer printout of key information for each patient and brief status reports at shift change.

Sample Worksheet—cont'd

B. State and sequence objectives in terms of specific resources, time lines, strategies, and responsible parties.

1. By May 1, S.O.P. committee representatives will meet with all nursing staff (on all three shifts) to define problem, identify solutions, and seek staff involvement.

2. By May 15, staff will complete short survey to determine overall willingness to adopt specific options for change in report method.

3. By June 1, S.O.P. committee will communicate most acceptable options with rationale and then field staff comments (survey results).

4. By June 7, S.O.P. committee and nurse manager will conduct sessions at staff meetings to update progress on two possible solutions.

5. On June 20 or September 1, staff will begin new shift report method for the transition between each shift change.

C. Identify unexpected occurrences and potential actions to handle.

1. Lack of general agreement on new shift report method: Reassess problems, solution(s), and associated legal–ethical issues with staff.

2. Reluctance/harmful resistance of staff members: Identify at beginning and during change process and use appropriate strategies to prevent sabotage of change process (communication ⟶ manipulation ⟶ coercion).

D. State methods for measuring the progress and outcome of the change process.

Ongoing/Process	Outcome/Summative
1. Survey of 6 to 10 questions to poll attitudes and abilities to support one or more options for new shift report method.	1. Conduct discussions with individual RNs/LPNs [LVNs] on all three shifts at random to assess knowledge of all patients on unit after change has been implemented for one to five weeks.
2. Informal interviews of RNs/LPNs [LVNs] during change process that include random attendance/discussion.	

Section III: Evaluation and Revision

A. State to what degree outcome(s) was met.

After 6 weeks of full implementation, evaluation measures with staff and attendance at all three shift report times show almost all staff knowledgeable about all unit patients. Patient, family, and provider information needs met more quickly and accurately.

B. Indicate ways to improve the change process or outcome quality after outcome evaluated.

Conduct quality study at monthly intervals to attain threshold of 95% consistently for 6 months at minimum. Build in more frequent points of seeking input from and giving feedback to staff (each shift initially, then weekly) related to movement toward outcome, with recognition provided for achievement and effort. Provide redirection for inability and unwillingness.

Understanding and Designing Organizational Structures

INTRODUCTION

Technology, which is defined as all the work required to carry out the nursing care of patients, has a major effect on the design of the organizational structure. The technology is determined by the type of setting, (e.g., critical care, long-term care, rehabilitation, home care, hospice). A primary factor to be considered is the amount of autonomy required in decision making. In settings where patients' conditions are unstable and unpredictable, structures are needed that provide for a great deal of independence in decision making. In community settings where access to higher levels for decision making is not available, a structure providing independence in decision making is also required. A good fit is required between organizational structure and technology.

Making decisions at the level that patient care is occurring provides many advantages to patients and their nurses. When decision making is delegated to this level, there has to be some means of ensuring that patients are treated equally and that one patient is not provided with advantages that are not granted to another. Agency guidelines for care established by nurses providing the care are one method of ensuring that all clients are treated equally.

ACTIVITY 9-1

Describe and illustrate with concrete examples the relationship between technology and structure, for example, how does one influence the other, how does organizational structure vary in different types of institutions, and what are resultant technology demands?

ACTIVITY 9-2

Describe a decentralized organization and list the positive factors of working in such an organization. Describe chaos that might occur in a completely decentralized organization and methods that could be used to avoid such chaos.

ACTIVITY 9-3

Obtain at least two organizational charts. Compare them in terms of their missions. Describe the placement, authority, and reporting for nursing.

ACTIVITY 9-4

The new chief nursing officer for the Cady Institute is reviewing several theories and philosophies in preparation for implementing one that can carry the organization through the twenty-first century. In perusing the literature, it became apparent that the concept of shared governance was most appealing because it seemed consistent with the mission of the institution as well as that of the nursing division. You have been appointed to the new committee that has been formed to review the requirements to be considered before this change. As a responsible member of this committee deliberating the proposed change, you have been requested to review the literature and cite at least three advantages and three disadvantages for this proposal.

Advantages of shared governance:

1.

2.

3.

Disadvantages of shared governance:

1.

2.

3.

Having completed this assignment, you report your findings to the committee at large. The committee then requests you to compare shared governance to participatory management and formulate a response supporting either management style.

You respond, "I have listed the pros and cons of each type of governance for your consideration before recommending adoption of one or the other."

Participatory management has the following advantages:

1.

2.

3.

Participatory management has the following disadvantages:

1.

2.

3.

The reasons you give reflect that you have also compared the advantages and disadvantages of participatory management.

YOUR RECOMMENDATION:

I recommend that (select one) be adopted for the following reasons:

My recommendation was based on the following considerations (please describe each in one or two sentences):

1. How does the educational level of staff affect the decision?

2. What style(s) of managerial leadership are preferred?

3. How are nursing staff members demonstrating autonomy?

Collective Action

INTRODUCTION

These activities ask you to reflect on those skills that will contribute to your success in collective action within the practice of nursing. Activity 10-1 begins with the Personal You and will influence your performance within the Professional You context. The remaining activities give you an opportunity to consider your role within nursing practice.

ACTIVITY 10-1

1. You have developed many interpersonal skills within your life. List three interpersonal skills that are essential for nurses to achieve collective action.
    1.
    2.
    3.

2. In the space provided, describe activities that will help you refine these skills.

3. Identify other skills that you think will assist you in collective action within your nursing practice.

ACTIVITY 10-2

Eden Valley is a community hospital. That is, it is an institution that operates solely within the community in which it is located. It is experiencing financial pressures. The options it is considering include selling to a national company, joining a multihospital group in the surrounding area, or trying to preserve its identity. Employees, including nurses, are experiencing stress related to the uncertainty. Employees in other job categories are unionized. Several nurses believe that it is a good time to consider organizing a staff union. They contact the state nurses' association (SNA) to discuss their concerns.

1. What factors will influence the establishment of a union?

2. What factors will be a barrier to the establishment of a union?

3. Identify goals for establishing a union.

4. What criteria are important in the selection of a union?

ACTIVITY 10-3

Obtain a copy of a collective bargaining contract between nurses and their employer. (If there are no contracts for nurses in your area, obtain a copy of a collective bargaining contract used by another group.) Identify three features of the contract that are important to you. Identify any features of the contract that are objectionable to you.

Contract Features

Features important to you:

1.

2

3.

Features objectionable to you:

1.

2.

3.

ACTIVITY 10-4

Nurses can no longer ignore or be uninformed about the business side of healthcare delivery. Knowledge of the facilities in which you practice and trends in the industry are necessary to make informed decisions. Imagine you have been informed that the hospital must decrease the number of registered nurses because of the new business practices designed to reduce costs and thus approximate insurance payment levels. From your perspective and those of your nurse colleagues, the hospital is doing fine. Identify three sources of public information related to an organization's financial health. Who would you contact to assist you in obtaining the information?

ACTIVITY 10-5

Read two articles related to the 1994 Supreme Court decision that struck down the nursing exception used by the National Labor Relations Board (NLRB) to determine supervisory status and the February 1996 ruling by the NLRB that upheld the nonsupervisory status of nurses in Anchorage. These decisions reflect two versions of the same ruling. Identify the implications for nurses within each decision.

ACTIVITY 10-6

Identify three subcultures within your current practice setting. The subcultures may be in nursing or not or within your unit or not. Describe three characteristics of each subculture.

1.
   a)

   b)

   c)

2.
   a)

   b)

   c)

3.
   a)

   b)

   c)

Managing Quality and Risk

INTRODUCTION

Planning is necessary to improve quality and decrease risk. Total quality management (TQM) and continuous quality improvement (CQI) programs will help improve the quality of care provided in an institution. Planning is an essential part of these programs, and the planning time is well spent. The occurrence of incidents may be costly for the institution. Decreasing those risks will decrease costs, improve the quality of care you provide, and improve patient satisfaction.

ACTIVITY 11-1

1. Form groups of four. Each group member will conduct his or her own interview with a healthcare professional regarding quality improvement. Select interviewees from the institutions in which you work or have clinical experience. Ask the interviewees to address quality improvement in their institution. You will want to interview people at different levels of the organization to gain a broad perspective of everyone's understanding of the process. Suggested people to interview include the head nurse, staff nurse, unit secretary, physician, director of quality improvement, and people from other departments.

2. After interviewing these people, reflect on and answer the following questions:
   a) Did each person give you a similar picture of the quality improvement process? Why or why not?

   b) If there were differences, were they significant? Why or why not? (If the differences are significant, they can affect how well the quality improvement process works.)

   c) Discuss the interviews in your groups and determine what similarities and differences you found.

ACTIVITY 11-2

Use the following steps to apply quality improvement principles to your own practice.

1. Identify a process or procedure that you perform routinely and wish to improve.

2. Using a flowchart, delineate each step of the procedure.

3. Collect data that show your present ability to do this process or procedure.

4. Set a measurable standard of excellence for this procedure. Use established standards if available, but remember to also determine what your customers value and expect.

5. Develop a plan to improve your practice to meet this standard. This could include further reading, education, or consultation with peers.

6. Collect data to document your improvement in this procedure.

7. When you successfully meet your performance standard, reward yourself.

ACTIVITY 11-3

Obtaining information from your customers is very important when assessing quality of care. Ask five patients about quality of care. Be certain to obtain the nurse manager's concurrence first. The following are some suggested questions to use in your interview:

1. What was most satisfying about the care you have received?

2. What was least satisfying about the care you have received?

3. Have there been any delays in the care that was provided (pain medication delayed, meal tray served late, call light not answered)?

4. Who was most attentive to your specific needs (physician, nurse, nursing assistant, housekeeper)?

5. What would you like to see changed?

6. What would you like to see stay the same?

7. Would you recommend this institution to others?

8. Is there anything else you would like to share regarding the quality of care you have received?

ACTIVITY 11-4

Obtain a copy of the form used in an institution to report incidents or occurrences. Review the related policy and procedure. Interview a nurse manager or staff nurse regarding the following if the policy and procedure handbook does not provide the information.

1. What happens to the occurrence report after it is completed by the reporting individual?

2. What types of incidents are to be reported?

3. What is the most frequently occurring incident?

4. How is corrective action taken after an occurrence has taken place?

Managing Information and Technology: Caring and Communicating With Computers

INTRODUCTION

These exercises will help you use the information presented in the chapter. The first activity can be used to help you think about your current practice from an information perspective. This exercise should help you understand the process to develop an evidence-based practice.

The second activity helps you subscribe to the student nurse listserv. Other list addresses are also provided for you. Try a few of them; they all provide valuable information for students and nurses in practice.

The third activity will help you find information on the Internet. A list of search engines and instructions for accessing them is provided. Be sure to use the help function to learn more about using these engines.

ACTIVITY 12-1

Evidence-Based Practice

Think about a specific patient population you work with often. Choose a problem or condition that you encounter in that population for which you do not know what therapy the evidence suggests (i.e., what the literature recommends for effective treatment). Go to the library's online reference databases and enter the Cochrane Library Database. (If you need assistance, talk with the librarian at the reference desk in the library.)

First-Time Users
The Cochrane Library contains databases, records, documents, Medical Subject Headings (MeSH), and search history screens. Review any content that you would like by placing your cursor over the highlighted text and clicking once. When you are finished, click the Back button on your browser (as many times as needed) to get to the screen containing the Cochrane Databases.

All Users
1. Enter in the search term box the problem or condition (keep the terms concise) for which you want to know what the literature recommends for effective treatment and then click the search button. The number of "hits" will be listed. Click on the highlighted text. Read through your list of "hits." Click on one or more pertinent reviews and find the recommended therapies. Print out key reviews if you would like.
   Note: If the "hits" are too broad, you can try narrowing your search (see search techniques under the Help option).

2. The next time you are in the clinical setting, find an expert clinician and ask him or her about his or her experience with whatever the recommended therapy was for the selected problem or condition. Does actual practice vary from recommended research evidence? If they differ, ask the clinician if he or she has tried the recommended approach and what the clinician's assessment of actual and recommended practices is. Reflect on what you have heard and read. Developing expertise comes from the integration of theoretical and practical knowledge.

ACTIVITY 12-2

Using a Listserv

Using one of the search engines in Activity 12-3, enter the term "SNURSE-L" to link to the site and to subscribe to the SNURSE-L listserv. Be sure to save the instructions returned to you by email. They explain how to unsubscribe to the listserv when you are finished using it. Read the messages for a few days to see what other students are saying. This is called *lurking*. You will notice that there are many responses and additions to a topic of interest. These messages become a "thread." When you are comfortable and have something to contribute, you may send a message to the list by clicking the reply button. Do *not* use all capital letters in your reply; this is considered to be shouting (rude); keep your messages short and to the point.

1. Did you have problems subscribing to the listserv? Were you able to find help?

2. Once you were subscribed, what information did you find useful for you? What information did you provide that was interesting and informative for others?

3. Did the listserv members respond to you?

4. Click on the print button to make a copy of your latest message.

Listserv Addresses

5. Remember to send subscribe and unsubscribe commands to the server address. Send the command message to the designated address. Be sure to type the commands subscribe or unsubscribe (see the example screen) in your message.

ACTIVITY 12-3

The Internet contains so much information that sometimes you may be unable to find what you are looking for. Search engines were developed to search through millions of websites to find exactly what you need. Following is a list of some common search engines and their functions.

Search Engine	Address (called the *URL*)	Description
AltaVista	www.altavista.digital.com	Fast searches, indexes every word on millions of pages. If information is on the web, you'll find it here.
Ask Jeeves	www.askjeeves.com	Can ask questions in "plain language."
Google	www.google.com	Comprehensive access; rated highly by users.
Lycos	www.lycos.com	Unique options will work around misspellings. Is an older useful site.
Webcrawler	www.webcrawler.com	Handles searches in an orderly and logical manner. Reviews and recommends the best websites. Not as fast as some others.
Yahoo	www.yahoo.com	Well-organized categories, easy to find and useful information, finds only keywords. A good place to start.

Go to your school computer laboratory and ask the personnel to show you how to access the Internet (if you do not already know how). These examples illustrate the use of the browser Netscape; if you are using Microsoft Explorer or another browser, your screen may look different.

1. Access your browser and enter the address (called the *uniform resource locator* or *URL*) of one of the search engines listed previously. Search for information that you need for patient education or for a paper that you are writing. What did you find? Was there too much information? Try searching for the keyword diabetes or cystic fibrosis. What did you find? Click the print icon on the tool bar to print and keep your findings.

2. Use the Internet to access the Centers for Disease Control and Prevention (CDC). Type the URL for the CDC in the address bar: www.cdc.gov/. When the CDC home page opens, click on an icon (picture) or underlined topic and follow the links. Use the Back and Forward buttons on the toolbar to move between the pages.

3. Check some of the statistics. Find information that might be useful in writing a paper about HIV or diabetes. Find health information for travelers.

4. Do you know how to write a reference for information that you find on the Internet? Check with your library for the latest APA format for citing electronic information because this is now an accepted form of reference. You can also access the website containing this information. The URL is www.nyct.net/~beads/weapas/.

Managing Costs and Budgets

INTRODUCTION

This section provides additional opportunities to consider in how to manage both costs and budgets.

ACTIVITY 13-1

1. You are a staff nurse in an ambulatory care clinic that is making a transition from fee-for-service reimbursement to capitation. Review the incentives for cost control in both methods of reimbursement. How are they different? How will this change affect the nursing practices in the clinic? What will be the important considerations when caring for patients under capitation?

2. Torrell Medical Center (TMC) grants all full-time employees 10 paid holidays and 12 paid vacation days annually. In addition, the Nursing Department experiences 6.4 average annual sick days and 1.6 other paid and nonpaid days off (e.g., bereavement, jury duty, education) per employee.
   a. How many productive hours are worked per full-time employee?

   b. One of TMC's medical-surgical units is expanding its capacity from 38 to 45 beds. The average daily census is anticipated to increase by 4 patients. The unit's average patient care standard is 5.4 hours of nursing care per patient day. How many *additional* FTEs will be needed as a result of the proposed expansion?

3. How is productivity measured on the unit or at the agency where you practice? What is the process for monitoring productivity? What is the role of staff nurses in monitoring and improving productivity?

4. For the past 3 months nursing salaries have exceeded the budgeted amount by 10%. Is this a positive or negative variance? How would you begin to investigate this variance? What factors might contribute to it? Which factors are controllable by the nurse manager? Are unfavorable or negative variances always a problem? Why or why not?

ACTIVITY 13-2

Do this exercise with a partner. Develop charts or other graphic ways to illustrate the following activities.

Scenario: Expansion!

You have been informed that because of your statistical justification efforts, administration has recognized the need for more monitored beds. This means that your department will expand from its current 11 beds to 20 monitored beds. As a nurse manager, you are initially very pleased about this expansion, but then you feel dismay because you will have a lot of work to do and only a little time in which to accomplish it. You also have an additional 12 FTEs to add to your current 20.5 FTEs. The current staffing mix is as follows:

RN FTEs = 12 (10 full-time and 4 part-time)

LPN (LVN) FTEs = 3.5 (2 full-time and 3 part-time)

Nursing assistant FTE's = 1.5 (6 work every other weekend and 1 works the Friday along with her weekend)

Nursing aide FTEs = 1.0 (full-time, works only Monday to Friday)

Unit clerk FTEs = 2.5 (2 full-time, work 9 to 5:30 during the week and every other weekend, and 1 part-time, works 6 PM to 10 PM Monday through Friday)

The additional 12 FTEs include all support personnel (unit clerks, nursing assistants, and aides as well as RNs and LPNs [LVNs]).

Establish the following:

1. List three goals for the new expanded unit. Include patient outcomes such as discharge criteria, acuity level, and patient teaching.

   a)

   b)

   c)

2. Make a list that differentiates the allocation of FTEs of caregivers and support personnel. Some of the support personnel may also be listed as caregivers, such as nursing assistants and/or unit clerks who are cross-trained as nursing aides. Consider the following when doing the allocation:
   a) There are nine more patients who require care.
   b) There are times when there is no unit clerk available, and the daytime clerks have to work overtime to cover the period from 5:30 to 6:00 PM.
   c) Who will be observing nine additional monitors? Would you want to consider a monitor tech or cross-training some of the other available personnel?
   d) Consider patient outcomes—will your patients be on the monitor during their entire stay in the unit and when the monitor is discontinued they are transferred, or will they remain on the unit until discharge and require a lower level of care?
   e) Currently the acuity level is higher than the original staffing plan was designed for, which is resulting in the nursing staff working overtime on a daily basis.

3. Decide how many part-time versus full-time positions you will need to accomplish the goals set forth in element 1.

Remember that when a part-time person works overtime, it is not usually paid at time and a half and they frequently are asked to contribute more to receive benefits.

4. Determine the minimum number of staff necessary for all three shifts. Keep in mind that the staffing ratio on your unit is currently one RN or, in some cases, LPN (LVN) to four patients. Take into account that full-time staff on your unit currently work 12-hour shifts and every third weekend.

5. Discuss with your partner and develop a clear rationale to demonstrate your understanding of overbudgeted hours and overtime.

CHAPTER **14** WORKBOOK

Consumer Relationships

INTRODUCTION

An awareness of how consumer relations affect the provision of nursing care is essential. Consumers are faced with many changes in the healthcare delivery system. When patients enter the healthcare system, they lose a significant amount of control. The following exercises are designed to help you identify how nurses can promote positive experiences with healthcare.

ACTIVITY 14-1

Mr. Irons is transferred to your unit after having a myocardial infarction (MI). He is the CEO at Interplast, an internationally known plastics manufacturer specializing in healthcare supplies. One report stated he has been very unhappy because of the limitations that have been placed on him in the intensive care unit (ICU) and is happy to go to the telemetry unit so that he can "carry on with his life." Mr. Irons has made arrangements for a laptop computer to be brought in and his secretary to be present for 4 hours a day. The staff has expressed concern regarding how wise it is for him to work while recovering from an MI and have witnessed many "type A" behaviors.

You are the nurse manager of the unit, and when you return from a meeting, you have a message to call the vice president for nursing regarding a patient complaint. When you call her, you are told that Mr. Irons has called the hospital administrator and demanded that a nurse on the unit be fired. His physician wants the "usual" procedures used. You have been asked to investigate the situation.

Upon investigation you find that Mr. Irons is very upset because the nurse has been attempting to do some patient education regarding reducing stress and providing time for relaxation. He believes that he rests adequately at night and if he does not take care of business there will be serious consequences at his company. The staff nurse is upset and fearful of being fired. The physician has ordered diazepam (Valium) for the patient.

Review the textbook pages promoting successful consumer relationships: service, advocacy, teaching, and leadership. Then answer the following questions.

1. How can your staff effectively provide services for Mr. Irons? List four ways.

   a)

   b)

   c)

   d)

2. If Mr. Irons refuses to collaborate with the staff in the plan of care, cite three effective ways to support staff regarding Mr. Irons' demands.
   a)

   b)

   c)

3. How are you going to respond to the vice president for nursing and to the hospital administration? Cite three critical areas to include in your response.
   a)

   b)

   c)

4. How will you handle Mr. Irons' demand for the staff nurse to be fired? Cite your approach and give supportive rationale for your selection.

   Approach:

   Rationale:

5. How will you be an advocate for Mr. Irons?

   Approach:

   Rationale:

ACTIVITY 14-2

Some institutions have designated patient representatives who act as ombudsmen (advocates) for the hospital and the patient. (These persons may also be designated as "risk managers.") They are often first in line and highly skilled in handling patient complaints. Consider how a person in such a position may effectively respond to Mr. Irons' concern. Make a list of at least three possible actions the patient representative could take.

1.

2.

3.

Compare your responses with at least two other classmates. Were your responses the same? Different? What would you do?

1.

2.

3.

Give rationale for each of these actions.

1.

2.

3.

ACTIVITY 14-3

(Refer to Activity 14-1.)

Role-Play

Time limit: 3 to 5 minutes

1. Divide into small groups of five to seven students. Two students will role-play while the others observe.

    Role-players for Mr. Irons and the staff nurse: Don't be afraid to express feelings of anger, fear, disappointment, and so forth. Think about how you would respond (both in words and in feelings) if you were the person.

    Observers make notes about (1) what is said, (2) what may be said differently, and (3) body language of the role-players.

2. Discuss what was observed. (*Note:* Be open to make and receive recommendations regarding the nurse role-play from your peers. This is your chance to receive nonthreatening feedback from your peers before confronting this possible situation clinically.)

3. Role-play repeat: After completing one role-play, two other members of the group rotate roles and complete the same process. Everyone should have the opportunity to have played at least one role, either nurse or patient.

    Other possible role combinations include the following: Mr. Irons and hospital administrator; nurse manager and vice president for nursing; Mr. Irons and nurse manager; nurse manager and staff nurse (the one Mr. Irons wants fired); nurse manager and Mr. Irons' physician; you, the ombudsman, and any one of the aforementioned persons.

4. Identify how it would feel to be in the role you are assigned. For example, as the patient, you want to make your own decisions; as the staff nurse, you feel concerned because you know the patient's behavior may be detrimental to his health.

    I felt:

5. Discuss the feelings that were identified as a group. For example, as the nurse manager, while you were discussing the situation with the vice president for nursing you felt defensive.

   List five suggestions generated by the group to avoid defensiveness.
   a)

   b)

   c)

   d)

   e)

6. Consider what responses would have made you feel better. For example, you become angry while talking to Mr. Irons and tell him you are going to have his doctor talk to him. With the assistance of the group, list five ways that this might have been said differently.
   a)

   b)

   c)

d)

e)

ACTIVITY 14-4

It is the practice of some institutions to have patient care conferences. The goals of these conferences are to handle problems that may occur and to design a plan to provide quality care for the patient. It is also a good time to support your peers, who may be having difficulties in providing care when there are problems.

You are responsible for leading a patient care conference and outlining a plan of care for Mr. Irons. Outline your plans for the conference. The patient should be involved in decisions made regarding the provision of care. Will you invite Mr. Irons to attend your patient care conference? Why? (Provide rationale.)

How will you involve Mr. Irons in his plan of care in the future? Identify five ways.
1.

2.

3.

4.

5.

ACTIVITY 14-5

(Refer to Activity 14-4)

Form a group of five to seven people and compare and discuss your individual responses. Develop group responses and provide rationale, using the space provided to write out your rationale and plan in detail.

Care Delivery Strategies

INTRODUCTION

Healthcare delivery has been significantly affected by many factors. Managed care and financing reforms will continue this rapid transformation in care delivery strategies. Identifying characteristics, strengths, and liabilities of each system will enable the nurse to match the care delivery strategy with the agency's philosophy, goals, and organizational and financial structure.

ACTIVITY 15-1

You are the charge nurse on a 10-patient subacute care unit. There are two RNs, one LPN/LVN, and one nursing assistant working today. Each care delivery strategy has different functions for care providers (e.g., in primary care, RNs have different functions than in the functional method). Describe the role of each care provider in each of the following care delivery strategies.

Case Method

RN no. 1 role:

RN no. 2 role:

LPN/LVN role:

Nursing assistant role:

Functional Method

RN no. 1 role:

RN no. 2 role:

LPN/LVN role:

Nursing assistant role:

Team Nursing

RN no. 1 role:

RN no. 2 role:

LPN/LVN role:

Nursing assistant role:

Primary Nursing

RN no. 1 role

RN no. 2 role:

LPN/LVN role:

Nursing assistant role:

Nurse Case Management

RN no. 1 role:

RN no. 2 role:

LPN/LVN role:

Nursing assistant role:

ACTIVITY 15-2

As a nurse manager, you know that each care delivery strategy has advantages for the manager, staff, and the patient and family. For each care method, describe two advantages and two disadvantages for the nurse manager, the staff nurse, and the patient and family.

ACTIVITY 15-3

Cite two care delivery strategies that would require a different staff mix to make them work. Describe the alterations in the staff composition that you would make.

ACTIVITY 15-4

As a baccalaureate-prepared nurse, which care delivery method would you be satisfied to work in? State a rationale for your selection. What if you were a nurse with an associate degree?

Which care delivery strategy would your chief financial officer favor? Why?

Staffing and Scheduling

INTRODUCTION

Staffing any nursing division is complex and challenging. Calculating staffing needs includes many factors, all of which are compounded whenever the number of staff and the appropriate mix are challenged, such as during a time of high demand for nurses. Some key factors are the average census, length of stay, complexity of care, legal and accreditation expectations, and staff qualifications. Balancing the needs of a given division in terms of the care needed with the needs and expectations of staff is a challenge all managers face. Institutional policies and contracts and state laws, rules, and regulations influence decisions.

ACTIVITY 16-1

You are the manager of a medical-surgical unit. The unit has 32 beds and an occupancy rate of 75%. The desired staffing mix consists of four RNs, two LPNs/LVNs, and two nursing assistants on the 7 AM to 3 PM shift; three RNs, one LPN/LVN, and two nursing assistants on the 3 PM to 11 PM shift; and two RNs, one LPN/LVN, and one nursing assistant on the 11 PM to 7 AM shift. Using the formulas from the textbook (see Chapter 16), determine how many FTEs of each category of employees will be necessary to cover the staffing expectations. Remember, this division will operate 24 hours every day, including weekends and holidays.

Key factors:

The employment benefits include the following:

   7 holidays per year

   10 sick days per year

   15 vacation days per year

   Every other weekend off

Determine the following:

   Number of RN FTEs needed: ___

   Number of LPN/LVN FTEs needed: ___

   Number of nursing assistant FTEs needed: ___

Using this same staffing pattern, determine what percentage of staff is allocated to each shift.

   Allocated to 7 AM to 3 PM: ___%

   Allocated to 3 PM to 11 PM: ___%

   Allocated to 11 PM to 7 AM: ___%

   TOTAL: 100%

ACTIVITY 16-2

Using the 32-bed unit just described, determine to what average daily census (ADC) a 75% occupancy rate equates. Now assume that the actual patient days in the past month were 836. Using the formula in Box 16-4 of the text, calculate the real ADC. Finally, assume that during the past month there were 102 discharges. Determine the average length of stay.

ACTIVITY 16-3

You have called a staff meeting and have encouraged the staff to bring concerns regarding staff satisfaction. The focus of this meeting is to consider a new approach of self-scheduling. Before looking at how such an approach could actually be implemented, you want staff to consider the pros and cons of the current approach (a managerial function) with the pros and cons of the potential approach (a self-scheduling approach). Complete the following chart to illustrate and clarify the dilemmas, benefits, issues, and problems associated with each.

(+) Self-Scheduling
1. Staff control over schedule

2.

3.

4.

5.

(−) Self-Scheduling
1. Peer negotiation regarding the schedule

2.

3.

4.

5.

(+) Managerial Scheduling
1. Efficiency

2.

3.

4.

5.

(−) Managerial Scheduling
1. Staff complaints

2.

3.

4.

5.

Now assume that you and your group decide to initiate self-scheduling on a trial basis. Before initiating this new approach, you will need to write some guidelines for self-scheduling. Review the chart above for ideas.

Guidelines for Self-Staffing (Proposed)

1. May only schedule Friday or Monday off with a weekend off one time per month.

2.

3.

4.

5.

Selecting, Developing, and Evaluating Staff

INTRODUCTION

The following exercises provide an opportunity for you to identify personal preferences for various types of appraisals, as well as the strengths and weaknesses for methods commonly used. You may wish to critique an appraisal from a system in which you are currently employed or where you have had clinical experience. Finally, you may develop and critique typical dialogues among professionals. Behaviors that foster empowerment and disempowerment, whether verbal or nonverbal, should be identified.

ACTIVITY 17-1

Design a performance appraisal process that you believe would help you grow professionally.

Which of the performance appraisal types listed would be a part of your preferred process? In the spaces that follow, identify the strengths and limitations of each. State a rationale for each regarding how the process could help you professionally.

a) *Graphic rating scales* provide feedback that can:

Strengths:
Limitations:
b) *Forced distribution* provides feedback that can:

Strengths:
Limitations:
c) *Peer review* provides feedback that can:

Strengths:
Limitations:
d) *Management by objectives* provides feedback that can:

Strengths:
Limitations:

e) *Behaviorally Anchored Rating Scales* provide feedback that can:

Strengths:
Limitations:

State three performance criteria that should be included in your process.
a)
b)
c)

Meet with one to three peers to construct a performance appraisal form incorporating each of the performance criteria that you have identified.

Share the group process that has been developed with a person responsible for appraising you, or someone who would. Will that person agree to use your process to assist you to grow professionally? Remember, because your organization uses a particular system does not preclude the use of an *additional* system!

ACTIVITY 17-2

Assess the state of performance appraisal in a clinical organization (setting) by using the checklist below.
_____ 1. Does your organization have a formal performance appraisal system? (If "no," see last item on this list.)
_____ 2. Does it use graphic rating scales?
_____ 3. Does it use forced distribution?
_____ 4. Does it include peer review?
_____ 5. Is it based on management by objectives?
_____ 6. Are the objectives based on a strategic plan?
_____ 7. Does it include a behaviorally anchored rating scale?
_____ 8. Does it influence compensation?
_____ 9. Does it serve as the basis for discipline?
_____10. Is it used to determine training needs?
_____11. Does it increase role clarity?
_____12. Do appraisal meetings occur at least quarterly?
_____13. Is the system based on up-to-date position descriptions/criteria?
_____14. Is there a clearly defined training process for appraisers?
_____15. Every organization has an appraisal process! If your organization has no formal process, you can be sure that an informal process exists. Your performance is assessed!

Cite three examples of criteria used in the informal system in the organization.
1.

2.

3.

What is your opinion regarding the workings of the informal system of appraisal in your organization?

How does the informal system of performance appraisal reflect the values, climate, or culture of the setting? Cite two ways.

1.

2.

ACTIVITY 17-3

Examine and analyze typical dialogues among nurses, managers, and other healthcare professionals. Cite three instances of both empowering and disempowering behaviors.

Empowering behaviors
1.

2.

3.

Disempowering behaviors
1.

2.

3.

Cultural Diversity in Healthcare

INTRODUCTION

The purposes of the exercises in this section are, first, to help you examine your own cultural attitudes to determine how they influence your behavior, and second, to compare and contrast your cultural beliefs and practices with those of others who come from a different cultural background.

ACTIVITY 18-1

Cultural Diversity Exercise: Cultural Awareness

1. Describe the differences among the terms *culture, race,* and *ethnicity.*

2. List at least six common characteristics usually associated with the middle-class American culture.
    a)
    b)
    c)
    d)
    e)
    f)

3. Describe common characteristics found in the culture of Western scientific medical practice (e.g., belief in medical model, germ theory).

4. Identify the four most prominent cultural groups in your area.
    a)
    b)
    c)
    d)

Choose two groups for an in-depth study. Identify the groups in relation to their health beliefs/customs in the areas of birth and death, and their use of folk healers or folk medicines.

5. Determine four similarities and four differences between the "folk medicine" and "Western, scientific medicine" systems. (You may need to think broadly.)

Similarities	Differences
a)	a)
b)	b)
c)	c)
d)	d)

ACTIVITY 18-2

Cultural Values Checklist

The following is a short checklist regarding culturally determined values, attitudes, and beliefs, especially as they pertain to healthcare. You must choose to strongly agree, agree, disagree, or strongly disagree with each statement as it is written. This requires that you be as introspective as possible to determine where you stand on each of the issues presented. Please remember that there is no right or wrong answer, just individual attitudes and beliefs. By answering as honestly as possible, this exercise will help you be more conscious of your own culturally determined beliefs.

Read each statement carefully, then circle the answer that most closely reflects your beliefs regarding each statement.

SA = Strongly agree   A = Agree   D = Disagree   SD = Strongly disagree

1. Only a small percentage of Americans use alternative forms of healing other than traditional medical science.

   SA   A   D   SD

2. People can change the outcome of serious medical conditions with prayer.

   SA   A   D   SD

3. True grief is expressed with loud sobbing and copious crying.

   SA   A   D   SD

4. Life support should be removed from a person who is brain-dead with no possible hope for recovery.

   SA   A   D   SD

5. Patients should be allowed to have family members at their bedside 24 hours a day.

   SA   A   D   SD

6. Family members should donate a deceased person's organs (as appropriate) so that others may be helped.

   SA   A   D   SD

7. Good health is largely determined by a person's diet, exercise, and other similar activities.

   SA   A   D   SD

8. Nurses should question a physician if the nurse is unsure of the rationale behind the physician's orders.

   SA   A   D   SD

9. To obtain a good patient history, the nurse must document the information as the patient is speaking to make sure that none of the information is missed.

   SA   A   D   SD

10. Family members should not be allowed to perform support tasks, such as bathing the patient, while the patient is hospitalized.

    SA   A   D   SD

11. To be an effective communicator, it is important to maintain good eye contact with people.

    SA   A   D   SD

12. If an employee is not performing satisfactorily, the manager should speak directly to that person, even if it involves giving straightforward criticism.

    SA   A   D   SD

13. Patting an employee on the back is a friendly gesture to say "thanks for a job well done."

    SA   A   D   SD

14. Providing psychosocial care is an important part of being a nurse and nurse manager.

    SA   A   D   SD

For each of the 14 statements in the previous checklist, identify one cultural group that would agree with the statement and one that would not:

1. AGREE _____ DISAGREE _____
2. AGREE _____ DISAGREE _____
3. AGREE _____ DISAGREE _____
4. AGREE _____ DISAGREE _____
5. AGREE _____ DISAGREE _____
6. AGREE _____ DISAGREE _____
7. AGREE _____ DISAGREE _____
8. AGREE _____ DISAGREE _____
9. AGREE _____ DISAGREE _____
10. AGREE _____ DISAGREE _____
11. AGREE _____ DISAGREE _____
12. AGREE _____ DISAGREE _____
13. AGREE _____ DISAGREE _____
14. AGREE _____ DISAGREE _____

Meet in groups of three or four students to discuss your responses to this exercise. Determine three areas of commonality and three areas of difference among members of your group.

Areas of commonality:
1.
2.
3.

Areas of difference:
1.
2.
3.

ACTIVITY 18-3

One responsibility of a family is to provide healthcare for its members by helping them stay well and taking care of members who are ill. Health-promotion activities and care given during illness vary greatly among families. Each function is very much influenced by the family's cultural orientation. Friedman (1992) describes six stages of family health/illness interactions that greatly influence each individual's response to healthcare. These stages are health promotion, illness recognition, care seeking, healthcare system, acute response, and adaptation to illness/recovery.

It is important to note that the family will not make contact with the healthcare delivery system until at least the fourth stage of this interaction continuum. Therefore the family may have engaged in various health activities before they ever have contact with anyone in a professional setting.

The Family Health/Illness Practices Inventory is designed to increase awareness of family and cultural values that shape health and illness practices. It is a tool that can increase self-awareness of the cultural factors that shape your current approach to healthcare. When used as an interview tool, it can increase awareness of other cultural perspectives regarding healthcare.

Complete your own Family Health/Illness Practices Inventory. Try to remember what it was like for you as a child growing up and answer the questions based on what your family did before you became a nurse.

Family Health/Illness Practices Inventory

Questions to ask:
1. Health promotion:
   Cite three health promotion/disease prevention activities done by your family.
   a)
   b)
   c)
   Did you consider your parents to be healthy, frail, sickly? What about your siblings?
   How did your family define *health?*

2. Illness recognition:
   Who was the primary person in the family responsible for determining whether a family member was ill?
   Who was primarily responsible for determining what should be done about the illness?
   Who in the family was seen as the "health expert"?

3. Care seeking:
   Who did the family turn to for information regarding the illness if the family was unable to resolve the problem on its own?
   Did the family discuss the problems with extended family members, neighbors, or friends, or go straight to a health professional?

4. Healthcare system:
   Did the family use folk practitioner/healers?
   Where was the initial contact with the healthcare delivery system made (e.g., healer, private physician, clinic, hospital)?
   Who in the family was responsible for deciding where to seek help?

5. Acute response:
   What did it mean to be "sick" in your family?

   What behaviors were expected of the sick person and of other family members in relation to the sick member?

   If it was a serious illness or crisis, how did the family cope?

   Who was seen as the leader in times of crisis?

   What happened if the traditional leader was sick?

6. Adaptation to illness/recovery:
   Did anyone in the family have a chronic illness?

   How did that affect the other family members?

   Who did the family depend on for support (physical, emotional)?

   After completing your own Family Health/Illness Practices Inventory, interview someone from a different cultural background. Explain that you are trying to learn more about how different cultures and families view health and illness. Assure the person that the information will be kept confidential, or seek out a classmate whose cultural background is different from yours and mutually compare and discuss your responses.

REFERENCE

Friedman, M. (1992). *Family nursing: Theory and practice* (3rd ed.). Norwalk, CT: Appleton & Lange.

Building Teams Through Communication and Partnerships

INTRODUCTION

Teamwork is the name of the game these days. In almost every type of institution there is an emphasis on building and maintaining effective teams. Despite this focus on teamwork, many of us still have old habits and beliefs about being effective individuals. Remember all those times you decided, and others encouraged you, to "do it yourself." "Be strong and handle it alone!" Now the emphasis has changed to cooperating and collaborating. These workbook exercises aim to increase your understanding of what produces high-performing teams. You will learn the power of focusing your attention on commitment to a particular task. You will also discover how to maintain the cohesiveness of a group and how individualist behaviors affect groups.

ACTIVITY 19-1

1. List at least five criteria for effective teamwork.
   a)
   b)
   c)
   d)
   e)

2. Recall a team you have observed. Identify what was missing from the team's performance. Apply criteria to your observations and experience in the group.

3. Based on your reading of Chapter 19 and various articles, list three specific ways to enrich team performance.
   a)
   b)
   c)

4. Identify and commit to at least two new actions you could take to improve your role as a team member. Write them down and set deadline dates.

   a) I will _____ by _____
   b) I will _____ by _____

ACTIVITY 19-2

Examine a work group that you are familiar with, either currently or from the past. Select two people you have worked with: one person with whom you enjoyed working and one with whom you were very reluctant to work. For each person, list two behaviors that are characteristic of that person's interactions with others.

Person I usually enjoyed working with:	**Person I was usually reluctant to work with:**
1.	1.
2.	2.

Next, respond to the following:

Do you demonstrate behaviors from either list?   YES   NO

Would you fall exclusively in one list or the other?   YES   NO

Cite two examples of your behavior to support your answer.
1.
2.

In considering the person you were reluctant to work with, cite two positive behaviors for him/her:
1.
2.

In what ways could you encourage growth and expansion of those behaviors?
1.
2.

What could this person contribute to a team?
1.
2.

ACTIVITY 19-3

Make a list of your strengths and limitations as a team member and as a team leader.

Team member	**Team leader**
Strengths	
1.	1.
2.	2.
3.	3.

Team member	**Team leader**
Limitations	
1.	1.
2.	2.
3.	3.

Now examine each of these and determine how each enhances or interferes with the team process.

Conflict: The Cutting Edge of Change

INTRODUCTION

The following activity assumes you have completed and scored the Conflict Self-Assessment (see Chapter 20) and responded to the questions in Boxes 20-5, 20-7, 20-9, 20-11, and 20-13. Effective conflict resolution and polarity management lead to effective leadership for change.

ACTIVITY 20-1

After you have read Chapter 20 in the text, complete and score the Conflict Self-Assessment in the text. Next, write out your responses to the self-assessment questions for each of the five approaches to conflict on pages 356, 357, 358, and 360 of the text (avoiding, accommodating, competing, compromising, and collaborating), focusing only on conflicts in your professional life. (If you are not yet in a professional position, you might instead focus on conflicts during your "career" as a student.) Use the Conflict Reflection Form that follows to focus your thinking. What new behaviors have you committed to for the future?

Conflict Reflection Form

Look at your scores on the Conflict Self-Assessment and responses to the five sets of self-assessment questions in the textbook. Reflect on how you act during conflict (professional and/or personal). Be honest with yourself without being critical.
1. How do you tend to balance the following polarities related to conflict?

    a) Unassertiveness and assertiveness?

    b) Uncooperativeness and cooperativeness?

    c) Avoidance and involvement?

    d) Escalation and minimization of any conflict?

    e) Rigid control and loose improvisation?

    f) Revelation and concealment of information?

    g) Intellectual and emotional reactions?

2. Which two approaches to conflict resolution do you tend to underemphasize? Why?
    a)
    b)
3. Which two do you tend to use most often? Why?
    a)
    b)

4. How might you be overemphasizing some approaches? Are they situation specific, or are they just the ones you rely on? Why?

5. When and how might you be matching approaches effectively to the particular nature of conflicts in which you are involved?

6. When and how might you be matching approaches ineffectively with the particular nature of conflicts in which you are involved?

ACTIVITY 20-2

Playing Twenty Questions: Conflict Analysis

Reflect on past and present conflicts in which you have been directly involved. Choose one conflict to focus on, particularly if it seems to be reappearing with the same or with other people. Check the text to determine whether it is a polarity. If it is, choose another conflict that is not a polarity. Then write out your responses to each of the 20 questions below.

Defining the Conflict
  1. Who was the conflict between? How were they affected?
     Who:
     How:

     Who:
     How:
  2. Who else was affected and how?
     Who:
     How:

  3. What was the actual conflict? What were the perceived incompatibilities?

Conflict Process Analysis
  Frustration Stage
  4. What did you feel at the beginning and in the early stages of the conflict?

  5. Why did you feel this way?

  6. How did you act as a result of these feelings?

7. What do you think the other people felt at the beginning and in the early stages of the conflict?

8. Why do you think they felt this way?

9. How did they act as a result of these emotions?

10. After the conflict moved into the conceptualization stage (see the following), what other emotions or changes in your initial emotions occurred? Why?

Conceptualization Stage

11. What did you think the real conflict (or issue, fight, disagreement, etc.) was? Why?

12. What do you now believe that the other people believed the conflict (or issue, fight, disagreement, etc.) was? Why?

13. Where did you and others have serious differences: facts and information, goals and objectives, means and methods of action, and/or standards and values?

14. Describe why you had the following differences:
    a) Exposure to different data?

    b) Different interpretations of the information?

    c) Differences in your roles and position?

    d) Different values and beliefs?

    e) Cultural differences?

    f) Different directions from someone else?

15. After the conflict moved into the action stage, what new views of the conflict (conceptualizations) were created by those involved? Why?

Action

16. How did you act specifically (and which of the five approaches to conflict were tried)? Why?

17. How did the other people act? Why?

18. After the conflict clearly was in the outcome stage, were there any new actions by anyone that were aimed at resolving this conflict or in changing any of the outcomes that follow?

Outcomes

19. What happened to the quality of task accomplishment and efficiency of action as a result of the actions taken? Why?

20. What happened to the quality of the relationships among those involved?

ACTIVITY 20-3

Imagine that you will be in a conflict in the future similar to the one you just analyzed in Activity 20-2. Knowing what you do about this past conflict, your tendencies to approach conflict (review the self-assessments in Chapter 20), and the five different approaches to conflict, write out a short scenario below (including all four stages of the process) describing how you could act to resolve the conflict.

Delegation: An Art of Professional Practice

INTRODUCTION

Delegation is a critical strategy for nurses to accomplish their work. It requires that nurses know many facts about patients, other workers, legal and ethical implications, and what the research suggests. This chapter provided key information for making appropriate delegation decisions. Once you understand the basics, skills can be developed for determining assignments from two perspectives: One requires knowing about specific patients in terms of some criteria, and the other requires hypothesizing what to anticipate in an unknown patient population. The following activities are designed to help you apply what you have learned in this chapter.

ACTIVITY 21-1

Arrive for your next clinical assignment 1 or 2 hours early. Using the actual patients on your unit, or in your population actively served, and the projected staffing, apply the factors for delegation for the anticipated tasks. Complete this assignment for at least five patients who have multiple tasks to be accomplished. Use the AACN criteria for delegation as one set of criteria to determine assignment. Then use Table 21-2 as a screening activity to determine whether your original conclusions were consistent with the answers you provided to the questions from Table 21-2. Which elements of the criteria and the questions were most difficult to assess? Why? When the assignments are actually made, compare your decisions about care with those actually made. Finally, ask the nurses responsible for those five patients how a decision was reached about delegation. If the nurses do not address factors such as how long the delegatee has worked with the nurses, be sure to ask. Also ask if the nurses know the type of training the delegatee has had. Then ask what one factor is the most important to each individual in deciding what to delegate.

ACTIVITY 21-2

Select a partner. Each of you should choose an uncommon (and preferably previously unstudied) chronic disease condition. In the space provided, identify the condition and your literature source. Next, identify what tasks you believe would be typical for a patient with that condition. Then list what care tasks you would delegate to a new nursing assistant. Identify what to ask. Provide rationale and a method of evaluating your decision. Include in your rationale statement how intense the supervision is likely to be.

Condition:

Source:

Delegated tasks:

Questions:

Rationale:

Method of evaluation:

CHAPTER 22 WORKBOOK

Managing Personal/Personnel Problems

INTRODUCTION

Successfully managing personal/personnel problems is a crucial element of the role of a nurse manager. To master this role function requires that the manager be able to accurately identify personnel problems, develop intervention strategies, implement those strategies, and then evaluate the effectiveness of the interventions. The exercises in this section will help you develop the assessment and intervention skills necessary to successfully manage personnel problems.

ACTIVITY 22-1

Personal/Personnel Problems: Chemical Dependency

1. Review the following documents:
   a) Your state board of nursing's policy and procedures regarding chemically impaired nurses
   b) The American Nurses Association *Code of Ethics for Nurses*
   c) A healthcare agency's policy and procedures regarding chemically dependent employees
   d) A healthcare agency's policy regarding employee drug screening

2. Define the differences between substance dependence and substance abuse.

   Substance dependence is:

   Substance abuse is:

3. List three factors leading to substance abuse in employees.
   a)
   b)
   c)

4. List five of the most common types of abused substances.
   a)
   b)
   c)
   d)
   e)

5. Describe four signs and symptoms of dependence/abuse that may be evident in a chemically impaired employee.
   a)
   b)
   c)
   d)

6. Write a short paragraph either supporting or contesting the following statements regarding chemically impaired healthcare employees.
   a) Substance dependence/abuse is a disease and therefore not fully under the control of the affected person. Substance abusers should be treated, not punished.

   b) Nurses and other healthcare professionals, with their knowledge about drugs and their social contract with patients, should be held to higher standards than the general population.

7. Obtain a copy of personnel policies from an agency in which you have clinical experience. Analyze the policy in relation to the following factors, recording your answers in the space provided.
   a) Is the *Diagnostic and Statistical Manual* (DSM-IV) definition used to define substance dependence/abuse in the agency policy?

   b) Is there a policy for reporting suspected or known impaired employees? If so, what is the role of the nurse manager? of the staff nurse?

   c) Does the policy include plans for intervention and treatment? Is an employee assistance program (EAP) provided for employees? What is the manager's role in intervention?

   d) Does the policy include a notification procedure? If so, who within the agency administration is to be notified? What is the policy for notifying the state board of nursing if the impaired worker is a nurse?

   e) List three key elements that you think should be included in an "ideal" agency policy.

   f) Does the return-to-work section of the policy identify how the recovering nurse will be monitored?

   g) Are there conditions within the policy to address how a relapse will be handled?

ACTIVITY 22-2

Personal/Personnel Problems: Mandatory Drug Testing for Healthcare Professionals

1. Review a copy of the following documents:
   - An agency's policy and procedure regarding chemically dependent employees
   - An agency's policy regarding employee preemployment and on-the-job drug screening
   - Your state board of nursing's policy and procedures on reporting suspected chemically dependent nurses

- The American Nurses Association *Code of Ethics for Nurses*. (Determine their policy statement regarding substance abuse.)
- An agency's policies on nondiscrimination in employment under the Americans with Disabilities Act

2. Prepare to debate the issue of mandatory drug testing for healthcare employees. Read the following debating statement. Prepare five key points to argue for each side (pro and con) of the issue, drawing support for your arguments from the list of readings in item 1 above: *Approximately 70% of all cases handled by state boards of nursing are related to chemically impaired nurses, and nurses have entered into a social contract with their patients to provide safe care; therefore, mandatory random drug testing should be done on all practicing nurses.*

	Pro	**Con**
a)		
b)		
c)		
d)		
e)		

ACTIVITY 22-3

1. Read about the legal, regulatory, and ethical issues related to termination of an employee. Refer to the following reading as a guide.
   Curtin, L. (1996). Ethics, discipline, and discharge. *Nursing Management, 27*(3), 51-52.
2. Review an agency's policies and procedures for terminating employees.
3. Read the following scenario below. Carefully weigh the pros and cons of each termination decision, considering the legal, ethical, and personal factors that enter into your decision.

Downsizing Scenario

You are a nurse manager in an agency that is experiencing financial difficulties. This problem affects more than just your agency. You are located in a county that is economically depressed, and unemployment is high. You have just received the budget for the next financial year and note that you have lost one full-time position, meaning you must lay off one of your full-time nurses. Because of a poor economic situation, it is not possible to transfer within the agency and the layoff will most likely be a permanent one. Also, no other agencies in the area are hiring, although some jobs may be available through a staffing pool or on a contingency basis. You must decide which of the following three employees to lay off. This is a nonunion agency, each of the nurses has the same number of years of service with the hospital, and all have had very similar performance evaluations for the last 3 years.

Nurse A: Nancy is 50 years old and entered nursing later in life after raising a family of four. She is married to the hospital's chief of staff, and some of the younger nurses on the unit resent her "country club" attitude. They think she is not really serious about nursing and only works to escape being bored. Nancy does a good job but does have some difficulty working with other staff nurses. You personally like Nancy a great deal. She is closer to you in age and life experience than the other staff nurses, and you find yourself turning to her for advice and support. Nancy has confided in you that she really enjoys her new-found career. She says that for the first time in her life she has an identity of her own instead of always being somebody's daughter, spouse, or mother. Nancy has missed 4 days of work in the last 6 months, two times to take her mother to the doctor for evaluation of Alzheimer's disease, one because her husband unexpectedly told her that she had to accompany him to an important hospital social event, and one time she called in sick.

Nurse B: John is 35 years old and the only male nurse on your unit. He has suffered a great deal of personal crises and losses in the past 2 years. His 2-year-old son has Down syndrome, and his 10-year-old son was killed in an automobile accident last year. Six months ago his father died unexpectedly from a heart attack. John has confided in you that he is really struggling with these personal losses. He is especially having difficulty with losing his son because he says he will never be able to do all the "father/son" things with his 2-year-old son that would have been possible with the older son. John says he just doesn't feel the same kind of bond with either his 2-year-old son or his 6-year-old daughter. John also states that he's having difficulty with his wife. Their relationship is very strained and stressful. He's not sure if the marriage will survive. He says that he has been very depressed over all of these crises and has sought professional counseling. He also tells you in confidence that the psychiatrist has him on antidepressants to help him cope. John has missed 4 days of work in the last 6 months. All of them have been on Mondays. He says that the depression has at times made it difficult for him to start another week.

Nurse C: Carrie is 33 years old and very well liked by her peers. She is an informal leader in the group. You personally don't like Carrie very much. She was working on the unit before you became manager, and she has constantly challenged you since you arrived. She is argumentative and resistant to change, but she always ends up doing what you have asked her to do. You worry about the effect that she has on unit morale. Yet you note that none of the staff nurses has ever reported having difficulties working with her. Nine months ago Carrie seriously injured her back when a patient she was ambulating started to fall. Carrie saved the patient from injury, but was on medical leave for 6 weeks because of the incident. Her recovery may have been hindered by the fact that she is 40 pounds overweight. Because of her back injuries, she often requests that she be assigned to charge (desk) duty. Other staff nurses have offered to give her their charge duty or volunteered to help her with patient care if she needs any assistance. Carrie has missed 4 days in the past 6 months, 2 days on two separate instances, both for complaints of back pain.

Which nurse will you lay off?
List two reasons to terminate or retain each of the nurses.
Nancy: 1.
        2.

John: 1.
        2.

Carrie: 1.
        2.

Indicate one personal, ethical, and legal issue that may be raised in terminating each of the three nurses.

Nancy: Personal:
        Ethical:
        Legal:

John: Personal:
        Ethical:
        Legal:

Carrie: Personal:
        Ethical:
        Legal:

Role Transition

INTRODUCTION

Roles in healthcare are changing rapidly. Are you in the midst of a role transition or are you anticipating the transition from nursing student to "real nurse"? No matter which situation you are in, Activities 23-1 and 23-2 can provide valuable insight. Thoughtful responses to the questions will help you clarify the roles of a nurse manager, your strengths, and areas for improvement.

ACTIVITY 23-1

1. Read Chapter 23 and complete the "Roles Assessment" on pages 404-405. In that assessment you are asked to analyze job responsibilities, opportunities to contribute and grow professionally, lines of communication, and expectations of others around the nurse manager. Talk to two staff nurses and ask each of them, "What are the two most important roles that a nurse manager must fulfill?"

1. a)

   b)

2. a)

   b)

Ask a nurse manager, "What are the two most important roles that you must fulfill?"

   a)

   b)

Compare the responses of the staff nurses and the nurse manager:

Similarities:

Differences:

Conflicts:

Share your impressions with two or three peers. Synthesize the information each of you has received from the staff nurses and managers. Identify as a group the similarities and differences in how staff nurses and nurse managers view the manager role. What conflicts exist between these perspectives?

Similarities:

Differences:

Conflicts:

Discuss responses with your peers and others (managers, staff) and have them assist in clarifying the multiple roles and expectations.

2. What roles and responsibilities excite you? Why?

3. Which ones seem to demand a "risk and stretch" for you? Why?

4. Which roles and responsibilities would you rather not have? Why?

ACTIVITY 23-2

Complete the self-assessment on page 410. As requested in the assessment, talk with a mentor of yours and compare your perspective of yourself with the mentor's perspective. You also could use some of the sentence completions that follow as additional items on which to focus.

1. One recent example of my success in providing leadership is:

2. I am especially proud of my ability to:

3. The part of my work I especially like is:

4. I believe in my capability to manage difficult:

5. I am very responsible in relation to:

6. A goal I have met in the past year of which I am most proud is:

7. I think my supervisor would evaluate my effectiveness as:

8. My colleagues would describe me as:

9. I accomplish the most when I:

10. One thing I am more successful with this year is:

Self-Management: Stress and Time

INTRODUCTION

The following activities afford the reader opportunities to put the principles described in Chapter 24 into action. The first activity invites you to analyze how stress and time management are related. Identifying your own coping skills and seeking more positive ways of managing stress are the focus of the second activity. The third exercise invites you to use your time management skills to plan a successful meeting.

ACTIVITY 24-1

Self-Management

1. Consider your last clinical day. Complete a time log for the entire day, from rising in the morning to going to sleep at night. Include the approximate amount of time you spent on each nursing task during the clinical day.
2. Identify those activities that took longer than expected by underlining those items.
3. Analyze the description in terms of the time management skills of goal setting, prioritization, organization (O), use of time tools (T), and dealing with information (I). Label each with the corresponding letters.
4. Identify periods of the day that were stressful by bracketing the time.
5. Analyze the stressful activities in relation to why they were stressful (S) and how you dealt with the stress. Label stressful items with an "S," and to the right, describe how you responded.
6. Analyze the appropriateness of a peer's stress management strategies.
7. Review the principles of self-management in Chapter 24 and identify how the day might have been made to be less stressful.

ACTIVITY 24-2

Stress

Use the following questions as a guide to understanding how you perceive stress, respond to it, and attempt to gain mastery.

1. Think about a recent situation in which you experienced a high level of distress. Indicate how you responded:

Emotionally

Behaviorally

Physically

Review what you have written and identify whether your coping strategies were negative (N) or positive (P), labeling each accordingly.

Consider an alternative approach for those coping strategies you have identified as negative.

2. Describe a situation in which you were in conflict with another person. How was that situation influenced by your expectations and behavior? Could the conflict have been avoided or resolved differently?

ACTIVITY 24-3

Meeting Management

Examine the Tips box on how to manage a meeting at the end of Chapter 24. Given the list of agenda items below, organize a 2-hour meeting to address them all. List them in an agenda with specific time limits for each item. Be prepared to give the rationale for the specific order you choose. When would you hold this meeting? What site might you choose for this meeting?

Agenda Items

a) Discuss how to make team meetings more effective
b) Decide on a new schedule format
c) Share the news
d) Discuss new possibilities for continuous improvement on the unit
e) Decide when to hold a shift party
f) Review last meeting's minutes
g) Revise a report form
h) Discuss agenda items for the next meeting
i) Give out assignments
j) Answer questions

CHAPTER **25** WORKBOOK

Power, Politics, and Influence

INTRODUCTION

Who would you say is the most important person at your place of employment? Give it some thought before you respond. Is it the president or chief executive officer? Is it the person who makes the most money? Is it the person who supervises the most employees? Is it the person who has the authority to fire or demote you? Is it the physician with the most influence? Is it the patient who threatens to sue you? This chapter examines the nature, effect, and uses of power in nursing management.

ACTIVITY 25-1

1. Review the definitions of power in the box on page 435 (Types or Bases of Social Power). Write a short personal example fitting each definition:
   a) Expert:

   b) Information:

   c) Legitimate:

   d) Coercive:

   e) Reward:

   f) Referent:

   g) Connection:

2. Now reread the introduction. Who is the most powerful person at your hospital? Explain why the most powerful person could be you, the nurse.

ACTIVITY 25-2

Read the following case, considering the different types of power. Reflect on the behaviors listed for Tracy, the emergency room charge nurse in the case.

Clinical Case Study

Tracy Starr (RN, BSN, CEN), the charge nurse in a very busy emergency room, was exhausted at the end of a 12-hour shift. Sixty-six patients had been triaged, assessed, cared for, counseled, educated, admitted, transferred, and/or discharged. One patient died. Some of the nursing responsibilities/behaviors carried out by Tracy on this shift included the following:

____ a) Took/gave shift report every 4 hours

____ b) Assigned staff to patient care responsibilities

____ c) Assigned staff to nonnursing responsibilities such as ordering supplies, room checks, and testing emergency equipment

____ d) Oriented two new medical students to department protocols and expectations

____ e) Requested assistance from the nursing supervisor to obtain ICU beds for two critical patients

____ f) Called the children's protective agency to request emergency placement for three abandoned children brought in by the police

____ g) Yelled over the phone at a newspaper reporter who insisted on obtaining details of a recent accident

____ h) Assisted a staff nurse to support very distressed family members whose elderly parent had just died

____ i) Talked to the coroner for 10 minutes by phone

____ j) Cared for five patients whose nurse left for a dinner break

____ k) Assisted three staff members who were restraining an out-of-control, intoxicated patient

____ l) Intervened between a staff nurse and physician who disagreed about a patient care issue

____ m) Promised to talk privately to an angry unit secretary later in the shift if there was time

____ n) Gathered all staff together at 11 PM to thank them for their hard work and good care

Write out short responses to the following questions about the case.

1. Determine all of the bases of power that Tracy exhibited. (Place the number of the power base that she used at the left side of each statement above.) Label each one according to the chapter definition: *1,* expert; *2,* information; *3,* legitimate; *4,* coercive; *5,* reward; *6,* referent; and *7,* connection.

2. How did this nurse empower the staff? Cite two ways.
   a)

   b)

3. Cite two missed opportunities for empowerment that you saw.
   a)

   b)

4. Visualize this nurse and write your description of her. What does Tracy look like?

How does Tracy speak to people?

What values does Tracy embody?

What influential person in your life does Tracy remind you of?

ACTIVITY 25-3

Empowerment is defined in Chapter 25 as the "process by which we facilitate the participation of others in decision making and taking action within an environment where there is an equitable distribution of power." Empowerment is power sharing and a form of feminine leadership. All of the following can be powerful attributes of a professional nurse. Rank them in order of importance to you by numbering them in the blanks provided (1 being most important).

____ 1. Professional knowledge, specialized knowledge
____ 2. Technological competence
____ 3. Professional experience
____ 4. Problem-solving skills
____ 5. Comfort with conflict resolution
____ 6. Ability to communicate clearly with colleagues
____ 7. A commitment to organizational philosophy and mission
____ 8. Above-average financial compensation
____ 9. A sense of humor
____10. Positive feelings of work satisfaction

Give this same list to a nursing colleague and to a nonnursing colleague and ask them to rank these items. Compare all three rankings. What similarities and differences exist?
Similarities:

Differences:

ACTIVITY 25-4

1. Meet in groups of three or four. Discuss the responses you wrote for the questions about the case in Activity 25-2 featuring Tracy Starr, RN.

2. What "power tools" were most effective in this example?
   a)

   b)

   c)

   d)

3. Describe the "coalition building" behaviors Tracy demonstrated.
   a)

   b)

   c)

4. Discuss the following assertion and its implication for your future in nursing and in nursing management: "Collegiality demands mutual respect, not friendship!" Are friendship and being a respected manager mutually exclusive? Why or why not? Is friendship with colleagues essential to you for effective working relationships? Why or why not?

ACTIVITY 25-5

Meet in groups of five or six. Combine your group rankings from Activity 25-3 (or make arrangements to combine the entire class's rankings).

1. What conclusions can you draw from this exercise? Identify, describe, and explain at least three differences that exist among the rankings by nurses.
   a)

   b)

   c)

2. What can you conclude? Identify at least three conclusions.
   a)

   b)

   c)

3. Do differences exist between the nurse rankings and the nonnurse rankings? Discuss specific similarities, differences, and conclusions.

Similarities:

a)

b)

Differences:

a)

b)

Conclusions:

a)

b)

ACTIVITY 25-6

Complete this exercise in a group of four to six. You are committed to the concept of healthcare for all. A bill is proposed in your state legislature to extend limited healthcare benefits, a combination of low-cost insurance and Medicaid, to the working poor who do not have access to healthcare insurance through their employers. Identify three powerful behaviors that you can use to support the passage of this bill that will operationalize an important aspect of health policy.

a)

b)

c)

Career Management: Putting Yourself in Charge

INTRODUCTION

Career management takes thought, time, and energy. The alternative to managing your own career is to experience whatever comes your way and hope for the best. Developing your career is related not only to securing a "good" position but also to planning your career in the way that you wish to proceed to meet your short- and long-term goals. It means being proactive for yourself.

This chapter identified specific strategies to launch a career and to keep it on a positive trajectory. The following activities are designed to use the elements presented in the chapter to create commonly used documents to market yourself in a manner that will enable you to "stand out among the rest."

ACTIVITY 26-1

1. You are in the last days of your undergraduate nursing program with many career options open to you. You have had diverse opportunities throughout your educational program that make you marketable for a variety of positions. Using the facts that you have compiled in your data collection system, create a résumé for each of the positions you are considering: (1) staff nurse in a surgical intensive care unit that accommodates many trauma patients, (2) staff nurse for a high-risk perinatal unit that cares for indigent patients who have had minimal prenatal care, and (3) staff nurse in the ambulatory surgery center that admits patients in the morning and discharges them later in the day after their surgery.

ACTIVITY 26-2

1. It is 6 months since your graduation from your nursing program. Update your data collection system, entering elements that have occurred since graduation. Complete a curriculum vitae (CV), which you are required to submit with your graduate school application.

ACTIVITY 26-3

1. Your nurse manager has selected you as a candidate to be interviewed for one of the mentorship positions on your unit. She tells you that the organization is developing a mentorship program for nursing service. The intent of this program is to mentor new staff as they join the organization. It is an honor to be considered for this position, and you must interview with a panel of nursing staff, nurse administrators, and nurse educators. If you are selected to be a mentor, you will attend mentor development classes and receive an adjustment to your base salary. You have been asked to submit a cover letter as a means of introducing yourself to the committee. Prepare your cover letter and practice interviewing for the position with one of your classmates.

Leading Through Professional Associations

INTRODUCTION

Leaders can be found in a variety of settings, including clinical, policy, research, and management settings. That an individual is a good manager does not necessarily mean that the individual would be a good leader. Leadership traits are acquired in a variety of ways, one of which is through professional associations. How can nurses learn leadership skills? Professional organizations provide the opportunities to engage in leadership activities and encourage professional growth. The activities here are designed to assist you in developing these skills.

ACTIVITY 27-1

1. How do you define or describe a professional association? an organization? Are there any differences? similarities?

2. Do you know faculty or co-workers who are members or officers of an association? Who? Which associations?

3. Have you explored opportunities within your local, state, and national student nurses' association (www.nsna.org)?

ACTIVITY 27-2

1. In the space provided, make a list of benefits that you might receive by joining your nursing association.

Benefits to Joining an Organization

2. Create a brief outline of your 1-year, 5-year, and 10-year goals and career plan.
   1 year:

   5 years:

   10 years:

a) What barriers have you identified that you think may prevent you from accomplishing the goals you have identified?

1 year:

5 years:

10 years:

b) Write a list of goals that you have for personal and professional development (e.g., make a public speech, write an article, hold an officer position, conduct research, be a manager).

c) Do you have any concerns about getting involved in a professional association? If so, what (e.g., fear that organization will require too great of a time commitment)?

d) Speak with faculty members/co-workers about their ideas and what they value and the benefits they receive through membership.

ACTIVITY 27-3

1. Read at least two articles concerning professional nursing organizations. Using the Internet, access the American Nurses Association: www.nursingworld.org.

2. Research at least one specialty nurse organization on the Internet and attend a meeting (e.g., Emergency Nurses Association).

3. Find out when the local association meeting is and attend one. Check the dates of the state conventions because there are invaluable opportunities for new graduates and they are often offered to students at special, reduced rates. List specific opportunities. Designate whether a reduced rate is available for students and/or new graduates.

Index

Page numbers followed by f indicate figure; b, box; t, table.